Health and Human Rights in a Changing World

Health and Human Rights in a Changing World is a comprehensive and contemporary collection of readings and original material examining health and human rights from a global perspective. Editors Grodin, Tarantola, Annas, and Gruskin are well-known for their previous two volumes (published by Routledge) on this increasingly important subject to the global community. The editors have contextualized each of the five parts with foundational essays; each reading concludes with discussion topics, questions, and suggested readings. This book also includes Points of View sections—originally written perspectives by important authors in the field.

Part I is a Health and Human Rights Overview that lays out the essential knowledge base and provides the foundation for the following parts.

Part II brings in notions of concepts, methods, and governance framing the application of health and human rights, in particular the Human Rights-based Approaches to Health.

Part III sheds light on issues of heightened vulnerability and special protection, stressing that the health and human rights record of any nation, any community, is determined by what is being done and not done about those who are most in need.

Part IV focuses on addressing system failures where health and human rights issues have been documented, recognized, even at times proclaimed as priorities, and yet insufficiently attended to as a result of State denial, unwillingness, or incapacity.

Part V examines the relevance of the health and human rights paradigm to a changing world, underscoring contemporary global challenges and responses.

Finally, a **Concluding Note** brings together the key themes of this set of articles and attempts to project a vision of the future.

"This is the most complete compendium on health and human rights—a much neglected and under-researched, but essential dimension of global health. It addresses both theoretical enquiries and very practical issues for a wide range of health practitioners."

Peter Piot, MD, PhD, Professor of Global Health and Director, London School of Hygiene & Tropical Medicine, UK, former Under Secretary-General of the United Nations, former Executive Director of the UN specialized agency UNAIDS

"*Health and Human Rights in a Changing World* documents the growing significance of the linkages between health and human rights during the past two decades. This comprehensive anthology attests to the widening scope and diversity of topics and approaches in the health and human rights field. The book offers a valuable resource for those teaching a course on the subject or desirous of widening their knowledge of the health and human rights field."

Audrey R. Chapman, PhD, Healey Professor of Medical Ethics, University of Connecticut School of Medicine, USA

Health and Human Rights in a Changing World

Edited by
Michael A. Grodin, Daniel Tarantola,
George J. Annas, and Sofia Gruskin

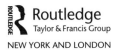
Routledge
Taylor & Francis Group

NEW YORK AND LONDON

First published 2013
by Routledge
711 Third Avenue, New York, NY 10017

Simultaneously published in the UK
by Routledge
2 Park Square, Milton Park, Abingdon, Oxon OX14 4RN

Routledge is an imprint of the Taylor & Francis Group, an informa business

Library of Congress Cataloging in Publication Data
   Health and human rights in a changing world / edited by Michael Grodin ... [et al.].
   p. ; cm.
   Consists of articles reprinted from various sources.
   Includes bibliographical references and index.
   Summary: "This anthology, compiled by four of the top scholars in the field,
   gives a global view of public health. The editors begin with an introduction
   to public health and move on to legal, economic, and political implications.
   The editors also include contextual essays for each of the four sections"
   —Provided by publisher.
   I. Grodin, Michael A.
   [DNLM: 1. Human Rights—Collected Works.
   2. Public Health—Collected Works.
   3. Health Policy—Collected Works. WA 5]
   362.1—dc23
   2012036203

ISBN: 978–0–415–50398–3 (hbk)
ISBN: 978–0–415–50399–0 (pbk)
ISBN: 978–0–203–57629–8 (ebk)

Typeset in Utopia
by Swales & Willis Ltd, Exeter, Devon

Printed and bound in the United States of America by Sheridan Books, Inc. (a Sheridan Group Company).

To those who, in their lives, professional environments and classrooms, are exploring the rich and promising field of health and human rights.

CONTENTS

PART IV: ADDRESSING SYSTEM FAILURES

ACKNOWLEDGMENTS

This textbook owes first and foremost to the authors of the quality articles and book chapters assembled here which project broad and diverse insight into the relationships between health and rights. We acknowledge particularly the contribution of world leaders in health and human rights who, responding enthusiastically and with extreme diligence to our invitation, have expressed their personal *Point of View* on issues at the heart of their work. Our gratitude goes to Mckenna Longacre, Boston University's Health and Human Rights Fellow and the senior administrator of this project, who had a vital role in all parts of the book's production. Special thanks to Matthew Brennan for his expert technical assistance. This book would not have been completed without the administrative and editorial support of Chelsea Moore, Emily Klotz, Alicia Orta, Erin Duffy, Fanny Petit, Siri Khalsa, and Lynn Squillace. We are indebted to the Deans and Heads of our respective universities and schools, including the University of New South Wales Faculty of Medicine School of Public Health and Community Medicine, the Institute of Global Health of the University of Southern California, and especially to Dean Robert Meenan of the Boston University School of Public Health. We also greatly appreciate the support of their staff all through the process of producing this book. Finally, our thanks are directed to past and present students who taught us as much as they learned from us, and to future students who, we hope, will find in this book inspiration and commitment to further advance health and human rights.

Introduction

How is the field of Health and Human Rights to be understood and used to foster both human rights and the health of populations? And what has happened in the past two decades that might shed a new light on the emergence, meaning and importance of the health and human rights conundrum framed under the leadership of Jonathan Mann in the mid-1990s?[1] These two decades witnessed the end of the 20th century promising to some the end of the world and human life, or at the least a massive collapse of electronic communication networks, while foretelling to others a 21st century and a new millennium of peace, security, justice and equitable global economic opportunities. As we, survivors of the 20th millennium, will testify, neither of these happened. Markedly, the end of the Cold War in the early 1990s and of apartheid in South Africa in 1994 opened an empty space for democracy and human rights to blossom.[2] Following was the birth or rebirth of national constitutions in which human rights were entrenched, and the emergence of health and human rights movements and scholarship. Recognizing the central role of human rights in human development, the United Nations, along with some Official Development Agencies and International Non-governmental Organizations (INGOs), undertook to "mainstream human rights" across their policies and programs, including within health and development agencies. Even global corporations responded to the 1999 appeal from the United Nations Secretary General Koffi Annan to join a Global Compact intended to stimulate "corporate citizenship" and align their operations and strategies with ten universally accepted principles in the areas of human rights, labor, environment and anti-corruption, all with significant implications not only for rights but for health. For those concerned with health and human rights, the future was indeed promising.

Over the past two decades, the role of NGOs has become increasingly critical to the health and human rights agenda at every level. There are now approximately 40,000 internationally operated NGOs, cutting across humanitarianism, development, environmental conservation and the constellation of concerns falling within the orbit of health and human rights. In general, their orientation is either operational or advocacy based, and their activities range from development, exposure, education, and advocacy to environmental protection. Many of these NGOs or civil society movements would identify human rights as their primary concern, others health, and human development and its ecology. Beyond their strong focus on local action, NGOs have grown to play major roles in the health arena and the human rights arena, but have to a lesser extent come together to work on health and human rights. Many still operate within the narrow boundaries of one or the other domains with little attempts or capacity to work across them. Several, however, including those with a human rights orientation such as Amnesty International and the Center for Reproductive Rights, and those with more of a health orientation such as Médecins Sans Frontières (MSF), OXFAM, CARE International, Save the Children, World Vision and the People's Health Movement, to only cite a few, have defined their health and human rights agendas and are actively contributing to—and occasionally challenging—the efforts of the United Nations in this area.

There are a number of reasons that NGOs have emerged as key players and often leaders on the global health and human rights stage. First and foremost, NGOs have the benefit of specificity in their cause, a certain degree of autonomy in their operations as compared to governmental organization and a characteristic personal investment, passion and commitment. Furthermore, efforts at the governmental level have, by and large, fallen short of projected goals.

NGOs dedicated to humanitarian health, medicine and emergency relief have played major roles in increasing the public's knowledge of the tragic health consequences of armed conflicts and natural disasters. These include the Red Cross Movement, MSF, Doctors of the World, the International Rescue Committee, Partners in Health, Physicians for Human Rights and several others operating frequently in extremely hazardous situations. It seemed natural for these groups to supplement their physician-focused bioethics language and approach with the language of human rights, especially health and human rights. Human rights and bioethics have not merged, but the ways in which they complement each other is well-illustrated in the health-related work of these NGOs. Yet, in situations of open conflicts, humanitarian NGOs have had to struggle with the constant dilemma of having to choose between silently and resiliently caring for victims as consistent with medical ethics or denouncing the blatant human rights violations they witness when public disclosure may expose the sustainability of their medical work and the safety of their staff to retaliations by local authorities. This dilemma, and the inherent tension between human rights and ethical imperatives, continues to plague the humanitarian field, and ever more so as the very nature of conflicts continues to evolve. Indeed, the last few decades have been marked by the eruption of civil wars, open international conflicts and other forms of collective violence in the Great Lakes region of East Africa and in West Africa, Central and East Asia and the Balkans. A persisting trend noted since World War II is the growing prominence of intra-state collective conflicts and the relative recess of inter-state conflicts.[3] Among the implications of these trends are that the International Geneva Conventions[4] which impose obligations of restraint and care concerning civilian populations, prisoners of war and the wounded in military conflict are unlikely to be adhered to by warring parties which do not hold State status. A further implication of this evolving trend is that "*in many of today's conflicts, civilians have become the main targets of violence. It is now conventional to put the proportion of civilian casualties somewhere in the region of 75%.*"[5] The 2011–2012 "Arab Spring" uprisings demonstrated how, invoking human rights, civil society could successfully challenge undemocratic governments with real immediate transformative impacts, even as these need to be monitored and assessed over time as societal changes set in.

The turn of the new Millennium brought firm hopes of greater peace, justice and security, a more equitable distribution of resources across the globe, changes in global and national governance and the progress of democracy, all inspired by human rights principles and a universal aspiration for better health and well-being. To date, unsurprisingly, these hopes have not (yet) been realized. Among the many obstacles to change, perhaps most of concern for the long term has been the global financial crisis affecting primarily and immediately high-income economies with an anticipated delayed impact on developing countries. "The world economy is teetering on the brink of another major downturn," says a May 2012 UN report on the World Economic Situation and Prospects. The report discusses "several policy directions which could avoid a double-dip recession, including: optimal design of fiscal policies to stimulate more direct job creation and investment in infrastructure, energy efficiency and sustainable energy supply, and food security; stronger financial safety nets; better coordination between fiscal and monetary policies; and the provision of sufficient support to developing countries in addressing the fallout from the crisis and the coordination of policy measures at the international level."[6] It is hoped that the voice of developing countries will be heard as responses are brought to bear on a global financial crisis which, in the long run, is likely to affect disproportionately and catastrophically the least advanced economies.

Already, the last two decades have witnessed a great volatility of international aid with significant implications for health and human rights. Aid peaked in 1992 over $60 billion to fall 6% to $56.4 billion in 1999, rose again in subsequent years to an unprecedented $137 billion in 2010 to fall again by 2.7% to $133.5 billion in 2011 as a result of the global financial crisis. To be noted is that this assistance represents only 0.31 per cent of the combined gross national income of members of the Development Assistance Committee of the Organization for Economic Co-operation and Development (OECD), far from the 0.7% threshold they had committed to in the 1990s.[7, 8]

The last two decades have also been marked by the rise of terrorism and the overwhelming response to what has been characterized as an "asymmetrical threat." The United States government post-9/11 greatly diminished its support for human rights protections, and adopted a US-centric, self-defense posture that permitted massive human rights violations to occur in the name of national security, including torture and arbitrary detention. These actions have threatened to destroy the country's credibility on human rights, and it is no longer able to effectively condemn, or even critique, massive human rights violations of other major powers, including China and Russia. Within the US, the 9/11 tragedy has also resulted in weariness of the International Criminal Court (ICC), not least by the US Congress that opposed the US joining the court, by fear that its armed forces and government officials might find themselves in the dock of the ICC. That the ICC is the "permanent Nuremberg" that the US fought so long to establish, but now will not even join, is tragic.

Fortunately, concerted responses to global health disparities, some designed with creative funding mechanisms, new oversight structures and supported by unprecedented amounts of financial resources have also emerged in the last 20 years. Indeed, by 2000, the deepening economic and health divide between affluent and low income countries, and within all of them the expanding disparity between the rich and the poor, had become so apparent that all could agree nothing short of a bold, massive and coordinated investment in health could improve the situation. Several initiatives were launched in the advent of the 21st century to curb poverty and ill health, a turning point which can rightly be cited as a landmark in global health. Three major global initiatives emerged within a few years: the Millennium Development Goals (MDGs, 2000), the foundation of the Global Alliance for Vaccines and Immunization (GAVI, 2000) and the creation of the Global Fund to fight AIDS, Tuberculosis and Malaria (GFATM, 2001). Each of these deserves a brief commentary here as they have responded to a revitalized interest in curbing global health and rights inequities.

The Millennium Development Declaration in 2000 by the United Nations General Assembly and the universal adoption of the MDG Goals were a bold attempt to alleviate poverty drastically within 15 years.[9] Along with poverty alleviation, some aspects of health were central to this endeavor either explicitly in the form of specific MDGs or implicitly as a condition for, and the outcome of, the realization of all other MDGs. Regrettably, it took several years to spell out the human rights dimensions of the MDGs, and even once spelled out, there was no link to the MDG accountability mechanisms, despite the fact that the Declaration from which they were born was explicit about these links. Nevertheless, as a human development framework, the MDGs have helped shape official development assistance and have remained very present in national and international agendas. The links between the MDGs and human rights have now been made explicit and as the Office of the High Commissioner for Human Rights (OHCHR) puts it: "*Governments that pursue development hand-in-hand with human rights stand a better chance of reaching the Millennium Development Goals (MDGs).*"[10] As we move towards a post-2015 agenda, one which will no doubt reflect the successes but also the failures of the MDGs, we must ensure sustained attention to human rights in the development and implementation of the new goals and framework.

The GAVI Alliance was also launched in 2000, at a time when the coverage of childhood immunizations failed to reach one in every five children in the poorest parts of the world. With a US$750 million initial commitment from the Bill & Melinda Gates Foundation, the vision of giving these children access to existing vaccines as well as newly developed ones against the leading killer diseases of children under the age of five was formed. By 2010, 288 million children had been immunized against life-threatening diseases and more than five million future deaths had been averted (2010 WHO estimation). Ever since it was founded, GAVI has remained rather silent about the connections between immunization and human rights. However, it states: "*If immunisation coverage is an index of how a child's right to basic health is respected, then the UN Convention on the Rights of the Child (CRC) is currently failing children in developing countries.*"[11] All is in the "if." Progress in immunization over the last decade has created a need to go beyond what GAVI can achieve. In 2012, the World Health Assembly (65th WHA, 2012) adopted a Global Action Plan to further scale-up immunization, complete the eradication of poliomyelitis and embark on control and elimination of measles and rubella. The WHA resolution underscores a principle laid out in the plan . . . "*Recognizing the importance of immunization as one of the most cost-effective interventions in public health which should be recognized as a core component of the human right to health.*"

In addition, in 2000 the World Health Organization (WHO) presented to the G8 summit in Okinawa a proposal to embark on a "massive effort to tackle infectious diseases" and create "a new mechanism to take proven interventions to scale."[12] Following consultations with donors, other UN agencies and foundations, the Global Fund to fight AIDS, Tuberculosis (TB) and Malaria (GFATM) became operational two years later. The mechanism would achieve internationally agreed targets to cut TB and malaria mortality by 50%, and HIV infection by 25% at a projected cost of $25 billion within five years. Within the following decade, the GFATM had committed US$22.6 billion in 150 countries to support large-scale prevention, treatment and care programs against the three diseases. Over time, human rights language, concepts and priorities found themselves sporadically within the work of the GFATM. The GFATM strategy was reformulated in 2012, however, now includes an explicit strategic direction to "Promote and protect human rights in the context of the three diseases . . . by ensuring that the Global Fund does not support programs that infringe human rights, increases investments in programs that address human rights-related barriers to access, and integrate human rights considerations throughout the grant cycle."[13] The extent to which these commitments will be reflected in funded proposals will depend on country capacity to incorporate human rights implementation and monitoring in their respective plan of action.

The emergence of these initiatives has brought unprecedented attention and resources to important public health issues—there are today more than 70 global health ventures underway—but the general failure to link them up-front to health and human rights concepts, methods and practice represents missed opportunities. Some human rights language appears here and there in relevant strategic statements, often limited to the prevention and redress of discrimination as may occur in the context of the chosen targeted diseases, but not extending human rights analyses and approaches to other dimensions that could add power and clarity to strategic designs. For example, value would be added to these initiatives at little extra cost to document the impacts of these initiatives not only on one or few but all MDGs. Omitting to examine systematically how these initiatives actually promote and protect the human rights to gender equality, to empowerment through participation, to education, to privacy and to other facets of human development does not bode well for their long-term sustainability. For narrowly targeted initiatives to survive political shifts and withstand donor volatility, they have to show not only that they successfully produce the intended health outcomes, but that they also have a desirable impact on other aspects of health and development, including the progressive realization of human rights.

Other significant developments have marked the evolution of global health in the last decade. Recognizing the positive that has and will result from these should not be misconstrued as deliberate oversight of the seriousness of the problems these developments are intended to respond to, often late and with insufficient political commitment and resources. Among these is the scaling-up since 2002 of access to HIV/AIDS care and treatment in the most affected parts of the world. By 2012, such treatment is reaching almost half of the eligible population in sub-Saharan Africa, the other half still not having access due to health system failures or the lack of resources. Childhood mortality has declined significantly, thanks to the expansion of immunization and more effective child care and nutrition. Worldwide, mortality in children younger than five years has dropped from 11.9 million deaths in 1990 to 7.7 million deaths in 2010 but disparities persist both across and within countries, including the United States.[14] The "Global Strategy for Women's and Children's Health" launched in 2010 sets out a plan for working together to "save women and children." It was developed under the auspices of the United Nations General-Secretary, Ban Ki-moon, and is supported by The Partnership for Maternal, Newborn & Child Health. The Global Strategy was launched at the time of the UN Leaders' Summit for the Millennium Development Goals (MDGs) in 2010, with some US$40 billion pledged towards women's health and children's health and the achievement of MDGs 4 & 5—to reduce child mortality and improve maternal health albeit with no explicit attention to rights in its formulation and approaches. Important, therefore, was the call shortly thereafter to eliminate preventable maternal mortality and morbidity through women's empowerment, which, in the context of the slow progress towards the related MDG 5, recalled the numerous declarations and plans of action since the 1994 Cairo conference as these, sadly, had had limited impacts on maternal mortality trends in the most affected countries.[15] Such shortcomings can be attributed to system failures whereby public health and human rights concerns are well documented, publicly acknowledged, recognized as global priorities in various international declarations, resolutions and national policies, and yet insufficiently attended to. The gaps between stated intents and actions in the realm of equitable health, social and economic development and human rights will remain a chronic challenge both within and across all countries, regardless of their level of income.

The first decade of the millennium has made it plain that if old threats to public health were still present, newly emerging epidemics were adding their toll to human health and national economies. SARS, avian flu H5N1, and swine flu H1N1 spread across the world, not always as massively as was feared, but always with a particular impact on disadvantaged communities. Multiple drug-resistant TB and more recently extensively drug-resistant TB are now spreading in communities where access to early diagnosis and first-line treatment is poorly implemented, for example in prison populations among others. The health and human rights implications of such rising threats, as well as of the responses brought against them, will have serious implications for human health, social harmony and faltering economies going forward. In 2005, the WHO produced new International Health Regulations upholding the principle that "*The implementation of these Regulations shall be with full respect for the dignity, human rights and fundamental freedoms of persons.*"[16] But they are silent about how, in practice, this principle is to be applied and monitored. The post-9/11 "*War on terrorism*" has amply illustrated how arbitrary derogations on human rights can be made under the pretence of protecting security and, in the case of bioterrorism, public health. Furthermore, the war and terrorism metaphors have been widely adapted to disease prevention and treatment, with the result that human rights have often been seen as expendable in the context of a potential global pandemic or a bioterrorist attack, the mantras "*saving lives*" and "*national security*" often replacing that of human rights and human dignity.

Many other public health and human rights issues that have come to light in the last decade could be added to this list: the unabated promotion of tobacco particularly in low and medium economies in spite of the 2005 WHO Framework Convention on Tobacco Control which reaffirms the right of all people to the highest standard of health, and is the first treaty negotiated under the auspices of the World Health Organization; the distress of health systems faced with structural decay and the erosion of human resources for health; the continuing neglect of non-communicable diseases in developing countries in the shadow of large-scale responses to selected communicable diseases; and the weakening or absence of equitable health insurance systems.[17] In the USA alone, nearly 50 million, or 16.3% of Americans were uninsured in 2012, with the lack of insurance affecting disproportionately Black and Hispanic communities and, among them, children. Steps are now underway to provide reasonable health care insurance to most of the United States population, as a result of a US Supreme Court decision, but the devil is of course in the details.

There have also been significant developments in the international human rights field during the last two decades, particularly during the most recent one. One of the most important has been the inauguration of the above-mentioned International Criminal Court, where those accused of war crimes and crimes against humanity can be tried. There have been other structural and political changes as well. Structurally, the UN human rights machinery underwent a reform leading to the creation of the Human

Rights Council, an inter-governmental body within the United Nations system made up of 47 States responsible for the promotion and protection of all human rights around the globe. Since 2006, the Universal Periodic Review, a new mechanism to improve the human rights situation in all countries and address human rights violations wherever they occur, has been put in place and often includes inquiry and discussion of health related issues. Two international human rights treaties with significant implications for health-related work came into force: the International Convention for the Protection of All Persons from Enforced Disappearance (2006) and most importantly the International Convention on the Rights of Persons with Disabilities (2006). Several General Comments have been issued by various treaty monitoring bodies in which they lay out their interpretation of the content of human rights provisions. Particularly relevant to the theme of this book are General Comments on: the Right to the Highest Attainable Standard of Health (2000); Derogations during a State of Emergency (2001); the Right to Water (2002); HIV/AIDS and the Right of the Child (2003); and Adolescent Health (2003).[18] And after forty years of negotiations, a Declaration on the Rights of Indigenous Peoples finally came into being (2007). The Declaration establishes a universal framework of minimum standards for the survival, dignity, well-being and rights of the world's indigenous peoples. It is hoped, with guarded optimism, that it will not take such a long time to move it to the status of an international human rights treaty.

These developments have, unfortunately, not occurred in an environment of unfailing state support and commitment to the promotion and protection of human rights. In fact, earlier commitments to human rights by states seem to have receded. Such has been the case with regards to sexual and reproductive rights where it seemed after the spate of international conferences happening in the mid-1990s that these rights were not only understood by the international community, but recognized as a priority. The move away from demographic models of population control towards a reproductive rights model which recognized respect, protection and fulfilment of rights as key to sustainable development was welcomed in the mid-1990s not only by advocates and progressive states but by the very people whose lives are affected by these decisions around the world and by the ways in which resources are therefore allocated. And positive changes did happen, in law and policy, in programmatic directions and in health outcomes. Increasingly, however, the so-called "*sensitive*" issues raised by attention to sexual and reproductive rights (e.g., young people's sexuality, homosexuality, abortion, the fertility intentions of HIV positive people and other key populations) are being overtaken by an increasingly conservative national and global climate. There is the very real concern that these issues are slowly and deliberately being taken off the global agenda—with potentially enormous repercussions for the health and rights of millions of people around the globe.

In spite of the aforementioned setbacks, the past decade has seen mounting interest in countries around the world to integrate human rights norms and standards into their health and development efforts. Hand in hand with this is the increasing role a number of countries are playing in the global economy and their desire to comply with global norms, standards and practices. Work in health and human rights requires the strengths of a range of disciplines, departments and schools, including public health, medicine, law, economics, international relations, communications, philosophy and the social sciences. These linkages are generating new ideas and approaches, including growth of academic centers with an explicit focus on the linkages between health and human rights, and increases in the number of courses being taught around the world with an explicit health and human rights focus. NGOs, governments and academic institutions around the globe are beginning to engage in this field in their research and programmatic work. This has resulted in increased attention to working across disciplines in order to advance fruitful conceptual work, empirical research and applied programs. Both conceptual and empirical work have been translated into tools in a growing variety of settings which has generated useful debate about their value amongst those concerned with these issues. Perspectives, concepts and semantics pertaining to health and human rights are not always consistent across disciplinary boundaries but differences reflect the intrinsic dynamism of this evolving field.

Altogether, the evolution of the world in the last two decades has been marked by half-successes and blatant failures. From an optimistic point of view, awareness, stated commitments and some actions in support of health and human rights agendas have multiplied since the launching of the movement in-spite of—and occasionally prompted by—civil, political, social, economic and cultural events that have exposed the world's vulnerability to human rights violations and ill health. From a less optimistic point of view, however, the values, norms and standards relevant to health and human rights remain weak elements in policy formulation and program development. The weakest links remain national and international governance mechanisms. States should be the prime actors in promoting and protecting health and human rights, and they should con-sciously deliver their obligations on both accounts and be willingly and transparently accountable. Unfortunately, as Albert Camus put it: "By definition, a government has no conscience. Sometimes it has a policy, but nothing more." It is our hope that you will find this book of use in exploring the world of health and human rights. That is as much as we can reasonably ask of you, but we also hope and believe that some of you will be inspired by the readings and work happening in this field. Revolted by the health, injustice and poverty problems that persist, you will have the option of being a passive passenger of this planet or instead choose to strive to ensure better policy, quality research and relent-less action to help make the world a better place for all of us and future generations.

ABOUT THIS TEXTBOOK

This textbook brings together carefully chosen texts of high scholarly quality, the vast majority of which have appeared in peer-reviewed journals or academic books in the last decade. They were chosen to best reflect knowledge gains and conceptual developments born out of experience, debates and research. Our selection of arti-cles was unfortunately constrained and somewhat skewed by the lack of literature on the subject from health and human rights writers in developing countries. The reader must rest assured that, as contributions from these authors expand, they will appear in their rightful place in further editions of this book. This book has both similarities and differences to the past two *Health and Human Rights* Readers.[19, 20] Like them, it includes the most important and relevant new publications we could find in the field. Unlike them, it is written as a textbook to be used in classroom-based instruction on health and human rights.

This book consists of five parts and a concluding note:

Part I is a health and human rights overview laying-out the essential knowledge base and providing the foundation for the following parts.

Part II brings in notions of concepts, methods and governance framing the application of health and human rights, in particular human rights-based approaches to health.

Part III sheds light on issues of heightened vulnerability and special protection, stressing that the health and human rights record of any nation, and any community, is determined by what is being done and not done about those who are most in need.

Part IV takes a focus on addressing system failures, where health and human rights issues have been documented, recognized, even at times proclaimed as priorities, and yet insufficiently attended to as a result of state denial, unwillingness or incapacity.

Part V examines the relevance of the health and human rights paradigm to a changing world, underscoring contemporary global challenges and responses.

Finally, a **Concluding Note** brings together the key themes of this set of chapters and attempts to project a vision of the future.

Each part of the book includes an introductory text and selected publications deemed to have achieved excellence in scholarly terms. Also included are short **Points of View** which give voice to leaders in the health and human rights field, creating a space to hear their thoughts and ideas in a personal, informal fashion.

Each chapter is followed by questions suggested to stimulate thinking and debate about the contents of the chapters and beyond. Also included are suggested additional readings to stimulate discussion that project views that may be consistent or at variance with those in the piece to which they are attached. Additionally, proposed topics for discussion appear at the end of each part to help frame group reflecton and interaction around the theme to which each part is devoted.

To save precious space, align the lay-out of chapters throughout the book, facilitate reading, and encourage students to search data bases and consult original sources of articles herein presented, explanatory footnotes have been removed. These can be found in the original publications, all of which are listed in the credits section at the end of this book and accessible from libraries and/or through the internet.

We wish you pleasant and fruitful reading, and invite you to take an active part in advancing the health and human rights action and research agenda.

REFERENCES

1. Gruskin S, Mills EJ, Tarantola D, History, principles, and practice of health and human rights, *The Lancet*, 4 August 2007, Vol. 370, 9585: 449–455.
2. Tarantola D (2008) A perspective on the history of health and human rights: from the Cold War to the Gold War, *Journal of Public Health Policy* 29(1): 42–53.
3. Jung D, Schlichte K, *From Inter-State War to Warlordism. Changing Forms of Collective Violence in the International System*; in: *Ethnicity and Intra-State Conflict. Types, causes and peace strategies*, Wiberg H and Sherrer, eds, Aldershot: Ashgate, 1999, pp. 35–51.

4. Geneva Conventions, Federal Departement of Foreign Affairs, Switzerland, http://www.eda.admin.ch/eda/en/home/topics/intla/humlaw/gecons.html

5. Annan K, Intervention, Ditchley Foundation Lecture, 26 June 1998 cited in: Roberts, A., Lives and Statistics: Are 90% of War Victims Civilians? *Survival* vol. 52, no 3 (June-July 2012): pp. 115–136.

6. United Nations, Development and Analysis Division: World Economic Situation and Prospects 2012, Update as of mid-2012 http://www.un.org/en/development/desa/policy/wesp/wesp_archive/2012wespupdate.pdf retrieved 25–06–2112

7. United Nations, Development and Analysis Division: World Economic and Social Survey 2010 http://www.un.org/en/development/desa/policy/wess/wess_archive/2010wess_overview_en.pdf

8. OECD http://www.oecd.org/document/49/0,3746,en

9. The Millennium Development Goals and Human Rights, OHCHR, http://www.ohchr.org/EN/Issues/MDG/Pages/FoundationforEngagement.aspx

10. Office of the U.N. High Commissioner for Human Rights, http://www.ohchr.org/EN/Issues/MDG/Pages/FoundationforEngagement.aspx

11. The GAVI Alliance, http://www.gavialliance.org/

12. The massive effort to tackle infectious diseases: a key to global prosperity, Round Table Meeting: Challenges for Development, http://www.who.int/director-general/speeches/2000/english/20000720_tokyo.html

13. The Global Fund Strategy, http://www.theglobalfund.org/en/library/documents/ retrieved 25–06–2012

14. Rajaratnam JK, Marcus JR, Flaxman AD, Wang H, Levin-Rector A, Dwyer L, Costa M, Lopez AD, Murray CJL. Neonatal, postneonatal, childhood, and under-5 mortality for 187 countries, 1970–2010: a systematic analysis of progress towards Millennium Development Goal 4. *The Lancet*. 24 May 2010, Vol. 375: 1988–2008.

15. United Nations Economic and Social Council, Commission on the Status of Women, 2010, http://www.un.org/womenwatch/daw/beijing15/outcomes/L%206%20_%20MM.Advance%20unedited.pdf

16. The International Health Regulations, art.3.1, 2005, http://whqlibdoc.who.int/publications/2008/9789241580410_eng.pdf

17. Iibrahim M, Damasceno I, Hypertension in Developing Countries, *The Lancet*, 11 August 2012, Vol. 380, 9841, 611–619.

18. OHCHR, General Comments, http://www2.ohchr.org/english/bodies/treaty/comments.htm

19. Mann, J M, Grodin, M A, Gruskin, S, Annas, G J, eds, *Health and Human Rights: A Reader*, London: Routledge, 1999.

20. Gruskin, S, Grodin, M A, Marks, S P, Annas, G J, eds, *Perspectives on Health and Human Rights*, London: Routldege, 2005.

PART I

*H*ealth and Human Rights Overview

Introduction

History is always important, even when it's a young history. Health and human rights is now widely recognized as a field of inquiry but this was not always the case. This first part of the book provides key pieces which have helped to promote clear thinking about the linkages between health and human rights, and to establishing the conceptual rigor of the field of health and human rights as we know it today.

It has been two decades since publication of the first chapter by Jonathan Mann and colleagues in 1994 set the basis for development of what is now understood to be the field of health and human rights. Since the early stages of the women's health, mental health, reproductive health, and indigenous health movements it has been asserted that public health policies and programs must be cognizant and respectful of human rights norms and standards. It was also thought that lack of respect for human rights hampered the effectiveness of public health policies and programs. Under Mann's leadership, an important first step in developing the health and human rights field was to draw attention, in particular, to the connections between the rights of people living with HIV and an effective public health response. Drawing on insights from the AIDS field, this piece presents the start of the conceptual work that has since emerged on the linkages between health and rights. As a result of this first piece, different approaches and areas where health and human rights were already being linked began to be heard and debated, courses to sensitize new generations of public health and other professionals to the value of exploring these linkages were started, and the conceptual and empirical development of the field began.

Within a short time, the question of "why" health and human rights had shifted to "how." How to do it in practice and what it meant to link these areas of research and study. Even as many thought the relationships between health and human rights made intuitive sense, it took development of a "health and human rights" language and the explicit naming of the connections between health and human rights to underpin and legitimize the conceptual, analytical, and empirical work that followed. Two pieces are included here which introduce this history. The chapter by Gruskin, Mills and Tarantola emphasizes the role that health professionals can play in reducing and preventing human rights violations, as well as in ensuring that health-related policies and practices promote rights. It discusses the changing views of human rights, with particular attention to HIV, and propose further development of the right to health through increased practice, evidence, and action. The piece that follows by Tarantola and Gruskin also draws from the experience gained in the global response to AIDS, and goes on to summarize ways in which key dimensions of public health and of human rights intersect and may be used as a framework for health policy analysis, development, and evaluation. Kirby then provides a compelling and personal set of insights on the history of the health and human rights movement.

As the field is still new, efforts are needed to ensure a rigorous and coherent approach to scholarship, which not only establishes the theoretical foundations for the field but also demonstrates tangible impacts. The piece by Paul Hunt, the former Special Rapporteur on the Right to the Highest Attainable Standard of Health, and his colleague Gunilla Backman, builds on established conceptual work in both the human rights and public health arenas to show how practical application of *the right to the highest attainable standard of health* can result in an effective and integrated health system. By systematically applying the recognized components of the right to health across the "building blocks" that together are understood by the World Health Organization and others to constitute a functioning health system, this article begins to bridge theory and practice.

To illuminate the distinct contributions offered by linking human rights to health, engagement with the various frameworks concerned with justice in health is necessary. In particular, the distinct relationship between bieoethics and the health field has highlighted important synergies with human rights, as well as places where each provide distinct contributions. Initially, there was the need to clarify why those engaged in health, as broadly defined, had to be concerned with human rights—as it was thought that ethics offered all that was needed for those with an interest in justice and health. At the outset of the health and human rights movement, Jonathan Mann argued that ethics was the natural language of medicine and human rights, the natural language of public health—and this formulation seemed just right. The Andorno article on "bioethics at UNESCO" outlines the controversies behind the new Universal Declaration of Bioethics and Human Rights, a major accomplishment by 180 nations. The UNESCO challenge is to recognize that while human rights are universal, and ethics more situational, there are commonalities and that, as the world shrinks and global health becomes more prominent, it makes sense to try to agree upon global bioethical standards that are consistent with human rights.

The first major document incorporating human rights principles into an area of direct concern to health professionals was the Nuremberg Code. We include an edited version of General Telford Taylor's opening statement at the 1946–7 trial of the Nazi doctors which led to articulation of the Code in the Judgment to provide a true piece of "living history." The Nazi Doctors were being tried for crimes against humanity and war crimes involving the murder and torture of concentration camp prisoners in a variety of barbaric human "experiments." The Code stands to this day as the most authoritative statement of rules for the proper conduct of research on human subjects, and is one the first clear articulations of the relationship between human rights and bioethics, and arguably as the birth of bioethics itself.

We close this part with a piece by Annas which takes a wide-ranging view introducing and reflecting on links between emergence of the health and human rights movement, with the fields of bioethics and social justice. Each has distinct value and, as Annas demonstrates, the differences in the paradigms they represent in particular with respect to means of observance, action, and enforcement if brought together explicitly have the potential to strengthen the work of all concerned with health and well-being. Drawing on popular culture and well-known references, and using examples drawn from the world of clinical research trials, as well as the nefarious impacts of globalization on health and rights, to make his points, Annas provides an intellectually grounded and entertaining argument for strengthening work in global health through explicit and conscious attention to human rights by governments, NGOs, and even transnational corporations.

Taken together, these pieces clarify the value of application of human rights norms and standards, both individually and in relation to other theoretical constructs, to address the underlying determinants of health, improve the delivery of health services, and ultimately impact health outcomes. Work in health and human rights is, by necessity, interdisciplinary. It requires the strengths of a range of disciplines, departments and schools, including public health, medicine, law, economics, international relations, communications, philosophy and the social sciences. The emphasis on the "AND" in "health and human rights" is at the forefront of bringing together this range of disciplines to advance fruitful conceptual work, empirical research, and applied programs. The ultimate goal has to be to generate cutting-edge scholarship on the links between health and human rights, and ultimately to yield the critical insights that can illuminate the forces and factors that shape—and the work that can be done to improve—population health around the world.

TOPICS FOR DISCUSSION

1. Consider the historical evolution of the health and human rights movement, and its initial groundings in various health topics. Why do you think that it was not until the HIV pandemic that global attention to the links between health and rights began to be understood and acted upon?
2. Name some current examples of human rights violations that have a significant impact on health. Consider both short- and long-term implications.
3. Cite some examples of policies or programs raising concerns about rights being infringed upon.
4. Take one health topic (e.g. tuberculosis, the rise of non-communicable disease, or the provision of abortion services), and consider the differences between application of a human rights lens, a social justice lens, and a bioethics framework as to how you would analyze and address the topic.

CHAPTER 1

Health and Human Rights

Jonathan M. Mann, Lawrence O. Gostin, Sofia Gruskin, Troyen Brennan, Zita Lazzarini and Harvey V. Fineberg

Health and human rights have rarely been linked in an explicit manner. With few exceptions, notably involving access to health care, discussions about health have rarely included human rights considerations. Similarly, except when obvious damage to health is the primary manifestation of a human rights abuse, such as with torture, health perspectives have been generally absent from human rights discourse.

Explanations for the dearth of communication between the fields of health and human rights include differing philosophical perspectives, vocabularies, professional recruitment and training, societal roles, and methods of work. In addition, modern concepts of both health and human rights are complex and steadily evolving. On a practical level, health workers may wonder about the applicability or utility ("added value"), let alone necessity of incorporating human rights perspectives into their work, and vice versa. In addition, despite pioneering work seeking to bridge this gap in bioethics,[1,2] jurisprudence,[3] and public health law,[4,5] a history of conflictual relationships between medicine and law, or between public health officials and civil liberty advocates, may contribute to anxiety and doubt about the potential for mutually beneficial collaboration.

Yet health and human rights are both powerful, modern approaches to defining and advancing human well-being. Attention to the intersection of health and human rights may provide practical benefits to those engaged in health or human rights work, may help reorient thinking about major global health challenges, and may contribute to broadening human rights thinking and practice. However, meaningful dialogue about interactions between health and human rights requires a common ground. To this end, following a brief overview of selected features of modern health and human rights, this chapter proposes a provisional, mutually accessible framework for structuring discussions about research, promoting cross-disciplinary education, and exploring the potential for health and human rights collaboration.

MODERN CONCEPTS OF HEALTH

Modern concepts of health derive from two related although quite different disciplines: medicine and public health. While medicine generally focuses on the health of an individual, public health emphasizes the health of populations. To oversimplify, individual health has been the concern of medical and other health care services, generally in the context of physical (and, to a lesser extent, mental) illness and disability. In contrast, public health has been defined as, ". . . [ensuring] the conditions in which people can be healthy."[6] Thus, public health has a distinct health-promoting goal and emphasizes prevention of disease, disability and premature death.

Therefore, from a public health perspective, while the availability of medical and other health care constitutes one of the essential conditions for health, it is not synonymous with "health." Only a small fraction of the variance of health status among populations can reasonably be attributed to health care; health care is necessary but clearly not sufficient for health.[7]

The most widely used modern definition of health was developed by the World Health Organization (WHO): "Health is a state of complete physical, mental and social well-being and not merely the absence of disease or infirmity."[8] Through this definition, WHO has helped to move health thinking beyond a limited, biomedical and pathology-based perspective to the more positive domain of "well-being." Also, by explicitly including the mental and social dimensions of well-being, WHO radically expanded the scope of health, and by extension, the roles and responsibilities of health professionals and their relationship to the larger society.

The WHO definition also highlights the importance of health promotion, defined as "the process of enabling people to increase control over, and to improve, their health." To do so, "an individual or group must be able to identify and realize aspirations, to satisfy needs, and to change or cope with the environment."[9] The societal dimensions of this effort were emphasized in the Declaration of Alma-Ata (1978), which described health as a ". . . social goal whose realization requires the action of many other social and economic sectors in addition to the health sector."[10]

Thus, the modern concept of health includes yet goes beyond health care to embrace the broader societal dimensions and context of individual and population well-being. Perhaps the most far-reaching statement about the expanded scope of health is contained in the preamble to the WHO Constitution, which declared that "the enjoyment of the highest attainable standard of health is one of the fundamental rights of every human being."[11]

MODERN HUMAN RIGHTS

The modern idea of human rights is similarly vibrant, hopeful, ambitious and complex. While there is a long history to human rights thinking, agreement was reached that all people are "born free and equal in dignity and rights"[12] when the promotion of human rights was identified as a principal purpose of the United Nations in 1945.[13] Then, in 1948, the Universal Declaration of Human Rights was adopted as a universal or common standard of achievement for all peoples and all nations.

The preamble to the Universal Declaration proposes that human rights and dignity are self-evident, the "highest aspiration of the common people," and "the foundation of freedom, justice and peace." "Social progress and better standards of life in larger freedom," including the prevention of "barbarous acts which have outraged the conscience of mankind," and, broadly speaking, individual and collective well-being, are considered to depend upon the "promotion of universal respect for and observance of human rights."

Several fundamental characteristics of modern human rights include: they are rights of individuals; these rights inhere in individuals because they are human; they apply to all people around the world; and they principally involve the relationship between the state and the individual. The specific rights which form the corpus of human rights law are listed in several key documents. Foremost is the Universal

Declaration of Human Rights (UDHR), which, along with the United Nations Charter (UN Charter), the International Covenant on Civil and Political Rights (ICCPR)—and its Optional Protocols—and the International Covenant on Economic, Social and Cultural Rights (ICESCR), constitute what is often called the "International Bill of Human Rights." The UDHR was drawn up to give more specific definition to the rights and freedoms referred to in the UN Charter. The ICCPR and the ICESCR further elaborate the content set out in the UDHR, as well as setting out the conditions in which states can permissibly restrict rights.

Although the UDHR is not a legally binding document, nations (states) have endowed it with great legitimacy through their actions, including its legal and political invocation at the national and international level. For example, portions of the UDHR are cited in numerous national constitutions, and governments often refer to the UDHR when accusing other governments of violating human rights. The Covenants are legally binding, but only on the states which have become parties to them. Parties to the Covenants accept certain procedures and responsibilities, including periodic submission of reports on their compliance with the substantive provisions of the texts.

Building upon this central core of documents, a large number of additional declarations and conventions have been adopted at the international and regional levels, focusing upon either specific populations (such as the International Convention on the Elimination of All Forms of Racial Discrimination, entry into force in 1969; the Convention on the Elimination of All Forms of Discrimination Against Women, 1981; the Convention on the Rights of the Child, 1989) or issues such as the Convention Against Torture and Other Cruel, Inhuman or Degrading Treatment or Punishment, entry into force in 1987; the Declaration on

the Elimination of All Forms of Intolerance and of Discrimination Based on Religion or Belief, 1981.

Since 1948, the promotion and protection of human rights have received increased attention from communities and nations around the world. While there are few legal sanctions to compel states to meet their human rights obligations, states are increasingly monitored for their compliance with human rights norms by other states, nongovernmental organizations, the media and private individuals. The growing legitimacy of the human rights framework lies in the increasing application of human rights standards by a steadily widening range of actors in the world community. The awarding of the Nobel Peace Prize for human rights work to Amnesty International and to Ms. Rigoberta Menchu symbolizes this extraordinary level of contemporary interest and concern with human rights.

Since the late 1940s, human rights advocacy and related challenges have gradually extended the boundaries of the human rights movement in four related ways. First, the initial advocacy focus on civil and political rights and certain economic and social rights is expanding to include concerns about the environment and global socioeconomic development. For example, although the right to a "social and international order in which (human rights) can be fully realized" (UDHR, Article 28) invokes broad political issues at the global level, attention to this core concept as a right has only grown in recent years.

Second, while the grounding of human rights thinking and practice in law (at national and international levels) remains fundamental, wider social involvement and participation in human rights struggles is increasingly broadening the language and uses of human rights concepts.

Third, while human rights law primarily focuses on the relationship between individuals and states, awareness is increasing that other societal institutions and systems, such as transnational business, may strongly influence the capacity for realization of rights, yet they may elude state control. For example, exploitation of natural resources by business interests may seriously harm rights of local residents, yet the governmental capacity to protect human rights may be extremely limited, or at best indirect, through regulation of business practices and laws which offer the opportunity for redress. In addition, certain individual acts, such as rape, have not been a traditional concern of human rights law, except when resulting from systematic state policy (as alleged in Bosnia). However, it is increasingly evident that state policies impacting on the status and role of women may contribute importantly, even if indirectly, to a societal context which increases women's vulnerability to rape, even though the actual act may be individual, not state-sponsored.

Finally, the twin challenges of human rights promotion (hopefully preventing rights violations; analogous to health promotion to prevent disease) and protection (emphasizing accountability and redress for violations; analogous to medical care once disease has occurred) have often been approached separately. Initially, the United Nations system highlighted promotion of rights, and the nongovernmental human rights movement tended to stress protection of rights, often in response to horrific and systematic rights violations. More recently, both intergovernmental and nongovernmental agencies have recognized and responded to the fundamental interdependence of rights promotion and protection.

In summary, despite tremendous controversy, especially regarding the philosophical and cultural context of human rights as currently defined, a vocabulary and set of human rights norms is increasingly becoming part of community, national and global life.

A PROVISIONAL FRAMEWORK: LINKAGES BETWEEN HEALTH AND HUMAN RIGHTS

The goal of linking health and human rights is to contribute to advancing human well-being beyond what could be achieved through an isolated health- or human rights-based approach. This chapter proposes a three-part framework for considering linkages between health and human rights; all are interconnected, and each has substantial practical consequences. The first two are already well documented, although requiring further elaboration, while the third represents a central hypothesis calling for substantial additional analysis and exploration.

First, the impact (positive and negative) of health policies, programs and practices on human rights will be considered. This linkage will be illustrated by focusing on the use of state power in the context of public health.

The second relationship is based on the understanding that human rights violations have health impacts. It is proposed that all rights violations, particularly when severe, widespread and sustained, engender important health effects, which must be recognized and assessed. This process engages health expertise and methodologies in helping to understand how well-being is affected by violations of human rights.

The third part of this framework is based on an overarching proposition: that promotion and protection of human rights and promotion and protection of health are fundamentally linked. Even more than the first two proposed relationships, this intrinsic linkage has strategic implications and potentially dramatic practical consequences for work in each domain.

The First Relationship: The Impact of Health Policies, Programs and Practices on Human Rights

Around the world, health care is provided through many diverse public and private mechanisms. However, the responsibilities of public health are carried out in large measure through policies and programs promulgated, implemented and enforced by, or with support from, the state. Therefore, this first linkage may be best explored by considering the impact of public health policies, programs and practices on human rights.

The three central functions of public health include: assessing health needs and problems; developing policies designed to address priority health issues; and assuring programs to implement strategic health goals.[14] Potential benefits to and burdens on human rights may occur in the pursuit of each of these major areas of public health responsibility.

For example, assessment involves collection of data on important health problems in a population. However, data are not collected on all possible health problems, nor does the selection of which issues to assess occur in a societal vacuum. Thus, a state's failure to recognize or acknowledge health problems that preferentially affect a marginalized or stigmatized group may violate the right to non-discrimination by leading to neglect of necessary services, and in so doing, may adversely affect the realization of other rights, including the right to "security in the event of . . . sickness (or) disability . . .", or to the "special care and assistance" to which mothers and children are entitled (UDHR, Article 25).

Once decisions about which problems to assess have been made, the methodology of data collection may create additional human rights burdens. Collecting information from individuals, such as whether they are infected with the human immunodefi-

ciency virus (HIV), have breast cancer, or are genetically predisposed to heart disease, can clearly burden rights to security of person (associated with the concept of informed consent) and of arbitrary interference with privacy. In addition, the right of nondiscrimination may be threatened even by an apparently simple information-gathering exercise. For example, a health survey conducted via telephone, by excluding households without telephones (usually associated with lower socioeconomic status), may result in a biased assessment, which may in turn lead to policies or programs that fail to recognize or meet needs of the entire population. Also, personal health status or health behavior information (such as sexual orientation, or history of drug use) has the potential for misuse by the state, whether directly or if it is made available to others, resulting in grievous harm to individuals and violations of many rights. Thus, misuse of information about HIV infection status has led to: restrictions of the right to work and to education; violations of the right to marry and found a family; attacks upon honor and reputation; limitations of freedom of movement; arbitrary detention or exile; and even cruel, inhuman or degrading treatment.

The second major task of public health is to develop policies to prevent and control priority health problems. Important burdens on human rights may arise in the policy-development process. For example, if a government refuses to disclose the scientific basis of health policy or permit debate on its merits, or in other ways refuses to inform and involve the public in policy development, the rights to "seek, receive and impart information and ideas . . . regardless of frontiers" (UDHR, Article 19) and "to take part in the government . . . directly or through freely chosen representatives" (UDHR, Article 21) may be violated. Then, prioritization of health issues may result in discrimination against individuals, as when the major health problems of a population defined on the basis of sex, race, religion or language are systematically given lower priority (e.g., sickle cell disease in the United States, which affects primarily the African-American population; or more globally, maternal mortality, breast cancer and other health problems of women).

The third core function of public health, to assure services capable of realizing policy goals, is also closely linked with the right to non-discrimination. When health and social services do not take logistic, financial, and socio-cultural barriers to their access and enjoyment into account, intentional or unintentional discrimination may readily occur. For example, in clinics for maternal and child health, details such as hours of service, accessibility via public transportation and availability of daycare may strongly and adversely influence service utilization.[15]

It is essential to recognize that in seeking to fulfill each of its core functions and responsibilities, public health may burden human rights. In the past, when restrictions on human rights were recognized, they were often simply justified as necessary to protect public health. Indeed, public health has a long tradition, anchored in the history of infectious disease control, of limiting the "rights of the few" for the "good of the many." Thus, coercive measures such as mandatory testing and treatment, quarantine, and isolation are considered basic measures of traditional communicable disease control.[16]

The principle that certain rights must be restricted in order to protect the community is explicitly recognized in the International Bill of Human Rights: limitations are considered permissible to "(secure) due recognition and respect for the rights and freedoms of others and of meeting the just requirements of morality, public order and the general welfare in a democratic society"

(UDHR, Article 29). However, the permissible restriction of rights is bound in several ways. First, certain rights (e.g., right to life, right to be free from torture) are considered inviolable under any circumstances. Restriction of other rights must be: in the interest of a legitimate objective; determined by law; imposed in the least intrusive means possible; not imposed arbitrarily; and strictly necessary in a "democratic society" to achieve its purposes.

Unfortunately, public health decisions to restrict human rights have frequently been made in an uncritical, unsystematic and unscientific manner. Therefore, the prevailing assumption that public health, as articulated through specific policies and programs, is an unalloyed public good that does not require consideration of human rights norms must be challenged. For the present, it may be useful to adopt the maxim that health policies and programs should be considered discriminatory and burdensome on human rights until proven otherwise.

Yet this approach raises three related and vital questions. First, why should public health officials be concerned about burdening human rights? Second, to what extent is respect for human rights and dignity compatible with, or complementary to public health goals? Finally, how can an optimal balance between public health goals and human rights norms be negotiated?

Justifying public health concern for human rights norms could be based on the primary value of promoting societal respect for human rights as well as on arguments of public health effectiveness. At least to the extent that public health goals are not seriously compromised by respect for human rights norms, public health, as a state function, is obligated to respect human rights and dignity.

The major argument for linking human rights and health promotion is described below. However, it is also important to recognize that contemporary thinking about optimal strategies for disease control has evolved; efforts to confront the most serious global health threats, including cancer, cardiovascular disease and other chronic diseases, injuries, reproductive health, infectious diseases, and individual and collective violence, increasingly emphasize the role of personal behavior within a broad social context. Thus, the traditional public health paradigm and strategies developed for diseases such as smallpox, often involving coercive approaches and activities which may have burdened human rights, are now understood to be less relevant today. For example, WHO's strategy for preventing spread of the human immunodeficiency virus (HIV) excludes classic practices such as isolation and quarantine (except under truly remarkable circumstances) and explicitly calls for supporting and preventing discrimination against HIV-infected people.

The idea that human rights and public health must inevitably conflict is increasingly tempered with awareness of their complementarity. Health policy-makers' and practitioners' lack of familiarity with modern human rights concepts and core documents complicates efforts to negotiate, in specific situations and different cultural contexts, the optimal balance between public health objectives and human rights norms. Similarly, human rights workers may choose not to confront health policies or programs, either to avoid seeming to undervalue community health or due to uncertainty about how and on what grounds to challenge public health officials. Recently, in the context of HIV/AIDS, new approaches have been developed, seeking to maximize realization of public health goals while simultaneously protecting and promoting human rights.[17] Yet HIV/AIDS is not unique; efforts to harmonize health and human rights goals are clearly possible in other areas. At present, an effort to identify human rights burdens created by public health policies, programs and practices, followed by negotiation towards an optimal balance whenever public health and human rights goals appear to conflict, is a necessary minimum. An approach to realizing health objectives that simultaneously promotes—or at least respects—rights and dignity is clearly desirable.

The Second Relationship: Health Impacts Resulting from Violations of Human Rights

Health impacts are obvious and inherent in the popular understanding of certain severe human rights violations, such as torture, imprisonment under inhumane conditions, summary execution, and "disappearances." For this reason, health experts concerned about human rights have increasingly made their expertise available to help document such abuses.[18] Examples of this type of medical-human rights collaboration include: exhumation of mass graves to examine allegations of executions;[18] examination of torture victims;[20] and entry of health personnel into prisons to assess health status.[21]

However, health impacts of rights violations go beyond these issues in at least two ways. First, the duration and extent of health impacts resulting from severe abuses of rights and dignity remain generally underappreciated. Torture, imprisonment under inhumane conditions, or trauma associated with witnessing summary executions, torture, rape or mistreatment of others have been shown to lead to severe, probably lifelong effects on physical, mental and social well-being.[22] In addition, a more complete understanding of the negative health effects of torture must also include its broad influence on mental and social well-being; torture is often used as a political tool to discourage people from meaningful participation in or resistance to government.[23]

Second, and beyond these serious problems, it is increasingly evident that violations of many more, if not all, human rights have negative effects on health. For example, the right to information may be violated when cigarettes are marketed without governmental assurance that information regarding the harmful health effects of tobacco smoking will also be available. The health cost of this violation can be quantified through measures of tobacco-related preventable illness, disability and premature death, including excess cancers, cardiovascular and respiratory disease. Other violations of the right to information, with substantial health impacts, include governmental withholding of valid scientific health information about contraception or measures (e.g., condoms) to prevent infection with a fatal virus (HIV).

As another example, the enormous worldwide problem of occupation-related disease, disability and death reflects violations of the right to work under "just and favorable conditions" (UDHR, Article 23). In this context, the World Bank's identification of increased educational attainment for women as a critical intervention for improving health status in developing countries powerfully expresses the pervasive impact of rights realization (in this case to education, and to non-discrimination on the basis of sex) on population health status.[24]

A related, yet even more complex problem involves the potential health impact associated with violating individual and collective dignity. The Universal Declaration of Human Rights considers dignity, along with rights, to be inherent, inalienable and universal. While important dignity-related health impacts may include such problems as the poor health status of many indigenous peoples, a coherent vocabulary and framework to characterize dignity and different forms of dignity violations are lacking. A taxonomy and an epidemiology of violations of dignity may uncover an enormous field of previously suspected, yet thusfar unnamed and therefore undocumented damage to physical, mental and social well-being.

Assessment of rights violations' health impacts is in its infancy. Progress will require: a more sophisticated capacity to document and assess rights violations; the application of medical, social science and public health methodologies to identify and assess effects on physical, mental and social well-being; and research to establish valid associations between rights violations and health impacts.

Identification of health impacts associated with violations of rights and dignity will benefit both health and human rights fields. Using rights violations as an entry point for recognition of health problems may help uncover previously unrecognized burdens on physical, mental or social well-being. From a human rights perspective, documentation of health impacts of rights violations may contribute to increased societal awareness of the importance of human rights promotion and protection.

The Third Relationship: Health and Human Rights—Exploring an Inextricable Linkage

The proposal that promoting and protecting human rights is inextricably linked to the challenge of promoting and protecting health derives in part from recognition that health and human rights are complementary approaches to the central problem of defining and advancing human well-being. This fundamental connection leads beyond the single, albeit broad mention of health in the UDHR (Article 25) and the specific health-related responsibilities of states listed in Article 12 of the ICESCR, including: reducing stillbirth and infant mortality and promoting healthy child development; improving environmental and industrial hygiene; preventing, treating and controlling epidemic, endemic, occupational and other diseases; and assurance of medical care.

Modern concepts of health recognize that underlying "conditions" establish the foundation for realizing physical, mental and social well-being. Given the importance of these conditions, it is remarkable how little priority has been given within health research to their precise identification and understanding of their modes of action, relative importance, and possible interactions.

The most widely accepted analysis focuses on socioeconomic status; the positive relationship between higher socioeconomic status and better health status is well documented.[25] Yet this analysis has at least three important limitations. First, it cannot adequately account for a growing number of discordant observations, such as: the increased longevity of married Canadian men and women compared with their single (widowed, divorced, never married) counterparts;[26] health status differences between minority and majority populations which persist even when traditional measures of socioeconomic status are considered;[27] or reports of differential marital, economic and educational outcomes among obese women, compared with non-obese women.[28]

A second problem lies in the definition of poverty and its relationship to health status. Clearly, poverty may have different health meanings; for example, distinctions between the health-related meaning of absolute poverty and relative poverty have been proposed.[29]

A third, practical difficulty is that the socioeconomic paradigm creates an overwhelming challenge for which health workers are neither trained nor equipped

to deal. Therefore, the identification of socioeconomic status as the "essential condition" for good health paradoxically may encourage complacency, apathy and even policy and programmatic paralysis.

However, alternative or supplementary approaches are emerging about the nature of the "essential conditions" for health. For example, the Ottawa Charter for Health Promotion (1986) went beyond poverty to propose that, "the fundamental conditions and resources for health are peace, shelter, education, food, income, a stable eco-system, sustainable resources, social justice and equity."[9]

Experience with the global epidemic of HIV/AIDS suggests a further analytic approach, using a rights analysis.[30] For example, married, monogamous women in East Africa have been documented to be infected with HIV.[31] Although these women know about HIV and condoms are accessible in the marketplace, their risk factor is their inability to control their husbands' sexual behavior, or to refuse unprotected or unwanted sexual intercourse. Refusal may result in physical harm, or in divorce, the equivalent of social and economic death for the woman. Therefore, women's vulnerability to HIV is now recognized to be integrally connected with discrimination and unequal rights, involving property, marriage, divorce and inheritance. The success of condom promotion for HIV prevention in this population is inherently limited in the absence of legal and societal changes which, by promoting and protecting women's rights, would strengthen their ability to negotiate sexual practice and protect themselves from HIV infection.[32]

More broadly, the evolving HIV/AIDS pandemic has shown a consistent pattern through which discrimination, marginalization, stigmatization and, more generally, a lack of respect for the human rights and dignity of individuals and groups heightens their vulnerability to becoming exposed to

HIV.[33, 34] In this regard, HIV/AIDS may be illustrative of a more general phenomenon in which individual and population vulnerability to disease, disability and premature death is linked to the status of respect for human rights and dignity.

Further exploration of the conceptual and practical dimensions of this relationship is required. For example, epidemiologically-identified clusters of preventable disease, excess disability and premature death could be analyzed to discover the specific limitations or violations of human rights and dignity which are involved. Similarly, a broad analysis of the human rights dimensions of major health problems such as cancer, cardiovascular disease and injuries should be developed. The hypothesis that promotion and protection of rights and health are inextricably linked requires much creative exploration and rigorous evaluation.

The concept of an inextricable relationship between health and human rights also has enormous potential practical consequences. For example, health professionals could consider using the International Bill of Human Rights as a coherent guide for assessing health status of individuals or populations; the extent to which human rights are realized may represent a better and more comprehensive index of well-being than traditional health status indicators. Health professionals would also have to consider their responsibility not only to respect human rights in developing policies, programs and practices, but to contribute actively from their position as health workers to improving societal realization of rights. Health workers have long acknowledged the societal roots of health status; the human rights linkage may help health professionals engage in specific and concrete ways with the full range of those working to promote and protect human rights and dignity in each society.

From the perspective of human rights, health experts and expertise may contribute usefully to societal recognition of the benefits and costs associated with realizing, or failing to respect human rights and dignity. This can be accomplished without seeking to justify human rights and dignity on health grounds (or for any pragmatic purposes). Rather, collaboration with health experts can help give voice to the pervasive and serious impact on health associated with lack of respect for rights and dignity. In addition, the right to health can only be developed and made meaningful through dialogue between health and human rights disciplines. Finally, the importance of health as a precondition for the capacity to realize and enjoy human rights and dignity must be appreciated. For example, poor nutritional status of children can contribute subtly yet importantly to limiting realization of the right to education; in general, people who are healthy may be best equipped to participate fully and benefit optimally from the protections and opportunities inherent in the International Bill of Human Rights.

CONCLUSION

Thus far, different philosophical and historical roots, disciplinary differences in language and approach, and practical barriers to collaboration impede recognition of important linkages between health and human rights. The mutually enriching combination of research, education and field experience will advance understanding and catalyze further action around human rights and health. Exploration of the intersection of health and human rights may help revitalize the health field as well as contribute to broadening human rights thinking and practice. The health and human rights perspective offers new avenues for understanding and advancing human well-being in the modern world.

REFERENCES

1. Beauchamps DE, "Injury, Community and the Republic," *Law, Medicine and Health Care* 17, no. 1 (Spring 1989): 42–49.
2. Ronald Bayer, Arthur L. Caplan and Norman Daniels, eds., *In Search of Equity: health needs and the health care system*, from The Hastings Center series in ethics (New York: Plenum Press), 1983.
3. Ronald Dworkin, *Taking Rights Seriously* (Cambridge: Harvard University Press), 1978.
4. Scott Burris, "Rationality Review and the Politics of Public Health," *Villanova Law Review* 34(1989): 1933.
5. Lawrence Gostin, "The Interconnected Epidemics of Drug Dependency and AIDS," *Harvard Civil Rights-Civil Liberties Law Review* 26, no. 1 (Winter 1991): 113–184.
6. Institute of Medicine, *Future of Public Health*, (Washington DC: National Academy Press) 1988.
7. The International Bank for Reconstruction and Development, *World Development Report 1993: Investing in Health* (NY: Oxford University Press), 1993.
8. World Health Organization, *Constitution*, in *Basic Documents*, 36th ed. (Geneva, 1986).
9. *Ottawa Charter for Health Promotion*, presented at first International Conference on Health Promotion (Ottawa, November 21, 1986).
10. *Declaration of Alma-Ata*, "Health for All" Series No. 1 (Geneva: World Health Organization, September 12, 1978).
11. *Supra* note 8.
12. *Universal Declaration of Human Rights*, adopted and proclaimed by UN General Assembly Resolution 217A(III) (December 10, 1948).
13. *United Nations Charter*, signed at San Francisco, 26 June 1945, entered into force on 24 October, 1945.
14. *Supra* note 6.
15. Emily Friedman, "Money Isn't Everything," *Journal of the American Medical Association* 271, no. 19 (May 18, 1994): 1535–1538.
16. American Public Health Association, *Control of Communicable Disease in Man*, 15th ed., (Washington, DC: APHAL 1990).
17. International Federation of Red Cross and Red Crescent Societies, *AIDS, Health and Human Rights: A manual* (in press).
18. Geiger HL and Cook-Deegan RM, "The role of physicians in conflicts and humanitarian crises: Case studies from the field missions of Physicians for Human Rights, 1988–1993," *JAMA* 270 (1993): 616–620.
19. Physicians for Human Rights, *Final Report of UN Commission of Experts.* UN document #S/1994/674 (May 27, 1994).
20. Mollica RF and Caspi-Yavin Y, "Measuring torture and torture-related syndromes," *Psychological Assessment* 3, no. 4 (1991): 1–7.
21. Timothy Harding, "Prevention of Torture and Inhuman or Degrading Treatment: Medical Implications of a New European Convention" *The Lancet* 1, no. 8648 (May 27, 1989): 1191–1194.
22. Anne E. Goldfield, Richard F. Mollica, Barbara H. Pesavento, et al., "The physical and psychological sequelae of torture; symptomatology and diagnosis," *JAMA* 259, no. 18 (May 13, 1988): 2725–2730.
23. Metin Basoglu, "Prevention of Torture and Care of Survivors: An integrated approach," *JAMA* 270, no. S (August 4, 1993): 607.
24. *Supra* note 7.
25. Dutton DB and Levine S, "Overview, methodological critique, and reformulation," in JP Bunker, OS Gomby and BH Kehrer, eds., *Pathways to Health. The role of social factors* (Menlo Park, CA: Henry J. Kaiser Family Foundation), 1989.
26. J. Epp, *Achieving Health for All: a framework for health promotion*, (Ottawa: Health and Welfare Canada, 1986)
27. Schoendorf KC, Hogue CL Kleinman JC, and Rowley D, "Mortality among infants of black as compared with white college-educated parents," *NEJM* 326(1992): 1522–6.
28. Gortmaker S, Must A, Perrin JM et al., "Social and economic consequences of overweight in adolescence and young adulthood," *NEJM* 329(1993): 1008–1012.
29. Ichiro Kawachi et al., "Income Inequality and Life Expectancy: Theory, Research and Policy/' *Society and Health Working Paper Series* May 1994, no. 94–2 (Boston: The Health Institute, New England Medical Center and Harvard School of Public Health), 1994.
30. Global AIDS Policy Coalition, "Towards a New Health Strategy for AIDS: A Report of the Global AIDS Policy Coalition" (Cambridge, MA: Global AIDS Policy Coalition, June 1993).
31. Said H. Kapiga, et al., "Risk Factors for HIV Infection among Women in Dar-er-Salaam, Tanzania" *JAMA* 7, no. 3 (1994): 301–309.
32. Jacques du Guerny and Elisabeth Sjoberg, "Inter-relationship between gender relations and the HIV/AIDS epidemic: some considerations for policies and programmes," *AIDS* 7 (1993): 1027–1034.
33. *Supra* note 30.
34. Jonathan M. Mann, Daniel J.M. Tarantola and Thomas W. Netter, *AIDS in the World*, (Cambridge: Harvard University Press), 1992.

QUESTIONS

1. The World Health Organization (WHO) defines health as "a state of complete physical, mental and social well-being and not merely the absence of disease or infirmity." How would you define well-being? Discuss how this definition relates to the language and uses of human rights mentioned in the text.

2. Consider the Universal Declaration of Human Rights. Which human rights would seem most important to achieving health as defined here and why?

3. The authors state that the "prioritization of health issues may result in discrimination against individuals, as when the major health problems of a population defined on the basis of sex, race, religion, or language are systematically given a lower priority." What are some examples of this type of neglected health issue? How would attention to human rights alter what are determined to be priority issues?

FURTHER READING

1. D'Oronzio, Joseph, C., The Integration of Health and Human Rights: An Appreciation of Jonathan M. Mann. *Cambridge Quarterly of Healthcare Ethics* 2001; 10: 231–40.
2. Marks, S., The Evolving Field of Health and Human Rights: Issues and Methods. *Journal of Law, Medicine & Ethics* 2002; 30: 739.
3. Marks, S., *Health and Human Rights: Basic International Documents*, 2nd ed. Francois-Xavier Center for Health and Human Rights, Harvard University Press, Cambridge MA (2006)
4. Rosales, Cecilia B., M.D., M.S., Coe, K., Ortiz, S., Gámez, G., & Stroupe, N., Social Justice, Health, and Human Rights Education: Challenges and Opportunities in Schools of Public Health. *Public Health Reports* 2012; 127: 126.

POINT OF VIEW

Eleanor Roosevelt Drives By

The Honorable Michael Kirby AC CMG

AN EPIPHANY DOWN UNDER

Where did it all begin? At least, where did it begin for me? In 1944 Australia was in the midst of a deadly struggle for survival. The danger of enemy invasion could not be discounted. Our military forces were fighting in the jungles and islands, shoulder to shoulder with the armed forces of the United States of America. I was in my first year of education, attending a kindergarten, conducted in a church hall near one of the main arterial roadways circling Sydney. Along the roadway, a seemingly endless parade of khaki coloured vans, bearing the white and red insignia of the Red Cross, could be seen on their way to the new Repatriation General Hospital at Concord, the suburb of my parental home.

On one particular day, the school children were all brought out to line the footpath. An important visitor was passing by on the way to the big new hospital. That edifice had been constructed with American aid to provide care and treatment to American and Australian soldiers wounded in the War. The visitor was the wife of Franklin D. Roosevelt, President of the United States. Eleanor Roosevelt was in Australia briefly to show the President's support for the war effort. We were commandeered to show our thanks. So we all waved flags and cried out as this great lady was driven past us. I wonder if our eyes ever met. If they had, I would have been proud. She was a special person. She was Eleanor Roosevelt. I was 6 years of age.

A bit more than a year later, the allies had won the War. A strange mushroom-shaped cloud invaded my consciousness. Soon after, in August 1945 every Australian school child received a round bronze medal, as big as a penny. It was the "V.P. medal"—Victory in the Pacific. Four years after that victory another event occurred. By now I was at a different school, well and truly embarked on the journey of education. Our teacher, Mr Redmond came into the boys only class with a packet containing an unusual gift. It was unusual in three respects. First, it had within it a large number of small pamphlets of miniature size, all bearing the blue insignia of the new United Nations Organisation, with which we school children were becoming more familiar. It was an odd shape, being oblong rather than square. And they were printed on airmail paper: a rarity in those days of post war reconstruction and austerity.

Our teacher began explaining the purpose of the documents, which was called the *Universal Declaration of Human Rights* (UDHR).[1] He mentioned that it had been drafted by a committee, chaired by the famous lady whose name I remembered, Eleanor Roosevelt. Moreover, it had been adopted by the General Assembly when an Australian, Dr. Herbert V. Evatt, was in the chair as President of the Assembly. We knew that he was an important man. In fact, he was our country's foreign minister. Before the War he had been a Justice of the High Court. However, he had resigned to re-enter politics at a time when the country was in peril. We were told that the purpose of the UDHR was to express and re-enforce the basic rights that people everywhere enjoyed. Only if those rights were guaranteed and protected, would human beings escape the dangers of another war and the catastrophe of that mushroom cloud. Amazing how the lessons of youth can enter the imagination of a child and remain in the consciousness for 60 years and more.

Amongst the principles stated in the UDHR (and there were many) were those expressed in Article 25. Eleanor Roosevelt had a strong attachment to this because she knew, from her husband and family, the importance of health and the challenge of disability:

> 25.1 Everyone has the right to a standard of living adequate for the health and wellbeing of himself and his family ... and medical care and necessary social services and the right to security in the event of ... sickness, disability ... [and] circumstances beyond his control.

Our teacher told us how, in Australia, we had as recently as 1946 adopted one of the very rare amendments to our 1901 Constitution, so as to permit the establishment of a publicly funded national health scheme, so that the Federal Parliament could make provisions for "maternity allowances, widows' pensions, child endowment, unemployment, pharmaceutical, sickness and hospital benefits, medical and dental services ... benefits to students and family allowances" (Australian Constitutions S51(xxiiiA)).

Later, I was to learn that the provisions of the Universal Declaration were converted into binding treaty language in two International Covenants adopted by the United Nations. One of these, the International Covenant on Economic Social and Cultural Rights (ICESCR) which came into force in January 1976, contained, in Article 12, an elaborate principle expressing the aspiration of a right to health.

Years after this Covenant was adopted, after I had been elected a Commissioner of the International Commission of Jurists (ICJ) in Geneva, I came to know the ICJ commissioner elected from Canada: Professor John Humphrey of McGill University in Quebec. In quiet moments, John Humphrey would tell me of what it was like working with Eleanor Roosevelt, for he had been a key person in the Secretariat of the United Nations, then based at Lake Success near New York. He had helped with the first draft. Truly, he had been present at the creation of the new world order, essential for peace and justice for all humanity. I am a child of those times. I grew up believing in the values written down by Eleanor Roosevelt. I still do. Not just for Australians. Or Americans. For everyone.

HEALTH FOR ALL: INSTITUTIONAL

It was all very well, Eleanor Roosevelt and John Humphrey proclaiming health for all. But how could this bold aspiration ever be translated into action for ordinary people? Particularly for poor, marginalised and disadvantaged people? Sickness has always been with us, back to biblical times. Is it not just something we have to learn to live with? Could the world afford the expense included in health for all?

A lawyer and a judge (even a judge of a final court) can occasionally make contributions to this macro problem. One of the last decisions I delivered before concluding my service as a judge on the High Court of Australia in February 2009, concerned a challenge by a medical practitioner to features of the Australian Medicare system. A doctor contended that it amounted to, or authorised, a form of "civil conscription," which was expressly prohibited by the grant of power afforded to the Federal Parliament by the Australian people. Obviously, with that grant came the necessities of administration and auditing of the huge sums of federal money involved. The difficulty was presented of drawing a line between the inherent necessities of control and its consequential impositions. By a majority, in which I participated, the Court rejected the medical practitioner's challenge (Wong v The Commonwealth of Australia). Decisions like this, however contentious, whilst important for people in a particular country cannot really touch the huge global challenges presented for affording the best attainable health care to human beings everywhere. But that had been Eleanor Roosevelt's aspiration.

On a global level, the United Nations duly established the World Health Organisation (WHO), an agency with a mandate to tackle health across borders. This agency has played a key role in advancing international co-operation so as to eradicate endemic diseases. In my lifetime, substantially with the aid of WHO, diseases such as smallpox have been eradicated and polio contained in ways that would have been impossible in early centuries.

When new and dangerous diseases have manifested themselves, WHO has played a leadership role in mobilising the response of the international community. It has done this in the case of *Ebola*; and new strains of influenza (popularly known as "swine flu" and "chicken flu"). It was an initiative of WHO that established the Global Programme on AIDS (GPA), under an inspired international civil servant Jonathan Mann, in 1987. From Geneva, in 1988, Dr. Mann invited me to join with others in the initial Global Commission on AIDS. This was established to advise WHO and national governments on the response that should be presented to the AIDS epidemic and specifically to the Human Immunodeficiency Virus (HIV). Without a pharmaceutical cure or a safe and reliable vaccine, innovative steps had to be taken to address the unexpected epidemic. I was privileged to participate in that global commission with the two scientists credited with identifying HIV, Luc Montagnier (France) and Robert Gallo (USA). Also a member of the Commission was Professor June Osborn (USA). She established the principle that every strategy had to be measured against the gold standard of the best empirical data. Dr. Mann insisted that universal human rights were an essential ingredient in fighting HIV/AIDS. Only by this means would there be any chance of getting into the heads of those whose decisions were essential for the ways HIV was transmitted.

Later (1993–1996) UN Secretary-General Boutros Boutros Ghali appointed me his Special Representative for human rights in Cambodia. In the aftermath of the genocide of the Khmer Rouge regime, I identified the "right to health" and to be free of infection by HIV as central considerations which the United Nations and Cambodian Government had to tackle. Initiatives taken at that time contributed to the fall in the rate of infection. Yet, globally, HIV infections have continued to spread. More than 30 million human beings have died of AIDS since it was first identified. More than 34 million are today living with HIV and AIDS. Beneficial anti-retroviral drugs can radically improve lives, reduce infectablity and increase economic and personal welfare. In the current circumstances of the Global Financial Crisis, however, the funds necessary to provide such drugs to all in need of them are uncertain. United Nations targets are not being met. Will people who live in rich countries with effective public health systems be treated? Will people in other countries, through inability to secure and maintain access to pharmaceuticals, lose their lives?

At least, when AIDS came along, the world confronted the new challenges, substantially as a global family. To reduce tensions and competition between United Nations agencies, a joint body, UNAIDS was created to give leadership and so as to mobilise every agency and all available resources. Other global health initiatives predicated on reducing mortality and morbidity due to tuberculosis, malaria, preventable childhood infections and malnutrition have emerged in the 21st century. But what of other life-threatening conditions? Especially conditions predominating in developing countries? What of maternal morbidity and mortality and the growing burden of non-communicable disease? Are these less important because less well known or their impacts better mitigated in the wealthier countries of the world?

HEALTH FOR ALL: ATTAINING THE DREAM

Because Eleanor Roosevelt's dream of universal access to essential health care has increasingly been seen as an attribute of our shared human rights, the United Nations Human Rights institutions over the past 20 years have increasingly given attention to this feature of global human rights. Yet against the enormity of the challenge to fulfil the aspirations of the Universal Declaration and the Covenants that grew out of it, even the initiatives that have been undertaken seem paltry. So what can be done to step up the momentum to achieve health for all and true fulfilment, sixty years later, of Eleanor Roosevelt's hopes for humanity?

We now have instruments of the international community and rules of international law. We have specialised agencies and institutions that harness the aspirations of humanity. We have experts who advise on how we can embrace the rational

and optimistic attributes of human nature. And avoid the peril of war, genocide and cruel discrimination. No nation can tackle these challenges alone. The health of men, women and children is something so basic that we can all understand it and grasp its necessity when we reflect on our own lives and those of our loved ones. Expression of the theory and concepts is essential to stimulate us into action. The examples of practical measures are necessary to show the benefits that action can produce and that change can occur.

These high aspirations were probably going through the mind of Eleanor Roosevelt, that great champion of humanity and of human dignity, as her car approached Concord in Sydney, Australia in 1944. The young school children waved to her. Even they knew that she was an important messenger that the future need not be like the past. And that it was a duty of new generations to make it so.

NOTE

1. UDHR, adopted and proclaimed by the General Assembly of the United Nations, resolution 217A (III), 10 December 1948.

Michael Kirby is Commissioner of the Global Commission on HIV and the Law of the United Nations Development Programme (2010–2012). Former Justice of the High Court of Australia (1996–2009). Former President of the International Commission of Jurists (1995–1998). Member of the UNESCO International Bioethics Committee (1996–2005). Member of the UNAIDS Reference Group on HIV and Human Rights (2003–).

CHAPTER 2

History, Principles and Practice of Health and Human Rights

Sofia Gruskin, Edward J. Mills and Daniel Tarantola

INTRODUCTION

Blatant violation of human rights affecting the health of both individuals and populations continues. Examples include the torture of detainees in Abu-Ghraib prison in Iraq;[1] systematic rapes and murders in the Balkans,[2] Rwanda,[3] Chechnya,[4] and Darfur;[5] physician involvement in torture,[6] botched executions;[7] inhumane experimentation;[8] and questionable interrogation techniques in the so-called war on terror.[1,9,10] Such violations of human rights can be engineered by or endorsed by governments, institutions of power, and individuals. These deplorable violations exist alongside more subtle activities that also have severe and long lasting effects on health and human rights such as absence of basic healthcare systems;[11] policies keeping medicines unaffordable;[12] and tolerance of discrimination against groups such as injecting drug users,[13] people with mental-health disorders,[14,15] illegal immigrants,[16] or homeless people.[17] The continuing and foreseeable absence of access to effective care for most people living with most diseases in poor countries can also be viewed as a violation of human rights.[18] Therefore human rights should be imperative in delivery of care and implementation of public-health programmes.

Three main relations between health and human rights exist: the positive and negative effects on health of promotion, neglect, or violation of human rights; the effect of health on the delivery of human rights; and the effects of public health policies and programmes on human rights.[19] Despite the advances in the study and advocacy of health and human rights we still do not fully understand the nature of these relationships, how they interact, or their value to medicine and public health practice. In this chapter we address the public health aspects of these relations, and highlight where further research and action are needed.

A BRIEF HISTORY OF HEALTH AND HUMAN RIGHTS

Since the Nuremberg trials and the creation of the UN more than 50 years ago, interest in the association between health and human rights has grown. Until the beginning of the AIDS epidemic in the 1980s and the end of the Cold War, these two issues evolved along parallel but distinctly separate tracks,[20] perhaps as a consequence of the state-centric (i.e., greater political concern for general state and public interests than for specific individuals or communities) view of the world that prevailed in the second half of the 20th century. However, governments have a responsibility both to deliver essential health and social services, and to enable people and their families to achieve better health by respecting human rights.

In the past 20 years, the HIV/AIDS pandemic and reproductive and sexual health concerns have been instrumental in clarifying the ways that health and rights connect. These issues encompass law and policymaking, and have established the roles and boundaries of responsibility held by state and non-state stakeholders for the conditions that constrain or enable health and for delivery of health and related services.[21] The first worldwide public health strategy to explicitly engage with human rights concerns took place in the late 1980s, when Jonathan Mann directed the Global Program on AIDS at WHO.[22] Although this strategy was partly motivated by moral outrage at abuses suffered by people living with HIV, the inclusion of human rights was primarily because evidence was emerging that showed that discrimination was driving people away from prevention and care programmes.[23]

Elimination of such discrimination was expected to encourage people not only to fully exert their rights, but also to come forward for voluntary counselling, testing, and treatment of opportunistic infections. Uptake of these services would in turn help them safeguard their dignity, improve their health and wellbeing, and motivate them to adopt behaviours that would restrict further spread of infection. That this strategy—upholding human-rights principles—was set forth by WHO, an inter-governmental organisation with responsibilities for promotion of rights conferred by the UN Charter, placed it in the realm of international law.[24] As a result, governments and inter-governmental organisations were made publicly accountable for their public health and human rights actions (or inactions).

Since the 1980s, responses to the HIV pandemic have drawn attention to the rights of the most vulnerable people and societies, and the need to prevent discrimination in both law and practice.[25]

A series of international conferences held by the UN, beginning in the early 1990s, further solidified the dual obligations of governments to the health and human rights of their people.[21] These conferences brought together emotions and values, but also the experiences of local, national, and international practitioners (physicians, nurses, and other health workers), advocates, and policymakers. The 1997 Program for Reform, designed by Kofi Annan, then UN Secretary General, highlighted the promotion of human rights as a core activity of the UN, which was another important step in moving issues of health and human rights from rhetoric to implementation, action, and accountability.[26]

Almost all development agencies, organisations and UN programmes,[27] albeit to varying degrees of success, now pay attention to human rights in their work in health. Additionally, many governments are beginning to integrate their human rights obligations into their health-related activities, both in high-income and low-income countries.[28] In addition to members of affected populations, medical practitioners have also contributed to bringing human rights into health through their advocacy and practice.[29,30] Nonetheless, integration of human rights in health efforts clearly still has a long way to go.

HUMAN RIGHTS AND HEALTH POLICY

The links between human rights and health are best understood by referring to the preface to the WHO constitution, which states that health is the "state of complete physical, mental, and social wellbeing and not merely the absence of disease or infirmity" and "the highest attainable level of health is the fundamental right of every human being."[31] Governments are therefore responsible for enabling their populations to achieve better health through respecting, protecting, and fulfilling rights (i.e., not violating rights, preventing rights violations, and creating policies, structures, and resources that promote and enforce rights).[32] This responsibility extends beyond the provision of essential health services to tackling the determinants of health such as, provision of adequate education, housing, food, and favourable working conditions. These items are both human rights themselves and are necessary for health.[33,34] The relation of people with their environment is complex and the fulfilment—or absence— of human rights and their effects on the main determinants of health needs much investigation.

Human rights encompass civil, political, economic, social, and cultural rights. These rights are cast in international law, through many treaties and declarations, beginning with the UN Universal Declaration of Human Rights in 1948.[35–41] These documents highlight the importance of promotion and protection of human rights as a prerequisite to health and wellbeing. Although one can devote attention and resources to one specific right, or to a category of closely connected rights, all rights are interdependent and interrelated,[42] and as a result individuals rarely suffer neglect or violation of one right in isolation.

Economic, social, and cultural rights, such as education and food, are relevant to health, as are such civil and political rights as those relating to life, autonomy, information, free movement, association, equality, and participation. Recognition of the legal and political obligations that connect economic, social, and cultural rights, as well as civil and political rights, continues to grow. The right to the highest attainable standard of health therefore builds on, but is by no means limited to, Article 12 of the UN International Covenant on Economic, Social, and Cultural Rights (ICESCR).[43] It transcends almost every other right.

THE RIGHT TO HEALTH IN INTERNATIONAL LAW

The right to the highest attainable standard of health—often referred to as the right to health—is most prominently connected to the ICESCR.[43] It stipulates that:

The states parties to the present covenant recognise the right of everyone to the enjoyment of the highest attainable standard of physical and mental health. The steps to be taken by the states parties to the present covenant to achieve the full realisation of this right shall include those necessary for:

(a) the provision for the reduction of the stillbirth rate and of infant mortality and for the healthy development of the child;
(b) the improvement of all aspects of environmental and industrial hygiene;
(c) the prevention, treatment, and control of epidemic, endemic, occupational, and other diseases;
(d) the creation of conditions which would assure to all medical service and medical attention in the event of sickness.

Although the right to health forms the legal basis for much of the present work in health and human rights, if written today it would probably place greater emphasis on health rather than sickness and on health systems rather than provision of medical care. Addressing the effects of discrimination, gender-related or otherwise, on health and delivery of services is well covered by other rights, again showing how human rights are intertwined.[44]

The legal obligation of states to respect health-related rights is only one part of the picture, because rights are also used to guide policies and programmes for health and wellbeing. They enable a broad response to health and development by national and international stakeholders with responsibilities that reach beyond the health sector. Thus, although international treaties, enriched by declarations and related documents, have legal implications, they importantly can also inform the development of policies and programmes in all states, whether or not a state has signed to be legally bound by the relevant treaty.

APPLYING HUMAN RIGHTS TO HEALTH

The idea of health and human rights as a subject of study is fairly new, and we need to recognise the different ways in which advances in health and human rights can be achieved. Human rights feature in many different ways in the health work of international nongovernmental organisations, governments, civil society groups, and individuals. These ways can be broadly categorised as advocacy, application of legal standards, and programming (including service delivery).[45] Some stakeholders use one approach; others use a combination in their work. We use HIV/AIDS as the main example to show the effectiveness of these approaches, although examples in reproductive health,[46] mental health,[47] disability,[48] neglected diseases,[49] or other serious health issues could effectively serve as illustrations.

Development of new treatments and the investment of substantial and increasing resources to offer these treatments to people living with HIV have resulted in access to treatment and care for some people. These people gain substantial duration and quality of life, allowing them to participate actively in political, civil, economic, social, and cultural activities. By contrast, despite global initiatives to increase access in resource-poor places, progress has been slow and remains below expectations.[50]

Advocacy and Bearing Witness

The model of health and human rights is often used in campaigns for changes in health-related policy and practice. Early campaigns as a response to some governments' complacency in dealing with AIDS illustrated the success of this approach and set a precedent for health campaigns around the world.[51,52] The focus of activism is often on recognition and exposure of governmental obligations, establishing the amount of government action or inaction that contributes to existing violations, looking at how a government deals or does not deal with identified problems, and recommending solutions.

Since the turn of the century, the pharmaceutical industry has lowered the price of antiretroviral drugs in low-income countries to less than ten percent of their cost in 2000,[53] mainly because of pressure framed around the right to access treatment, exercised on them by nongovernmental organisations, the mass media among others. Although this development brought opportunities for greater access to antiretroviral drugs, national and international work is still needed for these drugs to reach the people who need them, especially those living in low-income and middle-income countries.[54] The most recent international agreements to provide universal access, the human rights obligations of states to make such services available, and the obligations of wealthy countries to engage in international assistance and cooperation[40] puts additional obligations on wealthy countries to help poor ones to achieve these goals. These obligations can be used as an effective advocacy strategy.

Médecins Sans Frontières and Médecins Du Monde have both shown the important parts that individual health practitioners can play in international crises. These groups were founded on the premise that health practitioners and the communities sponsoring them have an international duty to maintain health, especially that of disadvantaged people living in regions affected by warfare or natural disasters. Such principles have grown to include the response to HIV/AIDS and situations of chronic extreme poverty.[55] These organisations were born of civil society in the late 1960s, inspired by the belief that clinicians, other health professionals, and volunteers could improve the health of poor and vulnerable people whose governments were failing to do so, either by design or incapacity.

Although not initially intended as the launch of a health and human rights movement, the emergence and growing influence of these groups and those that have followed, has drawn attention to the universal value of health and the duty of care providers, other humanitarian workers, and the international community to intervene when human rights are ignored. A recurring dilemma confronting these organisations is whether sustainable health action should be associated with documentation and denouncements of witnessed human rights violations, as these activities could both limit their ability to provide health services to the populations they serve, and

jeopardise the safety of their workers.[56] Of note, the international appeals from nongovernmental organisations and some relief agencies, in such situations as that of the Great Lakes area in Africa in the 1990s, in which a late and weak international response resulted in greater chaos and many casualties that could have been prevented.

Application of Legal Standards

In a strictly legal sense, applying human rights to health means using internationally accepted and nationally agreed upon norms, standards, and accountability mechanisms within healthcare systems and in the work of national and international health, economic, and developmental policymakers.[57] Legal mechanisms can sometimes also provide channels of redress for individuals whose rights have been violated in the context of public health interventions. In South Africa and several Latin American countries, the human rights provisions of national constitutions (e.g., the rights to life, to health, and to benefit from scientific progress) have been interpreted to enable claims for access to antiretroviral medicines.[58] In Latin America, individuals supported by nongovernmental organisations, have undertaken 13 successful lawsuits to date against their governments for access to antiretroviral drugs. In fact, in Argentina, one such success resulted in assurances of provision of care for 15,000 people.[58] Treatment Action Campaign in South Africa used the courts to ensure that the government was ordered to provide programmes in public clinics for reduction of mother-to-child transmission of HIV.[59] Although these efforts have resulted in positive changes in the law, advocacy is still needed to move these obligations into practice; thus emphasising how advocacy, and application of the law are interrelated.

Rights in Delivery of Care and Programming

Even though many organisations describe their approach to health as rights-based, we have no one definition of what this entails.[60] All such organisations seem generally concerned with ensuring that vulnerable populations are provided with the services that they need, but in practice these organisations have used different approaches to the incorporation of rights into different stages of the programming cycle; from situation analysis, to planning, implementation, monitoring, and assessment.[61] The core components of rights-based approaches include: examining the laws and policies under which programmes take place; systematically integrating core human rights principles such as participation, non-discrimination, transparency, and accountability into policy and programme responses; and focusing on key elements of the right to health—availability, accessibility, acceptability, and quality when defining standards for provision of services.[60]

HIV testing serves as a useful example to illustrate the link between health and rights in programming. Although voluntary HIV testing has been advocated by international agencies since the start of the pandemic[62] and is seen in many national laws and policies, the requirement for testing to be voluntary has recently been debated. The present argument is that people knowing their HIV status is more important than whether they voluntarily seek testing, because they will be able to accurately inform their partners of their HIV status, modify their behaviours, and seek treatment if available.[63] Consequently, an approach known as routine provider-initiated HIV testing is becoming increasingly common in healthcare settings—an approach that, without careful guidance, can consist largely of assuming that patients agree to be tested unless they express objection and opt out of taking the test. UNAIDS and WHO have released guidance to support the adaption of national policies to account for this new trend.[64, 65]

This seemingly well-intended approach will need careful monitoring and assessment to ascertain whether HIV tests are being routinely offered or routinely imposed, and whether in either case, the individual has informed choice and power to opt in or opt out of being tested.[66] Future work in this areas needs evidence, rather than ideology, to establish whether these conditions help people access HIV care services, and maintain contact with such services. Attention to principles of rights such as non-discrimination, participation of affected communities, and accountability for potential positive and negative effects of adopting routine HIV testing could help to measure its effectiveness in terms of both rights and health. When a government (most recently China[67] and Lesotho[68]—and both with the support of WHO) decides to screen an entire section of the population for HIV with disregard for domestic law, human rights principles, and international norms while providing little access to care for those testing positive, we face a complex challenge. How regard for human rights translates into policy formulation, programming, and service delivery continues to be debated.[69, 70]

A rights-based approach to programming needs interventions to be implemented in ways that improve health, and that efforts to reach national and international targets, for example, in relation to the numbers of people on treatment, do not result in the neglect or violation of human rights. Although application of human rights will not establish if priority should be given to prevention or treatment, consideration of human rights will ensure that attention is given not only to the outcomes of health interventions, but also to the ways they are implemented.[21] For example, an increase in uptake of HIV-testing services could be due to an increase in the availability of high-quality voluntary counselling and testing services, but on the other hand it could also be due to the introduction of mandatory testing for certain population groups.[71] Although both interventions would seem to lead to the same short-term outcome, without regard for the reasons behind the increase in HIV testing the problems of any strategy will not be seen, which could threaten both human rights and public health in the long term.

CONCERNS FOR THE FUTURE

Government roles and responsibilities are increasingly delegated to non-state actors (e.g., biomedical research institutions, health insurance companies, health management organisations, the pharmaceutical industry, and care providers) whose accountability is defined poorly and monitored inadequately. No objective measures are available of the commitment and capacity of governments to ensure that actions taken by the private sector and other players, including civil society, are informed by and comply with human rights. Likewise, as the discipline of health and human rights grows, its relevance and effectiveness will depend partly on the ability to understand cultural constraints. Even when countries commit to respect for human rights, health workers need to be educated about how to incorporate human rights principles into their work, and this should be done equally at schools of medicine, schools of public health, and nursing schools. We expect that as the number of health professionals involved with human rights increases, the practice of health and human rights will also develop.

STEPS FORWARD

Attention to human rights can be a way to enhance the value and effects of health work by health policymakers, programme developers, health practitioners, and students. Nonetheless, three topics urgently need that further work. The first is the development of adequate monitoring instruments that measure both health and human rights concerns; the second is building evidence of the effects of application of the health and human rights frameworks to health practice; and the third is the creation of a research agenda to advance our understanding of the associations between health and human rights.

Because health and human rights is a new subject, so too are the ways to measure whether a clinical scenario or public-health decision is ultimately successful in upholding human rights. Efforts are needed to assess the effectiveness of existing methods of assessment and indicators of human rights concerns, and the extent to which these indicators need to be changed. Eventually we will know how the incorporation of human rights can effect the effectiveness of policies and programmes.[72] We need to gain such knowledge quickly to allow us to develop an evidence base that shows the value of attention to rights for health as well as the negative effects on health of both grievous and subtle human rights violations. Until such a time, efforts to systematically review and collate existing information about the effects of human rights on health should be recognised as an urgent need.[47,73]

Public health efforts that consider human rights are more likely to be effective than those that neglect or violate rights.[74,75] Integration of human rights in international health systems is increasingly driven by the recognition that the respect, protection, and fulfillment of human, civil, political, economic, social, and cultural rights, is necessary—not because they are the binding legal obligations of governments, but because they are essential for improvement of the health status of individuals and populations. We need to strengthen and build upon the available information and education about human rights ideas and processes. We also need to share information and cooperate with those working on health and those working on human rights.[76,77] This cooperation might need institutional change and capacity building within governmental systems, international organisations, civil society stakeholders, and individuals. Increased understanding of human rights is not only of value in itself, but also provides those involved in health planning and care with the necessary means to create conditions that enable people to achieve optimum health.

REFERENCES

1. Miles SH. Abu Ghraib: its legacy for military medicine. Lancet 2004; 364: 725–29.
2. Gent RN. Balkan briefing. Abuses of human rights in the Kosovo region of the Balkans. J Epidemiol Community Health 1999; 53: 594–96.
3. Verwimp P. Death and survival during the 1994 genocide in Rwanda. Popul Stud (Camb) 2004; 58: 233–45.
4. Parfitt T. Russian soldiers blamed for civilian rape in Chechnya. Lancet 2004; 363: 1291.
5. Depoortere E, Checchi F, Broillet F, et al. Violence and mortality in West Darfur, Sudan (2003–04): epidemiological evidence from four surveys. Lancet 2004; 364: 1315–20.
6. How complicit are doctors in abuses of detainees? Lancet 2004; 364: 637–38.
7. Koniaris LG, Zimmers TA, Lubarsky DA, Sheldon JP. Inadequate anaesthesia in lethal injection for execution. Lancet 2005; 365: 1412–14.
8. Warrick P. Heimlich's Audacious Maneuver. Los Angeles Times Oct 30, 1994.
9. Farberman R. A stain on medical ethics. Lancet 2005; 366: 712.
10. Hargreaves S, Cunningham A. The politics of terror. Lancet 2004; 363: 1999–2000.
11. WHO. World health survey results. Geneva: World Health Organization, 2005.
12. Lynch T. Medication costs as a primary cause
13. Wood E, Spittal PM, Small W, et al. Displacement of Canada's largest public illicit drug market in response to a police crackdown. CMAJ 2004; 170: 1551–56.
14. Kennedy PJ. Why we must end insurance discrimination against mental health care. Harvard J Legis 2004; 41: 363–75.
15. Pinfold V, Byrne P, Toulmin H. Challenging stigma and discrimination in communities: a focus group study identifying UK mental health service users' main campaign priorities. Int J Soc Psychiatry 2005; 51: 128–38.
16. Ku L, Matani S. Left out: immigrants' access to health care and insurance. Health Aff (Millwood) 2001; 20: 247–56.
17. Ritchey FJ, La Gory M, Mullis J. Gender differences in health risks and physical symptoms among the homeless. J Health Soc Behav 1991; 32: 33–48.
18. WHO. Antiretroviral therapy coverage in low- and middle-income countries, by region. Situation as of June 2005. Geneva: World Health Organization, 2005.
19. Mann JM, Gostin L, Gruskin S, et al. Health and human rights. Health Hum Rights 1994; 1: 6–23.
20. Freeman M. Human Rights: an interdisciplinary approach. Cambridge: Polity, 2002.
21. Gruskin S, Tarantola D. Health and human rights. In: Detels R, McEwan J, Beaglehole R, Tanaka H, eds. Oxford Textbook on Public Health, 4th ed. Oxford: Oxford University Press, 2001.
22. WHO. Global strategy for the prevention and control of AIDS, Res. WHA40.26, World Health Organization World Health Assemb., 40th Sess. 1987.
23. Mann JM, Tarantola D. Responding to HIV/AIDS: A Historical Perspective, 2. Health and Human Rights 1998; 5: 5–8.
24. Gruskin S, Tarantola D. Droits de l'homme et santé, la synergie. In: Hazan YR, Chastonay P, eds. Santé et Droits de l'Homme, Paris: Collection Médecine Société, 2004.
25. UNAIDS. The Global Strategy Framework on HIV/AIDS, 2001.
26. UN. Renewing the United Nations: a programme for reform, report of the Secretary-General, U.N. GAOR, 51st Session, Agenda Item 168, U.N. Doc. A/51/950. 1997.
27. UN. Coordination of the policies and activities of the specialized agencies and other bodies of the United Nations system related to the coordinated follow-up to and implementation of the Vienna declaration and programme of action, report of the Secretary-General, U.N. ESCOR, 1998 Sess., Agenda Item 4, PP U.N. Doc. E/1998/60. 1998.

of nonadherence in the elderly. Consult Pharm 2006; 21: 143–46.

28. Hunt P. Report of the Special Rapporteur on the right of everyone to the enjoyment of the highest attainable standard of physical and mental health, Paul Hunt. Addendum. MISSION TO UGANDA. 2006. UN Doc. E/CN.4/2006/48/Add.2. 2006.

29. PHR. Health action AIDS campaign call to action. Physicians for Human Rights, Partners in Health; Record: Newsletter of Physicians for Human Rights. Vol XVIII, Number 1, Jan, 2005.

30. Captier C. MSF's principles and identity—the challenges ahead. 05/12/2005. Médecins Sans Frontières. 2005.

31. WHO. Constitution of the World Health Organization, adopted by the International Health Conference, New York, June 19–July 22, 1946, and signed on 22 July 1946 by the representatives of 61 States. World Health Organization, 1946.

32. Eide A. Economic, social and cultural rights as human rights. In: Eide A, Krause C, Rosas A, eds. Economic, social and cultural rights: a textbook. Dordrecht: Martinus Nijhoff, 1995.

33. Martikainen P, Stansfeld S, Hemingway H, Marmot M. Determinants of socioeconomic differences in change in physical and mental functioning. Soc Sci Med 1999; 49: 499–507.

34. Brunner E, Shipley MJ, Blane D, Smith GD, Marmot MG. When does cardiovascular risk start? Past and present socioeconomic circumstances and risk factors in adulthood. J Epidemiol Community Health 1999; 53: 757–64.

35. UN. Universal declaration of human rights. G.A. Res. 217A (III), UN GAOR, Res. 71, UN Doc. A/810. New York: United Nations, 1948.

36. UN. United Nations convention against torture and other cruel, inhuman, or degrading treatment or punishment, G.A. Res. 39/45, UN GAOR, 39th Sess., Supp. No. 51, at 197, UN Doc. A/39/51. New York: United Nations, 1985.

37. UN. United Nations convention on the elimination of all forms of discrimination against women, G.A. Res. 34/180, UN GAOR, 34th Sess., Supp. No. 46, at 193, UN Doc. A/34/46. New York: United Nations, 1979.

38. UN. United Nations convention on the elimination of all forms of racial discrimination, UN G.A. Res. 2106A(XX). New York: United Nations, 1965.

39. UN. United Nations convention on the rights of the child (CRC), G.A. Res. 44/25, UN GAOR, 44th Sess., Supp. No. 49, at 166, UN Doc. A/44/25. New York: United Nations, 1989.

40. UN. International covenant on economic, social and cultural rights (ICESCR). New York, United Nations, 1966. United Nations General Assembly resolution 2200 (XXI), UN GAOR, 21st Session, Supp. No. 16, at 49, UN Doc. A/6316, entered into force 3 January 1976. New York: United Nations, 1976.

41. UN. International covenant on civil and political rights (ICCPR). New York, United Nations, 1966. United Nations General Assembly resolution 2200A (XXI), 21 UN GAOR Supp. No. 16, at 52, UN Doc. A/6316, entered into force 23 March 1976. New York: United Nations, 1976.

42. World Conference on Human Rights, Vienna, Austria (June 14–25). 1993.

43. UN. Article 12, International covenant on economic, social and cultural rights, adopted and opened for signature, ratification and accession by United Nations General Assembly Resolution 2200 A(XXI). New York: United Nations, 1966.

44. Committee on Economic, Social and Cultural Rights. The right to the highest attainable standard of health: 11/08/2000. E/C.12/2000/4, CESCR General Comment 14. Twenty-second session Geneva, 25 April–12 May 2000 Agenda item 3.

45. Gruskin S. Is there a government in the cockpit: a passenger's perspective or global public health: the role of human rights. Temple Law Review 2004; 77: 313–34.

46. Shaw D, Faundes A. What is the relevance of women's sexual and reproductive rights to the practising obstetrician/gynaecologist? Best Pract Res Clin Obstet Gynaecol 2006; 20: 299–309.

47. Mills EJ, Singh S, Holtz TH, et al. Prevalence of mental disorders and torture among Tibetan refugees: a systematic review. BMC Int Health Hum Rights 2005; 5: 7.

48. Focht-New V. Beyond abuse: health care for people with disabilities. Issues Ment Health Nurs 1996; 17: 427–38.

49. Hunt P. The human right to the highest attainable standard of health: new opportunities and challenges. Trans R Soc Trop Med Hyg 2006; 100: 603–7.

50. Editorial, Predicting the failure of 3 by 5. Lancet 2005; 365: 1597.

51. Fauci AS. HIV and AIDS: 20 years of science. Nat Med 2003; 9: 839–43.

52. Stockdill BC. Activism against AIDS: at the intersections of sexuality, race, gender and class. Boulder: Lynne Rienner Publishers, 2002.

53. Fleshman M. Drug price plunge energizes AIDS fight: Africa and the United Nations mobilizing political leadership. Africa Recovery 2001; 15 1.

54. Trouiller P, Olliaro P, Torreele E, et al. Drug development for neglected diseases: a deficient market and a public-health policy failure. Lancet 2002; 359: 2188–94.

55. Doctors call for specialized HIV/AIDS treatment for children. AIDS Policy Law 2004; 19: 5.

56. Terry F. Condemned to Repeat? The paradox of humanitarian action. Ithaca: Cornell University Press, 2002.

57. Gruskin S. What are health and human rights? Lancet 2004; 363: 329.

58. Hogerzeil HV, Samson M, Vidal Casanovas J, Rahmani-Oncora L. Is access to essential medicines as part of the fulfillment of the right-to-health enforceable through the courts? Lancet 2006; 368: 305–11.

59. Gernholtz L. Preventing mother-to-child transmission: landmark decision by South African court. Can HIV AIDS Policy Law Rev 2002; 6: 20–24.

60. UNAIDS. Introduction to best practice guide and draft dos and don'ts documents. issue paper for the fifth meeting of the UNAIDS reference group on HIV and human rights, prepared by the Reference Group Secretariat. New York: Joint United Nations programme on AIDS, 2005.

61. Report of the Second Interagency Workshop on Implementing a Human Rights-Based Approach in the Context of UN Reform, May 5–7, 2003.

62. UNAIDS/WHO Policy Statement on HIV Testing. June 2004.

63. Flanigan TP, Beckwith C, Carpenter CC. Public health principles for the HIV epidemic. N Engl J Med 2006; 354: 877–78; author reply 877–78.

64. WHO/UNAIDS. Guidance on provider-initiated HIV testing and counseling in health facilities. Geneva: World Health Organization May 30, 2007.

65. Tarantola D, Gruskin S. New guidance on recommended HIV testing and counselling. Lancet 2007; 370: 202–03

66. Gruskin S. Bangkok 2004. Current issues and concerns in HIV testing: a health and human rights approach. HIV/AIDS Policy and Law Review 2004; 9: 99–103.

67. Parry J. China's pragmatic approach to AIDS. Bull World Health Organ 2006; 84: 261–62.

68. Mills EJ, Chong S. Lesotho embarks on universal HIV testing. HIV/AIDS Policy and Law Review 2006; 11: 27–28.

69. De Cock KM, Mbori-Ngacha D, Marum E. Shadow on the continent: public health and HIV/AIDS in Africa in the 21st century. Lancet 2002; 360: 67–72.

70. Gruskin S, Loff B. Do human rights have a role in public health work? Lancet 2002; 360: 1880.

71. Rennie S, Behets F. Desperately seeking targets: the ethics of routine HIV testing in low-income countries. Bull World Health Organ 2006; 84: 52–57.

72. Rights-Based Responses to HIV: Human Rights Indicators. Issue Paper for the Fifth Meeting of the UNAIDS Reference Group on HIV and Human Rights, prepared by the Reference Group Secretariat. UNAIDS 2005.

73. Braveman P, Gruskin S. Poverty, equity, human rights and health. Bull World Health Organ 2003; 81: 539–45.

74. Menon-Johansson AS. Good governance and good health: The role of societal structures in the human immunodeficiency virus pandemic. BMC Int Health Hum Rights 2005; 5: 4.

75. International Council of AIDS Service Organisations. HIV/AIDS and Human Rights Stories from the Frontlines. June 1999.

76. Mills EJ, Robinson J, Attaran A, et al. Sharing evidence on humanitarian relief. BMJ 2005; 331: 1485–86.

77. Gruskin S, Tarantola D. HIV/AIDS, Health and human rights. In: Lamptey P, Gayle H, Mane P, eds. HIV/AIDS prevention and care programs in resource-constrained settings: a handbook for the design and management of programs. Research triangle park: Family Health International, 2001.

QUESTIONS

1. The chapter notes that "Economic, social, and cultural rights, such as education and food, are relevant to health, as are such civil and political rights as those relating to life, autonomy, information, free movement, association, equality, and participation." Take the Universal Declaration of Human Rights and consider each right noted there. Discuss the implications of each right for health and well-being.

2. Government responsibility for health extends beyond the provision of health services, and includes tackling the determinants of health such as education,

housing, food, and favorable working conditions. How far should this go? Consider a government that has to set priorities within the limits of a shrinking budget. How should priorities for spending on health be determined?

3. As government resources shrink and the influence of the private sector grows, describe the potential implications for the health of individuals and populations that pharmaceutical companies, and other multi-national corporations and institutions do not have the legal obligations imposed on governments to promote and protect human rights in their actions. What difference, if any, do you think this makes for ensuring rights are upheld in how healthcare is delivered?

FURTHER READING

1. Gruskin, S., Tarantola D., Health and Human Rights. In Detels, R., McEwan, J., Beaglehole, R., Tanaka, H., eds., *Oxford Textbook on Public Health*, 4th ed. Oxford: Oxford University Press, 2001.
2. Yamin Alicia, E., The Right to Health under International Law and Its Relevance to the United States. *American Journal of Public Health*, 2005; 95: 1156–61.
3. Mann, J.M., & Tarantola, D., Responding to HIV/AIDS: A Historical Perspective. *Health and Human Rights*, 1998; 5: 5–8.
4. Tarantola, D. & Gruskin, S., Human Rights Approach to Public Health Policy. In Heggenhougen, Kris and Quah, Stella, eds., *International Encyclopedia of Public Health*, Vol 3. San Diego: Academic Press, 2008, 477–486.

CHAPTER 3

Human Rights Approach to Public Health Policy

Daniel Tarantola and Sofia Gruskin

INTRODUCTION

The origin and justification for human rights, whether anchored in natural law, positive law, or other theories and approaches laid out by various authors, as well as their cultural specificity and actual value as international legal commitments, remains subject to ongoing lively debate. Theoretical and rhetorical discourses continue to challenge and enrich current understanding of the relevance of human rights for policy and governance. Nonetheless, human rights have found their way into public health and play today an increasing role in the shaping of health policies, programs, and practice.

Health and human rights are not distinct but intertwined aspirations. Viewed as a universal aspiration, the notion of health as the attainment of physical, mental, and social well-being implies its dependency on and contribution to the realization of all human rights. From the same perspective, the enjoyment by everyone of the highest attainable standard of physical and mental health is in itself a recognized human right. From a global normative perspective, health and human rights are closely intertwined in many international treaties and declarations supported by mechanisms of monitoring and accountability (even as

their effectiveness can be questioned) that draw from both fields.

With respect to health specifically, it is arguably viewed as an important prerequisite for and desirable outcome of human development and progress. Health is

> ... directly constitutive of the person's well-being and it enables a person to function as an agent—that is, to pursue the various goals and projects in life that she has reason to value.
>
> (Anand, 2004: 17–18)

Health is also the most extensively measured component of well-being; it benefits from dedicated services and is commonly seen as a sine-qua-non for the fulfillment of all other aspirations. It may also be ... "a marker, a way of keeping score of how well the society is doing in delivering well-being" (Marmot, 2004: 37).

Health and human rights individually occupy privileged places in the public discourse, political debates, public policy, and the media, and both are at the top of human aspirations. There is hardly a proposed political agenda that does not refer to health in its own right, as well as justice, security, housing, education, and employment opportunities—all with relevance to health. These aspirations are often not framed as human rights but the fact that they are contained in human rights treaties and often translated into national constitutions and legislations provides legal support for efforts in these areas.

Incorporating human rights in public health policy therefore responds to the demands of people, policy makers, and political leaders for outcomes that meet public aspirations. It also creates opportunities for helping decipher how all human rights and other determinants of well-being and social progress interact. It allows progress toward these goals to be measured and shapes policy directions and agendas for action.

This chapter highlights the evolution that has brought human rights and health together in mutually reinforcing ways. It draws from the experience gained in the global response to HIV/AIDS, summarizes key dimensions of public health and of human rights and suggests a manner in which these dimensions intersect that may be used as a framework for health policy analysis, development, and evaluation.

HUMAN RIGHTS AS GOVERNMENTAL OBLIGATIONS

Human rights constitute a set of normative principles and standards which, as a philosophical concept can be traced back to antiquity, with mounting interest among intellectuals and political leaders since the seventeenth century (Tomushat, 2003). The atrocities perpetrated during World War II gave rise, in 1948, to the Universal Declaration of Human Rights (United Nations, 1948) and later to a series of treaties and conventions that extended the aspirational nature of the UDHR into instruments that would be binding on states under international human rights law. Among these are the International Covenant on Civil and Political Rights (ICCPR) and the International Covenant on Economic, Social, and Cultural Rights (ICESCR), both of which came into force in 1976.

Human rights are legal claims that persons have on governments simply on the basis of their being human. They are "what governments can do to you, cannot do to you and should do for you" (Gruskin, 2004). Even though people hold their human rights throughout their lives, they are nonetheless often constrained in their ability to fully realize them. Those who are most vulnerable to violations or neglect of their rights are also often those who lack sufficient power to claim the impact of the lack of enjoyment of their rights on their well-being, including their state of personal health. Human rights are intended to be inalienable (individuals cannot lose these rights any more than they can cease being human beings); they are indivisible (individuals cannot be denied a right because it is deemed less important or nonessential); they are interdependent (all human rights are part of a complementary framework, one right impacting on and being impacted by all others) (United Nations, 1993). They bring into focus the relationship between the State—the first-line provider and protector of human rights—and individuals who hold their human rights simply for being human. In this regard, governments have three sets of obligations toward their people (Eide, 1995):

- They have the obligation to respect human rights, which requires governments to refrain from interfering directly or indirectly with the enjoyment of human rights. In practice, no health policy, practice, program, or legal measure should violate human rights. Policies should ensure the provision of health services to all population groups on the basis of equality and freedom from discrimination, paying particular attention to vulnerable and marginalized groups.

- They have the obligation to protect human rights, which requires governments to take measures that prevent non-state actors from interfering with human rights, and to provide legal means of redress that people know about and can access. This relates to such important non-state actors as private healthcare providers, pharmaceutical companies, health insurance companies and, more generally, the health-related industry, but also national and multinational enterprises whose actions can impact significantly on lifestyle, labor, and the environment such as oil and other energy-producing companies, car manufacturers, agriculture, food industry, and labor-intensive garment factories.
- They have the obligation to fulfill human rights, which requires States to adopt appropriate legislative, administrative, budgetary, judicial, promotional, and other measures toward the full realization of human rights, including putting into place appropriate health and health-related policies that ensure human rights promotion and protection. In practice, governments should be supported in their efforts to develop and apply these measures and monitor their impact, with an immediate focus on vulnerable and marginalized groups.

Government responsibility for health exists in several ways. The right to the highest attainable standard of health appears in one form or another in most international and regional human rights documents, and equally importantly, nearly every article of every document can be understood to have clear implications for health.

The Right to Health

The right to the highest attainable standard of health builds on, but is by no means

Table 3.1 The right to highest attainable standard of health, Article 12 of the International Covenant on Economic, Social and Cultural Rights

1. The States Parties to the present Covenant recognize the right of everyone to the enjoyment of the highest attainable standard of physical and mental health
2. The steps to be taken by the States Parties to the present Covenant to achieve the full realization of this right shall include those necessary for:

   a. The provision for the reduction of the stillbirth rate and of infant mortality and for the healthy development of the child
   b. The improvement of all aspects of environmental and industrial hygiene
   c. The prevention, treatment, and control of epidemic, endemic, occupational and other diseases
   d. The creation of conditions which would assure to all medical service and medical attention in the event of sickness

From United Nations (1966a) *Article 2, International Covenant on Economic, Social and Cultural Rights.* United Nations General Assembly Resolution 2200A [XX1], 16/12/1966, entered into force 03/01/1976 in accordance with Art 17. New York: United Nations.

limited to, Article 12 of the ICESCR (Table 3.1). Rights relating to autonomy, information, education, food and nutrition, association, equality, participation, and nondiscrimination are integral and indivisible parts of the achievement of the highest attainable standard of health, just as the enjoyment of the right-to-health is inseparable from all other rights, whether they are categorized as civil and political, economic, social, or cultural. This recognition is based on empirical observation and on a growing body of evidence that establishes the impact that lack of fulfillment of any and all of these rights has on people's health status: Education, nondiscrimination, food and nutrition epitomizing this relationship (Gruskin and Tarantola, 2001). Conversely, ill-health constrains the fulfillment of all rights as the capacity of individuals to claim and enjoy all their human rights depends on their physical, mental, and social well-being.

The right-to-health does not mean the right to be healthy as such, but the obligation on the part of the government to create the conditions necessary for individuals to achieve their optimal health status. In addition to the ICESCR, the right-to-health is further elaborated in CERD (Convention on the Elimination of all forms of Racial Discrimination, 1965); in CEDAW (Convention on the Elimination of all forms of Discrimination Against Women, 1979), and CRC (Convention on the Rights of the Child art 24, 1989) and in a range of regional human rights documents.

In May 2000, the United Nations Committee on Economic, Social, and Cultural Rights adopted a General Comment further clarifying the substance of government obligations relating to the right to health (UN Committee on Economic, Social and Cultural Rights, 2000). In addition to clarifying governmental responsibility for policies, programs and practices impacting the underlying conditions necessary for health, it sets out requirements related to the delivery of health services including their availability, acceptability, accessibility, and quality. It lays out directions for the practical application of Article 12 and proposes a monitoring framework. Reflecting the mounting interest in determining international policy focused on the right to health, the UN Commission on Human Rights appointed in 2002 a Special Rapporteur whose mandate concerns the right of everyone to the enjoyment of the highest attainable standard of physical and mental health. The Special Rapporteur's role is to undertake country visits, transmit communications to states on alleged violations of the right to health, and submit annual reports to the Commission and the UN General Assembly. Accordingly, through publication review and country visits, the Special Rapporteur has explored policies

and programs related to such issues as maternal mortality, neglected medicines, and reproductive health as they connect to human rights (Hunt, 2007).

All international human rights treaties and conventions contain provisions relevant to health as defined in the preamble of the Constitution of the World Health Organization (WHO), repeated in many subsequent documents and currently adopted by the 191 WHO Member States: Health is a "state of complete physical, mental, and social well-being, and not merely the absence of disease or infirmity." The Constitution further stipulates that "The enjoyment of the highest attainable standard of health is one of the fundamental rights of every human being without distinction of race, political belief, economic or social condition." The Constitution was adopted by the International Health Conference held in New York from 19 June to 22 July 1946, signed on 22 July 1946 by the representatives of 61 States (World Health Organization, 1946), and entered into force on 7 April 1948. Amendments adopted by the Twenty-sixth, Twenty-ninth, Thirty-ninth and Fifty-first World Health Assemblies (resolutions WHA26.37, WHA29.38, WHA39.6 and WHA51.23) came into force on 3 February 1977, 20 January 1984, 11 July 1994 and 15 September 2005, respectively, and are incorporated in the present text.

THE EMERGENCE OF A NEW PUBLIC HEALTH

The focus of public health from its inception in the eighteenth century through the mid-1970s remained on combating disease and some of its most blatant social, environmental, and occupational causes. The state acted as a benevolent provider of services and the source of policies, laws, regulations, and practices generally based on the disease prevention and control model emphasizing risk- and impact-reduction strategies through immunization, case finding, treatment, and changes in domestic, environmental, and occupational hygiene.

In 1978, the Alma-Ata conference solidified a new international health agenda (Litsios, 2002). The aim of achieving Health for All by the Year 2000 was put forward, and this was to be achieved through a Primary Health Care (PHC) approach. Invoking the human right to the highest attainable standard of health, the Declaration of Alma-Ata called on nations to ensure the availability of the essentials of primary health care, including education concerning health conditions and the methods for preventing and controlling them; promotion of food supply and proper nutrition; an adequate supply of safe water and basic sanitation; maternal and child health care, including family planning; immunization against major infectious diseases; prevention and control of locally endemic diseases; appropriate treatment of common disease and injuries; and provision of essential drugs (Declaration of Alma-Ata, 1978).

The 1980s also witnessed the recognition that health was not merely determined by social and economic status but was dependent on dynamic social and economic determinants that could be acted upon through policy and structural changes. In 1986, the Ottawa Charter on Health Promotion helped sharpen the vision of the relationships between individual and collective health and its social, economic, and other determinants (Ottawa Charter for Health Promotion, 1986). The Charter spelled out the fundamental conditions and resources for health as peace, shelter, education, food, income, a stable ecosystem, sustainable resources, social justice, and equity. All of these prerequisites could have been framed as human rights. Probably to stay clear from political controversy that could have been divisive and best been addressed in a United Nations forum, however, the Charter did not explicitly bring human rights or state obligations into play.

The late 1980s and the 1990s saw growing attention being directed in the policy discourse to human rights and to their particular implications for health, and this resulted from several factors. First, the ICCPR and IESCR entered into force in 1976, and in the 1980s the UN Committees responsible for the monitoring of their implementation had begun to decipher their actual meaning and core contents, making the obligations of governments explicit and measurable. Second, the decay of the world geopolitical block ideologies of the late 1980s and the advent of economic neoliberalism created a space for alternate paradigms to help shape public policy and international relations. Human rights entered the scene of geopolitical reconstruction and became common parley after the Glasnost and the fall of the Berlin Wall, in 1989, regardless of whether in reality they were used or abused by new political leaders. Third, the connection between human rights and health was increasingly being shaped around focal causes in various social and political movements. This resulted in the creation of NGOs, some of which engaged in human rights work (responding to torture in particular), others in advocacy around reproductive health and rights issues, while others provided health assistance in armed conflicts and natural disasters, all with the intent of positively impacting on policy and practice. Fourth, and particularly important for the ways this contributed to the integration of human rights concepts into health policy, the emergence of AIDS in 1981, and the recognition of HIV as a global pandemic, resulted in a variety of human rights violations by those seeking to address this mounting public health problem. As traditional disease control policies that had marked the earlier history of public health were put in place by state authorities, with a few exceptions, community-based and advocacy organizations, supported by academic groups, voiced the necessity for policies that afforded greater protections for the rights of people living with or vulnerable to HIV.

Until this time, the focus of public health had generally been to promote the collective physical, mental, and social well-being of people, even if in order to achieve public health goals, policies had to be implemented that sacrificed individual choice, behavior, and action for the common good. This was, and continues to be, exemplified by the principles and practices that guide the control of such communicable diseases as tuberculosis, typhoid, or sexually transmitted infections, where quarantine or other restrictions of rights are imposed on affected individuals. In a number of instances, in particular where health policy addressed communicable diseases and mental illness, restrictions of such rights as privacy, free movement, autonomy, or bodily integrity have been imposed by public health authorities with the commendable intention to protect public health even without valid evidence of their intended public health benefit. The current resurgence of this issue in the context of systematic testing for HIV in health facilities or within entire populations, advocated by some in order to enhance the early access to care and treatment by people found infected, illustrates that disease control methods blind to human rights have by no means vanished. Insufficient attention has been devoted to assessing and monitoring the impact of such policies on the life of people whose rights were being restricted or denied, and to the negative consequences such impositions can have on their willingness to participate supportively in public health efforts that concern them. Public health abuses have also been exemplified by policies which result in the excessive institutionalization of people with physical or mental impair-

ments where alternate care and support approaches have not been adequately considered. In the fields of disability and in mental health, in a number of countries national policies have been found to be discriminatory and, in the case of mental health, at times when carried out in practice to amount to inhuman and degrading treatment. And far from uncommon was— and remains—something often invisible to policy but invidious if not adequately addressed, discrimination in the health-care setting on the basis of health status, gender, race, color, language, religion, or social origin, or any other attribute that can influence the quality of services provided to individuals by or on behalf of the State.

HIV AND GENESIS OF THE INTEGRATION OF HUMAN RIGHTS INTO HEALTH PRACTICE

Cognizant of the need to engage HIV-affected communities in the response to the fast-spreading epidemics in order to achieve their public health goals, human rights were understood as valuable by policy makers not for their moral or legal value but to open access to prevention and care for those who needed these services most, away from fear, discrimination and other forms of human rights violations, and as a way to ensure communities that needed to be reached did not go underground. The deprivation of such entitlements as access to health and social services, employment, or housing imposed on people living with HIV was understood to constrain their capacity to become active subjects rather than the objects of HIV programs, and this was recognized as unsound from a public health perspective.

The evolution of thinking about HIV/AIDS moved from the initial recognition of negative effects of human rights violations among people living with HIV to principles that guided the formulation of a global strategy on HIV/AIDS and, beyond, to the application of these principles to other health issues. In the decade that followed the emergence of AIDS, tremendous efforts were made to induce behavior change through policies that supported intensified, targeted prevention efforts. Everywhere, the initial approaches to HIV had been focused on the reduction of risk of acquiring HIV infection through policies that supported the creation of protective barriers: The use of condoms, early diagnosis and treatment of sexually transmitted infections, and reduction in the number of sexual partners. Some of these efforts were successful on a small scale, in particular where communities were educated and cohesive, as was the case for communities of gay men on the East and West Coasts of the United States, Western Europe, and Australia. Less immediately successful were interventions in communities under immediate social or economic stress and those hampered in their ability to confront HIV/AIDS as a result of strong cultural and other barriers. In sub-Saharan African countries, for example, early interventions related to condoms and other prevention methods, even when sup- ported by national-level policy, were confronted with denial and rejection. Gender-related discrimination was often at the core of resistance to change. Stigma and discrimination directed toward people living with HIV or people whose behaviors were associated with a risk of acquiring and transmitting infection (sex workers, injecting drug users, as well as people defined by their racial or ethnic characteristics) also created obstacles to reaching those who, even perhaps more than others, needed open access to prevention and care. For these reasons, the protection of human rights and combating discrimination became important underlying principles of the first Global Strategy on HIV/AIDS formulated by WHO in 1987 (World Health Organization, 1987).

The risk-reduction strategies of the late 1980s confronted several obstacles in implementation. One was the practical difficulty of scaling up successful approaches to national or international levels. Another was the poor results achieved from applying models proven successful in some settings to different social and cultural environments: Clearly, one size did not fit all. Empirical evidence showed that even as the capacity of individuals to minimize or modulate their risk of exposure to HIV was closely related to specific behaviors or situations, these were in turn influenced by a variety of other factors. In 1992, a risk-vulnerability analysis and reduction model was put forward, positing that in order to successfully impact on risk-taking behaviors, it was necessary to recognize and act on factors that determined the likelihood of individuals engaging in such behaviors (Mann and Tarantola, 1992). A broader perspective suggesting the need for an expanded response to HIV began to emerge, bridging risk, as measured by the occurrence of HIV infection, to risk-taking behaviors, and to their vulnerability determinants. Vulnerability factors could be categorized for simpler analysis as individual (linked to personal history and status, agency, knowledge, or skills); societal (linked to social, economic, and cultural characteristics of the community within which people lived or had lived, including the policy and legal environment); and program-related (dependent on the capacity and approach of programs—health and social in particular) and the extent to which they responded appropriately to people's needs and expectations and assured their participation (Mann and Tarantola, 1996).

While the linkages between health outcomes and health determinants was already very present in the public health discourse, the mounting HIV epidemic made clear the need for policy to simultaneously address a wide and complex assembly of health outcome and determinants touching many facets of society. Simply listing these determinants born out of the established and empirical evidence was overwhelming. There was a need to categorize these determinants in a logical fashion and in a way that would allow them to be taken up by different sectors engaged in human development. The human rights framework was very well suited to this purpose in that it allowed vulnerability factors to be categorized as civil, political, social, economic, or cultural, and each of these factors, recognized through research or empirical evidence, could be easily linked to one or more specific human rights. This expanded approach helped clarify the related responsibilities of different sectors, thereby expanding the scope of public policy change and possible interventions. Importantly, these interventions could build on commitments already expressed, and obligations subscribed to, by governments under international human rights law. From an initial focus on nondiscrimination toward people known or assumed to live with HIV/AIDS, human rights was now helping guide the analysis of the roots, manifestations, and impacts of the HIV epidemics. Stemming from an instrumental approach rather than moral or legal principles, the response to HIV had exposed the congruence between sound public health policy and the upholding of human rights norms and standards (Mann et al., 1994).

The analytical and action-oriented risk and vulnerability framework that linked HIV to the neglect or violations of human rights and the call for needed structural and societal changes grounded in solid policy were important features of the 1994 Paris Summit Declaration on HIV/AIDS (UNAIDS, 1999) and later served as one of the founding principles of the 1996 UNAIDS global strategy and its subsequent revisions (UNAIDS, 1996). These ideas are also apparent in the Declaration of Com-

mitment which emerged from the 2001 United Nations General Assembly.

International activism and a series of international political conferences that took place in this period facilitated similar changes in the approach taken to a wide range of diseases and health conditions, in particular with respect to reproductive and sexual health issues (Freedman, 1997). The 1994 Cairo International Conference on Population and Development was a watershed in recognizing the responsibility of governments worldwide to translate their international-level commitments into national laws, policies, programs, and practices that promote and do not hinder sexual and reproductive health among their populations. National laws and policies were thus open to scrutiny to determine both the positive and negative influences they could have on sexual and reproductive health programming, information, services, and choices. Human rights concerns, including legal, policy, and practice barriers that impact on the delivery and use of sexual and reproductive health services thereafter became a valid target for international attention.

HUMAN RIGHTS AND HEALTH POLICY IN THE NEW MILLENNIUM: KEY CONCEPTS

As, from a theoretical perspective, the interaction between health and human rights was drawing increased attention from policy makers in an expanding array of health-related domains, two issues were and continue to be cited as creating obstacles to the translation of theory into practice. The first is that the realization of the right to health cannot be made real in view of the structures, services, and resources it requires. The second, often cited by those concerned with communicable disease control, is that the protection of human rights should not be the prime concern of policy makers when and where such public health threats as emerging epidemics call for the restriction of certain individual rights. As these two obstacles are often used and misused to question the validity of the health and human rights framework, they are discussed briefly below.

Progressive Realization of Health-Related Human Rights

In all countries, resource and other constraints can make it impossible for a government to fulfill all rights immediately and completely. The principle of progressive realization is fundamental to the achievement of human rights as they apply to health (United Nations, 1966a), and applies equally to resource-poor countries as to wealthier countries whose responsibilities extend not only to what they do within their own borders, but also their engagement in international assistance and cooperation (United Nations, 1966b).

Given that progress in health necessitates infrastructure and human and financial resources that may not match existing or future needs in any country, the principle of progressive realization takes into account the inability of governments to meet their obligations overnight. Yet, it creates an obligation on governments to set their own benchmarks, within the maximum of the resources available to them, and to show how and to what extent, through their policies and practices, they are achieving progress toward the health goals they have agreed to in international forums such as the World Health Assembly, as well as those they have set for themselves. In theory, States account for progress in health (or lack thereof) through a variety of mechanisms that include global monitoring mechanisms, as well as national State of the Health of the Nation reports or similar forms of domestic public reporting.

Human Rights Limitations in the Interest of Public Health

There remains a deeply rooted concern of many in the health community that application of a health and human rights approach to health policy will deprive the State from applying such measures as isolation or quarantine or travel restrictions when public health is at stake. Public health and care practitioners alike, acting on behalf of the State, are used to applying restrictions to individual freedom in cases where the enjoyment of these rights creates a real or perceived threat to the population at large. Recently, the SARS and Avian flu epidemics have demonstrated that such restrictions can also be applied globally under the revised International Health Regulations (IHR), the only binding agreement thus far under the auspices of WHO (World Health Organization, 2005). They stipulate that WHO can make recommendations on an ad hoc, time-limited, risk-specific basis, as a result of a public health emergency of international concern, and that implementation of these Regulations "shall be with full respect for the dignity, human rights and fundamental freedoms of persons." The human rights framework recognizes that these are situations where there can be legitimate and valid restriction of rights, and this under several circumstances relevant to the creation of health policies: Public emergencies and public health imperatives. Public emergencies stipulate that in time of a public emergency that threatens the life of the nation and the existence of which is officially proclaimed, the States Parties to the present Covenant may take measures derogating from their obligations under the present Covenant to the extent strictly required by the exigencies of the situation, provided that such measures are not inconsistent with their other obligations under international law and do not involve discrimination solely on the ground of race, color, sex, language, religion, or social origin (Art 49, ICCPR). Public health imperatives give governments the right to take the steps they deem necessary for the prevention, treatment, and control of epidemic, endemic, occupational, and other diseases (Art 16, ICCPR).

Public health may therefore justify the limitation of certain rights under certain circumstances. Policies that interfere with freedom of movement when instituting quarantine or isolation for a serious communicable disease—for example, Ebola fever, syphilis, typhoid, or untreated tuberculosis, more recently SARS and pandemic influenza—are examples of limitation of rights that may be necessary for the public good and therefore may be considered legitimate under international human rights law. Yet arbitrary restrictive measures taken or planned by public health authorities that fail to consider other valid alternatives may be found to be both abusive of human rights principles and in contradiction with public health best practice. The limitation of most rights in the interest of public health remains an option under both international human rights law and public health laws, but the decision to impose such limitations must be achieved through a structured and accountable process. Increasingly, such consultative processes are put in place by national authorities to debate over the approach taken to public health issues as they arise, such as in the case of immunization, disability, mental health, HIV, smoking, and more recently pandemic influenza preparedness.

Limitations on rights are considered a serious issue under international human rights law—as noted in specific provisions within international human treaties—regardless of the apparent importance of the public good involved. When a government limits the exercise or enjoyment of a right, this action must be taken only as a last resort and will only be considered legitimate if the following criteria are met:

1. The restriction is provided for and carried out in accordance with the law.
2. The restriction is in the interest of a legitimate objective of general interest.
3. The restriction is strictly necessary in a democratic society to achieve the objective.
4. There are no less intrusive and restrictive means available to reach the same goal.
5. The restriction is not imposed arbitrarily, i.e., in an unreasonable or otherwise discriminatory manner (United Nations, 1984).

The restriction of rights, if legitimate, is therefore consistent with human rights principles. Both principles of progressive realization and legitimate limitations of rights are directly relevant to public health policy as they can inform decisions on how to achieve the optimal balance between protecting the rights of the individual and the best interest of the community. Examples of the impact of human rights violations and protection on public health are set out below. Discrimination—a frequent, severe, and persistent issue confronted both in society and in the healthcare setting—has been chosen to illustrate how public health can be hampered by the neglect of human rights and enhanced by their incorporation in public health policy.

PUBLIC HEALTH POLICY AND NONDISCRIMINATION

Discrimination can impact directly on the ways that morbidity, mortality, and disability—the burden of disease—are both measured and acted upon. In fact, the burden of disease itself discriminates: Disease, disability, and death are not distributed randomly or equally within populations, nor are their devastating effects within communities. Tuberculosis, for example, is exploding in disenfranchised communities, in particular among prison inmates and people already affected by HIV and subjected to dual discrimination both in their communities and in the healthcare setting.

Far from uncommon, discrimination in health systems, including health centers, hospitals, or mental institutions, may further contribute to exacerbating disparities in health. A few examples of myriads that could be cited are named here. Undocumented migrant workers receive poor or no treatment for fear of having to justify their civil status. Documented migrant workers, refugees, and asylum seekers and their families may not avail themselves of services that have not been designed to suit their culture and respond to their specific needs. People with hemophilia have been given unsafe blood products on the premise that this adds only a marginal risk to their lives. People with physical or mental disabilities receive substandard care; they are unable to complain or if they do, they fare poorly in legal action (Moss et al., 2007). Discrimination in health systems concerns not only diseases that are already stigmatized, such as AIDS, hepatitis B and C, tuberculosis, and cancer, but also others, such as diabetes and cardiovascular diseases, which could be alleviated if equal treatment within societies and within healthcare settings became the norm. A health and human rights approach to policy development concerning health systems requires that state authorities refrain from enacting discriminatory policies and provide information, education, training, and support to their staff toward eliminating discrimination in public health practice and within the workforce.

Discrimination can also be at the root of unsound human development policies and programs that may impact directly or indirectly on health. For example, an infrastructure development project may require the displacement of entire populations and fail to pay sufficient attention to the new environment to which these populations will have to adjust. In the developing world, when the health impact of large-scale development programs at the local level is considered, it is often from the perspective of the possible further spread of such infectious diseases as malaria and other waterborne diseases. The psychological capacity of displaced communities to relocate and rebuild new lives or the long-term physical and social consequences of such displacement are seldom factored into the equation.

The ongoing international movement toward poverty alleviation has emphasized the critical importance of health in the fight against poverty. The eight Millennium Development Goals (MDGs)—which set targets for 2015 to halve extreme poverty, halt the spread of HIV/AIDS, and improve health and education—have been agreed to by all the world's countries and all the world's leading development institutions (United Nations, 2005). Arguably, all MDGs have a linkage to health either by their direct bearing on health outcomes and the needed services (e.g., through efforts to reduce child and maternal mortality, HIV, malaria, and other diseases) or by underscoring principles central to public health policy (e.g., gender equality) or else by calling for the creation of policies addressing the underlying conditions for progress in health (e.g., education, environmental sustainability, and global partnerships).

PUBLIC HEALTH POLICY AND THE VALUE OF HEALTH AND HUMAN RIGHTS

Human rights and public health policy intersect in a number of ways, which, for practical purposes, can be regrouped into three broad categories: The national and international context within which policy is developed; the outcome of public policy; and the process through which it is developed, applied, and monitored.

Context

A distinction exists between public policy affecting health (most of them do) and public health policy (often emerging from public health governmental authorities or on their initiative). Policies affecting health—for example, those related to gender, trade, intellectual property, the environment, migration, education, housing, or labor—are contingent upon national laws and international treaties or agreements which often overlook—by omission or commission—their potential health consequences. As the Health Impact Assessment of development and social policies gained credence in the 1990s, the development of a human rights assessment for the formulation and evaluation of public health policies emerged (Gostin and Mann, 1999). Health Impact Assessment (HIA), applying different methods, has become more frequently practiced to guide policy options both nationally and internationally. While the aim of such exercises is to forecast the health impact of a single or alternative policies or programs (including those related to infrastructure, financing, service delivery, transportation, or production and many others), the impact of such policies and programs on both health and human rights remains to be adequately tested. Much work is currently ongoing toward the development of a health and human rights Impact Assessment for which assessment methods and health and human rights indicators are required.

An example where such an impact assessment might have been useful was when a number of countries—industrialized and developing alike—applied for membership of the World Trade Organization when such a membership implied for the signatory country to become party to the Agreement on Trade Related Aspects of Intellectual Property Rights (TRIPS). The constraints imposed by TRIPS on developing countries with regards to intellectual protection of pharmaceuticals in particular only became evident in the late 1990s as new, proven therapies for HIV/AIDS were reaching the international market. Civil society movements and some international organizations embarked on an active campaign to overcome the constraints set by TRIPS to the production or importation of generic medicines by developing countries needing them most. It was not until 2002, however, that WHO and WTO jointly produced a document on WTO agreements and public health (World Health Organization and World Trade Organization, 2002). In most developing countries, Ministries of Health had not been consulted, been equipped to assess, or had underestimated, the possible health impacts of the new trade and intellectual property agreement they were signing on to as new members of the WTO. This was and continues to be a painful reminder of the oversight or deliberate neglect of the possible health consequences of public policy guided by other agendas, international trade in this case.

Public health policy should seek the optimal synergy between health and human rights, building on the premise that the optimal quality of a public health policy is attained when the highest possible health outcome and the fullest realization of human rights are both attained. This requires a close interaction between public health professionals, human rights practitioners and representatives of affected communities. The response to HIV has been shaped by such an interaction with significant positive impact—at least in the short term—in such countries as Australia, Sweden, Thailand, Brazil, or

Uganda. Where misconceptions about either sound public health or human rights have distorted HIV policies and programs, the epidemic has continued to strive, as illustrated by the situation in South Africa or China.

As it is generally formulated and monitored by the State, public health policy should operate in the context of the obligations the State has subscribed to under international human rights treaties and national law. Central to these obligations are those to respect, protect, and fulfill all human rights, including the rights to participate in public affairs and policy making, equality, nondiscrimination, and dignity.

Outcome and Impact

Both public health policy and human rights emphasize the importance of outcome and impact, crudely measured in public health terms by the reduction of mortality, morbidity and disability, and the improvement of quality of life, along with economic measurement enabling an assessment of the value for money of particular policies or programs that can guide priority setting. The extent to which outcome includes the fulfillment of human rights is seldom factored in. For example, one would like to see the value of policies that promote sex education in school measured not only in terms of reduction of teenage pregnancy or the incidence of sexually transmitted diseases, but how the right of the child to information is fulfilled in this way and how it impacts on further demands for other health-related, life-saving information. Likewise, when assessing the outcome and impact of policies that prioritize childhood immunization programs, one would want to know not only how immunization makes people healthier, both early and later in their childhood, but also how such public health policies will advance the right of the child to growth and development and her right to education by improving her attendance to and performance at school.

Measuring the outcome and impact of health and health-related policies from a combined health and human rights perspective implies measurement indicators that are neither fully developed nor tested. One of the constraints is that measuring health and human rights on the national, aggregate level is not sensitive to disparities that may exist within the nation, for example as a result of discrimination.

Process

The human rights to information, assembly, and participation in public affairs— including policy making—imply, among other practical steps, the engagement of communities in decisions affecting their health. As highlighted earlier, the history of health and human rights has amply established that community representation in decision-making bodies increases the quality and impact of public health measures. An important issue is to determine who can legitimately speak on behalf of concerned communities. In the last two decades, stimulated by the response to HIV in particular, nongovernmental organizations, and more broadly civil society, have played key roles in drawing attention to policies that were or could be detrimental to health (e.g., restrictions in access to medicines, denial of sex education of young people, access to harm reduction methods among substance users, promotion of tobacco products in young people, marginalized communities and low-income countries, environmental degradation, marketing of unhealthy foods). While state machineries are increasingly cognizant of the growing need for transparency in policy development, civil society is likely to sustain its contribution to such a process, and this through active monitoring by national-level NGOs and such international groups as Amnesty International, Human Rights Watch, or Physicians for Social Responsibility.

IN CONCLUSION

This chapter has attempted to lay out the principles underlying the application of health and human rights principles to public health policy, and it has done so by recalling the historical emergence of these concepts and the opportunities they provide for new approaches to policy development.

Health and human rights, together and independently from each other, have achieved today a degree of prominence in the political and public discourse never witnessed before. The fields of health and rights are illuminated today by their commonalties, no longer by their differences. Both are obligations of governments toward their people; and each supports and requires the fulfillment of the other.

Overall, health and human rights provide a framework for all aspects of policy and program development. In practice, human rights considerations are often built into public health policy through the application of what are today called rights-based approaches. The practical application of these principles is a subject of active and rich debates. Rights-based approaches to health are but some of the attempts currently being made to offer practical guidance to health policy makers and other stakeholders in health and human rights toward translating these principles into health policies, programs, and interventions. Through further reflection, practice and research, public health and human rights practitioners can further establish how and to what extent the promotion and protection of health and human rights interact. In the search for a world where the attainment of the highest standard of physical, mental, and social well-being necessitates, and reinforces, the dignity, autonomy, and progress of every human being, the broad goals of health and human rights are universal and eternal. They give us direction for our understanding of humanity and practical tools for use in our daily work.

REFERENCES

Anand S (2004) The concerns for equity in health. In: Anand S, Peter F, and Sen A (eds.) *Public Health and Ethics*, pp. 17–18. Oxford, UK: Oxford University Press.

Anonymous (1978) Declaration of Alma-Ata, International Conference of Primary Health Care. Alma-Ata: USSR, 6–12 September 1978. http://www.who.int/hpr/NPH/docs/declaration_almaata.pdf.

Burris SC, Swanson JW, Moss K, Ullman MD, and Ranney LM (2006) Justice disparities: Does the ADA enforcement system treat people with psychiatric disabilities fairly? *Maryland Law Review*.

Eide A (2001) Economic, social and cultural rights as human rights. In: Eide A, Krause C, and Rosas E (eds.) *Economic, Social, and Cultural Rights: A Textbook*, pp. 9–28. The Hauge, The Netherlands: Kluwer Law International.

Freedman L (1997) Human rights and the politics of risk and blame: Lessons from the international reproductive health movement. *Journal of the American Medical Women's Association* 52(4): 165–168.

Gostin L and Mann J (1999) Toward the development of a human rights impact assessment for the formulation and evaluation of public health policies. In: Mann J, Gruskin S, Grodin M, and Annas G (eds.) *Health and Human Rights: A Reader*, pp. 54–71. New York: Routledge.

Gruskin S (2004) Is there a government in the cockpit: A passenger's perspective or global public health: The role of human rights. *Temple Law Review* 77: 313–334.

Gruskin S and Tarantola D (2001) Health and human rights. In: Detels R, McEwen J, Beaglehole R, and Tanaka H (eds.) *The Oxford Textbook of Public Health*, 4th ed. Oxford, UK: Oxford University Press.

Hunt P (2007) *Report of the Special Rapporteur on the Right of Everyone to the Enjoyment of the Highest Attainable Standard of Physical and Mental Health*. Human Rights Council 4th session, A/HRC/28, 17 January 2007. pp. 15–21.

Litsios S (2002) The long and difficult road to Alma-Ata: A personal reflection. *International Journal of Health Services* 32: 709–732.

Mann J and Tarantola D (1992) Assessing the vulnerability to HIV infection and AIDS. In: Mann J,

Tarantola D, and Netter T (eds.) *AIDS in the World*, pp. 557–602. Cambridge, MA: Harvard University Press.

Mann J and Tarantola D (1996) Societal vulnerability: Contextual analysis. In: Mann J and Tarantola D (eds.) *AIDS in the World II*, pp. 444–462. London: Oxford University Press.

Mann JM, Gostin L, Gruskin S, Brennan T, Lazzarini Z, and Fineberg H (1994) Health and human rights. *Health and Human Rights* 1(1): 58–80.

Marmot M (2004) Social causes of inequity in health. In: Anand S, Peter F, and Sen A (eds.) *Public Health and Ethics*, p. 37. Oxford, UK: Oxford University Press.

Ottawa Charter for Health Promotion (1986) *First International Conference on Health Promotion: The Move Towards a New Public Health.* November 17–21, 1986, Ottawa, Ontario, Canada. WHO/HPR/HEP/95.1.

Tomuschat C (2003) *Human Rights, Between Idealism and Realism.* New York: Oxford University Press.

UNAIDS (1996) *Global Strategy*, 1996/2001. Geneva, Switzerland: United Nations Joint Programme on HIV AIDS.

UNAIDS (1999) *From Principle to Practice: Greater Involvement of People Living with or Affected by HIV/AIDS (GIPA) UNAIDS/99.43E.*

United Nations (1948) *Universal Declaration of Human Rights. G.A. Res. 217A (III) UN GAOP, Res 71, UN Doc.A/810.* New York: United Nations.

United Nations (1966a) *Article 2, International Covenant on Economic, Social and Cultural Rights. United Nations General Assembly Resolution 2200A [XX1],* 16/12/1966, entered into force 03/01/1976 in accordance with Art 17. New York: United Nations.

United Nations (1966b) *Article 2, International Covenant on Civil and Political Rights. United Nations General Assembly Resolution 2200A [XX1],* 16/12/1966, entered into force 23/03/1976 in accordance with Article 49. New York: United Nations.

United Nations (1984) *The Siracusa principles on the limitation and derogation provisions. In: The International Covenant on Civil and Political Rights.* Annex to UN Document E/CN.4/1985/4 of 28/09/1984. New York: United Nations.

United Nations (1993) *Vienna Declaration and Programme of Action (A/CONF.157/23).*

United Nations (2001) *Declaration of Commitment on HIV/AIDS: Global Crisis-Global Action. Resolution adopted by the General Assembly. United Nations.* New York (A/S-26/L.2).

United Nations (2005) *UN Millennium Project 2005. Investing in Development: A Practical Plan to Achieve the Millennium Development Goals.* New York: United Nations Development Programme.

United Nations Committee on Economic, Social and Cultural Rights (2000) *General Comment 14 on the Right to the Highest Attainable Standard of Health.* New York: United Nations.

World Health Organization (1946) *Constitution of the World Health Organization.* Off. Rec. Wld Hlth Org., 2, 100. Geneva, Switzerland: World Health Organization.

World Health Organization (1987) *The Global Strategy for AIDS Prevention and Control. Geneva, Switzerland: World Health Organization;* unpublished document SPA/INF/87.1.

World Health Organization (2005) *Revisions of the International Health Regulations, endorsed by the Fifty-eighth World Health Assembly in Resolution 58.3.* Geneva, Switzerland: World Health Assembly 23/05/2005.

World Health Organization (2006) *Constitution of the World Health Organization Basic Documents. Forty-fifth edition.* Supplement, October 2006.

World Health Organization and World Trade Organization (2002) *WTO Agreements and Pubic Health, a joint study by the WHO and the WTO Secretariat, World Health Organization and World Trade Organization.* Geneva, Switzerland: World Health Organization.

QUESTIONS

1. The right to health imposes an obligation on governments to create the conditions necessary for individuals to achieve their optimal health status. Consider the differences between a very rich country and a very poor country. How would you define these conditions? To what extent are these conditions, or should be, the responsibility of the international community, of national governments or simply of each individual?

2. Imagine you are working within a Ministry of Health and are confronted with a new and apparently deadly communicable disease. There are limited data with respect to transmission and prevention, and no treatment is yet available. What actions will you take in the short term? In the long term? What human rights will you restrict and why? How will you justify these restrictions?

3. Are health and human rights concerns always synergistic? Are there times when human rights and public health concerns will be in opposition? Give examples of when you think this might happen and why. Take one example and consider what issues will need to be resolved in order to ensure rights and health can work together most usefully to support the health of a population.

FURTHER READING

1. World Health Organization, *25 Questions and Answers on Health and Human Rights*. Health and Human Rights Pubs, No. 1. Geneva, Switzerland: World Health Organization, 2002.
2. London, L., What is a Human Rights-based Approach to Health and does It Matter? *Health and Human Rights*, 2008; 10: 13–6 .
3. Pillay, N., Right to Health and the Universal Declaration of Human Rights. *Lancet*, 2008; 372: 2005–6. http://search.proquest.com/docview/199013669?accountid=12935
4. Yamin, A. E., Beyond Compassion: The Central Role of Accountability in Applying a Human Rghts Framework to Health. *Health and Human Rights*, 2008; 10 http://search.proquest.com/docview/58813390?accountid=12935

POINT OF VIEW

Health and Human Rights—A View from Nepal

Paul Farmer

On a map of the world and to a doctor's eye, Nepal is a rib-shaped slice of a country stretched laterally between two giants, hemmed in to the north by the Himalayas and to the south by India. In the words of anthropologist Dor Bahadur Bista, "Nepal is such a complex social conglomeration seeking perpetually to accommodate, if not synthesize, its diverse discrete parts." In spite of close to three centuries of national identity, groups defined variously by class, caste, ethnicity, language, region, and religion jostle for rights that people everywhere want: access to health care and education, the chance to make a decent living without risking life and limb. In much of the country, and among the poor, such risks are faced every day. Although the rules of feudalism have been abolished, landless poverty keeps millions in profound dependence. Some estimates peg the number of Nepalis who live on less than $2 a day as high as 80 percent.[1]

Physicians are trained to expect an often grim universality from pathophysiology. A bad chest x-ray looks familiar in Boston or Rwanda or Kathmandu; lungs and hearts sound the same across the globe; a fracture is a fracture is a fracture. Yet whether among the poor and marginalized in wealthy or developed countries or among the great majority in the world's poorest countries, the concept of justice in action—of actually delivering on lofty concepts regarding the right to food security, safe schools, housing, water, and health care—remains as powerful and important now as ever.[2] Perhaps more powerful: it's impossible to argue, in the 21st century, that any of these challenges are somehow technically insuperable. They're not, and we all know it.

A few years ago, a group of medical students, trainees of mine, founded Nyaya Health, working in partnership with local groups and public health authorities to promote the right to health and to help break the cycle of poverty and disease.[3] They opened a health center in a warehouse in a small town, and brought in Achham district's first biomedically trained doctor. Until recently, the district counted a quarter of a million souls but not a single physician.

Their work isn't easy. It's well over 100 degrees in summer and humid enough to make one wish for rain. Inside the clinics and wards, the mortal dramas are all too familiar. Women with third-trimester catastrophes. Abscesses from injuries. Rheumatic heart disease. Enteric fever. Childhood malnutrition and its companion diarrheal disease. All manner of waterborne ailments. Tuberculosis and AIDS. (Achham probably has Nepal's highest rates of these two chronic infections, long associated with poverty, gender-based disparities, and labor migration, all of which are also associated with conflict.[4]) Of course, there are non-communicable chronic diseases, too: congestive heart failure, renal insufficiency, many cancers, mental illness. It's a well-known catalogue, seen in every impoverished corner of the world.

Every one of these problems can be prevented or palliated or cured by the basics of modern medicine and public health. By basics I mean clean water and safer roads, of course, but also a fairly modest array of vaccines and diagnostics and treatments. In an era in which we talk glibly of "value for money" or "cost-effective interventions," it would be hard to argue that the work at hand in Achham doesn't offer a terrific bargain—to push the metaphor crassly—for those wishing to make a difference in a world driven by inequality and its attendant suffering.

Taking on the noxious synergy of poverty and disease is tedious and full of pitfalls and disappointments. But many have fought hard and made great sacrifices in order to insist on something as simple as a hospital in a place such as Achham district in far-western Nepal. Those sacrifices include the lives of six people killed during a demonstration in 1976; people in the region were agitating for a hospital and the protest turned violent. Six more people went to jail, some as far away as Kathmandu. Some of those who served time returned to see the hospital reborn and growing. The vigor of purpose in providing a preferential option for the poor has remained unwavering. The challenge we face is not lack of conviction, just as it is not lack of available technology. Delivering on the promise of the right to health care is, some have argued, the ranking human rights challenge of our time.

Over the past quarter-century, I have been asked a thousand variants of the following questions: "This work to provide health care as a right is a good thing, but is it sustainable? Can it ever be brought to scale?" And we've said a thousand times, especially to our own students, that it's possible to tell whether these questions are asked to start the conversation or to end it. For those seeking to start conversations about sustainability and scale, or about the right to health care, we have learned a great deal. To sustain such efforts requires

that a new generation of practitioners, policymakers, scholars, researchers, and advocates take up the mantle of human rights and global health equity. It requires investments in training on both sides of the great divide between rich and poor.[5] To bring such efforts to scale requires that we engage the public sector, since only governments can confer rights to those living within their borders.

If you do this work long enough—I've worked with the same people in Haiti and at Harvard for nearly thirty years—life starts to be defined by tension between the general and the specific, the universal and the particular, and is always linked to the mortal dramas mentioned above. These dramas can be hidden away, and often are, but they exist whether we acknowledge them or not. And yet, acknowledging injustice is not enough; linking knowledge to reparative action is what we're all called to do, together; it's the heart of the matter for all partners in health, lower case. As I have learned from Amartya Sen and from colleagues at Nyaya Health, the Sanskrit-based word *nyaya* means "justice in action"—it's perhaps a shorter and more elegant term for global health delivery and for human rights.[6] No single group can possibly bring services to all who need them. But the lives of those we never see or meet are just as valuable as the lives of those we meet directly, and their health just as much a right as our own.

REFERENCES

1. UNDP. *Human Development Report.* New York: Oxford University Press, 2003.
2. Farmer PE. *Pathologies of Power: Health, Human Rights, and the New War on the Poor.* Berkeley: University of California Press, 2005.
3. Maru DS-R, Sharma A, Andrews J, Basu S, Thapa J, et al. Global Health Delivery 2.0: Using Open-Access Technologies for Transparency and Operations Research. *PLoS Med,* 2009; 6(12): e1000158.
4. Collier L., Elliott H. et al. *Breaking the Conflict*

Trap: Civil War and Development Policy. Washington, DC: World Bank and Oxford University Press, 2003.

5. Furin J, Farmer P, et al. A Novel Training Model to Address Health Problems in Poor and Underserved Populations. *Journal of Health Care for the Poor and Underserved,* 2006; 17: 17–24.

6. Sen A. *The Idea of Justice.* Cambridge: Harvard University Press, 2009.

Paul Farmer is Kolokotrones University Professor, Harvard University; Chair, Department of Global Health and Social Medicine, Harvard Medical School; and Founding Director, Partners in Health, Boston, MA, USA.

CHAPTER 4

Health Systems and the Right to the Highest Attainable Standard of Health*

Paul Hunt and Gunilla Backman

The right to the highest attainable standard of health depends upon the interventions and insights of medicine and public health. Equally, the classic, long-established objectives of medicine and public health can benefit from the newer, dynamic discipline of human rights. At an abstract level, a few far-sighted people understood this when the World Health Organization (WHO) Constitution was drafted in 1946, and the Declaration of Alma-Ata was adopted in 1978, which is why both instruments affirm the right to the highest attainable standard of health. The Ottawa Charter of Health Promotion of 1986 also reflects the connections between public health and human rights.

However, these connections were general and abstract. At the time, the right to the highest attainable standard of health was only dimly understood and attracted limited support from civil society. It was little more than a slogan. Others have surveyed the evolution of health and human rights since Alma-Ata and Ottawa, and we will not repeat this exercise here.[1]

One vital part of this evolutionary process has been a deepening understanding of the right to the highest attainable standard of health. Although neglected in much of the literature, this fundamental human right must surely be the cornerstone of any consideration of health and human rights. Through the endeavours of innumerable organizations and individuals, the content of the right to the highest attainable standard of health is now sufficiently well understood to be applied in an operational, systematic and sustained manner. Crucially, this understanding is new: It dates from within the last ten years or so. Of course, much more work is needed to grasp all the implications of the right to the highest attainable standard of health, but it can no longer be seen (or dismissed) as merely a rhetorical device. In these circumstances, it is timely to revisit Alma-Ata, and examine health systems, from the new, operational perspective of the right to the highest attainable standard of health.

In any society, an effective health system is a core institution, no less than a fair justice system or democratic political system.[2] In many countries, however, health systems are failing and collapsing,[3] giving rise to an extremely grave and widespread human rights problem. At the heart of the right to the highest attainable standard of health lies an effective and integrated health system, encompassing medical care and the underlying determinants of health, which is responsive to national and local priorities, and accessible to all. Without such a health system, the right to the highest attainable standard of health can never be realized. It is only through building and strengthening health systems that it will be possible to secure sustainable development, poverty reduction, economic prosperity, improved health for individuals and populations, as well as the right to the highest attainable standard of health.

There is an analogy between, on the one hand, court systems and the right to a fair trial and, on the other hand, health systems and the right to the highest attainable standard of health. The right to a fair trial is widely recognized to have strengthened many court systems. It has helped to identify the key features of a fair court system, such as independent judges, trials without undue delay, the opportunity to call witnesses and make legal argument, legal aid for impecunious defendants in serious cases, and so on. The right to a fair trial has exposed unfair judicial processes and led to welcome reforms. Significantly, many features arising from the right to a fair trial have major budgetary implications.

In much the same way, the right to the highest attainable standard of health can help to establish effective, integrated and accessible health systems. If this is to happen, however, greater clarity is needed about the key features of a health system that arise from the right to the highest attainable standard of health.

Importantly, the right to the highest attainable standard of health is recognized in the constitution of many states.[4] Also, it is enshrined in numerous binding international human rights treaties, such as the International Covenant on Economic, Social and Cultural Rights (ICESCR) and the Convention on the Rights of the Child (CRC), which has been ratified by every state of the world, except for two (the United States of America (USA) and Somalia).

This chapter identifies some of the key right to health features of a health system. It considers health systems from the new, operational perspective of the right to the highest attainable standard of health. All of the features and measures identified here are already found in some health systems, recognized in some international health instruments (such as the Declaration of Alma-Ata), or advocated in the health literature. But they are not usually recognized as human rights issues. The chapter outlines how the right to the highest attainable standard of health underpins and reinforces an effective, integrated, accessible health system—and why this is important.[5]

A RIGHT TO HEALTH APPROACH TO STRENGTHENING HEALTH SYSTEMS

In the last decade, states, international organizations, international and national human rights mechanisms, courts, civil society organizations, academics and many others have begun to explore what the right to the highest attainable standard of health means and how it can be put into practice.[6] Health workers are making the most decisive contribution to this process.[7] Drawing upon this deepening experience, and informed by health good practices, this section briefly outlines the general approach of the right to the highest attainable standard of health towards the strengthening of health systems.

At the Centre: The Wellbeing of Individuals, Communities and Populations

A health system gives rise to numerous technical issues. Of course, experts have an indispensable role to play in addressing these technical matters. But there is a risk that health systems become impersonal, "top-down" and dominated by experts.

Additionally, as a recent WHO publication observes, "health systems and services are mainly focused on disease rather than on the person as a whole, whose body and mind are linked and who needs to be treated with dignity and respect."[8] The publication concludes, "health care and health systems must embrace a more holistic, people-centred approach."[9] This is also the approach required by the right to the highest attainable standard of health. Because it places the well being of individuals, communities and populations at the centre of a health system, the right to health can help to ensure that a health system is neither technocratic nor removed from those it is meant to serve.

Not Only Outcomes, but Also Processes

The right to the highest attainable standard of health is concerned with both processes and outcomes. It is not only interested in what a health system does (e.g., providing access to essential medicines and safe drinking water), but also how it does it (e.g., transparently, in a participatory manner, and without discrimination).

Transparency

Access to health information is an essential feature of an effective health system, as well as the right to the highest attainable standard of health. Health information enables individuals and communities to promote their own health, participate effectively, claim quality services, monitor progressive realization, expose corruption, hold those responsible to account, and so on. The requirement of transparency applies to all those working in health-related sectors, including states, international organizations, public private partnerships, business enterprises and civil society organizations.

Participation

All individuals and communities are entitled to active and informed participation on issues bearing upon their health. In the context of health systems, this includes participation in identifying overall strategy, policy-making, implementation and accountability. The importance of community participation is one of the principal themes recurring throughout the Declaration of Alma-Ata. Crucially, states have a human rights responsibility to establish institutional arrangements for the active and informed participation of all relevant stakeholders, including disadvantaged communities.[10]

Equity, Equality and Non-Discrimination

Equality and non-discrimination are among the most fundamental elements of international human rights, including the right to the highest attainable standard of health. A state has a legal obligation to ensure that a health system is accessible to all without discrimination, including those living in poverty, minorities, indigenous peoples, women, children, slum and rural dwellers, people with disabilities, and other disadvantaged individuals and communities. Also, the health system must be responsive to the particular health needs of women, children, adolescents, the elderly, and so on. The twin human rights principles of equality and non-discrimination mean that outreach (and other) programmes must be in place to ensure that disadvantaged individuals and communities enjoy, in practice, the same access as those who are more advantaged.

Equality and non-discrimination are akin to the critical health concept of equity. There is no universally accepted definition of equity, but one definition is "equal access to health-care according to need."[11]

All three concepts have a social justice component. In some respects, equality and nondiscrimination, being reinforced by law, are more powerful than equity. For example, if a state fails to take effective steps to tackle race discrimination in a health system, it can be held to account and required to take remedial measures. Also, if a health system is accessible to the wealthy but inaccessible to those living in poverty, the state can be held to account and required to take remedial action.

Respect for Cultural Difference

A health system must be respectful of cultural difference. Health workers, for example, should be sensitive to issues of ethnicity and culture. Also, a health system is required to take into account traditional preventive care, healing practices and medicines. Strategies should be in place to encourage and facilitate indigenous peoples, for example, to study medicine and public health. Moreover, training in some traditional medical practices should also be encouraged.[12] Of course, cultural respect is right as a matter of principle. But, additionally, it makes sense as a matter of practice. As Thoraya Obaid, Executive Director of the United Nations Population Fund (UNFPA), observes: "Cultural sensitivity . . . leads to higher levels of programme acceptance and ownership by the community, and programme sustainability."[13]

Medical Care and the Underlying Determinants of Health

The health of individuals, communities and populations requires more than medical care. For this reason, international human rights law casts the right to the highest attainable standard of physical and mental health as an inclusive right not only extending to timely and appropriate medical care, but also to the underlying determinants of health, such as access to safe water and adequate sanitation, an adequate supply of safe food, nutrition and housing, healthy occupational and environmental conditions, access to health-related education and information, including on sexual and reproductive health, and freedom from discrimination.[14] The social determinants of health, such as gender, poverty and social exclusion, are major preoccupations of the right to the highest attainable standard of health. In his work, for example, the first United Nations Special Rapporteur on the Right to Health consistently looked at medical care and the underlying determinants of health, including the impact of poverty and discrimination on health. In short, the right to the highest attainable standard of health encompasses the traditional domains of both medical care and public health. This is the perspective that the right to the highest attainable standard of health brings to the strengthening of health systems.

Progressive Realization and Resource Constraints

The right to the highest attainable standard of health is subject to progressive realization and resource availability. In other words, it does not make the absurd demand that a comprehensive, integrated health system be constructed overnight. Rather, for the most part, human rights require that states take effective measures to progressively work towards the construction of an effective health system that ensures access to all. The disciplines of medicine and public health take a similar position; the Declaration of Alma-Ata, for example, is directed to "progressive improvement."[15] Also, the right to health is realistic, it demands more of high-income than low-income states. That is to say, implementation of the right to health is subject to resource availability.

These two concepts—progressive realization and resource availability—have numerous implications for health systems, some of which are briefly explored later in this chapter. For example, because progressive realization does not occur spontaneously, a state must have a comprehensive, national plan, encompassing both the public and private sectors, for the development of its health system. The crucial importance of planning is recognized in the health literature, the Declaration of Alma-Ata, and General Comment No. 14 on the right to the highest attainable standard of health of the United Nations Committee on Economic, Social and Cultural Rights.[16]

Another implication of progressive realization is that an effective health system must include appropriate indicators and benchmarks, otherwise there is no way of knowing whether or not the state is improving its health system and progressively realizing the right to the highest attainable standard of health. Moreover, the indicators must be disaggregated on suitable grounds, such as sex, socio-economic status and age, so that the state knows whether or not its outreach programmes for disadvantaged individuals and communities are working. Indicators and benchmarks are already commonplace features of many health systems, but they rarely have all the elements that are important from a human rights perspective, such as disaggregation on appropriate grounds.[17]

A third implication arising from progressive realization is that at least the present level of enjoyment of the right to the highest attainable standard of health must be maintained. This is sometimes known as the principle of non-retrogression.[18] Although rebuttable in certain limited circumstances, there is a strong presumption that measures lowering the present enjoyment of the right to health are impermissible.

Finally, progressive realization does not mean that a state is free to choose whatever measures it wishes to take so long as they reflect some degree of progress. A state has a duty to adopt those measures that are most effective, while taking into account resource availability and other human rights considerations.

Duties of Immediate Effect: Core Obligations

Although subject to progressive realization and resource availability, the right to the highest attainable standard of health gives rise to some core obligations of immediate effect. A state has "a core obligation to ensure the satisfaction of, at the very least, minimum essential levels" of the right to the highest attainable standard of health.[19] What, more precisely, are these core obligations? Some are discussed later in this chapter. Briefly, they include an obligation to:

- Prepare a comprehensive, national plan for the development of the health system.
- Ensure access to health-related services and facilities on a non-discriminatory basis, especially for disadvantaged individuals, communities and populations; this means, for example, that a state has a core obligation to establish effective outreach programmes for those living in poverty.
- Ensure the equitable distribution of health-related services and facilities e.g., a fair balance between rural and urban areas.
- Establish effective, transparent, accessible and independent mechanisms of accountability in relation to duties arising from the right to the highest attainable standard of health.

Also, a state has a core obligation to ensure a minimum "basket" of health-related services and facilities, including essential food, to ensure freedom from hunger, basic sanitation and adequate water, essential medicines, immunization against the community's major infectious diseases, and sexual and reproductive health services including information, family planning, pre-natal and post-natal services, and emergency obstetric care. Some states have already identified a minimum "basket" for those within their jurisdiction. Some international organizations have also tried to identify a minimum "basket" of health services. This is a difficult exercise, not least because health challenges vary widely from one state to another and therefore, in practice, the minimum "basket" may vary between countries. In some countries the challenge is undernutrition, elsewhere it is obesity.

Much more work has to be done to help states identify the minimum "basket" of health-related services and facilities required by the right to the highest attainable standard of health. However, that vital task is not the purpose of this chapter. The aim here is to identify a number of additional, and frequently neglected, features arising from the right to the highest attainable standard of health, and informed by health good practices, that are required of all health systems. These include, for example, access on the basis of equality and non-discrimination, an up-to-date health plan, effective accountability for the public and private health sector, and so on.

Quality

All health services and facilities must be of good quality. For example, a health system must be able to ensure access to good quality essential medicines. If rejected in the North because they are beyond their expiry date and unsafe, medicines must not be recycled to the South. Because medicines may be counterfeit or tampered with, a state must establish a regulatory system to check medicine safety and quality. The requirement of good quality also extends to the manner in which patients and others are treated. Health workers must treat patients and others politely and with respect.

A Continuum of Prevention and Care with Effective Referrals

A health system should have an appropriate mix of primary (community-based), secondary (district-based) and tertiary (specialized) facilities and services, providing a continuum of prevention and care. The system also needs an effective process when a health worker assesses that their client may benefit from additional services, and the client is referred from one facility or department to another. Referrals are also needed, in both directions, between an alternative health system (e.g., traditional practitioners) and "mainstream" health system. The absence of an effective referral system is inconsistent with the right to the highest attainable standard of health.

Vertical or Integrated?

There is a longstanding debate about the merits of vertical (or selective) health interventions, which focus on one or more diseases or health conditions, and a comprehensive, integrated approach. By drawing off resources, vertical interventions can jeopardize progress towards the long-term goal of an effective health system. They have other potential disadvantages, such as duplication and fragmentation. However, in some circumstances, such as during a public health emergency, there may be a place for vertical intervention. When these circumstances arise, the intervention must be carefully designed, so far as possible, to strengthen and not undermine a comprehensive, integrated health system.

Coordination

A health system, as well as the right to the highest attainable standard of health, depends upon effective coordination across a range of public and private actors (including nongovernmental organizations) at the national and international levels. The scope of the coordination will depend upon how the health system is defined. But, however it is defined, coordination is crucial. For example, a health system and the right to the highest attainable standard of health demand effective coordination between various sectors and departments, such as health, environment, water, sanitation, education, food, shelter, finance and transport. They also demand coordination within sectors and departments, such as the Ministry of Health. The need for coordination extends to policy-making and the actual delivery of services.

Health-related coordination in many states is very patchy and weak. Alone, the Cabinet is an insufficient coordination mechanism for health-related issues. Other coordination mechanisms are essential.

Health as a Global Public Good: The Importance of International Cooperation[20]

Public goods are goods that benefit society as a whole. The concept of "national public goods," such as the maintenance of law and order, is well established. In an increasingly interdependent world, much more attention is being paid to "global public goods." They address issues in which the international community has a common interest. In the health context, global public goods include the control of infectious diseases, the dissemination of health research, and international regulatory initiatives, such as the WHO Framework Convention on Tobacco Control.

Although it remains very imprecise, the concept of "global public goods" confirms that a health system has both national and international dimensions.

The international dimension of a health system is also reflected in states' human rights responsibilities of international assistance and cooperation. These responsibilities can be traced through the Charter of the United Nations, the Universal Declaration of Human Rights, and several more recent international human rights declarations and binding treaties.[21] They are also reflected in the outcome documents of several world conferences, such as the Millennium Declaration, as well as numerous other initiatives, including the Paris Declaration on Aid Effectiveness (2005).

As a minimum, all states have a responsibility to cooperate on transboundary health issues and to "do no harm" to their neighbours. High-income states have an additional responsibility to provide appropriate international assistance and cooperation in health for low-income countries. They should especially assist low-income countries to fulfil their core obligations arising from the right to the highest attainable standard of health. Equally, low-income states have a responsibility to seek appropriate international assistance and cooperation to help them strengthen their health systems. The relationship between health "global public goods" and the human rights responsibility of international assistance and cooperation in health demands further study.

Striking Balances

Few human rights are absolute. Frequently, balances have to be struck between competing human rights. Freedom of information, for example, has to be balanced with the right to privacy. Moreover, there are often legitimate but competing claims arising from the same human right, especially in relation to those numerous rights that are subject to resource availability. In the context of health systems, finite budgets give rise to tough policy choices. Should the government build a new teaching hospital, establish more primary health care clinics, strengthen community care for people with disabilities, improve sanitation in the capital's slum, improve access to anti-retrovirals, or subsidize an effective but expensive cancer drug? Human rights do not provide neat answers to such questions, anymore than do ethics or economics. But human rights require that the questions be decided by way of a fair, transparent, participatory process, taking into account explicit criteria, such as the well being of those living in poverty, and not just the claims of powerful interest groups.[22]

Because of the complexity, sensitivity and importance of many health policy issues, it is vitally important that effective, accessible and independent mechanisms of accountability are in place to ensure that reasonable balances are struck by way of fair processes that take into account all relevant considerations, including the interests of disadvantaged individuals, communities and populations.

Monitoring and Accountability

Rights imply duties, and duties demand accountability. Accountability is one of the most important features of human rights— and also one of the least understood. Although human rights demand accountability, that does not mean that every health worker or specialized agency becomes a human rights enforcer. Accountability includes the monitoring of conduct, performance and outcomes. In the context of a health system, there must be accessible, transparent and effective mechanisms of accountability to understand how those with responsibilities towards the health system have discharged their duties. The

crucial role of monitoring and accountability is explored later in this chapter.

Legal Obligation

The right to the highest attainable standard of health gives rise to legally binding obligations. A state is legally obliged to ensure its health system includes a number of the features and measures signalled in the preceding paragraphs. The health system must have, for example, a comprehensive, national plan; outreach programmes for the disadvantaged; a minimum "basket" of health-related services and facilities; effective referral systems; arrangements to ensure the participation of those affected by health-decision making; respect for cultural difference; and so on. Of course, these requirements also correspond to health good practices. One of the distinctive contributions of the right to the highest attainable standard of health is that it reinforces such health good practices with legal obligation and accountability.

THE "BUILDING BLOCKS" OF A HEALTH SYSTEM

Informed by health good practices, the preceding section outlines the general approach of the right to the highest attainable standard of health towards the strengthening of health systems. This general approach has to be consistently and systematically applied across the numerous elements that together constitute a functioning health system. What are these functional elements of a health system? The health literature on this issue is very extensive. For its part, WHO identifies "six essential building blocks" which together make up a health system:[23]

- Health services (medical and public health)
- Health workforce

- Health information system
- Medical products, vaccines and technologies
- Health financing
- Leadership, governance, stewardship.

Each "building block" has generated a huge literature over many years. For present purposes, three short points demand emphasis. First, these are not only "building blocks" for a health system—they are also "building blocks" for realizing the right to the highest attainable standard of health. Like a health system, the right to health requires health services, health workers, health information, medical products, financing and stewardship.

Second, in practice, the "building blocks" might not have all the features required by the right to the highest attainable standard of health. For example, a country might have a health information system, one of the WHO "building blocks." But the information system might not include appropriately disaggregated data, which is one of the requirements of the right to health. In short, an essential "building block" might be in place, but without all the features required by international human rights law.

Third, the crucial challenge is to apply—or integrate—the right to the highest attainable standard of health, as well as other human rights, across the six "building blocks." The general approach outlined in the preceding section has to be consistently and systematically applied to health services, health workers, health information, medical products, financing and stewardship—all the elements that together constitute a functioning health system.

The systematic application of the right to health to the six "building blocks" is likely to have a variety of results. In some cases, a focus on the right to health will reinforce existing features of the "building blocks" that routinely receive the attention they deserve. In other cases, the application of the right will identify existing features of the "building blocks" that tend to be overlooked in practice and that require much more attention, such as the disaggregation of data on appropriate grounds. It is also possible that the application of the right may identify features that, although important, are not usually regarded as forming any part of the six "building blocks."[24]

APPLYING THE RIGHT TO HEALTH APPROACH TO ONE OF THE "BUILDING BLOCKS" OF A HEALTH SYSTEM

By way of illustration, this section begins to apply the right to the highest attainable standard of health to one of WHO's six "building blocks": leadership, governance and stewardship. This is "arguably the most complex but critical building block of any health system."[25] It encompasses many elements, including planning, monitoring and accountability.

Planning

Planning is one of the weakest features of the development and strengthening of health systems. With a few honourable exceptions, the record of health planning is poor, while the history of health planning is surprisingly short. Many states do not have comprehensive, up-to-date health plans. Where they exist, plans "often fail to be implemented and remain grand designs on paper. Elsewhere plans may be implemented but fail to respond to the real needs of the population."[26]

However, from the perspective of the right to the highest attainable standard of health, effective planning is absolutely critical. Progressive realization and resource availability—two inescapable components of the international right to health—cannot be addressed without planning.[27]

Recognizing the critical role of effective planning, the United Nations Committee on Economic, Social and Cultural Rights designated the preparation of a health "strategy and plan of action" as a core obligation arising from the right to the highest attainable standard of health. The Committee also encouraged high-income states to provide international assistance "to enable developing countries to fulfil their core . . . obligations," including the preparation of a health plan.[28] According to the Declaration of Alma-Ata: "All governments should formulate national policies, strategies and plans of action to launch and sustain primary health care as part of a comprehensive national health system and in coordination with other sectors."[29]

Health planning is complex and many of its elements are important from the perspective of the right to the highest attainable standard of health, including the following.

The entire planning process must be as participatory and transparent as possible. It is very important that the health needs of disadvantaged individuals, communities and populations are given due attention. Also, effective measures must be taken to ensure their active and informed participation throughout the planning process. Both the process and plan must be sensitive to cultural difference. One example where the participatory approach was used was in the village of San Jose de Secce and the communities of Oqopeqa, Punkumarqiri, Sanuq and Laupay in the Ayacucho district, Peru, where high maternal mortality rates were registered. It was estimated that 94 per cent of the women gave birth at home, compared to 6 per cent in the health centres. This was due to various barriers, such as because the state health services did not take account of local cultural conceptions of health and sickness. In an attempt to reduce the maternal mortality, a culturally-adapted project was introduced which provided sexual and reproductive health services and promoted a participatory approach between health workers and the community, including the traditional birth attendants (TBA). As a result, the delivery room and care given during prenatal checkups, delivery and the postnatal period, were made culturally acceptable, for example, by providing a bed as well as sturdy rope, so that the women could give birth squatting and gripping the rope, as they were accustomed to. The protocol for care outlined, among others, that the person attending the birth should speak Quechua and preferably be female. Further, in line with the beliefs in the communities, the protocol included the requirement to deliver the placenta to the family member present so that it could be buried, and the opportunity for the user to remain in the health facility for up to eight days. An evaluation after the measures had been taken demonstrated a great increase in deliveries at health centres.[30]

Prior to the drafting of the plan, there must be a health situational analysis informed by suitably disaggregated data. The analysis should identify, for example, the characteristics of the population (e.g., birth, death and fertility rates), their health needs (e.g., incidence and prevalence by disease), and the public and private health-related services presently available (e.g., the capacity of different facilities).

The right to the highest attainable standard of health encompasses an obligation on the state to generate health research and development that addresses, for example, the health needs of disadvantaged individuals, communities and populations. Health research and development includes classical medical research into drugs, vaccines and diagnostics, as well as operational or implementation research into the social, economic, cultural, political and policy issues that determine access to medical care and the effectiveness of public health interventions. Implementation research, which has an important role to play with a view to dismantling societal obstacles to health interventions and technologies, should be taken into account when drafting the national health plan.

The plan must include certain features such as clear objectives and how they are to be achieved, time-frames, indicators and benchmarks to measure achievement, effective coordination mechanisms, reporting procedures, a detailed budget that is attached to the plan, financing arrangements (national and international), evaluation arrangements, and one or more accountability devices. In order to complete the plan, there will have to be a process for prioritizing competing health needs.

Before their finalization, key elements of the draft plan must be subject to an impact assessment to ensure that they are likely to be consistent with the state's national and international legal obligations, including those relating to the right to the highest attainable standard of health. For example, if the draft plan proposes the introduction of user fees for health services, it is vital that an impact assessment is undertaken to anticipate the likely impact of user fees on access to health services for those living in poverty. If the assessment confirms that user fees are likely to hinder access, the draft plan must be revised before adoption, otherwise it is likely to be inconsistent with the state's obligations arising from the right to the highest attainable standard of health.[31]

Of course, planning is only the means to an end: an effective, integrated health system that is accessible to all. The main task is implementation. Evaluation, monitoring and accountability can help to ensure that all those responsible for implementation discharge their duties as planned, and that any unintended consequences are swiftly identified and addressed.

Monitoring and Accountability

As already discussed, monitoring and accountability have a crucial role to play in relation to human rights and health systems. Monitoring is a precondition of accountability. Accountability provides individuals and communities with an opportunity to understand how those with responsibilities have discharged their duties. Equally, it provides those with responsibilities the opportunity to explain what they have done and why. Where mistakes have been made, accountability requires redress. But accountability is not a matter of blame and punishment. It is a process that helps to identify what works, so it can be repeated, and what does not, so it can be revised. It is a way of checking that reasonable balances are fairly struck.

In the context of health systems, there are many different types of accountability mechanisms, including health commissioners, democratically elected local health councils, public hearings, patients' committees, impact assessments, maternal death audits, judicial proceedings, and so on. An institution as complex and important as a health system requires a range of effective, transparent, accessible, independent accountability mechanisms. The media and civil society organizations have a crucial role to play as well.

Accountability in respect of health systems is often extremely weak. Sometimes the same body provides health services, regulates and holds to account. In some cases, accountability is little more than a device to check that health funds were spent as they should have been. Of course, that is important. But human rights accountability is much broader. It is also concerned with ensuring that health systems are improving and the right to the highest attainable standard of health is being progressively realized, for all, including disadvantaged individuals, communities and populations.

In some states, the private health sector, while playing a very important role, is largely unregulated. Crucially, the requirement of human rights accountability extends to both the public and private health sectors. Additionally, it is not confined to national bodies; it also extends to international actors working on health-related issues.

Accountability mechanisms are urgently needed for all those—public, private, national and international—working on health-related issues. The design of appropriate, independent accountability mechanisms demands creativity and imagination. Often associated with accountability, lawyers must be willing to understand the distinctive characteristics and challenges of health systems, and learn from the rich experience of medicine and public health.

The issue of accountability gives rise to two related points. First, the right to the highest attainable standard of health should be recognized in national law. This is very important because such recognition gives rise to legal accountability for those with responsibilities for health systems. As is well known, the right is recognized in WHO's Constitution, as well as the Declaration of Alma-Ata. It is also recognized in numerous binding international human rights treaties. The right to the highest attainable standard of health is also protected by numerous national constitutions. It should be recognized in the national law of all states.

Second, although important, legal recognition of the right to the highest attainable standard of health is usually confined to a very general formulation that does not set out in any detail what is required of those with responsibilities for health. For this reason, a state must not only recognize the right to health in national law, but also ensure that there are more detailed provisions clarifying what society expects by way of health-related services and facili-

ties. For example, there will have to be provisions relating to water quality and quantity, blood safety, essential medicines, the quality of medical care, and numerous other issues encompassed by the right to the highest attainable standard of health. Such clarification may be provided by laws, regulations, protocols, guidelines, codes of conduct and so on. WHO has published important standards on a range of health issues. Obviously, clarification is important for providers, so they know what is expected of them. It is also important for those for whom the service or facility is intended, so they know what they can legitimately expect. Once the standards are reasonably clear, it is easier (and fairer) to hold accountable those with responsibilities for their achievement.

In summary, there is a legal obligation arising from the right to the highest attainable standard of health to ensure that health planning is participatory and transparent; addresses the health needs of disadvantaged individuals, communities and populations; and includes a situational analysis. Before finalization, key elements of the draft plan must be subject to an impact assessment, and the final plan must include certain crucial features. These (and there are others) are not just a matter of health good practice, sound management, justice, equity or humanitarianism. They are a matter of international legal obligation. Whether or not the obligations are properly discharged should be subject to review by an appropriate monitoring and accountability mechanism.

CONCLUSION

Like other human rights, the right to the highest attainable standard of health is a site of struggle.[32] It is not, and never will be, a substitute for struggle. In recent years, the contours and content of the right to the highest attainable standard of health have become clearer, making it possible to tease through its practical implications for health policies, programmes and projects. The right brings a set of analytical, policy and programmatic tools. As always, the right retains its powerful rhetorical, campaigning qualities. The right to the highest attainable standard of health should be seen as one important element in a multi-dimensional strategy for progressive social change.

Whether the right to the highest attainable standard of health can successfully shape health systems depends upon multiple variables. Progressive governments must be persuaded to integrate the right across their policy-making processes, in accordance with their legal obligations. WHO and other international organizations must be prevailed upon to champion the right to the highest attainable standard of health. Civil society organizations have to campaign around health and human rights. Judges and lawyers have to be willing to learn from health workers and find innovative ways to vindicate the right to the highest attainable standard of health. Health workers must grasp the potential of the right to the highest attainable standard of health to help them achieve their professional objectives. Human rights mechanisms must take this fundamental human right seriously and its meaning must be further clarified. More right to health tools must be fashioned. Disadvantaged individuals, communities and populations must apprehend that the right to the highest attainable standard of health empowers them by granting entitlements which place legal and moral obligations on others.

Today, there are numerous health movements and approaches, including health equity, primary health care, health promotion, social determinants, health security, continuum of care, biomedical, macroeconomics, and so on. All are very important. It is misconceived, however, to regard human rights as yet another approach with the same status as the others. Like ethics, the right to the highest attainable standard of health is not optional—and, like ethics, it recurs throughout all other approaches. The right to the highest attainable standard of health is the only perspective that is both underpinned by universally recognized moral values and reinforced by legal obligations. Properly understood, the right to the highest attainable standard of health has a profound contribution to make towards building healthy societies and equitable health systems.

REFERENCES

* This chapter is a shortened and revised version of the report of the UN Special Rapporteur on the right of everyone to the enjoyment of the highest attainable standard of physical and mental health, A/HRC/7/11, 31 January 2008. Also see Hunt and Backman, "Health Systems and the Right to the Highest Attainable Standard of Health," *Health and Human Rights: An International Journal*, Vol. 10, No. 1 (2008); and Backman and others, "Health Systems and the Right to Health: an Assessment of 194 Countries," *Lancet*, Vol. 372, No. 9655 (2008), at 2047–2085. In this chapter "the right to the highest attainable standard of health" or "the right to health" are used as short hand for the full formulation of the right.

1. See, for example, J. Mann, S. Gruskin, M. Grodin and G. Annas (eds), *Health and Human Rights: A Reader* (New York and London: Routledge, 1999); S. Gruskin, M. Grodin, G. Annas and S. Marks (eds.), *Perspectives on Health and Human Rights* (New York and London: Routledge, 2005); A. Yamin, 'Journeys towards the Splendid City', 26 *Human Rights Quarterly* (2004), at 519; the report of the UN Special Rapporteur on the right to the highest attainable standard of health, A/HRC/4/28, 17 January 2007; and P. Hunt, 'The Health and Human Rights Movement: Progress and Obstacles', *Journal of Law and Medicine* (2008) 15 JLM 714–724.

2. L. Freedman, 'Achieving the MDGs: Health Systems as core social institutions', 48 *Development* (2005), at 1.

3. World Health Organization, *Everybody's Business: Strengthening Health Systems to Improve Health Outcomes* (Geneva: WHO, 2007), at 1.

4. E. Kinney and B. Clark, 'Provisions for Health and Health Care in the Constitutions of the Countries of the World' 37 *Cornell International Law Journal* (2004) 285–355.

5. The literature reveals many definitions of a health system, each with carefully nuanced differences. In 2007, for example, WHO defined a health system as "all organizations, people and actions whose *primary intent* is to promote, restore or maintain health." Ibid. at 2 (italics in the original). For present purposes, there is no need to favour one definition over another because all the features and measures identified in this chapter should be part of any health system, however defined.

6. For surveys of the key international instruments and a selection of the case law, see the reports of the UN Special Rapporteur on the right of everyone to the enjoyment of the highest attainable standard of physical and mental health, E/CN.4/2003/58, 13 February 2003, and A/HRC/4/28, 17 January 2007.

7. Health workers include all those developing, managing, delivering, monitoring and evaluating preventive, curative and rehabilitative health in the private and public health sectors, including traditional healers.

8. WHO, *People at the Centre of Health Care* (Geneva: WHO, 2007), at v.

9. Ibid., at VII.

10. See H. Potts, *Human Rights in Public Health: Rhetoric, Reality and Reconciliation,* unpublished PhD thesis, Monash University, Melbourne, Australia, 2006. Also, participation in the context of the right to health has been explored in several reports of the UN Special Rapporteur on the right of everyone to the enjoyment of the highest attainable standard of physical and mental health, including E/CN.4/2006/48/Add.2 (on Uganda) and E/CN.4/2005/51 (on mental disability).

11. A. Green, *An Introduction to Health Planning for Developing Health Systems* (Oxford: Oxford University Press, 2007) at 64.

12. For more on indigenous peoples and the right to the highest attainable standard of health see, for example, the reports of the UN Special Rapporteur on the right of everyone to the enjoyment of the highest attainable standard of physical and mental health, A/59/422 and E/CN.4/2005/51/Add.3.

13. UNFPA, *Culture Matters* (Geneva: UNFPA, 2000), at v.

14. See, for example, Article 24 of the Convention on the Rights of the Child. Medical care includes dental care.

15. Paragraph VII(6).

16. For more on planning, see page 52.

17. For a human rights-based approach to health indicators, see the report of the UN Special Rapporteur on the right of everyone to the enjoyment of the highest attainable standard of physical and mental health, E/CN.4/2006/48, 3 March 2006.

18. Committee on Economic, Social and Cultural Rights (CESCR), *General Comment No. 14 on the right to the highest attainable standard of health,* 11 August 2000, UN Doc. E/C.12/2000/4, at para. 32.

19. Ibid., paras. 43–45.

20. This section draws extensively from United Kingdom Department of Health, *Health is Global: Proposals for a UK Government-Wide Strategy* (London: Department of Health, 2007) especially at 46.

21. See S. Skogly, *Beyond National Borders: States' Human Rights Obligations in International Cooperation* (Antwerp: Intersentia, 2006).

22. On prioritization, see the report of the UN Special Rapporteur on the right of everyone to the enjoyment of the highest attainable standard of physical and mental health, A/62/2/214, 8 August 2007.

23. WHO, *supra* note 3, at 3.

24. Such as ex-ante impact assessments (see paragraphs below on planning).

25. WHO, *supra* note 3, at 23.

26. Green, *supra* note 11, at 18.

27. See previous section on progressive realization and resource constraints.

28. General Comment No. 14, *supra* note 18, paras. 43–45.

29. Para. VIII.

30. P. Hunt and J. Bueno de Mesquita, *Reducing Maternal Mortality: The Contribution of the Right to the Highest Attainable Standard of Health* (2007).

31. See P. Hunt and G. MacNaughton, *Impact Assessments, Poverty and Human Rights: A Case Study Using the Right to the Highest Attainable Standard of Health,* 2006.

32. P. Hunt, *Reclaiming Social Rights: International and Comparative Perspectives* (Aldershot, UK: Dartmouth, 1996) at 186 and Yamin, *supra* note 1, at 528.

QUESTIONS

1. Given the limited resources of most states, do you agree with the list of core obligations noted here? Are these realistic? Are they too limited? Too large? What do you think should be included in a "minimum basket?" And why?

2. Consider the concept of progressive realization as this applies to strengthening and improving health systems, what should be the approach for deciding which issues are to be addressed immediately and which can be delayed until there are more resources? Who should have the authority to make such decisions and how should they be held accountable?

3. Choose one of the WHO identified "six essential building blocks" and apply the right-to-health approach outlined by the authors. Pay specific attention to strengths and weaknesses you see in applying the right-to-health approach to the chosen building block.

FURTHER READING

1. Cohn, J., Russell, A., Baker, B., Kayongo, A., Wanjiku, E., & Davis, P., Using Global Health Initiatives to Strengthen Health Systems: A Civil Society Perspective. *Global Public Health: An International Journal for Research, Policy and Practice,* 2011; 6: 687–702.
2. Ruger, J. P., *Health and Social Justice.* New York: Oxford University Press, 2010.
3. Anand, S., Fabienne P, & Sen, A., eds. *Public Health, Ethics, and Equity.* Oxford: Oxford University Press, 2004.

CHAPTER 5

Global Bioethics at UNESCO: In Defense of the Universal Declaration on Bioethics and Human Rights

Roberto Andorno

Former United Nations (UN) Secretary General Dag Hammarskjöld often said that the UN was not created to take humanity to heaven but to save it from hell. By this aphorism, he meant that although the UN has its weaknesses and limitations, it has an irreplaceable role in our conflictive world by promoting peace, respect for human rights, and social and economic development. The UN is imperfect because it mirrors the world, with its divisions and disagreements. Nevertheless, it is the only forum where humanity speaks in its entirety and where it is able to express, as best as it can, its collective hopes and convictions.

If we consider the specific domain of bioethics, Hammarskjöld's dictum could be applied to UN agencies that are engaged in this specialty. Although they are not able to guarantee that biomedical advances will always be used for the greatest well-being of humanity, they can at least contribute to prevent their use in a manner that would be contrary to human dignity and human rights. Among the means UN agencies use to achieve their goals (in this case, the promotion of responsible biomedical research and clinical practice), the "standard setting activity" is one of the most salient ones.

It is precisely in such a context and with such an expectation that the Universal Declaration on Bioethics and Human Rights was adopted on 19 October 2005, at the 33rd session of the General Conference of UN Education, Scientific, and Cultural Organisation (UNESCO), by representatives of 191 countries. It is interesting to point out that the drafting process was preceded by a report of an International Bioethics Committee (IBC) working group that considered the feasibility of such an instrument. The working group, chaired by Professors Leonardo De Castro (Philippines) and Giovanni Berlinguer (Italy), concluded by supporting the initiative and affirming the need to develop "a worldwide common sense to foster understanding and cohesion in relation to new ethical categories and new practical possibilities emerging from science and technology".[1] With this background in mind, the IBC, chaired at the time by Mrs Michèle Jean (Canada), prepared the preliminary draft declaration, after almost 2 years of discussions and public consultations with governmental and nongovernmental organisations. Justice Michael Kirby (Australia) chaired the drafting group, which was open to all IBC members. To ensure transparency in the process, the successive versions of the document were posted on the internet as they were being developed. In January 2005, the draft was examined by the Intergovernmental Bioethics Committee and, finally, it was revised in two successive meetings of governmental representatives, who introduced several amendments.[2]

Despite the great number of existing international guidelines, statements and declarations relating to bioethics, the new UNESCO Declaration makes its own remarkable contribution to this topic. It is worth mentioning that this is the first international legal, though non-binding, instrument that comprehensively deals with the linkage between human rights and bioethics. Regardless of the weaknesses inherent to this kind of instrument, the very fact that virtually all states reached an agreement in this sensitive area is in itself a major achievement. It should be noted that most international declarations and guidelines in this topic do not have the status of legal instruments because they have been issued by non governmental organisations such as the World Medical Association (WMA), the Council for International Organizations of Medical Sciences and other academic or professional institutions. Other documents, although adopted by intergovernmental bodies, cover only specific bioethical issues, such as the UN Declaration on Human Cloning of 2005[3] and the UNESCO Universal Declaration on the Human Genome and Human Rights of 1997, or are regional but not global instruments, such as the European Convention on Human Rights and Biomedicine of 1997.

It is important to indicate that the Declaration includes in its section II important substantive principles relating to bioethics, such as:

- Respect for human dignity and human rights (Article 3.1)
- Priority of the individual's interests and welfare over the sole interest of science or society (Article 3.2)
- Beneficence and non-maleficence (Article 4)
- Autonomy (Article 5)

- Informed consent (Article 6)
- Protection of persons unable to consent (Article 7)
- Special attention to vulnerable persons (Article 8)
- Privacy and confidentiality (Article 9)
- Equality, justice and equity (Article 10)
- Non-discrimination and non-stigmatisation (Article 11)
- Respect for cultural diversity and pluralism (Article 12)
- Solidarity and cooperation (Article 13)
- Access to healthcare and essential medicines (Article 14)
- Benefit sharing (Article 15)
- Protection of future generations (Article 16)
- Protection of the environment, the biosphere and biodiversity (Article 17).

Section III ("Application of the principles") is devoted to principles of a more procedural nature such as:

- The requirement for professionalism, honesty, integrity and transparency in the decision-making process regarding bioethical issues (Article 18)
- The need to establish independent, multidisciplinary and pluralist ethics committees (Article 19)
- The call for an appropriate risk assessment and management in the biomedical field (Article 20)
- The need for justice in transnational research (Article 21).

THREE BASIC FEATURES OF THE DECLARATION

At this point, three basic features of the declaration should be emphasised.

Firstly, the principles it contains are formulated in very general terms; the declaration does not give almost any definition of their precise meaning (which are only provided, to some extent, by the explanatory memorandum that accompanied the preliminary draft declaration). This method, which may surprise some, is in fact a common practice in law, in conformity with the old maxim "Omnis definitio in jure periculosa est". (Every definition in law is perilous.) Except for very technical terms, lawmakers normally prefer not to define precisely most of the words they use. Rather, they tend to leave that task to common understanding and, ultimately, to courts' interpretation, in order not to be constricted in advance by rigid definitions. In the case of the UNESCO Declaration, this strategy can also be explained for practical reasons, because it would have been impossible to reach a global agreement on the precise meaning of terms such as "human dignity", "autonomy", "justice", "benefit", "harm" or "solidarity", which have a long philosophical history and are, to some extent, conditioned by cultural factors. Thus, the generality in the formulation of the principles can ultimately be justified by the need to find a balance between the universalism of some bioethical norms and the respect for cultural diversity.

A second feature of the declaration relates to the nature of UNESCO itself as an intergovernmental body. This should not be forgotten because it would be a mistake to assess with purely academic criteria an instrument such as the declaration, which is not the exclusive product of academic work, but rather a kind of compromise between a theoretical conceptualisation made by experts and what is practically achievable given the political choices of governments. We need to keep in mind that governments, not independent experts, have the last word in every declaration or convention issued by UN agencies. This is not to say that the quality of such instruments is necessarily affected negatively by the requirements of governments. It is true that the IBC draft was more precise on several points than the version adopted by governmental representatives, as Justice Kirby himself has admitted.[4] Personally, I regret for instance that the recognition of the precautionary principle as a risk management tool for public health purposes has been removed from the final version of the document. On the other hand, I acknowledge that some of the amendments introduced by governmental representatives really enhanced the declaration, such as the more detailed provision regarding research on people unable to consent (Article 7) and the reference to human vulnerability (Article 8). What I intend to argue here is that the approach to bioethics followed by international instruments such as the new declaration is not only an academic but also a political one, and therefore must be assessed with different, broader criteria.

A third important characteristic of the declaration is its non-binding nature. Like any declaration adopted by UN agencies, the new UNESCO document makes up part of the so-called soft law instruments—that is, instruments that are weaker than conventions because they are not intended to oblige states to enact enforceable rules inspired by the common standards, but to encourage them to do so. This procedure permits states to take on commitments they otherwise would not have taken, because they assume just political obligations that are not legally binding. Furthermore, soft law instruments present the advantage of permitting countries to gradually become familiar with the proposed standards before they are confronted with the adoption of enforceable rules or with the development of a binding instrument—that is, a convention.[5] In addition, it is helpful to remember that, if the same non-binding standards are reaffirmed in successive declarations, in the course of time they may become binding rules, in the form of customary law and jurisprudential criteria, as it happened with the Universal Declaration of Human Rights of 1948.[6]

UNESCO'S INVOLVEMENT IN BIOETHICS

The following sections of this chapter will focus on two serious criticisms that have been levelled against the new declaration. The most fundamental one is the involvement of UNESCO itself in bioethics. The other one relates to the use of a human rights framework to achieve common standards in this discipline.

Regarding the first charge, it has been advanced that UNESCO would be in an "obvious attempt at meddling in the professional domain of another UN agency, WHO" and that "it is entirely unclear why UNESCO should concern itself with such a matter".[7] Similarly, it has been argued that "UNESCO is clearly overstepping its mandate and encroaching on that of the World Health Organization (WHO)".[8]

In response to these objections, it should be noted, first of all, that a clear-cut division of competences between UN agencies is not always as simple as it may seem at first glance, especially in issues that are at the intersection of different disciplines. Secondly, what is really unclear is why the only UN agency specialised in sciences (both natural and human sciences) and having served for decades as a forum for philosophical discussion on cross-cultural issues would be excluded from making any contribution to the normative guidance for life sciences. It is helpful to remember here that the purpose of UNESCO is, according to its Constitution, to promote "collaboration among nations through education, science and culture in order to further universal respect for justice, for the rule of law and for the human rights and fundamental freedoms".[9] Is it really then surprising that an organisation with such a mission may be interested in the establishment of some common standards for bioethics?

In addition, it is noteworthy that, since its foundation in the aftermath of the Second World War, UNESCO has been associated in the preparation of some 28 international conventions, 12 declarations and about 31 recommendations, including the Convention against Discrimination in Education (1960), the Universal Copyright Convention (1971), the Convention concerning the Protection of the World Cultural and Natural Heritage (1972), the Declaration on Principles of International Cultural Cooperation (1966), the Declaration on Race and Racial Prejudice (1978), the Declaration on the Responsibilities of the Present Generations Towards Future Generations (1997), the Recommendation on the Status of Scientific Researchers (1974), the Recommendation concerning the International Standardization of Statistics on Science and Technology (1978) and, more recently, the Convention on the Protection and Promotion of the Diversity of Cultural Expressions (2005). Why could the international community not take advantage of this long experience regarding sciences, its cross-cultural effect and its significance for human rights to set up global bioethical standards?

This is especially to be considered when one reflects on the fact that the UNESCO's strong involvement in bioethics is not new. It dates back at least to 1993, when the IBC was established on the initiative of Dr. Federico Mayor, Director-General of the organisation at that time. The first task of the Committee was the preparation of the preliminary draft of the Universal Declaration on the Human Genome and Human Rights, adopted in 1997. Thereafter, the IBC worked on the drafting of the International Declaration on Human Genetic Data, finalised in 2003. Additionally, since its creation, the IBC produced about 14 reports on various bioethical issues such as genetic counselling, ethics and neurosciences, confidentiality and genetic data, embryonic stem cells, ethics of intellectual property and genomics, and pre-implantation genetic diagnosis and germ-line interventions. In light of this, the question is: Are there many other global intergovernmental organisations that could claim the same level of experience at the intersection of sciences, ethics and human rights? The answer, at least at this stage, seems to be "no".[10, 11]

In reality, a conflict of competence between two or more UN agencies interested in this matter would be as absurd as a dispute between a philosopher and a doctor over the "ownership" of bioethics. Of course, bioethics does not belong in exclusivity to any of them. As it is by its very nature an interdisciplinary specialty, all related professions (and likewise, all related UN bodies) have the right—and the duty—to make their specific contribution to this emerging and complex domain. It is noteworthy that, in fact, UN agencies have already recognised their mutual interest in this matter and, on this ground, have established in 2003 the UN Inter-Agency Committee on Bioethics with the task of improving the coordination of activities in this area.

Concerning the WHO, there is no doubt that, as it is the specialised UN agency for health, it is to have a major role in the standard-setting activities in biomedical sciences. Nevertheless, as some experts have pointed out, clearly, WHO cannot manage this task alone, for the following reasons:

- The field is growing, rapidly encompassing more diverse and complex concerns, due to its interdisciplinary nature.
- WHO has very limited experience in international health lawmaking.
- Such a task would deplete the organisation's limited resources and undermine its ability to fulfill its well established and essential international health functions.
- Member states are highly unlikely to

limit their autonomy and freedom by granting to WHO alone such an expansive new mandate.
- Decentralisation of the international lawmaking enterprise presents great advantages that cannot be ignored.[12]

Furthermore, beyond the fact that UNESCO and WHO are, after all, composed of the same member states, there is a more substantial reason for favouring simultaneous participation of both UN agencies in the topic of bioethics: their standard-setting activities operate at different levels. While UNESCO tends to produce general normative frameworks of a predominantly philosophical and legal nature, WHO's guidelines are usually more technical and focused on specific health-related issues. Therefore, as the approach followed by both organisations is different, their respective engagement in this matter can perfectly coexist. Moreover, it is to be hoped that sincere efforts will be made to stimulate greater cooperation between both UN agencies, which could be extremely fruitful given their complementary expertise in this domain.

USE OF A HUMAN RIGHTS FRAMEWORK

Another criticism of the UNESCO declaration relates to the use of a human rights framework. It has been reasoned that "human dignity and human rights, both strong features of European enlightenment philosophy, pervades this Declaration" and that UNESCO "chose an ideological framework (human rights) that does not feature particularly prominently in professional bioethical analyses".[5]

In my opinion, these objections are misplaced. It is true that the current notion of human rights has its immediate origins in the insights of the European enlightenment philosophers. But this historical circumstance is not a good enough reason to discard the idea that human beings have inherent rights, just as it would not be enough to argue that Mozart or Bach were Europeans to deny the extraordinary beauty of their works. The relevant question is whether the notion that every human being has an inherent dignity and inherent rights makes sense, no matter where this idea comes from. My personal view on this is that the current widespread conviction that people have unconditional rights simply by virtue of their humanity is one of the major achievements of human civilisation, much more important than any scientific or technical development.

This does not mean to ignore the fact that in many Western nations there has been an excessive emphasis on rights and freedoms for the individual, sometimes to the detriment of family and community values, which are of paramount importance to most non-Western societies. Neither does it mean to disregard the great philosophical discussion on whether, or how, the recognition of universal human rights can be conciliated with cultural diversity. However, the truth is that today these controversies have lost much of their practical significance—firstly, because of the increasing number of non-Western states that are party to international human rights treaties; secondly, because human rights emerge from international law instruments with sufficient flexibility to be compatible with full respect for cultural diversity. Far from imposing one cultural standard, human rights instruments set up a minimum protection necessary for human dignity.[12, 13]

It has to be noted that, paradoxically, some of the most severe criticisms of the universality of human rights come from Western scholars. According to Amartya Sen,[15] these views are often based on a misconception of non-Western (largely Asian) societies, as if people in these countries had little or no interest in their rights and were only concerned with issues of social order and discipline (misconception which is of course well exploited by authoritarian regimes . . .). In this connection, it is revealing that the only two papers written by non-Western authors that appear in a journal special issue on the declaration openly contradict the pessimistic view of the journal editorial and have a favourable opinion of the human rights approach adopted by UNESCO.[16, 17] One of these papers[17] even argues that the universality of the principles of human dignity and human rights . . . is not emphasised enough by the Declaration!

Furthermore, the objection that the bioethical discourse is alien to a human rights approach is simply contrary to the facts: many, if not most, international policy documents relating to bioethics issued during the past two decades are framed on a rights-based approach and attach utmost importance to the notion of human dignity. A paradigmatic example in this respect is the Council of Europe's Convention on Human Rights and Biomedicine ("Oviedo Convention").[18] Nevertheless, this is not an exclusive feature of Western instruments. Indeed, about 200 worldwide declarations, guidelines, recommendations, opinions and codes relating to bioethics adopted by very different institutions could be cited in support of this assertion.[19] For illustrative purposes, a few examples can be mentioned. Firstly, the famous WMA Declaration of Helsinki on Research Involving Human Subjects (1964/2000),[20] which refers in explicit terms to the rights of participants (paragraphs 8, 21 and 22) and regards the protection of human dignity of research subjects as the first basic principle for medical research, along with respect for their life, health and privacy (paragraph 10).[21] Secondly, the UN Commission on Human Rights Resolution 2003/69 of 25 April 2003 entitled "Human rights and bioethics",[22] which strongly insists on the need to ensure the protection of human rights in this field and makes a recurring appeal to the "dignity of the human being". Thirdly, the various statements of the ethics committee of the Human Genome Organisation (HUGO),[23] which emphasise the need to "adhere to international norms of human rights" and to accept and uphold "human dignity and freedom".[24]

Why this reliance on human rights to set up global bioethical standards?

The first obvious reason is that, as biomedical activities deal with the most basic human prerogatives such as the right to life and to physical integrity, it is perfectly sound to have recourse to the umbrella of international human rights law to ensure their protection. Despite all its weaknesses, the existing human rights system, with its extensive body of international standards and wide range of mechanisms, represents a considerable achievement of our time. This is why it would be strange that a human rights framework could not be used to protect people from harm in the biomedical specialty.

A more practical reason for this phenomenon is that "there are few mechanisms available other than human rights to function as a global ethical foundation, a Weltethik".[25] In other words, "the human rights framework provides a more useful approach for analysing and responding to modern public health challenges than any framework thus far available within the biomedical tradition".[26]

Regarding the idea of human dignity, it can be said that, far from being a useless notion as some have argued,[27] it has a key role in international bioethics by providing the ultimate rationale for the norms relating to this discipline.[28] Certainly, the appeal to human dignity in international law is neither new nor specific to instruments dealing with biomedical issues. On the contrary, this notion is at the cornerstone of the universal human rights movement that emerged after the Second World War. However, recent international biolaw instruments emphasise the importance of human dignity in a more powerful way than traditional human rights law. Indeed, the contrast between the background role assigned to human dignity in international human rights instruments and the foreground role assigned to it in international biolaw could not be more impressive.[29]

The UNESCO Declaration[2] inscribes itself in this trend when it places at the top of its principles that of "human dignity, human rights and fundamental freedoms" (Article 3.1). Similarly, when it provides that "the interests and welfare of the individual should have priority over the sole interest of science or society" (Article 3.2). This provision of Article 3.2, which has surprisingly also been criticised,[7] is in fact included, with almost the same wording, in several international documents relating to bioethics, such as the WMA Declaration of Helsinki (Article 5),[18] the European Convention on Human Rights and Biomedicine (Article 2) and the UNESCO Declaration on the Human Genome and Human Rights (Article 10). Through this provision, the new UNESCO Declaration sought to emphasise a direct corollary of the principle of human dignity: that people should not simply become instruments for the benefit of science, because science is not an absolute, but only a means at the service of the human person. It is indeed hard to see what other bioethical principle could be more fundamental than this one.

CONCLUSION

The Universal Declaration on Bioethics and Human Rights is an important step in the search for global bioethical standards. Like any other international instrument of its kind, it is not free from shortcomings.

However, in view of the sensitive nature of bioethical issues, the simple fact that virtually all states reached a comprehensive agreement in this discipline is in itself a major achievement. Certainly, most of the declaration's principles are not original; they are derived from several existing international documents. This is why the greatest merit of this instrument is to gather those principles and to integrate them into a human rights framework. In sum, the purpose of the declaration is not to invent new bioethical principles or to provide the definitive solution to the growing list of bioethical dilemmas. Its main goal is much more modest: to assemble some basic standards to help states in their efforts to promote responsible biomedical research and clinical practice, in conformity with the principles of international human rights law.

REFERENCES

1. UNESCO IBC. *Report on the possibility of elaborating a universal instrument on bioethics*, 13 June 2003.
2. UNESCO 33rd General Conference, Paris, 19 October 2005.
3. United Nations. Declaration on Human Cloning. GA Res 59/280 of 8 March 2005.
4. Kirby M. UNESCO and universal principles on bioethics: what's next? In: *Twelfth session of the International Bioethics Committee (IBC), Abstracts or Texts of the Presentations of Speakers*. Paris: UNESCO, 2005, 9–19.
5. Lenoir N, Mathieu B. *Les normes internationales de la bioèthique*. Paris: PUF, 1998.
6. United Nations. Universal Declaration of Human Kights. GA Res 217 A (III) of 10 Dec 1948, UN Doc A/810 at 71.
7. Schuklenk U, Landman W. From the editors. *Developing World Bioethics*. Special Issue: Reflections on the UNESCO Draft Declaration on Bioethics and Human Rights, 2005; 5: iii–vi.
8. Williams J. UNESCO's proposed declaration on bioethics and human rights. A bland compromise. *Developing World Bioethics*. Special Issue: Reflections on the UNESCO Draft Declaration on Bioethics and Human Rights, 2005; 5: 210–5.
9. UNESCO Constitution, 16 November 1945 (Article 1).
10. Harmon S. The significance of UNESCO's universal declaration on the human genome and human rights. Scripted, *J Law Tech* 2005; 2: 18–47.
11. Taylor A. Globalization and biotechnology: UNESCO and an international strategy to advance human rights and public health. *Am J Law Med* 1999; 4: 479–542.
12. Taylor A. Governing the globalization of public health. *J Law Med Ethics* 2004; 32: 500–8.
13. Ayton-Shenker D. *The challenge of human rights and cultural diversity*, United Nations background note. New York: United Nations Department of Public Information, 1995.
14. Donnelly J. *Universal human rights in theory and practice*. Ithaca, NY: Cornell University Press, 1989.
15. Sen A. Universal truths: human rights and the westernizing illusion. *Harvard Int Rev* 1998; 20: 40–3.
16. Asai A, Oe S. A valuable up-to-date compendium of bioethical knowledge. *Developing World Bioethics*. Special Issue: reflections on the UNESCO draft declaration on bioethics and human rights, 2005; 5: 216–19.
17. Jing-Bao N. Cultural values embodying universal norms: a critique of a popular assumption about cultures and human rights. *Developing World Bioethics*. Special Issue: reflections on the UNESCO draft declaration on bioethics and human rights, 2005; 5: 251–7.
18. Andorno R. The Oviedo Convention: a European legal framework at the intersection of human rights and health law. *J Int Biotech Law* 2005; 2: 133–43.
19. University of Minnesota Human Rights Library, "Bioethics and Human Rights Links." http://www1.umn.edu/humanrts/links/bioethics.html (accessed 4 April 2006).
20. World Medical Association. Declaration of Helsinki on Ethical Principles for Medical Research Involving Human Subjects, as amended by the 52nd WMA General Assembly, Edinburgh, October 2000.
21. World Medical Association. Declaration of Helsinki on Ethical Principles for Medical Research Involving Human subjects, as amended by the 52nd WMA General Assembly, Edinburgh, October 2000.
22. United Nations Commission on Human Rights. Resolution 2003/69 on human rights and bioethics of 25 April 2003 (E/CN.4/2003/L.II/Add.7).
23. Human Genome Organisation's (HUGO) Ethics Committee. Statements.

24. Human Genome Organisation (HUGO) Ethics Committee.
25. Thomasma D. Proposing a new agenda: bioethics and international human rights. *Camb Q Healthc Ethics* 2001; 10: 299–310.
26. Mann J. Health and human rights. Protecting human rights is essential for promoting health [Editorial]. BMJ 1996; 312: 924–5.
27. Macklin R. Dignity is a useless concept. *BMJ* 2003; 327: 1419–20.
28. Andorno R. La notion de dignité humaine est-elle superflue en bioéthique? *Revue Génér Droit Méd* 2005; 16: 95–102.
29. Beyleveld D, Brownsword R. *Human dignity in bioethics and biolaw.* Oxford: Oxford University Press, 2002.

QUESTIONS

1. Medicine and public health are becoming more and more interrelated, especially as more and more of medicine is involved with screening and trying to prevent "life-style" diseases. Bioethics and human rights may be more symbiotic than overlapping, but nonetheless the UNESCO effort seems worthwhile. What are the two strongest arguments in favor of the UNESCO approach? What are the strongest arguments against it?

2. Human rights are universal; but can bioethics ever be universal? Think about this question in the context of abortion and the new reproductive technologies.

3. Are human rights and bioethics on a convergence course or are they rivals? In this context, it has been proposed that all British medical schools now teach global health towards 21 specific learning outcomes, five of which being on "human rights and ethics" (editorial, *The Lancet,* 2012: 379: 2033–35).

FURTHER READING

1. Smith, George P., *Law and Bioethics: Intersections along the Mortal Coil.* New York: Routledge, 2012.
2. Ashcroft, Richard E., Could Human Rights Supersede Bioethics? *Human Rights Law Rev.* 2010; 10: 639–660.
3. Faunce, Thomas, Will International Human Rights Subsume Medical Ethics? *J Medical Ethics* 2004; 31: 173–178.
4. Annas, George J., *American Bioethics: Crossing Health Law and Human Rights Boundaries.* New York: Oxford University Press, 2005.

CHAPTER 6

The Nuremberg Doctors' Trial
(a) Opening Statement of the Prosecution, Dec. 9, 1946

Telford Taylor

The defendants in this case are charged with murders, tortures, and other atrocities committed in the name of medical science. The victims of these crimes are numbered in the hundreds of thousands. A handful only are still alive; a few of the survivors will appear in this courtroom. But most of these miserable victims were slaughtered outright or died in the course of the tortures to which they were subjected.

For the most part they are nameless dead. To their murderers, these wretched people were not individuals at all. They came in wholesale lots and were treated worse than animals. They were 200 Jews in good physical condition, 50 gypsies, 500 tubercular Poles, or 1,000 Russians. The victims of these crimes are numbered among the anonymous millions who met death at the hands of the Nazis and whose fate is a hideous blot on the page of modern history.

The charges against these defendants are brought in the name of the United States of America. They are being tried by a court of American judges. The responsibilities thus imposed upon the representatives of the United States, prosecutors and judges alike, are grave and unusual. It is owed, not only to the victims and to the parents and children of the victims, that just punishment be imposed on the guilty, but also to the defendants that they be accorded a fair hearing and decision. Such responsibilities are the ordinary burden of any tribunal. Far wider are the duties which we must fulfill here.

These larger obligations run to the peoples and races on whom the scourge of these crimes was laid. The mere punishment of the defendants, or even of thousands of others equally guilty, can never redress the terrible injuries which the Nazis visited on these unfortunate peoples. For them it is far more important that these incredible events be established by clear and public proof, so that no one can ever doubt that they were fact and not fable; and that this Court, as the agent of the United States and as the voice of humanity, stamp these acts, and the ideas which engendered them, as barbarous and criminal.

We have still other responsibilities here. The defendants in the dock are charged with murder, but this is no mere murder trial. We cannot rest content when we have shown that crimes were committed and that certain persons committed them. To kill, to maim, and to torture is criminal under all modern systems of law. These defendants did not kill in hot blood, nor for personal enrichment. Some of them may be sadists who killed and tortured for sport, but they are not all perverts. They are not ignorant men. Most of them are trained physicians and some of them are distinguished scientists. Yet these defendants, all of whom were fully able to comprehend the nature of their acts, and most of whom were exceptionally qualified to form a moral and professional judgment in this respect, are responsible for wholesale murder and unspeakably cruel tortures. It is our deep obligation to all peoples of the world to show why and how these things happened. It is incumbent upon us to set forth with conspicuous clarity the ideas and motives which moved these defendants to treat their fellow men as less than beasts. The perverse thoughts and distorted concepts which brought about these savageries are not dead. They cannot be killed by force of arms. They must not become a spreading cancer in the breast of humanity. They must be cut out and exposed for the reason so well stated by Mr. Justice Jackson in this courtroom a year ago. "The wrongs which we seek to condemn and punish have been so calculated, so malignant, and so devastating, that civilization cannot tolerate their being ignored because it cannot survive their being repeated."

To the German people we owe a special responsibility in these proceedings. Under the leadership of the Nazis and their war lords, the German nation spread death and devastation throughout Europe. This the Germans now know. So, too, do they know the consequences to Germany: defeat, ruin, prostration, and utter demoralization. Most German children will never, as long as they live, see an undamaged German city.

To what cause will these children ascribe the defeat of the German nation and the devastation that surrounds them? Will they attribute it to the overwhelming weight of numbers and resources that was eventually leagued against them? Will they point to the ingenuity of enemy scientists? Will they perhaps blame their plight on strategic and military blunders by their generals?

If the Germans embrace those reasons as the true cause of their disaster, it will be a sad and fatal thing for Germany and for the world. Men who have never seen a German city intact will be callous about flattening English or American or Russian cities. They may not even realize that they are destroying anything worthwhile, for lack of a normal sense of values. To reestablish the greatness of Germany they are likely to pin their faith on improved military techniques. Such views will lead the Germans straight into the arms of the Prussian militarists to whom defeat is only a glorious opportunity to start a new war game. "Next time it will be different." We know all too well what that will mean.

This case, and others which will be tried in this building, offer a signal opportunity to lay before the German people the true cause of their present misery. The walls and towers and churches of Nuernberg were, indeed, reduced to rubble by Allied bombs, but in a deeper sense Nuernberg had been destroyed a decade earlier, when it became the seat of the annual Nazi Party rallies, a focal point for the moral disintegration in Germany, and the private domain of Julius Streicher. The insane and malignant doctrines that Nuernberg spewed forth account alike for the crimes of these defendants and for the terrible fate of Germany under the Third Reich.

A nation which deliberately infects itself with poison will inevitably sicken and die. These defendants and others turned Germany into an infernal combination of a lunatic asylum and a charnel house. Neither science, nor industry, nor the arts could flourish in such a foul medium. The country could not live at peace and was fatally handicapped for war. I do not think the German people have as yet any conception of how deeply the criminal folly that was nazism bit into every phase of German life, or of how utterly ravaging the consequences were. It will be our task to make these things clear.

These are the high purposes which justify the establishment of extraordinary courts to hear and determine this case and others of comparable importance. That murder should be punished goes without the saying, but the full performance of our task requires more than the just sentencing of these defendants. Their crimes were the inevitable result of the sinister doctrines which they espoused, and these same doctrines sealed the fate of Germany, shattered Europe, and left the world in ferment. Wherever those doctrines may emerge and prevail, the same terrible consequences will follow. That is why a bold and lucid consummation of these proceedings is of vital importance to all nations. That is why the United States has constituted this Tribunal.

I pass now to the facts of the case in hand. There are 23 defendants in the box. All but three of them—Rudolf Brandt, Sievers, and Brack—are doctors. Of the 20 doctors, all but one—Pokorny—held positions in the medical services of the Third Reich. To understand this case, it is necessary to understand the general structure of these state medical services, and how these services fitted into the overall organization of the Nazi State.

[The material on the organization of the military medical personnel, and where the individual defendants fit into it, has been deleted.]

CRIMES COMMITTED IN THE GUISE OF SCIENTIFIC RESEARCH

I turn now to the main part of the indictment and will outline at this point the prosecution's case relating to those crimes alleged to have been committed in the name of medical or scientific research. The charges with respect to "euthanasia" and the slaughter of tubercular Poles obviously have no relation to research or experimentation and will be dealt with later. What I will cover now comprehends all the experiments charged as war crimes in paragraph 6 and as crimes against humanity in paragraph 11 of the indictment, and the murders committed for so-called anthropological purposes which are charged as war crimes in paragraph 7 and as crimes against humanity in paragraph 12 of the indictment.

Before taking up these experiments one by one, let us look at them as a whole. Are they a heterogeneous list of horrors, or is there a common denominator for the whole group?

A sort of rough pattern is apparent on the face of the indictment. Experiments concerning high altitude, the effect of cold, and the potability of processed sea water have an obvious relation to aeronautical and naval combat and rescue problems. The mustard gas and phosphorous burn experiments, as well as those relating to the healing value of sulfanilamide for wounds, can be related to airraid and battlefield medical problems. It is well known that malaria, epidemic jaundice, and typhus were among the principal diseases which had to be combated by the German Armed Forces and by German authorities in occupied territories. To some degree, the therapeutic pattern outlined above is undoubtedly a valid one, and explains why the Wehrmacht, and especially the German Air Force, participated in these experiments. Fanatically bent upon conquest, utterly ruthless as to the means or instruments to be used in achieving victory, and callous to the sufferings of people whom they regarded as inferior, the German militarists were willing to gather whatever scientific fruit these experiments might yield.

But our proof will show that a quite different and even more sinister objective runs like a red thread through these hideous researches. We will show that in some instances the true object of these experiments was not how to rescue or to cure, but how to destroy and kill. The sterilization experiments were, it is clear, purely destructive in purpose. The prisoners at Buchenwald who were shot with poisoned bullets were not guinea pigs to test an antidote for the poison; their murderers really wanted to know how quickly the poison would kill. This destructive objective is not superficially as apparent in the other experiments, but we will show that it was often there.

Mankind has not heretofore felt the need of a word to denominate the science of how to kill prisoners most rapidly and subjugated people in large numbers. This case and these defendants have created this gruesome question for the lexicographer. For the moment we will christen this macabre science "thanatology," the science of producing death. The thanatological knowledge, derived in part from these experiments, supplied the techniques for genocide, a policy of the Third Reich, exemplified in the "euthanasia" program and in the wide-spread slaughter of Jews, Gypsies, Poles, and Russians. This policy of mass extermination could not have been so effectively carried out without the active participation of German medical scientists.

* * *

The 20 physicians in the dock range from leaders of German scientific medicine, with excellent international reputations, down to the dregs of the German medical profession. All of them have in common a callous lack of consideration and human regard for, and an unprincipled willingness to abuse their power over the poor, unfortunate, defenseless creatures who had been deprived of their rights by a ruthless and criminal government. All of them violated the Hippocratic commandments which they had solemnly sworn to uphold and abide by, including the fundamental principles never to do harm—"primum non nocere."

Outstanding men of science, distinguished for their scientific ability in Germany and abroad, are the defendants Rostock and Rose. Both exemplify, in their training and practice alike, the highest traditions of German medicine. Rostock headed the Department of Surgery at the University of Berlin and served as dean of its medical school. Rose studied under the famous surgeon, Enderlen, at Heidelberg and then became a distinguished specialist in the fields of public health and tropical diseases. Handloser and Schroeder are outstanding medical administrators. Both of them made their careers in military medicine and reached the peak of their profession. Five more defendants are much younger men who are nevertheless already known as the possessors of considerable scientific ability, or capacity in medical administration. These include the defendants Karl Brandt, Ruff, Beiglboeck, Schaefer, and Becker-Freyseng.

A number of the others such as Romberg and Fischer are well trained, and several of them attained high professional positions. But among the remainder few were known as outstanding scientific men. Among them at the foot of the list is Blome who has published his autobiography entitled *Embattled Doctor*, in which he sets forth that he eventually decided to become a doctor because a medical career would enable him to become "master over life and death."

* * *

I intend to pass very briefly over matters of medical ethics, such as the conditions under which a physician may lawfully perform a medical experiment upon a person who has voluntarily subjected himself to it, or whether experiments may lawfully be performed upon criminals who have been condemned to death. This case does not present such problems. No refined questions confront us here.

None of the victims of the atrocities perpetrated by these defendants were volunteers, and this is true regardless of what these unfortunate people may have said or signed before their tortures began. Most of the victims had not been condemned to death, and those who had been were not criminals, unless it be a crime to be a Jew, or a Pole, or a Gypsy, or a Russian prisoner of war.

Whatever book or treatise on medical ethics we may examine, and whatever expert on forensic medicine we may question, will say that it is a fundamental and inescapable obligation of every physician under any known system of law not to perform a dangerous experiment without the subject's consent. In the tyranny that was Nazi Germany, no one could give such a consent to the medical agents of the State; everyone lived in fear and acted under duress. I fervently hope that none of us here in the courtroom will have to suffer in silence while it is said on the part of these defendants that the wretched and helpless people whom they froze and drowned and burned and poisoned were volunteers. If such a shameless lie is spoken here, we need only remember the four girls who were taken from the Ravensbrueck concentration camp and made to lie naked with the frozen and all but dead Jews who survived Dr. Rascher's tank of ice water. One of these women, whose hair and eyes and figure were pleasing to Dr. Rascher, when asked by him why she had volunteered for such a task replied, "rather half a year in a brothel than half a year in a concentration camp."

Were it necessary, one could make a long list of the respects in which the experiments which these defendants performed departed from every known standard of medical ethics. But the gulf between these atrocities and serious research in the healing art is so patent that such a tabulation would be cynical.

We need look no further than the law which the Nazis themselves passed on the 24th of November 1933 for the protection of animals. This law states explicitly that it is designed to prevent cruelty and indifference of man towards animals and to awaken and develop sympathy and understanding for animals as one of the highest moral values of a people. The soul of the German people should abhor the principle of mere utility without consideration of the moral aspects. The law states further that all operations or treatments which are associated with pain or injury, especially experiments involving the use of cold, heat, or infection, are prohibited, and can be permitted only under special exceptional circumstances. Special written authorization by the head of the department is necessary in every case, and experimenters are prohibited from performing experiments according to their own free judgment. Experiments for the purpose of teaching must be reduced to a minimum. Medico-legal tests, vaccinations, withdrawal of blood for diagnostic purposes, and trial of vaccines prepared according to well-established scientific principles are permitted, but the animals have to be killed immediately and painlessly after such experiments. Individual physicians are not permitted to use dogs to increase their surgical skill by such practices. National Socialism regards it as a sacred duty of German science to keep down the number of painful animal experiments to a minimum.

If the principles announced in this law had been followed for human beings as well, this indictment would never have been filed. It is perhaps the deepest shame of the defendants that it probably never even occurred to them that human beings should be treated with at least equal humanity.

* * *

I said at the outset of this statement that the Third Reich died of its own poison. This case is a striking demonstration not only of the tremendous degradation of German medical ethics which Nazi doctrine brought about, but of the undermining of the medical art and thwarting of the techniques which the defendants sought to employ. The Nazis have, to a certain extent, succeeded in convincing the peoples of the world that the Nazi system, although ruthless, was absolutely efficient; that although savage, it was completely scientific; that although entirely devoid of humanity, it was highly systematic—that "it got things done." The evidence which this Tribunal will hear will explode this myth. The Nazi methods of investigation were inefficient and unscientific, and their techniques of research were unsystematic.

These experiments revealed nothing which civilized medicine can use. It was, indeed, ascertained that phenol or gasoline injected intravenously will kill a man inexpensively and within 60 seconds. This and a few other "advances" are all in the field of thanatology. There is no doubt that a number of these new methods may be useful to criminals everywhere and there is no doubt that they may be useful to a criminal state. Certain advance in destructive methodology we cannot deny, and indeed from Himmler's standpoint this may well have been the principal objective.

Apart from these deadly fruits, the experiments were not only criminal but a scientific failure. It is indeed as if a just deity had shrouded the solutions which they attempted to reach with murderous means. The moral shortcomings of the defendants and the precipitous ease with which they decided to commit murder in quest of "scientific results," dulled also that scientific hesitancy, that thorough thinking-through, that responsible weighing of every single step which alone can insure scientifically valid results. Even if they had

merely been forced to pay as little as two dollars for human experimental subjects, such as American investigators may have to pay for a cat, they might have thought twice before wasting unnecessary numbers, and thought of simpler and better ways to solve their problems. The fact that these investigators had free and unrestricted access to human beings to be experimented upon misled them to the dangerous and fallacious conclusion that the results would thus be better and more quickly obtainable than if they had gone through the labor of preparation, thinking, and meticulous preinvestigation.

A particularly striking example is the sea-water experiment. I believe that three of the accused—Schaefer, Becker-Freyseng, and Beiglboeck—will today admit that this problem could have been solved simply and definitively within the space of one afternoon. On 20 May 1944 when these accused convened to discuss the problem, a thinking chemist could have solved it right in the presence of the assembly within the space of a few hours by the use of nothing more gruesome than a piece of jelly, a semipermeable membrane and a salt solution, and the German Armed Forces would have had the answer on 21 May 1944. But what happened instead? The vast armies of the disenfranchised slaves were at the beck and call of this sinister assembly; and instead of thinking, they simply relied on their power over human beings rendered rightless by a criminal state and government. What time, effort, and staff did it take to get that machinery in motion! Letters had to be written, physicians, of whom dire shortage existed in the German Armed Forces whose soldiers went poorly attended, had to be taken out of hospital positions and dispatched hundreds of miles away to obtain the answer which should have been known in a few hours, but which thus did not become available to the German Armed Forces until after the completion of the gruesome show, and until 42 people had been subjected to the tortures of the damned, the very tortures which Greek mythology had reserved for Tantalus.

In short, this conspiracy was a ghastly failure as well as a hideous crime. The creeping paralysis of Nazi superstition spread through the German medical profession and, just as it destroyed character and morals, it dulled the mind.

Guilt for the oppressions and crimes of the Third Reich is widespread, but it is the guilt of the leaders that is deepest and most culpable. Who could German medicine look to keep the profession true to its traditions and protect it from the ravaging inroads of Nazi pseudo-science? This was the supreme responsibility of the leaders of German medicine—men like Rostock and Rose and Schroeder and Handloser. That is why their guilt is greater than that of any of the other defendants in the dock. They are the men who utterly failed their country and their profession, who showed neither courage nor wisdom nor the vestiges of moral character. It is their failure, together with the failure of the leaders of Germany in other walks of life, that debauched Germany and led to her defeat. It is because of them and others like them that we all live in a stricken world.

SOURCE

The full opening statement and opinion is published in: *Trials of War Criminals Before the Nuremberg Military Tribunal Under Control Council Law* 10, Vol. 1 (Washington D.C.: Superintendent of Documents, U.S. Government Printing Office, 1950); Military Tribunal, Case 1, *United States v. Karl Brandt et al.*, pp. 27–74.

The Nuremberg Doctors' Trial
(b) Excerpts from the Judgment, Aug. 19, 1947

Judges Harold Sebring, Walter Beals and Johnson Crawford

Military Tribunal I was established on 25 October 1946 under General Orders No. 6 issued by command of the United States Military Government for Germany. It was the first of several military tribunals constituted in the United States Zone of Occupation pursuant to Military Government Ordinance No. 7, for the trial of offenses recognized as crimes by Law No. 10 of the Control Council for Germany.

* * *

The trial was conducted in two languages— English and German. It consumed 139 trial days, including 6 days allocated for final arguments and the personal statements of the defendants. During the 133 trial days used for the presentation of evidence 32 witnesses gave oral evidence for the prosecution and 53 witnesses, including the 23 defendants, gave oral evidence for the defense. In addition, the prosecution put in evidence as exhibits a total of 570 affidavits, reports, and documents; the defense put in a total number of 901—making a grand total of 1471 documents received in evidence.

* * *

COUNTS TWO AND THREE

War Crimes and Crimes against Humanity. The second and third counts of the indictment charge the commission of war crimes and crimes against humanity. The counts are identical in content, except for the fact that in count two the acts which are made the basis for the charges are alleged to have been committed on "civilians and members of the armed forces [of nations] then at war with the German Reich ... in the exercise of belligerent control," whereas in count three the criminal acts are alleged to have been committed against "German civilians and nationals of other countries." With this distinction observed, both counts will be treated as one and discussed together.

Counts two and three allege, in substance, that between September 1939 and April 1945 all of the defendants "were principals in, accessories to, ordered, abetted, took a consenting part in, and were connected with plans and enterprises involving medical experiments without the subjects' consent ... in the course of which experiments the defendants committed murders, brutalities, cruelties, tortures, atrocities, and other inhuman acts." It is averred that "such experiments included, but were not limited to" the following:

a. *High-Altitude Experiments.* From about March 1942 to about August 1942 experiments were conducted at the Dachau concentration camp, for the benefit of the German Air Force, to investigate the limits of human endurance and existence at extremely high altitudes. The experiments were carried out in a low-pressure chamber in which the atmospheric conditions and pressures prevailing at high altitude (up to 68,000 feet) could be duplicated. The experimental subjects were placed in the low-pressure chamber and thereafter the simulated altitude therein was raised. Many victims died as a result of these experiments and others suffered grave injury, torture, and ill-treatment. The defendants Karl Brandt, Handloser, Schroeder, Gebhardt, Rudolf Brandt, Mrugowsky, Poppendick, Sievers, Ruff, Romberg, Becker-Freyseng, and Weltz are charged with special responsibility for and participation in these crimes.

b. *Freezing Experiments.* From about August 1942 to about May 1943 experiments were conducted at the Dachau concentration camp, primarily for the benefit of the German Air Force, to investigate the most effective means of treating persons who had been severely chilled or frozen. In one series of experiments the subjects were forced to remain in a tank of ice water for periods up to 3 hours. Extreme rigor developed in a short time. Numerous victims died in the course of these experiments. After the survivors were severely chilled, rewarming was attempted by various means. In another series of experiments, the subjects were kept naked outdoors for many hours at temperatures below freezing .... The defendants Karl Brandt, Handloser, Schroeder, Gebhardt, Rudolf Brandt, Mrugowsky, Poppendick, Sievers, Becker-Freyseng, and Weltz are

charged with special responsibility for and participation in these crimes.

c. *Malaria Experiments.* From about February 1942 to about April 1945 experiments were conducted at the Dachau concentration camp in order to investigate immunization for and treatment of malaria. Healthy concentration camp inmates were infected by mosquitoes or by injections of extracts of the mucous glands of mosquitoes. After having contracted malaria the subjects were treated with various drugs to test their relative efficacy. Over 1,000 involuntary subjects were used in these experiments. Many of the victims died and others suffered severe pain and permanent disability. The defendants Karl Brandt, Handloser, Rostock, Gebhardt, Blome, Rudolf Brandt, Mrugowsky, Poppendick, and Sievers are charged with special responsibility for and participation in these crimes.

d. *Lost (Mustard) Gas Experiments.* At various times; between September 1939 and April 1945 experiments were conducted at Sachsenhausen, Natzweiler, and other concentration camps for the benefit of the German Armed Forces to investigate the most effective treatment of wounds caused by Lost gas. Lost is a poison gas which is commonly known as mustard gas. Wounds deliberately inflicted on the subjects were infected with Lost. Some of the subjects died as a result of these experiments and others suffered intense pain and injury. The defendants Karl Brandt, Handloser, Blome, Rostock, Gebhardt, Rudolf Brandt, and Sievers are charged with special responsibility for and participation in these crimes.

e. *Sulfanilamide Experiments.* From about July 1942 to about September 1943 experiments to investigate the effectiveness of sulfanilamide were conducted at the Ravensbrueck concentration camp for the benefit of the German Armed Forces. Wounds deliberately inflicted on the experimental subjects were infected with bacteria such as streptococcus, gas gangrene, and tetanus. Circulation of blood was interrupted by tying off blood vessels at both ends of the wound to create a condition similar to that of a battlefield wound. Infection was aggravated by forcing wood shavings and ground glass into the wounds. The infection was treated with sulfanilamide and other drugs to determine their effectiveness. Some subjects died as a result of these experiments and others suffered serious injury and intense agony. The defendants Karl Brandt, Handloser, Rostock, Schroeder, Genzken, Gebhardt, Blome, Rudolf Brandt, Mrugowsky, Poppendick, Becker-Freyseng, Oberheuser, and Fischer are charged with special responsibility for and participation in these crimes.

f. *Bone, Muscle, and Nerve Regeneration and Bone Transplantation Experiments.* From about September 1942 to about December 1943 experiments were conducted at the Ravensbrueck concentration camp, for the benefit of the German Armed Forces, to study bone, muscle, and nerve regeneration, and bone transplantation from one person to another. Sections of bones, muscles, and nerves were removed from the subjects. As a result of these operations, many victims suffered intense agony, mutilation, and permanent disability. The defendants Karl Brandt, Handloser, Rostock, Gebhardt, Rudolf Brandt, Oberheuser, and Fischer are charged with special responsibility and participation in these crimes.

g. *Sea-Water Experiments.* From about July 1944 to about September 1944 experiments were conducted at the Dachau Concentration camp, for the benefit of the German Air Force and Navy, to study various methods of making sea water drinkable. The subjects were deprived of all food and given only chemically processed sea water. Such experiments caused great pain and suffering and resulted in serious bodily injury to the victims. The defendants Karl Brandt, Handloser, Rostock, Schroeder, Gebhardt, Rudolf Brandt, Mrugowsky, Poppendick, Sievers, Becker-Freyseng, Schaefer, and Beiglboeck are charged with special responsibility for and participation in these crimes.

h. *Epidemic Jaundice Experiments.* From about June 1943 to about January 1945 experiments were conducted at the Sachsenhausen and Natzweiler concentration camps, for benefit of the German Armed Forces, to investigate the causes of, and inoculations against, epidemic jaundice. Experimental subjects were deliberately infected with epidemic jaundice, some of whom died as a result, and others were caused great pain and suffering. The defendants Karl Brandt, Handloser, Rostock, Schroeder, Gebhardt, Rudolf Brandt, Mrugowsky, Poppendick, Sievers, Rose, and Becker-Freyseng are charged with special responsibility for and participation in these crimes.

i. *Sterilization Experiments.* From about March 1941 to about January 1945 sterilization experiments were conducted at the Auschwitz and Ravensbrueck concentration camps, and other places. The purpose of these experiments was to develop a method of sterilization which would be suitable for sterilizing millions of people with a minimum of time and effort. These experiments were conducted by means of X-ray, surgery, and 2 various drugs. Thousands of victims were sterilized and thereby suffered great mental and physical anguish. The defendants Karl Brandt, Gebhardt, Rudolf Brandt, Mrugowsky, Poppendick, Brack, Pokorny, and Oberheuser are charged with special responsibility for and participation in these crimes.

j. *Spotted Fever (Fleckfieber) Experiments.* From about December 1941 to about February 1945 experiments were conducted at the Buchenwald and Natzweiler concentration camps, for the benefit of the German Armed Forces, to investigate the effectiveness of spotted fever and other vaccines. At Buchenwald, numerous healthy inmates were deliberately infected with spotted fever virus in order to keep the virus alive; over 90 percent of the victims died as a result. Other healthy inmates were used to determine the effectiveness of different spotted fever vaccines and of various chemical substances. In the course of these experiments 75 percent of the selected number of inmates were vaccinated with one of the vaccines or nourished with one of the chemical substances and, after a period of 3 to 4 weeks, were infected with spotted fever germs. The remaining 25 percent were infected without any previous protection in order to compare the effectiveness of the vaccines and the chemical substances. As a result, hundreds of the persons experimented upon died. Experiments with yellow fever, smallpox, typhus, paratyphus A and B, cholera, and diphtheria were also conducted. Similar experiments with like results were conducted at Natzweiler concentration camp. The defendants Karl Brandt, Handloser, Rostock, Schroeder, Genzken, Gebhardt, Rudolf Brandt, Mrugowsky, Poppendick, Sievers, Rose, Becker-Freyseng, and Hoven are charged with special responsibility for and participation in these crimes.

k. *Experiments with Poison.* In or about December 1943 and in or about October 1944 experiments were conducted at the Buchenwald concentration camp to investigate the effect of various poisons upon human beings. The poisons were secretly administered to experimental subjects in their food. The victims died as a result of the poison or were killed immediately in order to permit autopsies. In or about September 1944 experimental subjects were shot with poison bullets and suffered torture and death. The defendants Genzken, Gebhardt, Mrugowsky, and Poppendick are charged with special responsibility for and participation in these crimes.

l. *Incendiary Bomb Experiments.* From about November 1943 to about January 1944 experiments were conducted at the Buchenwald concentration camp to test the effect of various pharmaceutical preparations on phosphorus burns. These burns were inflicted on experimental subjects with phosphorus matter taken from incendiary bombs, and caused severe pain, suffering, and serious bodily injury. The defendants Genzken, Gebhardt, Mrugowsky, and Poppendick are charged with special responsibility for and participation in these crimes.

In addition to the medical experiments, the nature and purpose of which have been outlined as alleged, certain of the defendants are charged with criminal activities involving murder, torture, and ill-treatment of non-German nationals as follows:

7. Between June 1943 and September 1944 the defendants Rudolf Brandt and Sievers . . . were principals in, accessories to, ordered, abetted, took a consenting part in, and were connected with plans and enterprises involving

the murder of civilians and members of the armed forces of nations then at war with the German Reich and who were in the custody of the German Reich in exercise of belligerent control. One hundred twelve Jews were selected for the purpose of completing a skeleton collection for the Reich University of Strasbourg. Their photographs and anthropological measurements were taken. Then they were killed. Thereafter, comparison tests, anatomical research, studies regarding race, pathological features of the body, form and size of the brain, and other tests were made. The bodies were sent to Strasbourg and defleshed.

8. Between May 1942 and January 1944 the defendants Blome and Rudolf Brandt ... were principals in, accessories to, ordered, abetted, took a consenting part in, and were connected with plans and enterprises involving the murder and mistreatment of tens of thousands of Polish nationals who were civilians and members of the armed forces of a nation then at war with the German Reich and who were in the custody of the German Reich in exercise of belligerent control. These people were alleged to be infected with incurable tuberculosis. On the ground of insuring the health and welfare of Germans in Poland, many tubercular Poles were ruthlessly exterminated while others were isolated in death camps with inadequate medical facilities.

9. Between September 1939 and April 1945 the defendants Karl Brandt, Blome, Brack, and Hoven ... were principals in, accessories to, ordered, abetted, took a consenting part in, and were connected with plans and enterprises involving the execution of the so-called "euthanasia" program of the German Reich in the course of which the defendants herein murdered hundreds of thousands of human beings, including nationals of German-occupied countries. This program involved the systematic and secret execution of the aged, insane, incurably ill, of deformed children, and other persons, by gas, lethal injections, and diverse other means in nursing homes, hospitals, and asylums. Such persons were regarded as "useless eaters" and a burden to the German war machine. The relatives of these victims were informed that they died from natural causes, such as heart failure. German doctors involved in the "euthanasia" program were also sent to the eastern occupied countries to assist in the mass extermination of Jews.

* * *

Counts two and three of the indictment conclude with the averment that the crimes and atrocities which have been delineated "constitute violations of international conventions . . . , the laws and customs of war, the general principles of criminal law as derived from the criminal laws of all civilized nations, the internal penal laws of the countries in which such crimes were committed, and of Article II of Control Council Law No. 10."

* * *

THE PROOF AS TO WAR CRIMES AND CRIMES AGAINST HUMANITY

Judged by any standard of proof, the record clearly shows the commission of war crimes and crimes against humanity substantially as alleged in counts two and three of the indictment. Beginning with the outbreak of World War II criminal medical experiments on non-German nationals, both prisoners of war and civilians, including Jews and "asocial" persons, were carried out on a large scale in Germany and the occupied countries. These experiments were not the isolated and casual acts of individual doctors and scientists working solely on their own responsibility, but were the product of coordinated policy-making and planning at high governmental, military, and Nazi Party levels, conducted as an integral part of the total war effort. They were ordered, sanctioned, permitted, or approved by persons in positions of authority who under all principles of law were under the duty to know about these things and to take steps to terminate or prevent them.

PERMISSIBLE MEDICAL EXPERIMENTS

The great weight of the evidence before us is to the effect that certain types of medical experiments on human beings, when kept within reasonably well-defined bounds, conform to the ethics of the medical profession generally. The protagonists of the practice of human experimentation justify their views on the basis that such experiments yield results for the good of society that are unprocurable by other methods or means of study. All agree, however, that certain basic principles must be observed in order to satisfy moral, ethical and legal concepts:

1. The voluntary consent of the human subject is absolutely essential. This means that the person involved should have legal capacity to give consent; should be so situated as to be able to exercise free power of choice, without the intervention of any element of force, fraud, deceit, duress, over-reaching, or other ulterior form of constraint or coercion; and should have sufficient knowledge and comprehension of the elements of the subject matter involved as to enable him to make an understanding and enlightened decision. This latter element requires that before the acceptance of an affirmative decision by the experimental subject there should be made known to him the nature, duration, and purpose of the experiment; the method and means by which it is to be conducted; all inconveniences and hazards reasonably to be expected; and the effects upon his health or person which may possibly come from his participation in the experiment.

    The duty and responsibility for ascertaining the quality of the consent rests upon each individual who initiates, directs or engages in the experiment. It is a personal duty and responsibility which may not be delegated to another with impunity.

2. The experiment should be such as to yield fruitful results for the good of society, unprocurable by other methods or means of study, and not random and unnecessary in nature.

3. The experiment should be so designed and based on the results of animal experimentation and a knowledge of the natural history of the disease or other problem under study that the anticipated results will justify the performance of the experiment.

4. The experiment should be so conducted as to avoid all unnecessary physical and mental suffering and injury.

5. No experiment should be conducted where there is an *a priori* reason to believe that death or disabling injury will occur; except, perhaps, in those experiments where the experimental physicians also serve as subjects.

6. The degree of risk to be taken should never exceed that determined by the humanitarian importance of the problem to be solved by the experiment.

7. Proper preparations should be made and adequate facilities provided to protect the experimental subject against

even remote possibilities of injury, disability, or death.

8. The experiment should be conducted only by scientifically qualified persons. The highest degree of skill and care should be required through all stages of the experiment of those who conduct or engage in the experiment.

9. During the course of the experiment the human subject should be at liberty to bring the experiment to an end if he has reached the physical or mental state where continuation of the experiment seems to him to be impossible.

10. During the course of the experiment the scientist in charge must be prepared to terminate the experiment at any stage, if he has probably cause to believe, in the exercise of the good faith, superior skill and careful judgment required of him that a continuation of the experiment is likely to result in injury, disability, or death to the experimental subject.

Of the ten principles which have been enumerated our judicial concern, of course, is with those requirements which are purely legal in nature—or which at least are so clearly related to matters legal that they assist us in determining criminal culpability and punishment. To go beyond that point would lead us into a field that would be beyond our sphere of competence. However, the point need not be labored. We find from the evidence that in the medical experiments which have been proved, these ten principles were much more frequently honored in their breach than in their observance. Many of the concentration camp inmates who were the victims of these atrocities were citizens of countries other than the German Reich. They were non-German nationals, including Jews and "asocial persons," both prisoners of war and civilians, who had been imprisoned and forced to sub-

mit to the tortures and barbarities without so much as a semblance of trial. In every single instance appearing in the record, subjects were used who did not consent to the experiments; indeed, as to some of the experiments, it is not even contended by the defendants that the subjects occupied the status of volunteers. In no case was the experimental subject at liberty of his own free choice to withdraw from any experiment. In many cases experiments were performed by unqualified persons; were conducted at random for no adequate scientific reason, and under revolting physical conditions. All of the experiments were conducted with unnecessary suffering and injury and but very little, if any, precautions were taken to protect or safeguard the human subjects from the possibilities of injury, disability, or death. In every one of the experiments the subjects experienced extreme pain or torture and in most of them they suffered permanent injury, mutilation, or death, either as a direct result of the experiments or because of lack of adequate follow-up care.

Obviously all of these experiments involving brutalities, tortures, disabling injury, and death were performed in complete disregard of international conventions, the laws and customs of war, the general principles of criminal law as derived from the criminal laws of all civilized nations, and Control Council Law No. 10. Manifestly human experiments under such conditions are contrary to "the principles of the law of nations as they result from the usages established among civilized peoples, from the laws of humanity, and from the dictates of public conscience."

Whether any of the defendants in the dock are guilty of these atrocities is, of course, another question.

Under the Anglo-Saxon system of jurisprudence every defendant in a criminal case is presumed to be innocent of an offense charged until the prosecution, by competent, credible proof, has shown his guilt to the exclusion of every reasonable doubt. And this presumption abides with a defendant through each stage of his trial until such degree of proof has been adduced. A "reasonable doubt" as the name implies is one conformable to reason—a doubt which a reasonable man would entertain. Stated differently, it is that state of a case which, after a full and complete comparison and consideration of all the evidence, would leave an unbiased, unprejudiced, reflective person, charged with the responsibility for decision, in the state of mind that he could not say that he felt an abiding conviction amounting to a moral certainty of the truth of the charge.

If any of the defendants are to be found guilty under counts two or three of the indictment it must be because the evidence has shown beyond a reasonable doubt that such defendant, without regard to nationality or the capacity in which he acted, participated as a principal in, accessory to, ordered, abetted, took a consenting part in, or was connected with plans or enterprises involving the commission of at least some of the medical experiments and other atrocities which are the subject matter of these counts.

* * *

NOTE

Judgment and sentencing were rendered in August, 1947. Fifteen of the 23 defendants were found guilty. Seven were found not guilty. One (Poppendick) was acquitted of the charges of having performed medical experiments but was found guilty of SS membership.

Karl Brandt, Gebhardt, Mrugowsky, Rudolf Brandt, and three nonphysicians-Sievers, Brack, and Hoven-were sentenced to death by hanging. Life imprisonment sentences were imposed on Handloser, Schroeder, Genzken, Rose, and Fischer. Herta Oberheuser, the only woman among the defendants, was sentenced to 20 years, as was Becker-Freysing. Beiglboeck was sentenced to 15 years, Poppendick to 10 years for SS membership. Rostock, Blome, Ruff, Romberg, Weltz, Schaefer, and Pokorny were acquitted and freed.

"The hangings took place on June 2, 1948. The scene was the prison at Landsberg, in the American zone. Here Hitler had been imprisoned while he wrote *Mein Kampf.* History records that the hangings took 62 minutes. Two black gallows were created in the prison courtyard. Karl Brandt was the only one of the seven who refused religious solace. The last words of the other murderers were not reported. In any event, 7 were hanged, only 4 of them physicians—7 out of the 23, and out of the many more who, as Dr. Mitscherlich's narrative makes clear, were involved in the Nazi medical crimes. It can never be said that the quality of American mercy had been strained" (A. Mitscherlich and F. Mielke, *Doctors of Infamy.* New York: Schuman, 1949, 146–148)

QUESTIONS

1. The trial of the major war criminals was called the International Military Tribunal and was conducted before a multinational tribunal made up of judges from the US, UK, France and the Soviet Union. After that trial was concluded in 1946, the US conducted 12 "subsequent trials" on its own. The first, and the best known, is this one, the "Doctors' Trial." Why do you think the prosecution chose physicians as the group to try first? The famous movie, *Judgment at Nuremberg* (1961) was based on the Judges Trial. You should watch it if you can. Are German judges and lawyers more culpable than physicians for the atrocities of the Third Reich?

2. Taylor says in his opening that this is a "murder and torture" trial. This is certainly true, but it is much more as the focus on medical ethics and human experimentation make clear. Why do you think Taylor decided to go beyond murder and torture and examine the ethics of human experimentation? Do physicians have special obligations not to violate human rights?

3. The "Nuremberg Code" appears at the end of the edited judgment. What is the legal status of the Nuremberg Code? Where does it appear in the International Covenant on Civil and Political Rights? What is the difference between the Nuremberg Code and the Nuremberg Principles (articulated in the IMT, the principles include that individuals can be held responsible for committing war crimes and crimes against humanity, and "obeying orders" is no excuse)?

FURTHER READING

1. Annas, George, J. & Grodin, Michael A., *The Nazi Doctors and the Nuremberg Code: Human Rights in Human Experimentation.* New York: Oxford University Press, 1992.

2. Schmidt, Ulf, *Justice at Nuremberg: Leo Alexander and the Nazi Doctors Trial.* Hampshire: Palgrave, 2004.

3. Katz, Jay, *Experimentation with Human Beings.* New York: Russel Sage, 1972.

4. Nuremberg Trials Project: A Digital Document Collection. Harvard Law School Library http://nuremberg.law.harvard.edu/php/docs_swi.php?DI=1&text=overview

CHAPTER 7

Global Health and Post-9/11 Human Right

George J. Annas

After 9/11 it became fashionable to ask, at least in the arena of global health, if human rights had any special relevance anymore. This question is still being asked as the second year of the Obama administration approaches. The president picked Joseph O'Neill's post-9/11 novel *Netherland* to read shortly after taking office. The novel's narrator, Hans van den Broek, simply refuses to consider many of the questions raised by the attack and our response to it. In his words:

> I found myself unable to contribute to conversations about the value of international law or the feasibility of producing a dirty bomb or the constitutional rights of imprisoned enemies or the efficacy of duct tape as a window sealant or the merits of vaccinating the American masses against smallpox or the complexity of weaponizing deadly bacteria or the menace of the neoconservative cabal in the Bush administration, or indeed any of the debates, each apparently vital, that raged everywhere—raged, because the debaters grew heated and angry and contemptuous . . . I had little interest. I didn't really care. In short, I was a political-ethical idiot.

Hans is, of course, not the only one who has lost interest in these topics. *Netherland* has deservedly been blessed with gushing reviews and a presidential endorsement.

Nonetheless, my own choice for pursuing a conversation about "the value of international law" in the context of global health is *Falling Man.* The conflicting perceptions of the value of international human rights are echoed in the decidedly mixed reviews Don DeLillo's *Falling Man*, garnered. The novel (like human rights?) has been described by reviewers as "frustratingly disjointed," "masterly polyphonic fizzling," "a terrible disappointment," "setting the standard," and "a display of cumulative brilliance." My own view is that the post-World War II human rights movement in general, and its much more recent health and human rights application to global health, sets the "standard" and even represents "a display of cumulative brilliance."

DeLillo's last great novel, *Underworld*, published in 1997, portrays the Cold War and its fallout as well as anything in fiction or nonfiction. Its cover, surely not meant to be purposely prophetic, pictures the twin towers on both the front and back (one a photo positive, the other a negative) with a church steeple and cross in front of them, and a bird of prey flying in their direction. The cover of *Falling Man* is self-consciously derivative. The front cover is illustrated by a blue sky as seen from above cloud cover; the back cover contains the same cloudscape with the twin towers breaking through. Both books are about our fear and confusion, followed by our death and decay, which we cover up—with more or less success—with consumption and by building massive monuments to ourselves. But *Falling Man* has more bite than *Underworld*, no doubt because of the fall of the towers. It is filled, as we are, with loss and self-destruction. Memory loss is its central obsession, but it is also filled with assorted ways and reasons to commit suicide in the midst of plenty. The main character of *Falling Man*, a survivor from the first tower, is almost universally described by reviewers as a shallow, middle-aged businessman (the typical American?). DeLillo describes his plight at the end of the novel (which ends where it begins, with the main character escaping from the tower, and observing what is happening): "He could not find himself in the things he saw and heard."

Human rights advocates usually don't have a hard time finding themselves, and their general quest is to change the things they see and hear. But they may see more blue sky than threatening clouds on the horizon, and may or may not have faded memories of the horrors of World War II that gave birth to modern human rights. Nonetheless, 9/11 changed the international human rights movement as well. Former Yale Law School Dean Harold Koh, for example, the leading human rights expert in the Obama administration, has perceptively identified four eras of human rights: (1) the *Era of Universalism* (1941–56), beginning with Roosevelt's Four Freedoms speech (freedom of speech and religion, freedom from want and fear), and containing the founding of the United Nations and the adoption of the UDHR; (2) the *Era of Institutionalization* (1965–76) when the treaties were adopted and the institutional structures of human rights were formed, mostly at the UN; (3) the *Era of Operationalization* (1976–89), with the

formation of national and regional human rights regimes, constitutional law applications, special reporters, and specialized nongovernmental organizations (NGOs); and finally (4) the *Era of Globalization* (1989–present). Koh divides the globalization of human rights into two periods: (1989–2001) the Age of Optimism, from the fall of the Berlin Wall to 9/11; and the Age of Pessimism from 9/11 to today.[1] He delineated these eras before the election of Barack Obama, and there is at least the hope that the Obama presidency could mark a turning point in the Age of Pessimism concerning human rights. Nonetheless, reasons for continued pessimism abound.

The United States used 9/11 as a rationale to abandon not only our rhetorical role of global leader in human rights (always contested by some), but also to abandon human rights itself as a professed guide to our own actions, adopting methods we had consistently condemned since World War II, including preemptive war, torture, cruel and humiliating treatment, indefinite detention, disappearances, and grave breaches of the Geneva Conventions. We became a human rights outlaw in promoting the use of torture, and our country is no longer credible as a moral, or even rhetorical, leader in this arena.[2]

This is disheartening. But does it mean that it is also time to abandon the nascent health and human rights movement as a potential fundamental underpinning for global health? I think not. In spite of our recent disgraceful and illegal behavior in the human rights arena labeled "civil and political rights," in the health portion of "economic, social, and cultural rights," as Solly Benatar and Renee Fox have argued, "the United States is the country with the most *potential* for favorably influencing global health trends"[3] (emphasis in original).

HEALTH AND HUMAN RIGHTS

Jonathan Mann is righty identified as the father of the (public) health and human rights movement. As he first noted, it is neither health nor human rights alone that provide the prospect of motivating a global public health movement, but the combination of health and human rights. Not only do negatives in one area exacerbate negatives in the other, positives in both amplify each other.[4]

World War II, arguably the first truly global war, led to a global acknowledgment of the universality of human rights and the responsibility of individuals and governments to promote them. Jonathan Mann also perceptively identified the HIV/AIDS epidemic as the first global epidemic because it is taking place at a time when the world is unified electronically and by swift transportation. Like World War II, this worldwide epidemic requires us to think in new ways and to develop effective methods to treat and prevent disease on a global level. Globalization is a mercantile and ecological fact; it is also a public health reality. The challenge facing medicine and public health, both before and after 9/11, is to develop a global language and a global strategy that can help to improve the health of all of the world's citizens.

To address the HIV/AIDS epidemic it has been necessary to deal directly with a wide range of human rights issues, including discrimination, the rights of women, privacy, and informed consent, as well as education and access to healthcare. Although it is easy to recognize that population-based prevention is required to effectively address the HIV/AIDS epidemic on a global level (as well as, for example, tuberculosis, malaria, and tobacco-related illness), it has been much harder to articulate a global public health ethic, and public health itself has had an extraordinarily difficult time developing its own ethical language. Because of its universality and its emphasis on equality and human dignity, the language of human rights is well suited for public health.

Similarly, Paul Farmer has asked, "What can a focus on health bring to the struggle for human rights?" and answered, "A 'health angle' can promote a broader human rights agenda in unique ways." Using the example of TB in Russian prisons, he noted that he and his colleagues would not have been invited in if they were seen as human rights workers. But as physicians with expertise in TB treatment, they were welcomed in the spirit of "pragmatic solidarity" which, Farmer noted, "may in the end lead to penal reform as well."[5]

Health and human rights experts Sofia Gruskin and Daniel Tarantola have made it crystal clear that the health and human rights movement is based on the human rights movement itself, including the corpus of human rights law articulated in international human rights treaties. As such, primary obligations to respect, protect, and fulfill human rights, including the right to health, fall on the governments of those countries that have signed these treaties and have adopted their own domestic laws to operationalize them. Most fundamentally, human rights law is itself founded on the principle of nondiscrimination: All people everywhere should be treated equally.[6] Women and children also merit special protection under the right to health, and their rights are also reinforced by specific treaties, the Convention on the Elimination of Discrimination Against Women (CEDAW), and the Convention on the Rights of the Child (CRC). Gruskin insists that human rights obligations are legal obligations that bind countries, and it is the legal dimension of the health and human rights field that distinguishes it from the more aspirational field of social justice.[7]

Gruskin is, I believe, quite correct. Nonetheless, as a public health advocate, she would likely agree that spending time mining for differences between the human rights and the social justice approaches, rather than seeking commonalities that can lead to public health action, is counterproductive. Human rights is action- and advocacy-oriented, characteristics that also commend it for global public health.

More than ten years ago I was asked to review a conference-generated book entitled *Ethics, Equity, and Health for All.* The 1997 conference was intended to develop an action plan to promote equity in health and was based on four principles for action: (1) take an inclusive approach to the governance of ethics and human rights in health; (2) give priority to the involvement of countries and groups that are underrepresented in ethics and human rights deliberations; (3) combine shorter- and longer-term efforts to incorporate ethical practice and respect for human rights in the applications of science and technology to health policy and practice; and (4) give priority to the development of human and institutional capacity to ensure sustainability of effort. These principles are reasonable, but the ultimate action plan suggested by the participants, perhaps unsurprisingly, was not. It called primarily for more work to "prepare working definitions of such key terms as ethics, equity, solidarity, [and] human rights, to take account of international . . . and cultural diversity."

Writing this chapter on global health reminded me of the conference, as well as of my initial thoughts about it. Just as books often end by suggesting other books, so conferences have a tendency to end by suggesting more conferences. I wrote at the time:

The conference wound up calling for more conferences. *Academic conferences have an important place in health and human rights work, but do we really need more conferences to define "equity, ethics, and human rights" in our world?* Aren't the inequalities gross enough and obvious enough to warrant direct attention to actions to deal with the problem itself, rather than to refine the "ethics" of approaching it? Moreover, strong theoretical works already exist that provide astute analyses of the relationships between equity (and ethics) and development. Of special note are two books by Amartya Sen, *On Ethics and Economics,* and *Inequality Reexamined.*[8] (emphasis added)

Today it is worth asking again, Do we really need more conferences (or books?) to define equity, ethics, and human rights before engaging in advocacy and direct health action? I remain skeptical. I think we can conference and write ourselves and the would-be beneficiaries of direct public health action to death. On the other hand, it must be recognized, as Sudhir Anand, Fabienne Peter, and Amartya Sen have suggested in their *Public Health, Ethics, and Equity,* that "the commitment of public health to social justice and to health equity raises a series of ethical issues which, until recently, have received insufficient attention."[9] Their book however, has not satisfied everyone. Bioethicists Madison Powers and Ruth Faden, for example, suggest that we do need more conferences and books, when they argue that "the foundational moral justification for the social institution of public health is social justice," and that "commentary on ethics and public health is, at best, thin."[10] Nor is their view idiosyncratic.

Jennifer Ruger has argued that although "global health inequalities are wide and growing . . . [and] pose ethical challenges for the global health community . . . we lack a moral framework for dealing with them," and suggests pursuing equality from a theory of justice.[11] Elsewhere, Ruger has suggested that on the specific question of the human right to health, "One would be hard pressed to find a more controversial or nebulous human right than the 'right to health'" (although she has also suggested that a philosophical justification for this right can be provided).[12] Others, including physician-anthropologist and activist Jim Kim, president of Dartmouth College, has argued that the human rights approach to health disparities and inequality is more rhetoric than reality, akin to singing "Kumbaya."[13]

It is easy to be cynical about or disenchanted with human rights. Law professor David Kennedy has catalogued the major critiques of human rights, noting that human rights can be legitimately critiqued for driving out other emancipatory possibilities, for framing problems and solutions too narrowly, for overgeneralizing and being unduly abstract, and for expressing a Western liberalism. Kennedy's list continues: human rights promises more than it can deliver, the human rights bureaucracy is itself part of the problem—it can strengthen bad government, and it can be bad politics in particular contexts. In his words, "The generation that built the human rights movement focused its attention on the ways in which evil people in evil societies could be identified and restrained. More acute now is how good people, well-intentioned people in good societies, can go wrong, can entrench and support the very things they have learned to denounce. Answering this question requires a pragmatic reassessment of our most sacred humanitarian commitments, tactics and tools."[14]

There is a measure of truth in all these observations, and effective action does require defined goals and specific actions to reach them. But as Joseph Kunz observed almost 60 years ago in regard the Universal Declaration of Human Rights, "In the field of human rights . . . it is necessary to avoid the Scylla of a pessimistic cynicism and the Charybdis of mere wishful thinking and

superficial optimism."[15] No other language than rights language seems as suitable for global health advocacy. All people have (inherent) human rights by definition, and people with rights can demand change, not just beg for it. And rights matter-and will matter even more as judicial structures to enforce them, like the International Criminal Court, continue to be established and nourished. Values of course underlie rights, but it would be incomprehensible to adopt a "Bill of Values" rather than a "Bill of Rights" to protect people.

In the language of contemporary human rights, governments don't simply have an obligation to act or not to act. Governments have obligations to *respect* the rights of the people themselves, to *protect* people in the exercise of their rights, and to *promote* and *fulfill* the rights of people. Of course, not all governments can immediately fulfill economic rights, like the right to health, because of financial constraints. International human rights law therefore provides that a government's obligation can be defined as working toward the "progressive realization" of these rights within their resource constraints. Some countries are so limited in their resources that they require assistance from the world community. The novel but potentially powerful right to development speaks to the obligations of the world community to provide that assistance, as do the goals of the UN's Millennium Declaration.

In public health, of course, it is well-recognized that many countries require the support of the world community to deal effectively with epidemic diseases, like SARS and the H1N1 flu, and that such support is in everyone's collective interests. Another development, the globalization of clinical research trials, provides a good example of the conflicting agendas and conflicts of interest that both call for and seek to avoid universal human rights norms.

THE GLOBALIZATION OF CLINICAL TRIALS

The globalization of clinical research trials calls for more effective ethical and legal rules to protect research subjects, as well as to guard the scientific integrity of the research.[16] Nonetheless, as the former editor of the *New England Journal of Medicine*, Marcia Angell, observed more than a decade ago in this context, "there appears to be a general retreat from the clear principles enunciated in the Nuremberg Code and the Declaration of Helsinki as applied to research in the Third World."[17] The situation has not improved.

Near the end of the Bush administration, the FDA decided that research studies submitted to it for review need no longer follow the Declaration of Helsinki, but instead could follow the less exacting, industry-sponsored, International Conference on Harmonization's Guidelines for Good Clinical Practice.[18]

There is another choice—the human rights choice as articulated in the Nuremberg Code. The Declaration of Helsinki is a statement of research ethics by physicians. But what is the legal status of the Nuremberg Code? Does it, like Helsinki and the Harmonization Guidelines, also represent a collection of bioethics rules that researchers can ignore with impunity? Or has the Nuremberg Code, and especially its uncompromising informed consent requirement, arrived at the status of international human rights norm that must be followed? Just as controversy over the US-sponsored 076 maternal-to-child HIV transmission interruption trials in Africa in the mid-1990s gave rise to a continuing debate about standard of care and benefit obligations, so another mid-1990s research trial in Africa has brought international research rules and the doctrine of informed consent back to center stage.

Four years after it occurred, the *Washington Post* broke the story of a 1996 medical experiment conducted by Pfizer researchers in Kano, Nigeria, during a meningitis epidemic. The story created a sensation, especially its lead, which described the slow death of a 10-year-old little girl known only as subject 6587-0069. The researchers monitored her dying without modifying her treatment, but simply followed the research protocol designed to test their potential breakthrough antibiotic, Trovan, on children. The *Post* noted that the story was hardly unique, their investigation having discovered corporation-sponsored experiments in Africa, Asia, Eastern Europe, and Latin America that were "poorly regulated," "dominated by private interests," and that "far too often betray" their promises to research subject and consumers.[19]

Following the expose, the families of the children-subjects in the Kano experiment brought suit against Pfizer in Nigeria, and later in the United States as well, charging Pfizer with conducting medical experiments without informed consent. The lawsuits initially met dogmatic and sometimes zealous resistance by judges in both the United States and Nigeria. Pfizer had successfully argued both that there was no international norm that required the company physicians to obtain informed consent to experimental drugs, and that in any event, any lawsuit against them by the subjects and their families should be tried in Nigerian, not US courts. Pfizer abandoned this latter claim in 2006 when a copy of an internal report by the Nigerian Ministry of Health on the experiment was made public. The report concluded, among other things, that the study violated Nigerian law, the Declaration of Helsinki, and the Convention on the Rights of the Child (CRC). Following the release of the report, the Nigerian government filed both a criminal and a civil suit against Pfizer in Nigeria. Pfizer settled the Nigerian cases in 2009 for $75 million.

More important in human rights terms than the Nigeria litigation, is the litigation in the United States, especially the 2009 opinion of the Second Circuit Court of Appeals, which reversed a lower court dismissal of the lawsuit and sent it back for trial.[20] In the area of human rights, the Second Circuit is best known for its 1980 opinion that a physician from Paraguay could sue the inspector general of police of Asuncion, Paraguay, in the United States for the murder and torture of his son in Paraguay under the Alien Tort Statute. The reason, according to the court, was because torture is universally condemned as a violation of international human rights law, and "The torturer has become—like the pirate and the slave holder before him—*hostis humani generis*, an enemy of all mankind."[21] To oversimplify (but not much), at issue in the Pfizer case before the Second Circuit was whether the researcher who experiments on humans without their informed consent violates a substantially similar international human rights law norm.

It is worth underlining that there has never been a trial in this case, and that the facts alleged by the Nigerian families may not be able to be proven in court. Nonetheless, for the purposes of deciding whether they should have their day in an American court, the Second Circuit had to assume the facts as alleged in the complaint are true. These allegations are primarily that, in the midst of a meningitis epidemic in Nigeria, Pfizer dispatched physicians to go to the Kano Infectious Disease Hospital to do a study on 200 sick children to compare the efficacy of their new drug, Trovan, with the FDA-approved antibiotic Rocephin. Trovan had never before been tested on children in its oral form. The experiment was conducted over a two-week period, then the Pfizer team precipitously left. In the court's words, "According to the appellants, the tests caused the deaths of eleven children, five of whom had taken Trovan and six of whom had taken the lowered dose of ceftriaxone, and left many others blind, deaf, paralyzed, or brain-damaged." The central allegation is that "Pfizer, working in partnership with the Nigerian government, failed to secure the informed consent of either the children or their guardians and specifically failed to disclose or explain the experimental nature of the study or the serious risks involved," or the immediate availability of alternative treatment by Médecins Sans Frontières (MSF) at the same facility.

The Supreme Court has cautioned lower courts to be conservative in determining whether a particular category of actions contravene "the law of nations" accepted by the "civilized world" as a norm of customary international law.[22] For the Second Circuit to permit this case to proceed it had to conclude that the requirement of informed consent to medical experiments on humans has become a norm of customary international law. The court so concluded because it found the informed consent requirement is sufficiently "(i) universal and obligatory, (ii) specific and definable, and (iii) of mutual concern," to be a customary international law norm that can support a claim under the Alien Tort Statute.

Perhaps of most interest from the global health perspective is that the court found the war crimes trials at Nuremberg, especially the Doctors' Trial, to provide the legal foundation for its conclusion. The major war crimes trial, the International Military Tribunal (IMT), was the only multinational trial at Nuremberg. Nonetheless, the court found that the US military trials that followed the IMT, including the Doctors' Trial, "effectively operated as extensions of the IMT." The Doctors' Trial, of course, produced the 1947 Nuremberg Code in the judgment, the first precept of which is the requirement for voluntary, competent, informed, and understanding consent of the research subject. In the court's words, "The American tribunal's conclusion that action that contravened the Code's first principle constituted a crime against humanity is a lucid indication of the international legal significance of the prohibition on nonconsensual medical experimentation." As important, the Nuremberg consent principle has been widely adopted in international treaties, including the International Covenant on Civil and Political Rights (ICCPR); the Geneva Conventions; and domestic law, as well as in nonbinding international ethics codes like the Declaration of Helsinki.

The court found that in addition to being universal, the Nuremberg norm is specific in its requirement (so researchers could understand it), and is of mutual concern among nations. To make this last point the court concluded that promoting global use of essential medicines can help reduce the spread of contagious disease, "which is a significant threat to international peace and stability." Contrariwise, conducting drug trials in other countries without informed consent "fosters distrust and resistance . . . to critical public health initiatives in which pharmaceutical companies play a key role." The example the court cited is the impact of local distrust of international pharmaceutical companies that caused the Kano boycott of the 2004 effort to stem a polio outbreak there that later spread across Africa, making global eradication of polio all the more difficult.[23]

Post-World War II ethical standards of clinical research have not effectively protected subjects or ensured scientific integrity. The Second Circuit's persuasive opinion that the doctrine of informed consent has attained the status of an international human rights norm that can be enforced in the world's courts should help persuade international corporations and researchers alike to take informed consent, and perhaps the other principles of the Nuremberg

Code, much more seriously. If so, it will provide a powerful example of the beneficial impact of human rights on the health and welfare of subjects in clinical trials. But could social justice do the job just as well or better? As I have already suggested, I don't think arguing for one approach or the other is terribly fruitful, and that working together is much more likely to promote the publics' health than working separately. In Senator Edward Kennedy's last letter to President Obama on healthcare, which the president read from in his September 2009 speech on the subject to a joint session of Congress), for example, Kennedy referenced both "fundamental principles of social justice" and making healthcare "a right and not a privilege" as complimentary rationales for universal access. It is, nonetheless, worth noting that even commentators who seem to believe social justice alone is the preferable frame for public health action can't help coming back to the health and human rights movement.

SOCIAL JUSTICE AND HUMAN RIGHTS

In their discussion of social justice and public health, Powers and Faden describe what they characterize as "one of the most compelling recent examples of work in public health on behalf of an oppressed group. . . ." The example is the documentation of the rights of women by Physicians for Human Rights (PHR) during pre-9/11 Taliban rule. The authors write, "Research conducted by the group Physicians for Human Rights provides powerful evidence that the denial of basic rights to women resulted not only in horrible injustices with regard to respect, affiliation, and personal security but also with regard to health."[24] Of course, this research project by PHR can be characterized as public health research and as documenting a major injustice to women. But neither characterization accurately describes what PHR itself thought it was doing.

PHR's name could not be more descriptive of their membership and their goals: Physicians for Human Rights. Nor could the subtitle of its' Taliban report be any more explicit: *The Taliban's War on Women: A Health and Human Rights Crisis in Afghanistan.* The first sentence of their report says it again: "This report documents the results of a three-month study of women's health and human rights concerns and conditions in Afghanistan by Physicians for Human Rights." The report continues: "Taliban policies of systematic discrimination against women seriously undermine the health and well-being of Afghan women. Such discrimination and the suffering it causes constitute an affront to the dignity and worth of Afghan women, and humanity as a whole."

PHR's report is extremely powerful and merits the praise it has received. Nonetheless, it is a report by a physician group, not a public health group, and it is a group dedicated to doing health and human rights work, here founded on the ICCPR and CEDAW, not engaged in social justice. Although primarily focused on health, the report also noted that "The Taliban's edicts restricting women's rights have had a disastrous impact on Afghan women and girls' access to education, as well as health care. One of the first edicts issued by the regime when it rose to power was to prohibit girls and women from attending school."[25]

Since the beginning of the ongoing post-9/11 war in Afghanistan, conditions for women have marginally improved, but much remains to be done. Leadership in human rights has been since its creation in the hands of a physician, Sima Samar, chair of the Afghan Independent Human Rights Commission. This is the first human rights commission in Afghanistan's history and it has a wide-ranging mandate, including the promotion of health and human rights, especially the health and human rights of women. When this Commission speaks of justice, it means bringing the perpetrators of war crimes in Afghanistan to justice. And when it speaks of health, it does so in the language of human rights, for example in its 2006 report on "Economic and Social Rights in Afghanistan." Of special note is the Commission's recommendation regarding women and children's health: "The Government should prioritize reproductive (prenatal and postnatal) and child healthcare, according to their obligations under international treaties to which Afghanistan is a party. Afghan women should have universal access to reproductive health care."[26]

It is easy for Americans to criticize the marginalization of human rights and health of women in other countries. But when the health of women in the United States is directly undermined by our government, silence seems the preferred response. Thus, when our Supreme Court ruled that it is constitutionally acceptable for Congress to make it a crime for a physician to use a specific medical procedure that the physician believes is the best one to protect his female patient's health, most commentary focused on abortion politics, rather than the health of women. Few noted that American physicians have never before been prohibited from using a recognized medical procedure, or that prohibiting its use only affected the health of women. The Taliban must have been smiling. As human rights expert Rebecca Cook noted in the broader context of abortion availability globally, "Whether it is discriminatory and socially unconscionable to criminalize a medical procedure that only women need is a question that usually goes not simply unanswered but unasked."[27]

GLOBALIZATION AND HUMAN RIGHTS

American bioethics has had a major positive impact on the way medicine is currently practiced in the United States, especially in the areas of care of dying patients, including advance directives and palliative care, and medical research, including federal regulations to protect research subjects and institutional review boards. It is noteworthy that these accomplishments all came by enacting specific laws related to health. American bioethics has not exhausted what it can usefully accomplish in these spheres, but has of late seen most of its efforts and energy devoted to the interrelated fields of abortion, embryo research, and cloning.

Given the decade-long embryo-centric US activity (Obama's national healthcare plan did produce renewed political interest in discussing "death panels"), I think it is fair to conclude that bioethics is likely to have a stunted future in the real world without a significant reorientation of its focus and direction. I suggest that the most useful reformulation involves recognition and engagement with two interrelated forces reshaping the world and simultaneously providing new frameworks for ethical analysis and action: globalization and public health.

In *American Bioethics,* I argued that the boundaries between bioethics, health law, and human rights are permeable, and border crossings are common. That these disciplines have often viewed each other with suspicion or simple ignorance tells us only about the past. They are most constructively viewed as integral, symbiotic parts of an organic whole, with a common birthplace: Nuremberg.[28]

Globalization, of course, does not depend upon physicians, ethicists, or lawyers, anymore than it depends upon health law, bioethics, or human rights. It does not even depend primarily upon the actions of governments. Rather, two relatively new players dominate globalization: the transnational corporation, and to a lesser extent, the NGO. Both, I think, can be use-fully viewed as new life forms on our planet that are increasingly evolving and changing our environment. A notable health-related example of an NGO is Médecins Sans Frontières (MSF), a humanitarian-human rights organization founded on the belief that access to medical care in emergencies transcend national borders and thus human rights workers cannot be constrained by borders but should cross them when necessary. MSF expands medical ethics to include physician action to protect human rights, blending these two fields and treating the law that protects government territorial boundaries as subordinate to the requirements of providing emergency care. Other human rights and health NGOs, like Physicians for Human Rights, view their primary mission as advocating for human rights.[29]

Transnational corporations deserve our attention because of their incredible potential to both help and harm the planet and its people. Corporations have historically seen at least part of their social responsibility as providing charity to the communities in which they have a large presence. They have, however, been quick to argue that this is purely voluntary and that the responsibility to provide direct services to people, including drugs and medical treatment, rests with the government. A nascent movement to articulate the human rights obligations of transnational corporations is now underway, both in the UN and among corporations themselves. It is too soon to tell whether the global recession, which required governments to rescue both large corporations and banks, will lead to a new recognition of the interdependence of governments and corporations, and thus of their complementary obligations to the people of the world.

Prior to the global financial meltdown, John Ruggie, the Special Representative of the Secretary-General on the issue of human rights and transnational corporations released his report on "Business and

Human Rights." The report identifies five avenues to introduce human rights law into corporate behavior (in order, from the strongest to the weakest): (1) the state's duty to protect its citizens against non-state actor human rights abuses; (2) corporate responsibility and accountability for international crimes (including the use of slave labor, child soldiers, and the use of torture) under complicity theories; (3) corporate responsibility for other human rights violations under international law (e.g., under the Universal Declaration of Human Rights, although this is currently "not necessarily legal in nature"); (4) "soft law" mechanisms, such as voluntary international agreements, like the Kimberley process, which seeks to prohibit international trade in "conflict diamonds"; and (5) self-regulation, in which at least some of the 77,000 transnational corporations and their 770,000 subsidiaries voluntarily adopt and follow human rights standards in their businesses.

Approximately 3,000 transnational corporations, including some major pharmaceutical companies, have joined the UN's Global Compact and committed themselves to its principles, the first two of which are that corporations should support and respect the protection of internationally proclaimed human rights, and that corporations should make sure that they are not complicit in human rights abuses. In the conclusion to his report, Ruggie makes three points that have special importance to global health: (1) "human rights and the sustainability of globalization are inextricably linked"; (2) corporations can be tried in "courts of public opinion" for human rights violations; and (3) "no single silver bullet can resolve the business and human rights challenge."[30]

In our current climate, where transnational corporations like Pfizer seem intent on fostering protection of intellectual property more than the protection of

people, is there any room for optimism? I think there is. This is because it is becoming critical for transnational corporations to respect human rights for their own sakes. As already discussed, for example, transnational corporations are becoming involved in human rights and bioethics because of their desire to do clinical trials around the world. Corporations may want to set their own rules. But most corporations recognize that they must follow generally accepted international norms of informed consent to conduct their clinical trials if they expect to use the results to have their products certified by government regulators. In short, in at least some cases, transnational corporations must adopt and follow human rights norms to accomplish their business goals. In addition, the human rights and bioethics issues that confront corporations continue to expand, and now include patenting, pricing, and access to their products by people who need them to survive or thrive, but who (either individually or through their governments) simply cannot afford them. These are basic human rights issues that have not been addressed by bioethics.

DeLillo would likely think that human rights and transnational corporations make too unlikely a combination to take seriously. In *Underground*, he saw the transnationals simply taking over from the exhausted Cold War governments. He pictured, for example, waste disposal done in secret by private corporations using underground nuclear explosions. One Kazakhstan company, named Tchaika (meaning seagull, a "nicer name" than rat or pig), is looking for an American broker to recruit US customers:

They want us to supply the most dangerous waste we can find and they will destroy it for us. Depending on the degree of danger, they will charge their customers—the corporation or government or municipality—between three hundred dollars and twelve hundred dollars per kilo. Tchaika is connected to the commonwealth arms complex, to bomb-design laboratories and the shipping industry. They will pick up waste anywhere in the world, ship it to Kazakhstan, put it in the ground and vaporize it. We will get a broker's fee.[31]

DeLillo may be right. And little progress is likely to be made in global health without the active engagement of the transnational corporations. This could be done either through private-public agreements, or by holding transnationals themselves accountable for not only respecting human rights, but also for protecting and fulfilling them in their spheres of business. In real life, Tchaika, for example, should be legally responsible for all the radiation-caused health consequences of its activities, and should therefore seek to prevent them. The currently contested question, of course, is whether transnationals should have obligations to help fulfill human rights as well, including the right to access to the potentially life-saving drugs whose supply and price they control.[32]

The hero of *Netherland,* Chuck Ramkisoon, tells Hans that his dream is to bring peace to the planet (or at least New York City) through cricket: "I'm saying that people, all people, Americans, whoever, are at their most civilized when they're playing cricket. What's the first thing that happens when Pakistan and India make peace? They play a cricket match."[33] Chuck is a dreamer, but has an abiding belief in the cornerstone of human rights: all human are fundamentally the same, and will recognize this fact when they get to know each other.

On a grander scale, Tony Blair entitled his thoughts on 9/11 in *Foreign Affairs,* "A Battle for Global Values." Much in his essay, especially about the continuing wars in Iraq and Afghanistan, is easy to disagree with. But his basic message is sound: We are not in a war that can be won by force of arms. "This is a battle of values [and] we have to show that our values are not Western, still less American or Anglo-Saxon, but values in the common ownership of humanity, universal values that should be the right of the global citizen." A name exists for those universal values that are the "right of the global citizen," and that name is human rights. Blair goes further, noting,

> The challenge now is to ensure that the agenda is not limited to security alone. There is a danger of a division of global politics into "hard" and "soft," with the "hard" efforts going after the terrorists, whereas the "soft" campaign focuses on poverty and injustice. That divide is dangerous because interdependence makes all these issues just that: interdependent. The answer to terrorism is the universal application of global values, and the answer to poverty and injustice is the same. That is why the struggle for global values has to be applied not selectively but to the whole global agenda.[34]

In the sphere of global health, another way to make Blair's point is, as Jonathan Mann put it, health and human rights are inextricably linked.

REFERENCES

1. Harold Koh, Oral Presentation ("Father Drinan's Revolution") at the announcement of the Robert F. Drinan, SJ., Chair in Human Rights, Georgetown University Law Center, October 23, 2006. An early version of this chapter, "Global Health and Post-9/11 Human Rights," was prepared for a May 2007, Workshop on "Values and Moral Experience in Global Health: Bridging the Local and the Global," held at Harvard University.
2. Annas, G.J., Human Rights Outlaws: Nuremberg, Geneva, and the Global War on Terror, *Boston University Law Review* 2007; 87: 427–66.
3. Benatar, S.R. and Fox, R.C., Meeting Threats to Global Health: A Call for American Leadership, *Perspectives in Biology and Medicine* 2005; 48: 344–61.
4. *See generally,* Jonathan Mann, Sofia Gruskin,

Michael Grodin, and George Annas, eds., *Health and Human Rights: A Reader,* New York: Routledge, 1999; Sofia Gruskin, Michael Grodin, George Annas, and Stephen Marks, eds. *Perspectives on Health and Human Rights,* New York: Routledge, 2005; and Mann, J., Health and Human Rights, *Lancet* 1996; 312: 924–25.

5. Farmer, P. and Gastineau, N., Rethinking Health and Human Rights: Time for a Paradigm Shift, *Journal of Law, Medicine & Ethics* 2002; 30: 655–66.

6. Gruskin, S. and Tarantola, D., Health and Human Rights (in) Sofia Gruskin et al., supra note 4 at 3–57.

7. Gruskin, S., What Are Health and Human Rights?, *Lancet 2004;* 363: 329.

8. Annas, G.J., The Rich Have More Money, *Health and Human Rights* 1998; 5: 180–85.

9. Sudhir Anand, Fabienne Peter, and Amartya Sen, eds., *Public Health, Ethics, and Equity,* Oxford: Oxford University Press, 2004. *See also,* Angus Dawson and Marcel Verweij, eds., *Ethics, Prevention, and Public Health,* Oxford: Oxford University Press, 2007; and Ronald Bayer, Lawrence O. Gostin, Bruce Jennings, and Bonnie Steinbock, eds., *Public Health Ethics: Theory, Policy, and Practice,* New York: Oxford University Press, 2007.

10. Madison Powers and Ruth Faden, *Social Justice: The Moral Foundations of Public Health and Health Policy,* New York: Oxford University Press, 2006.

11. Ruger, J.P., Ethics and Governance of Global Health Inequalities, *Journal of Epidemiology and Community Health* 2006; 60: 998–1003.

12. Ruger, J.P., Toward a Theory of a Right to Health: Capability and Incompletely Theorized Agreements, *Yale Journal of Law & the Humanities* 2006; 18: 273–326. On the "right to health" *see* General Comment No. 14: The Right to the Highest Attainable Standard of Health (Article 12 of the International Covenant on Economic Social and Cultural Rights; July 4, 2000) reprinted in Sofia Gruskin et al., supra note 4 at 473–95; Judith Asher, *The Right to Health: A Resource Manual for NGOs,* London: British Medical Association, 2004; Backman, G., Hunt, P., Khorla, R. et al., Health Systems and the Right to Health: An Assessment of 194 Countries, *Lancet* 2008; 372: 2047–85; Andrew Clapham and Mary Robinson, eds., *Realizing the Right to Health,* Zurich: Ruffer & Rub, 2009.

13. *Compare* Louis Henkin, *The Age of Rights,* New York: Columbia University Press, 1990.

14. Kennedy, D., The International Human Rights Movement: Part of the Problem?, *Harvard Human Rights Journal 2002;* 15: 101–40.

15. Kunz, J., The United Nations Declaration of Human Rights, *American Journal of International Law* 1949; 43: 316–22. For a persuasive argument that the rights set forth in the UDHR are inherent in human beings as humans. *See* Johannes Morsink, *Inherent Human Rights: Philosophical Roots of the Universal Declaration,* Philadelphia: University of Pennsylvania Press, 2009.

16. Glickman, S.W., McHutchison, J.G., Peterson, E.D., et al., Ethical and Scientific Implications of the Globalization of Clinical Research, *New England Journal of Medicine* 2009; 360: 816–23. This section, on the Pfizer litigation, is based on Annas, GJ., Globalized Clinical Trails and Informed Consent, *New England Journal of Medicine* 2009; 360: 2050–53.

17. Angell, M., The Ethics of Clinical Research in the Third World, *New England Journal of Medicine* 1997; 337: 847–49. *See generally,* Adriana Pertryna, *When Experiments Travel: Clinical Trials and the Global Search for Human Subjects,* Princeton: Princeton University Press, 2009.

18. Kimmelman, J., Weijer, C., and Meslin, E.M., Helsinki Discords: FDA, Ethics, and International Drug Trials, *Lancet* 2009; 373: 13–14.

19. Stephens, J., Where Profits and Lives Hang in the Balance; Finding an Abundance of Subjects and Lack of Oversight Abroad, Big Drug Companies Test Offshore to Speed Products to Market, *Washington Post,* December 17, 2000, A1.

20. *Abdullahi v. Pfizer,* 562 F.3d 163 (2d Cir. 2009).

21. *Filartiga v. Pena-Irala,* 630 F.2d 876 (2d Cir. 1980).

22. *Sosa v. Alvarez-Machain,* 542 U.S. 466 (2004).

23. *See, e.g.,* Roberts, L., Polio: Looking for a Little Luck, *Science* 2009; 323: 702–705.

24. Powers and Faden, supra note 10.

25. Physicians for Human Rights, *The Taliban's War on Women: A Health and Human Rights Crisis in Afghanistan.* Boston: Physicians for Human Rights 1998. *See also,* Audrey Chapman and Leonard Rubenstein, eds., *Human Rights and Health: The Legacy of Apartheid,* New York: American Association for the Advancement of Science, 1998.

26. *See* the Commission's website for this and other reports, www.aihrc.org.af. *See also* Samar, S., Despite the Odds: Providing Reproductive Health Care to Afghan Women, *New England Journal of Medicine* 2004; 351: 1047–49.

27. Cook, R., Gender, Health and Human Rights. *Health and Human Rights* 1995; 1: 350–66.

28. George J. Annas, *American Bioethics: Crossing Human Rights and Health Law Boundaries.* New York: Oxford University Press, 2005, 159–66.

29. Irene Khan summarized the situation regarding transnational corporations and human rights well in her foreword to Amnesty International's 2007 Annual Report, which she titled "Freedom from Fear": "Corporations have long resisted binding international standards. The United Nations must confront the challenge, and develop standards and promote mechanisms that hold big business accountable for its impact on human rights. The need for global standards and effective accountability becomes even more urgent as multinational corporations from diverse legal and cultural systems emerge in a global market" (at 4).

30. United Nations, Human Rights Council (4th sess. It. 2), *Business and Human Rights: Mapping International Standards of Responsibility and Accountability for Corporate Acts*, Feb. 19, 2007. For a more skeptical view *see*, Adriana Petryna, Andrew Lakoff, and Arthur Kleinman, eds., *Global Pharmaceuticals: Ethics, Markets,* *Practices*, Durham: Duke University Press, 2006.

31. Don DeLillo, *Underworld*, New York: Scribner, 1997, 788.

32. For an account of MSF's campaign to lower drug prices for the resource poor world *see* James Orbinski, *An Imperfect Offering: Humanitarian Action for the Twenty-First Century*, New York: Walker & Company, 2008, 351–79.

33. Joseph O'Neill, *Netherland*, New York: Pantheon Books, 2008, 211.

34. Blair, T., A Battle for Global Values, *Foreign Affairs* 2007, 79–90. It is worth noting that Telford Taylor used similar language describing the Nazi atrocities in his opening statement at the Doctors' Trial at Nuremburg: "The perverse thoughts and distorted concepts which brought about these savageries are not dead. They cannot be killed by force of arms. They must not become a spreading cancer in the breast of humanity. They must be cut out and exposed . . . ."

QUESTIONS

1. How do you think 9/11 impacted on the promotion and protection of international human rights? Do you think this change is permanent or temporary? Comment on the premise that there must be a balance between civil rights and security, and we must trade off at least some of our human rights for security from terrorists.

2. The author raises questions about the role of transnational corporations in human rights. What do you think the obligations of transnational corporations are in relation to health and human rights, and how might they be monitored and enforced? Can corporations be guilty of war crimes and crimes against humanity?

3. Do you think there are major differences between a social justice approach to health problems and a health and human rights approach? Explain.

FURTHER READING

Powers, Madison & Faden, Ruth, *Social Justice*. New York: Oxford University Press, 2006.

Annas, G.J., *Worst Case Bioethics: Death, Destruction and Public Health*, New York: Oxford University Press, 2010.

London, L., Kagee, A., Moodley, K., & Swartz, L., Ethics, Human Rights and HIV Vaccine Trials in Low-income Settings. *Journal of Medical Ethics*, 2012; 38: 286–293.

Bostrom, Nick & Cirkovic, Milan, eds., *Global Catastrophic Risks*. Oxford: Oxford University Press, 2008.

PART II

Concepts, Methods and Governance

Introduction

The field of health and human rights is relatively new. Despite increased attention begin-ning in the 1990s, efforts made to bring public health and human rights together have fallen short of the demand; there still exists a lack of methods and tools to evidence the relationships between health and rights. Globally, the principles of health and human rights have found their way to a variety of national, institutional and international poli-cies and programs. However, insufficient attention has been devoted to exploring and documenting the extent to which these intents have been translated into practice. States are historically more inclined to express statements of commitment than to induce real changes. Rapid progress must be made to acknowledge the mutually reinforcing rela-tionships between health and rights. Already, skepticism has grown in some sectors about the practicality and "value added" of such approaches. Commonly, in order to enact public policy or program changes advocated by civil society advocates, states give them, in particular academia, the task of producing the evidence supporting the proposed changes. The "burden of proof" of the "added value" of human rights rests on the shoulders of advocates, even though states have to uphold international human rights principles, norms and standards and deliver their related obligations. To respond to such demands requires experience, skills and financial resources that are chronically lacking in this domain within both government circles and civil society. To change this state of affairs and impact the quality of governance, the concepts and methods underly-ing the health and human rights conundrum must be exposed, improved, applied and disseminated.

The purpose of this part is to illustrate the interconnectedness of public health goals and human rights principles, as well as to provide conceptual and methodological frame-works. In doing this, we hope to stimulate interest among readers to engage in reflection, debate, practice, evaluation and research. Most of all, the following chapters have been selected to advance the understanding of health and human rights using new evidence and analytical frameworks. In this regard, it is worth noting that more evidence has been published to underscore the negative impacts of overt human rights violations than the positive impacts of the realization of rights. Establishing causation or even association between a documented human rights violation and its health outcomes is rarely an easy matter. Even more difficult to demonstrate is the attribution of a health outcome—posi-tive or negative—to the fulfilment of one or more human rights, or, conversely, that a desirable health outcome has contributed to progress in human rights. This invokes definitional and methodological questions such as: Which right should be invoked? Which particular health outcome? What criteria, indicators or descriptors would best reflect the enjoyment of human rights? How does one minimize confounders when uncontrolled contextual changes have occurred?

At the outset of this part, the chapter by Gruskin and Tarantola traces this evolution and its particular attention to underserved and marginalized populations. It sets out the reality of what linking health and human rights has meant to date, and discusses programmatic applications of "rights-based" approaches to health. Noting "the erosion of the distinctions between classes of rights lies at the heart of much of the ESC rights jurisprudence from the 1990s, including both national- and international-level jurisprudence relating to the right to health," Yamin examines the extent to which litigations around issues of access to medicines have demonstrated, against common beliefs, the justiciability of economic, social and cultural rights, the right to health in particular, and have impacted on public policy. Along the same line of thought, Hogertzeil and colleagues present a practical example of how international human rights principles, norms and standards can be brought to bear on public health policy. This work describes how the courts have helped enforce access to essential medicines in some countries and possibly deterred the violations of this normative component of the right to health in others. This is one of several chapters in this book that speak to how structural barriers to progress in health and human rights can be overcome. The newly established Global Commission on HIV and the Law, on which Dalhiwal comments, is an important global mechanism to "examine the impact of law on HIV responses, to catalyze action at the country level, and to create legal environments which protect and promote human rights." Even as the Commission's first report was being prepared and not formally released, greater attention was drawn in a number of countries to old, new and prospective laws impacting or likely to impact positively or negatively on the lives of people living with and vulnerable to HIV. Taken together, human rights-based approaches and the use of the law to enforce state obligations are avenues towards greater governmental responsiveness and accountability, and progress in both health and human rights.

Population health status and outcomes are determined more strongly by social and economic factors than by health-focused interventions. From this perspective, health, human rights and human development are symbiotic. An analytical and action-oriented framework linking these three domains is presented by Tarantola and colleagues. MDGs were intended to underscore the interconnectedness of development, health, and human rights in order to combat proverty. The human rights dimensions of these challenges seem to have come as an afterthought, even though the conceptors of the MDGs were UN entities charged to promote and monitor human rights. Langford proposes six ways to fix the MDGs by placing human rights squarely in the development equation, including in the ways development priorities are determined, framed, acted upon and accounted for. O'Malley notes the weak attention to human rights in both the MDGs and the report of the WHO Commission on the Social Determinants of Health, and calls for bold action to overcome "obstacles hindering action, including limitations in the evidence base, complexity of program design, limitations to national and international health governance, disconnects between the worlds of health and human rights, and of course power and politics." In turn, Pemberton and colleagues explain concretely how the human rights framework can help reduce child poverty and improve child survival rates more effectively than through narrowly designed public health and medical interventions. The authors argue that while child rights constitute a useful theoretical and political tool, some rights should have priority over others so that "child rights may move from the realms of rhetoric to those of tangible reality."

Documenting health and human rights processes and outcomes raises issues of assessment, both quantitatively and qualitatively. Responding to this need, several institutions (the UN OHCHR among others) have embarked on the development of monitoring and evaluation indicators which bring health and human rights together. To ensure that the internal and external validity of data is acceptable by both fields, such indicators need to satisfy several criteria. Some of the complexities in developing monitoring and evaluation indicators as well as the criteria that can be used to do this are highlighted by Gruskin and Ferguson. Importantly, these authors too emphasize the need for a bold move from rhetoric to practice through the practical use of monitoring and evaluation data to enhance accountability and advance policies and programs. Monitoring and evaluating human rights-based approaches to health is an open and challenging field of research and practice in which readers are strongly encouraged to engage.

Among evaluation methods that are under development, the incorporation of human rights in Health Impact Assessment (HIA) may be one tool to project the effects of public policies or programs on both health and human rights outcomes. Gay discusses the pros and cons of using health as an entry point and the main focus of HIA by examining the determinants of health and some projected health outcomes and, alternatively, using human rights as entry points, assessing their direct or indirect impacts on health outcomes through a Human Rights Impact Assessment (HRIA). While concerns regarding overextending the scope of HIA have been voiced by a number of authors in recent years, others have advocated establishing more strongly and assessing, from the outset of policy development, the interaction between health and human rights, and even extending it to human development, both conceptually and methodologically.

In light of the deepening global economic crises and the widening development gap, heath and human rights rhetoric must avoid isolating public health work from development and human rights. The expanding realization that health, development and human rights are intrinsically linked has been debated and written about extensively in the last two decades. Yet, existing international health governance structures and mechanisms have only partly succeeded in bridging the dual health and development gap. Has the time come to recast the concept of duty bearers and obligations in global health and restructure its governance? As Friedman and Gostin suggest, is there a need for a binding universal framework convention on global health that encompasses its human rights dimensions and defines the roles and responsibilities of all actors in global health to achieve "Health for All, Justice for All"?

TOPICS FOR DISCUSSION

1. What mechanisms would you consider effective in order to induce government awareness about, and commitment to, upholding their human rights and health obligations?

2. You are now going to role-play as you have been invited to take part in a policy development group in any country of your choice. You may wish to assign among yourselves the roles of a community representative, a human rights advocate, a public health leader, a representative of the Chamber of Commerce, or the head of government. How would you each state your position regarding a proposal to introduce and implement a new policy and program aimed at protecting children against passive tobacco smoking? If there are opposing views, what approaches would you suggest to achieve the best health and human rights outcome of such a policy and program with maximum support from all constituencies?

3. Having read the chapters of this part and some of its suggested readings, can you list and summarize some of the progress that has been achieved in moving from the rhetoric of health and human rights and the launching of the health and human rights movement to the application of concepts and methods in practice? Can you list and summarize some of the pitfalls that have hampered this progress? What are the main opportunities and barriers to inscribing health and human rights in development agendas and in governance?

CHAPTER 8

Bringing Human Rights into Public Health

Sofia Gruskin and Daniel Tarantola

INTRODUCTION

What role do human rights have in public health work? Since the early stages of the women's health, reproductive health, and indigenous health movements it has been asserted that public health policies and programs must be cognizant and respectful of human rights norms and standards. It has also been stated that lack of respect for human rights hampers the effectiveness of pubic health policies and programs. For the last decade or so, an interdisciplinary 'health and human rights' movement has been generating scholarship and inspiring programming intended to realize "the highest attainable standard of health" (UN International Covenant on Economic, Social, and Cultural Rights, 1966; Gruskin and Tarantola, 2001) with a particular focus on the most underserved and marginalized populations and human rights language has been integrated into numerous national and international public health strategies, such as those embraced by UNAIDS (2005, 2006). Yet moving beyond the rhetoric, there is still diversity of opinion as to what this means in practice.

Given that many public health practitioners are interested in the application of human rights to their work even as they are unsure what besides having a good heart

this means for their efforts, as a first step an understanding of some aspects of human rights is necessary. In the present chapter we attempt to set out what application of these concepts has meant to date in practice, discuss 'rights-based' approaches to health, and suggest questions and concerns for the future.

Although this chapter will not seek to incorporate bioethical frameworks into the discussion, it is important to recognize the long-standing relationship of those working in bioethics and those working in human rights in relation to health (see, e.g., UNESCO, 2005). The two fields are distinct, but they do overlap particularly in relation to instituting international guidelines for research via professional norm-setting modes. Human rights and ethics in health are closely linked, both conceptually and operationally (Mann, 1999; Gruskin and Dickens, 2006). Each provides unique, valuable, and concrete guidance for the actions of national and international organizations focused on health and development. Public health workers should appreciate their distinct value, but also the differences in the paradigms they represent in particular with respect to means of observance, action, and enforcement. The similarities and differences between bioethics and human rights frameworks for strengthening protections in relation to health are beginning to be explored but are outside the scope of the present chapter.

In the work of public health we have learned that explicit attention to human rights shows us not only who is disadvantaged and who is not, but also whether a given disparity in health outcomes results from an injustice. Human rights are now understood to offer a frame-work for action and for programming, as well as providing a compelling argument for government responsibility—not only to provide health services but also to alter the conditions that create, exacerbate, and perpetuate poverty, deprivation, marginalization, and discrimination (Gruskin and Braveman, 2005). A diverse array of actors are increasingly finding innovative ways to relate human rights principles to health-related work, thereby demonstrating how a human rights perspective can yield new insights and more effective ways of addressing health needs within country settings as well as in the policy and programmatic guidance offered at the global level.

APPROACHES TO BRINGING HUMAN RIGHTS INTO HEALTH WORK

Over time it has become clear that people tend to work in a variety of ways to further work on health and human rights, and that while some take health as an entry point, others take human rights and no one approach has primacy as the only way to make these connections. Despite this diversity, the frameworks within which they operate can be generally assigned to four broad categories: advocacy, legal, policy, and programs. We summarize each framework briefly as follows.

Advocacy Frameworks

Advocacy is a key component of many organizations' work in health and human rights. Work in the advocacy category can be described as using the language of rights to draw attention to an issue, mobilize public opinion and advocate for change in the actions of governments and other institutions of power. Advocacy efforts may call for the implementation of rights even if they are not yet in fact established by law, and in so doing serve to move governmental and inter-governmental bodies closer to legitimizing these issues as legally enforceable human rights claims. This means also linking of activists working on issues related to health (such as groups focused on violence against women, poverty and global trade issues), reaching out to policy makers and other influential groups, translating international human rights norms to the work and concerns of local communities, and supporting the organizing capabilities of affected communities to push for change in legal and political structures. An example of an advocacy approach is the People's Health Movement (PHM), a civil society initiative created in 2000, bringing together individuals and organizations committed to the implementation of the Alma-Ata Declaration on Primary Health Care (Declaration of Alma-Ata, 1978; The People's Health Charter, 2005). In 2006, The PHM launched a campaign "To promote the Health for All goal through an equitable, participatory and intersectoral movement and as a rights issue" (Right to Health and Health Care Campaign, 2006).

Legal Frameworks

This approach prioritizes the role of human rights law at international and national levels in producing norms, standards, and accountability in health-related efforts. This includes engaging with law in the formal sense, including building on the consonance between national law and international human rights norms, for example, to promote and protect the rights of people living with HIV/AIDS through litigation and other means. Pursuing legal accountability through national law and international treaty obligations often takes the form of analyzing what a government is or is not doing in relation to health and how this might constitute a violation of rights, seeking remedies in national and international courts and tribunals and focusing on transparency, accountability, and functioning norms and systems to promote and protect health-related rights. Examples of a legal approach include recent court cases in Latin America and in South Africa focused on access to antiretroviral therapy by people living with HIV, invoking in particular the right to life and the right to health (Carrasco, 2000; Nattrass, 2006). There, constitutional provisions and international human rights treaties were used to challenge the inaction or opposition of governments to the procurement and availability of drugs alleged to be beyond the economic means of the state or, in the case of South Africa, lacking scientific evidence of their safety and efficacy (Elliott, 2002; PAHO, 2006).

Policy Frameworks

This approach looks to instituting human rights norms and standards mostly through global and national policymaking bodies from health, economic, and development perspectives. These include human rights norms or language as it appears in the documents and strategies that emanate from these bodies as well as the approach taken to operationalize human rights work within an organization's individual programs and departments. In addition to the inclusion of human rights norms within recent global consensus documents such as the UN General Assembly Special Session on AIDS (UN, 2006), a large and growing number of national and international entities have formulated rights-based approaches to health in the context of their own efforts. Among

these are several official development assistance organizations and agencies, funds, and programs of the United Nations System. (These agencies include UNAIDS, UNICEF, UNDP, UNFPA, DFID, as well as Canadian CIDA and Swedish SIDA.)

Programmatic Frameworks

This approach is concerned with the implementation of rights in health programming. This includes the design, implementation, monitoring, and evaluation of health programs, including what issues are prioritized and why, at different stages of the work. Often these efforts are carried out by large international organizations, including both inter-governmental and nongovernmental entities. In general, work in this category refers to inclusion of key human rights components within programmatic initiatives and in daily practice such as ensuring attention to the participation of affected communities, nondiscrimination in how policies and programs are carried out, attention to the legal and policy context within which the program is taking place, transparency in how priorities were set and decisions were made, and accountability for the results. Examples with respect to this category are discussed in more detail below.

As the health and human rights field has become more strongly rooted in robust human rights principles and sound public health, it is appropriate that such different interpretations and applications to practice are coming forward. This has, however, unfortunately, in many ways fuelled the lack of clarity as to what added-value human rights offer to public health work. Despite significant differences, work which falls under these different rubrics is often amalgamated under what is called a 'rights-based approach' to health, and these are in themselves 'all over the map,' whether encompassing legal, advocacy, or programmatic efforts. One can say that it is a great accomplishment of all those who have fostered the dialogue around 'rights-based approaches to health' that this term is now being used to characterize such a wide range of activities. A great challenge is that the term is used in very different ways by different institutions and individuals. At worst, the inconsistencies in how 'rights-based approaches to health' are conceptualized threaten to undo major accomplishments. At best, the diversity in interpretation of what is meant by 'rights-based approaches to health' means the field is alive and well.

THE ELUSIVE RIGHTS-BASED APPROACH TO HEALTH

Ultimately much of the work to bring human rights into public health is looking at synergies and trade-offs between health and human rights and working, within a framework of transparency and accountability, toward achieving the highest attainable standard of health. Central in all settings are the principles of nondiscrimination, equality, and to the extent possible the genuine participation of affected communities. This does not mean a one-size-fits-all approach. In addition to differences in frameworks, the rights issues and the appropriateness of policies and programs relevant to one setting with one population might not be so in a different setting to another.

Initially conceptualized in the mid-1990s as a 'human rights based approach to development programming' by the United Nations Development Programme (UNDP, 1998), rights-based approaches have been applied to specific populations (e.g., children, women, migrants, refugees, and indigenous populations), basic needs (e.g., food, water, security, education, and justice), health issues (e.g., sexual and reproductive health, HIV, access to medicines), sources of livelihood (e.g., land tenure, pastoral development, and fisheries), and the work of diverse actors engaged in development activities (e.g., UN system, governments, NGOs, corporate sector). Even as health cuts across all of these areas and is regarded both as a prerequisite for and an important outcome of development, the understanding of what a rights-based approach actually means for public health efforts varies across sectors, disciplines, and organizations.

In order to define the core principles of rights-based approaches (RBAs) applicable across all sectors of development, including health, a "Common Understanding" was elaborated by the UN system in 2003 (UN, 2003). In short, it suggests that the following points are critical for identifying a rights-based approach: all programs should intentionally further international human rights; all development efforts, at all levels of programming, must be guided by human rights standards and principles founded in international human rights law; and all development efforts must build the capacity of "duty bearers" to meet obligations and/or "rights holders" to claim rights (UN, 2003 May).

UN Statement of Common Understanding of the Human Rights-Based Approach to Development

1. All programmes of development cooperation, policies and technical assistance should further the realisation of human rights as laid down in the Universal Declaration of Human Rights and other international human rights instruments.
2. Human rights standards contained in, and principles derived from the Universal Declaration of Human Rights and other international human rights instruments guide all development cooperation and programming in all sectors and in all phases of the programming process.
3. Development cooperation contributes to the development of the capacities of 'duty-bearers' to meet their obligations and/or of 'rights-holders' to claim their rights.

This common understanding has clear implications for the implementation of health policies and programs because it offers a common way of thinking although, even within the health domain, the interpretation of what these programs actually mean in practice remains far from universal. A review of public health programs termed 'rights based' by a range of UN system actors and their partners points to several areas relevant to what implementation of a rights-based approach to health might look like (Annotated Bibliography, n.d.). A rights-based approach to health makes explicit reference to human rights from the outset, does not invent the content of rights, and does not name the relevance of rights in retrospect; it emphasizes building capacity and does not use human rights norms as a way to name violations after they occur but as a way to prevent violations from occurring in the first place; and it is based on implementation of one or several core rights concepts, including nondiscrimination, participation, accountability, and transparency.

Anchoring public health strategies in human rights can enrich the concepts and methods used to attain health objectives by drawing attention to the legal and policy context within which health interventions occur, as well as bringing in rights principles such as nondiscrimination and the participation of affected communities in the design, implementation, monitoring, and evaluation of health systems, programs, and other interventions. In addition, it allows for governments and intergovernmental agencies to be held publicly accountable for their actions and inactions. The introduction of human rights into public health work is about approaches and processes and their application toward maximum public health gains. It does not mean how the work is done or what its ultimate outcome will be is preordained to be a certain way. For example, using human rights standards with a focus on health systems requires attention to their availability, accessibility, acceptability, quality, and outcomes among different population groups (General Comment no. 14, 2000). These terms have concrete implications:

- Availability demands that public health and health-care facilities, goods, and services, as well as programs be offered to the maximum availability of resources available to governments. These resources may originate from public funding sources or international aid.
- Accessibility requires that health facilities, goods, and services be attainable by everyone without discrimination, including gender and other recognized forms of discrimination as well as socioeconomic status, the community to which they belong, and the distance they live from an urban area.
- Acceptability calls for health facilities, goods, and services to be culturally and otherwise appropriate for the intended populations.
- Finally, health facilities, goods, and services must be scientifically and medically appropriate and of the optimal quality.

Although none of the above should be unfamiliar to those working in public health, the added value of a human rights approach to health is in systematizing attention to these issues, requiring that benchmarks and targets be set to guarantee that any targets set are realized progressively, and ensuring transparency and accountability for what decisions are made and their ultimate outcomes.

RIGHTS-BASED APPROACHES TO HEALTH IN PRACTICE

Bringing health and human rights together provides a framework within which the progress, success, or failure of a policy or program can be developed and evaluated against both public health and human rights benchmarks. In practice, the assessment, design, implementation, monitoring, and evaluation of any health policy, strategy, and program or intervention should incorporate the key components of a rights-based approach.

Public health and human rights practitioners are increasingly working to transform a commitment to health and rights into an agenda for action with respect to the development, design, implementation, monitoring, and evaluation of policies, programs, and interventions. Table 8.1 is given as an example of how the connections between sound public health and human rights norms and standards can be explicitly established and strengthened. It represents an attempt to outline a process whereby points of convergence and possible tensions between health and rights practices may emerge. It schematically divides the field into five elements, including policy and legal context; situation assessment and analysis; policy, program, or intervention design; implementation; and monitoring and evaluation. It proposes questions that would allow each of these elements to be examined from the perspective of key components of a rights-based approach selected for their relevance to both public health and human rights: participation, attention to the most vulnerable populations, nondiscrimination, and accountability. This table is merely intended to help systematize and present examples of the questions that a rights-based approach to health would ask at each stage of engagement. It is in no way intended to be exhaustive, and if used in practice would require adaptation with respect to the specific health or disability issue considered.

A rights-based approach to health therefore can guide choices about what should be done and how it should be done, for example when applied locally to an insti-tutional or community setting. As with other approaches applied to public health programming efforts, it aims to achieve congruence in responding to individual and collective health needs but also seeks to advance the promotion and protection of human rights. Applying a rights-based approach is only one tool in doing effective public health work. It does not, in and of itself, establish priorities among programs competing for resources, each of which arguably would improve health and the satisfaction of relevant rights, nor does it determine the best way to intervene once a particular intervention has been agreed upon. A rights-based approach will be strongest when used in conjunction with empirical assessment of the complex epidemiological, economic, management, and other information relevant to deciding how resources can most effectively be used and what kinds of improvements in population health should be emphasized.

CONCLUSION

Considerable progress has been achieved in the last decade in understanding and promoting rights-based approaches to health. The last few years, however, have seen a worrisome trend where, in some quarters, the inadequate success of public health strategies in areas ranging from HIV/AIDS to child survival is blamed on "unnecessary attention to human rights" (De Cock et al., 2002). Although those arguments may be vague, unfocused, and often based on misinterpretations of how human rights and health actually operate, the skepticism driving such arguments will need to be addressed in the coming years. Greater clarity about the central paradigms of health and human rights is essential to make this work more effective, as well as to enable the framing of counter-arguments that will not only be persuasive to the skeptics but useful to the public health community at large. A benefit then of considering different ways of conceptualizing and pursuing rights-based approaches to health alongside one another is that when considering different initiatives that claim to be 'rights-based' it is possible to get a clearer sense of what work is being done but also what work is needed to move the field of health and human rights in the direction of greater clarity. The idea is not to impose one definition of rights-based approaches to health over another, but rather to encourage a discussion about how efforts among different actors working in health and human rights can be better aligned. A preliminary step is to examine these differences rather than to obscure them.

Of critical importance is documentation of the effectiveness of rights-based approaches to health; that is, presentation of solid evidence of how human rights approaches to public health initiatives have actually strengthened those initiatives and informed sound public health practice rather than acting as deterrents. The rights-based approaches to health currently under way in a number of institutions should be examined and validated to ensure clarity in what are understood to be the strengths and limitations of the ways they bring human rights into governmental, nongovernmental, and international health work. Efforts are needed to collect and analyze data to demonstrate how human rights have been relevant to every aspect of public health programming ranging from the analysis of the health and health needs of a population to the ways health systems performance assessments are done. Research is then needed not only to expand the evidence already available that infringements on human rights negatively affect health, but that the enjoyment of human rights—all human rights—has beneficial impacts on health and well-being.

It is through such efforts that the ability to generate the evidence of the effectiveness of rights-based approaches to health will occur. The challenge is now to harness the power of human rights to improve the work of public health in all domains. This will require marshalling the skills and commitment of the entire public health community. While embracing the differences in how rights-based approaches are operationalized, the task is now to ensure that public health and human rights continue to come together in strong, powerful, and practical ways.

REFERENCES

Carrasco E (2000) Access to treatment as a right to life and health. International Conference on AIDS, 9–14; 13 July. Abst. no. TuOrE458.gateway.nlm.nih.gov/MeetingAbstracts/d102239925.html (accessed December 2007).

Declaration of Alma-Ata (1978) International Conference of Primary Health Care, Alma-Ata, USSR, 6–12 September 1978.

De Cock KM, Mbori-Ngacha D, and Marum M (2002) Shadow on the continent: public health and HIV/AIDS in Africa in the 21st century. *The Lancet* 360: 67–72.

Elliott R (2002) Inter-American Commission on Human Rights hold hearing on access to treatment in Latin America and the Caribbean. *Canadian HIV/AIDS Policy and Law Review* 17: 66.

General Comment No. 14. (2000) The right to the highest attainable standard of health (article 12 of the International Covenant on Economic, Social and Cultural Rights). E/C.12/2000/4, CESCR.

Gruskin S (2006) Rights-based approaches to health: Something for everyone. *Health and Human Rights* 19: 5–9.

Gruskin S and Braveman P (2005) Addressing social injustice in a human rights context. In: Sidel V and Levy B (eds.) *Social Injustice and Public Health*, pp. 405–417. London/New York: Oxford University Press.

Gruskin S and Dickens B (2006) Human rights and ethics in public health. *American Journal of Public Health* 96(11): 1903–1905.

Gruskin S and Tarantola D (2001) Health and human rights. In: Detels R and Beaglehole R (eds.) *Oxford Textbook on Public Health*, pp. 311–335. London/New York: Oxford University Press.

Mann JM (1999) Medicine and public health, ethics and human rights. In: Mann JM, Gurskin S, Grodin MA, and Annas GJ (eds.) *Health And Human Rights: A Reader*, pp. 439–452. New York: Routledge.

Table 8.1 Applying a rights-based approach to public health: Examples of questions to be addressed to ensure maximum congruence between public health and human rights

Public health elements	Human rights elements			
	Participation	*Attention to most vulnerable populations*	*Non-discrimination*	*Accountability*
1. Policy and legal context	Is participation of communities and interest groups supported by law and policy? Have communities been exposed to or disproportionately affected by the health issue in question, been invited to contribute to the drafting of policies concerning them?	Do policies refer to specific vulnerable populations with regards to health, disability, and social and economic determinants? Have the structures, processes and needed resources been made available to translate these policies and laws into practice?	Are policies and laws discriminatory with regards to ill health and its recognized social and economic determinants, practices, and impacts? Are there policies and laws that specifically oppose discrimination on the grounds of health or disability status and their recognized social determinants, practices, and impacts? Are there monitoring, claims, and redress mechanisms in place?	Have policies and laws been debated through political processes and in public fora? Are policies, programs, and interventions consistent with the law and human rights norms and standards? Have policies and laws been translated into decrees or other instruments to make them effective? Is a reporting mechanism in place to address claims of violations of policies and laws? Is a functioning judicial process in place to handle these claims? Have efforts been made to alert people about policies and laws specific relevant to them?
2. Analysis of the health situation of a particular population or of a specific public health problem	Have members of concerned governmental sectors, private sector, and civil society organizations participated in the design of the study?	Has the situation assessment recognized populations most vulnerable to ill health or disability and focused on assessing	Is the situation assessment in any way discriminatory in its aim, design, conduct, and analysis?	How and by whom will the results of the analysis be disseminated among political leaders, professional groups, communities, and the media? Will the situation

	Has attention been devoted to ensure that populations affected by ill health or their representatives have participated in the design of situation assessments?	their situation, needs and capacity? Have factors leading to increased vulnerability to ill-health and disability been appropriately mapped out and incorporated in the design of the situation analysis?		assessment be carried out by competent and trustworthy entities? Has the existing body of evidence informed the situation assessment design? Is the presentation of results sensitive to the risk of aggravating discrimination? If so, what mechanism has been put in place to minimize this risk?
3. Process of devising a public policy, program, or intervention	Has public information and consultation been included in the steps taken to devise the policy, program, or intervention? Have divergent views been taken into consideration before a final decision was reached?	Have communities particularly concerned with the health or disability issue participated in policy, program, or intervention design? What benefits and risks from the policy, program, or interventions could accrue to communities particularly vulnerable to or affected by the health or disability issue? Are sufficient attention and resources devoted to the meet the needs of vulnerable populations?	Is the design of the policy, program, or intervention, in any way discriminatory? Are there legitimate restrictions of rights being considered as part of the policy, program, or intervention? If so, what process has been put in place to legitimize such restrictions?	Is the development of policy, program, intervention openly discussed with vulnerable communities or their representatives? If restrictions of rights have been pronounced in the interest of public health, has there been a clear presentation of the reasons for and process applied to such decisions? Have the authorities responsible for designing the policy, program, or intervention been made known to the public? Does the policy, program, or intervention meet the criteria of availability, accessibility, acceptability, and quality

Table 8.1 (Continued)

Public health elements	Human rights elements			
	Participation	*Attention to most vulnerable populations*	*Non-discrimination*	*Accountability*
				in the way it responds to the needs of the population? Does the design of the policy, program, or intervention include targets and benchmarks to measure progress in relation to availability, accessibility, acceptability, and quality of services?
4. Implementation of policy, program, or intervention on health and disability	Are public information, education and participation effectively included in policy, program, or intervention implementation? Have actors in health systems and other relevant sectors been educated, trained, and equipped to implement the policy, program, or intervention in a health and human rights sensitive fashion?	Are particularly vulnerable or affected communities engaged in implementing the policy, program, or intervention? Is implementation of the policy, program, or intervention striving towards greater availability, accessibility, acceptability, and quality of services among these populations?	Is implementation of the policy, program, or intervention discriminatory in its application? In what forms is such discrimination perpetrated? In what setting and by what actors? How can discrimination in implementation of the policy, program, or intervention be combated? What plans have been made and resources allocated to combat active discrimination?	Does the implementation of the policy, program, or intervention meet the criteria of availability, accessibility, acceptability, and quality in the way it responds to the needs of the population?
5. A framework within which	Have targets been set and success	Have targets been set	Is the monitoring and evalua-	Is there a mechanism to monitor

the success or failure of a policy or program can be evaluated, against both public health and human rights benchmarks

and failure been defined with public participation?

and success and failure been defined with the participation of vulnerable or affected communities or their representatives?

Is implementation meeting the needs of these populations to the maximum of available resources?

Are monitoring and evaluation systems efficiently monitoring and evaluating availability, accessibility, acceptability, and quality of services among these populations?

tion system designed to detect causes, practices, and impacts of discriminatory actions?

Are claims on grounds of discrimination heard and taken into account in the monitoring and evaluation process?

and evaluate the implementation and impacts of the policy, program, or intervention according to set criteria of availability, accessibility, acceptability, and quality?

Have processes been planned and resourced to measure the impact of the policy, program, or intervention put in place?

Are these findings made public?

Are the impacts on health of any potential violations of human rights researched and documented?

Has the policy, program, or intervention contributed to the promotion of human rights, including the right to health?

Has the policy, program, or intervention contributed to progress in the realization of other human rights?

Are these findings used to inform needed changes or adjustments in policy, program, or interventions both within and outside the health sector?

Nattrass N (2006) *AIDS, Science and Governance: The Battle over Antiretroviral Therapy in Post-Apartheid South Africa.* AIDS and Society Research Unit, University of Cape Town, 19 March 2006.

PAHO (2006) Latin America Legislation and Milestones in Access to Antiretroviral Treatment in Latin America and the Caribbean.

Right to Health and Health Care Campaign (2006) *The People's Health Charter* (2000) Formulated and endorsed by the participants of the First People's Health Assembly, Dhaka, Bangladesh, December 2000.

UN (1966) *International Covenant on Economic, Social and Cultural Rights.* adopted 16 Dec. 1966, 993 U.N.T.S. 3 (entered into force 3 Jan. 1976), G.A. Res. 2200 (XXI), 21 U.N. GAOR Supp. (No. 16) at 49, UN Doc. A/6316 (1966). See art. 11.

UN (2003) *The Statement on a Common Understanding of a Human Rights Based Approach to Development Cooperation.* as agreed the Stamford Workshop and endorsed by the UNDG Programme Group.

UN (2003) *The Human Rights-based Approach to Development Cooperation Towards a Common Understanding among the UN Agencies ('Common Understanding')"* (outcome document from an interagency workshop on a Human Rights-based Approach in the context of UN reform 3–5 May 2003)

UN (2006) *Political Declaration on HIV/AIDS.* GA Res. 60/262, UN GAOR, 60th Sess., UN Doc. A/RES/60/262, (2006).

UNAIDS (2005) *Intensifying HIV Prevention.* UNAIDS policy position paper. UNAIDS/05.18E. August 2005.

UNAIDS (2006) *Scaling up Access to HIV Prevention, Treatment, Care and Support: The Next Steps.*

UNDP. Integrating human rights with sustainable human development. UNDP. January 1998.

UNESCO (2005) *Universal Declaration on Bioethics and Human Rights.* UNESCO Resolution adopted on the report of Commission III at the 18th plenary meeting, on 19 October 2005, Paris, France: UNESCO.

QUESTIONS

1. Consider the four frameworks suggested by the authors for bringing rights into public health work (advocacy, legal, policy and programs). Give examples of where you have seen each applied. How are or aren't these frameworks interrelated?

2. Rights-based approaches were first articulated in the context of development. What do you consider to be the implications of this for the growth of rights-based approaches to health?

3. Integrating health and human rights has many practical consequences for the practice of public health. Why do you think integrating human rights into public health work is a good idea? Please give examples of what integration might look like.

FURTHER READING

1. Gruskin, S., Is There a Government in the Cockpit: A Passenger's Perspective, or Global Public Health: The Role of Human Rights. *Temple Law Review*, 2004; 77: 313–334.

2. Pillay, N., Right to Health and the Universal Declaration of Human Rights. *Lancet,* 2008; 372: 2005–6. http://search.proquest.com/docview/199013669?accountid=12935

3. Miller, Carol & Thomson, Marilyn, *Case Studies on Rights-based Approaches to Gender and Diversity,* Gender and Development Network (2005). See in particular Case studies, p14–48 http://webcache.googleusercontent.com/search?q=cache:R5kr679xR9AJ:www.gadnetwork.org.uk/storage/gadn-publications/Case%2520Studies%2520on%2520Rights-based%2520Approaches%2520to%2520Gender%2520and%2520Diversity.pdf+&hl=en

POINT OF VIEW

Power, Suffering and Courts: Reflections on Promoting Health Rights through Judicialization

Alicia Ely Yamin

In general, the global phenomenon of health rights litigation emerged in the 1990s with the achievement of effective antiretroviral therapy for the treatment of HIV/AIDS. Even if litigation began earlier and included other aspects, it is fair to say that the trajectory of right-to-health litigation globally, as well as within the countries under study, was undoubtedly shaped by cases centering on HIV/AIDS medications, precisely because these cases presented a clear-cut argument for justiciability. First, HIV/AIDS cases implicated the right to life, which was clearly protected as a fundamental right even when the right to health was not. For example, in Costa Rica in 1992, the Constitutional Chamber of the high court refused to hear a case on ensuring access to antiretrovirals but five years later heard an almost identical case. By 1997, the Constitutional Chamber, citing such sources as *Morbidity and Mortality Weekly*, was convinced that recently developed antiretroviral combination therapies were indeed effective in turning what had been a death sentence into a chronic disease. The Court unanimously reversed itself and ordered the provision of antiretrovirals, stating, "What good are the rest of the rights and guarantees, the institutions and programs, the advantages and benefits of our system of liberties, if a person cannot count on the right to life and health assured?" (*García Alvarez v. Caja Costarricense de Seguro Social*, Judgment 5934 Sala Constitucional de la Corte Suprema de Jus-

ticia, [Sup. Ct. Const. Ch.] Exp. 5778–V-97 N. 5934–97 (1997)).

In the 1990s, HIV/AIDS cases simultaneously brought attention to what was perceived as a potentially major epidemiological threat and issues relating to the treatment of marginalized and excluded populations. The starkest threat by far [was] in South Africa. Yet, the sense of HIV being different or unprecedented in its status as a major public health problem is played out in many of the early judgments relating to antiretrovirals across multiple contexts. Also, the stigma and discrimination faced by affected populations meant that these cases often involved arguments regarding discrimination, which courts were familiar with addressing.

Further, contrary to many of the classical arguments against the justiciability of economic, social and cultural rights, these antiretroviral cases presented a clearly defined obligation (provision of a certain medication or combination of medications), a clear duty bearer (the ministry of health or equivalent institution), and a clear remedy. There was no need to sort out diffuse responsibility or to grapple with complex chains of causality: without these medications, the plaintiffs would die; with the medications, as some courts explicitly noted, there was the "Lazarus effect" whereby the patient could resume a "normal and productive life." And it was within the scope of the ministry of health's functions to provide the plaintiffs with these miraculous drugs.

However, it is not enough to point to the advent of effective antiretrovirals, as courts' role in securing treatment for HIV/AIDS has been highly variable. In Argentina, Brazil, Colombia, and South Africa, the 1980s and early 1990s ushered in new, emancipatory constitutions with robust enumerations of ESC rights, in addition to important structural reforms. In India, beginning in the 1970s, important judge-made reforms strengthened the role of the courts in a constitution that Jawaharlal Nehru had envisioned as a socially transformative document. In South Africa and Colombia, newly created constitutional courts took on iconic significance as actors using the law—previously understood popularly as entrenching oppression in South Africa and, at a minimum, condoning horrific inequity in Colombia—to advance greater social justice in their respective societies.

Across these countries, reforms that made for favorable legal opportunity structures included, for example, the establishment of a high court (or chamber of the high court in the case of Costa Rica) as a specialized tribunal overseeing a new "constitutional jurisdiction"; the loosening and, in some cases, almost complete abolition of standing requirements; and a notable move away from legal formalism. In some countries, the speed with which health cases could be resolved was also crucial to making litigation appealing; for example, the *tutela* mechanism in Colombia required claims to be resolved in under ten days; in Brazil, interim orders could be used to resolve constitutional health rights petitions in as little as forty-eight to seventy-two hours.

At the same time, the political organs of many of the governments under study were deeply influenced by neoliberal economic policies emanating from the so-called Washington Consensus. No domain was more affected by these neoliberal policies than the health sector. Structural adjustment programs reduced the availability and accessibility of health services through cuts in health spending and increased reliance on user fees; at the same time, they reduced household income, which in turn left people less able to pay for health services. Health-sector reforms implemented during this time emphasized privatization of services and allocation through market mechanisms, coupled with targeting for the very poor. Further, the World Trade Organization's Agreement on Trade-Related Aspects of Intellectual Property Rights, negotiated in the 1986–94 Uruguay Round, introduced intellectual property rules into the multilateral trading system, which also deeply affected access to medications and, in turn, the possibilities for people in the global South to enjoy their right to health.

In many countries in the global South, the political branches of government were forced to swallow the bitter medicine of structural adjustment even when, as in the case of South Africa, it openly conflicted with their ideologies. In others, such as Argentina and Colombia, governments seemed to embrace it with zeal, together with its implied neoliberal vision of modernity. However, high courts—if not the entire judiciaries—were well-placed to act as bulwarks against the hegemonic onslaught of neoliberalism, and they appear to have done so to greater or lesser extents, at least regarding health. Some degree of judicial independence and both respect for the rule of law and a tradition of judicial review was present in all of the countries studied here—with the arguable exception of Argentina under the Menem administration—and seems to be critical to enabling courts to play robust roles in the enforcement of programmatic rights, including the right to health, in the context of neoliberalism or any other pervasive ideology.

Together with other scholars, I have argued elsewhere that neoliberalism's push toward commodification, commercialization, and privatization undermines both the concept and enjoyment of a right to health, in addition to other ESC rights. Neoliberal economic paradigms are closely linked with narrow liberal—i.e., libertarian—conceptions of rights, which construe rights as negative shields against governmental interference and leave little space for positive claims on the government. In contrast, the erosion of the distinctions between classes of rights lies at the heart of much of the ESC rights jurisprudence from the 1990s, including both national- and international-level jurisprudence relating to the right to health.

Across these countries in the 1990s (and in India before), even when not directly influenced by international law, we see courts abandoning formalistic distinctions between negative and positive rights, and, in turn, fundamental rights (e.g., the right to life) and directive principles (e.g., the right to health in many constitutions). For example, the Constitutional Court of Colombia noted in a 1999 opinion unifying its jurisprudence on the right to health that justiciability is a fluid concept, more aptly applied to dimensions than to categories of rights. According to the Court, broad notions underlying ESC rights "tend to become transmuted into individual rights to the extent that elements are in place that permit an individual or groups of individuals to demand that the state complies with a specific obligation, thereby consolidating the generalized duty of assistance with the concrete reality for a specific person or group of persons" (Constitutional Court of Colombia, *Alvarez v. Estado Colombiano*, SU.819/99 (1999)).

The sometimes stark philosophical and ideological differences between the neoliberal policies often being executed by the executive branch and the conceptions of rights and society being promoted by the courts do not fully explain the phenomenon of health rights litigation. Rather, appealing legal opportunity structures, resulting from liberalized standing and low thresholds for bringing cases, were coupled with closed political avenues for reform across most of the countries under study. South Africa presents perhaps the starkest example in that former president Mbeki's AIDS denialism precluded an adequate political response to the country's HIV/AIDS epidemic. In turn, the courts seemed to be the only channel for redress in the face of both the multinational pharmaceutical industry's intellectual property practices and the government's recalcitrance.

The overall story of judicialization of health rights needs to be situated in a larger account of the matrix of the history and political economy of health. Global forces beyond the nation-state create the conditions that drive much of the access-to-treatment litigation. Examining the country level alone obscures the power dynamics in the global order and the upstream decisions that often determine patterns of health and access to care, types of litigation, and the ideological context for judicial assessments of governmental efforts.

In these contexts, the real question for health rights—and social policy more broadly—revolves not around absolute resources but around incorporating equity considerations into decision-making processes and institutional design at all levels (local, national, and international). It is not a question of remedying specific violations so much as changing decision-making processes to incorporate prospectively an equity lens, which goes beyond health specifically to also contemplate other social determinants from fiscal to labor to land policy. We should develop a far better understanding as to the contexts, courts are able to contribute meaningfully to processes for incremental institutional reform, as well as to bolder transformations in both the organization and conceptualization of health systems.

Adapted from A.E. Yamin, "Power Suffering and the Courts: Reflections on Promoting Health Rights through Judicialization" in A.E. Yamin and S. Gloppen eds, *Litigating Health Rights: Can Courts Bring More Justice to Health?* (Harvard University Press, Harvard Law School Human Rights Program Series; 2011).

Alicia Ely Yamin is Director, Program on the Health Rights of Women and Children, François-Xavier Bagnoud Center for Health and Human Rights; Lecturer, Department of Global Health and Population, Harvard School of Public Health; Joseph F. Flom Global Health and Human Rights Fellow, Harvard Law School, Boston, MA, USA; and Executive Editor, Critical Concepts, *Health and Human Rights: An International Journal.*

CHAPTER 9

Is Access to Essential Medicines a Part of the Fulfillment of the Right to Health Enforceable through the Courts?

Hans V. Hogerzeil, Melanie Samson, Jaume Vidal Casanovas
and Ladan Rahmani-Ocora

INTRODUCTION

Issues of human rights affect the relations between the State and the individual; they generate State obligations and individual entitlements. The promotion of human rights is one of the main purposes of the UN. For example, the WHO Constitution of 1946 says that "The enjoyment of the highest attainable standard of health is one of the fundamental rights of every human being without distinction of race, religion, political belief, economic or social condition." Article 25.1 of the Universal Declaration of Human Rights (1948) says that "Everyone has the right to a standard of living adequate for the health of himself and of his family, including food, clothing, housing and medical care and necessary social services."

The right to health is also recognized in many other international[1-3] and regional[4-6] treaties, especially the International Covenant on Economic, Social and Cultural Rights (ICESCR) of 1966, an international treaty that is binding on States parties (States that have acceded to, signed, or ratified an international treaty) and provides the foundation for legal obligations under the right to health. In the ICESCR, States parties "recognize the right of everyone to the enjoyment of the highest attainable standard of physical and mental health." In Article 12.2, the treaty lists several steps to be taken by States parties to achieve the full realisation of this right, including the right to: maternal, child, and reproductive health; healthy natural and workplace environments; prevention, treatment, and control of disease; and "the creation of conditions which would assure to all medical service and medical attention in the event of sickness." Article 12 thus constitutes an important standard against which to assess the laws, policies, and practices of States parties.

The implementation of the ICESCR is monitored by the Committee on Economic, Social and Cultural Rights, which regularly issues authoritative but non-binding General Comments, which are adopted to assist States in their interpretation of the ICESCR. In General Comment 3, the Committee confirms that States parties have a core obligation to ensure the satisfaction of minimum essential levels of each of the rights outlined in the ICESCR, including essential primary care as described in the Alma-Ata Declaration, which includes the provision of essential medicines.

General Comment 14 of May, 2000, is particularly relevant to access to essential medicines. Here the Committee states that the right to medical services in Article 12.2 (d) of the ICESCR includes the provision of essential drugs "as defined by the WHO Action Programme on Essential Drugs,"[7] According to the latest WHO definition, essential medicines are: "those that satisfy the priority health care needs of the population. Essential medicines are selected with due regard to disease prevalence, evidence on efficacy and safety, and comparative cost-effectiveness. Essential medicines are intended to be available within the context of functioning health systems at all times, in adequate amounts, in the appropriate dosage forms, with assured quality, and at a price the individual and the community can afford. The implementation of the concept of essential medicines is intended to be flexible and adaptable to many different situations; exactly which medicines are regarded as essential remains a national responsibility."[8]

Although the ICESCR acknowledges the limits of available resources and provides for progressive (as opposed to immediate) realisation of the right to medical services, States parties have an immediate obligation to take deliberate and concrete steps towards the full realisation of Article 12, and to guarantee that the right to health will be exercised without discrimination of any kind.

Most countries in the world have acceded to or ratified at least one worldwide or regional covenant or treaty confirming the right to health. For example, more than 150 countries have become State parties to the ICESCR, and 83 have signed regional treaties.[9] More than 100 countries have incorporated the right to health in their national constitution.

Some might argue that social, cultural, and economic rights are not enforceable through the courts, and some national courts have indeed been reluctant to intervene in resource allocation decisions of governments. Yet accountability and the possibility of redress are essential components of the rights-based approach. Being a State party to a human rights treaty that is internationally binding creates certain State obligations to its people. Do governments live up to these binding obligations in practice? If not, do individuals manage to obtain their rights? And if they do, which factors have contributed to their success?

This study analyses the question of whether access to essential medicines as part of the fulfilment of the right to health can be enforced through national courts (is justiciable) in low-income and middle-income countries. The study is part of a general attempt by WHO to integrate the promotion and protection of human rights into national policies and to support further mainstreaming of human rights throughout the UN.

METHODS

A systematic search was done to identify completed court cases in low-income and middle-income countries in which individuals or groups had claimed access to essential medicines with reference to the right to health in general, or to specific human rights treaties ratified by the government. Six different search methods were used. A general boolean search of the internet was done with variations in the keywords that were linked together (such as human rights, essential drugs, access to medicines). An email survey was sent to a group of the most prominent nongovernmental organisations (NGOs) working on the right to medicines that were noted from the internet search. The email requested assistance in finding information on cases, to which the Lawyers Collective in India responded with information. The following legal databases were accessed and searched: LexisNexis, Natlex, Ohada, Portal Droit

Francophonie, CSA Illumina, Electronic Information System for International Law, Westlaw database, Eurolex, and the Legal Information Institute. Other databases consulted were The Economic, Social and Cultural Rights database on the internet ESCR-NET, the Asian Legal Resource Centre database, the AllAfrica database, the European Court of Human Rights database (HUDOC), the International Commission of Jurists website, the Inter-American Court of Human Rights, and reports from the UN Human Rights regional offices. Individual country searches were done for all low-income and middle-income signatories to the International Covenant on Economic, Social and Cultural Rights. The World Legal Information Institute was used to locate each country's online national jurisprudence database. A further specific internet search was done on countries without any online national jurisprudence database, focusing on the country name and the search terms; this method considered each country in a thorough and systematic way.

Role of the Funding Source

The sponsor of the study had no role in study design, data collection, data analysis, data interpretation, or writing of the report. The corresponding author had full access to all data in the study and had final responsibility for the decision to submit for publication.

Table 9.1 Number of court cases per country

	Right to health enshrined in the constitution	International treaties enjoy constitutional rank	Successful cases claiming the right to health (cases referring to international treaties)		Unsuccessful cases claiming the right to health (cases referring to international treaties)	
			n	First case	n	First case
Argentina	No	Yes	8 (2)	1998	1 (1)	2003
Brazil*	Yes	No	3 (0)	2002		
Bolivia	Yes	Yes†	1 (0)	2003		
Colombia	Yes	Yes	28 (1)	1992	2 (0)	2001
Costa Rica	Yes	Yes	7 (5)	1994	3 (0)	1992
Ecuador	Yes	Yes	1 (1)	2004		
India	No	No	2 (0)	2000		
Nigeria	Yes	No			1 (1)	2001
Panama	Yes	No			2 (0)	1998
San Salvador	Yes	Yes	1 (1)	2001	1 (0)	2004
South Africa	Yes	Yes†	2 (1)	2002	2 (0)	1997
Venezuela	Yes	Yes	6 (3)	1997		
Total			59 (14)		12 (2)	

* Large number of new cases filed more recently. † Status not fully clear.

Table 9.2 Key characteristics* of 71 litigation cases in low-income and middle income countries on access to essential medicines as part of the fulfilment of the right to health

	Successful cases (n=59) claiming the right to health (cases referring to international treaties)		Unsuccessful cases (n=12) claiming the right to health (cases referring to international treaties)	
	n*	%	n*	%
Type of case				
Individual case	44 (8)	75%	6 (1)	50%
Public interest case	21 (9)	36%	6 (2)	50%
NGO-supported case	10 (5)	17%	4 (2)	33%
Disease aspects				
HIV/AIDS (prevention, diagnosis, treatment)	27 (8)	46%	7 (1)	58%
Cancer (e.g., leukaemia, breast, prostate)	6 (1)	10%	1 (0)	8%
Neurological (eg, trauma, Down's syndrome, epilepsy)	6 (0)	10%		
Surgery (e.g., renal and liver transplant)	5 (1)	8%		
Other (e.g., diabetes, multiple sclerosis, lupus erythematosus)	17 (4)	29%	5 (1)	42%
Defendant				
Social Security	33 (9)	56%	5 (0)	42%
Ministry of Health	18 (6)	31%	5 (1)	42%
Ministry of Defence	3 (0)	5%		
Health institution/hospital	4 (0)	7%	3 (1)	25%
Prison authority	2 (0)	3%		
Human rights treaties quoted				
Unspecified, all	8 (8)	14%	1 (1)	8%
International Covenant on Economic, Social and Cultural Rights	4 (4)	7%	1 (1)	8%
Regional Human Rights treaties	5 (5)	8%	2 (2)	17%
Universal Declaration of Human Rights	3 (3)	5%		
Universal Declaration of the Rights of the Child	2 (2)	3%		
Other aspects quoted				
Right to life	49 (11)	83%	6 (1)	50%
Physical integrity	16 (0)	27%	1 (0)	8%
Acquired right/non-interruption of treatment	11 (4)	19%	1 (0)	8%
Non-discrimination	7 (3)	12%	1 (1)	8%
Conclusions reached in successful cases				
Right to health is stronger than limitations in the national essential medicines list	22 (2)	37%		
Right to health is stronger than limitations in social security benefits	18 (2)	31%		
State has obligations towards the poor and disadvantaged	14 (2)	24%		
Judgment is extended to all individuals in similar circumstances	14 (5)	24%		
International treaties create obligations towards individuals	11 (9)	19%		
Government policies can be challenged in court	2 (1)	3%		

* Characteristics are not mutually exclusive.

Table 9.3 Main arguments quoted in unsuccessful cases (n = 12)

	n (%)	Country
National list of essential medicines upheld	4 (33%)	Argentina*, Colombia, Panama, South Africa
The medicine claimed was the wrong choice, lack of evidence on efficacy, or no need	3 (25%)	Costa Rica (2×), El Salvador
The medicine had been supplied in the mean time	2 (17%)	Colombia, Costa Rica
Court of Law not ready to decide on policy issues	1 (8%)	South Africa
Case dismissed on technical grounds	1 (8%)	Panama
Court refuses to hear the plaintiff because of fear of HIV infection	1 (8%)	Nigeria*

* Cases referring to international treaties signed by the government.

RESULTS

The systematic search identified 73 cases from 12 low-income and middle-income countries. In five cases, only a brief summary of the judgment was available. In three of these cases, information was still sufficient to include them in the analysis. The full analysis is therefore based on 71 cases, of which 59 were won and 12 were lost (Table 9.1). Of the cases included in the analysis, 14 successful and two unsuccessful cases specifically referred to one or more international human rights treaties signed by the government. The main characteristics of the cases are shown in Table 9.2. Arguments used in the unsuccessful cases are shown in Table 9.3. Full references and summary information for each case are available from the authors on request.

Of the 12 countries in which court cases were identified, 11 are State parties to the ICESCR; South Africa has signed but not ratified the ICESCR. In all countries except Argentina and India, the right to health is recognized in the constitution. In six countries the constitution includes a provision that international treaties signed by the State have constitutional rank, override domestic laws in case of conflict, or both (Table 9.1).

More than 90% of cases are from nine countries in Central and Latin America. Between 1991 and 1997, three countries (Colombia, Costa Rica, and Venezuela) had their first successful case; in the 7 years from 1998 to 2004 there were the first successful cases in seven other countries, including countries outside the Americas (South Africa and India). Most cases (50 cases, 70%) were individual; 27 (38%) were public interest cases, and 14 (20%) were supported by NGOs. In 61 (86%) cases the Social Security system or the Ministry of Health were the defendants. About half the cases related to potentially life-saving treatment of HIV/AIDS.

DISCUSSION

This study has shown that access to essential medicines as part of the fulfilment of the right to health could indeed be enforced through the courts in several low-income and middle-income countries, with most of the experience to date coming from Central and Latin America. The most important success factor has been that certain rights are enshrined in the national constitution. Key constitutional provisions seem to be those on the right to health and on defined State obligations with regard to health care services and social welfare. Human rights treaties ratified by the government have probably supported the creation of such constitutional provisions in the first place. When referred to in the courts they have usually provided additional force to such constitutional obligations, especially in the presence of a constitutional provision that international treaties supersede domestic law. One case in Argentina shows that international human rights treaties can also successfully be invoked in the absence of a constitutional right to health. In 80% of cases, the right to health was linked to the right to life. Most negative rulings were based on a recognition of the limitations specified in the national essential medicines list or social security benefits, although some courts also made their own analysis of the medical merits of the claim.

Our study has two limitations. First, the fact that most cases were seen in Central and Latin America (despite intensive and targeted efforts to identify cases from other regions) suggests that the observations and conclusions are probably more relevant in this region than in the rest of the world. A possible explanation for this finding is that social security is much more developed in the Americas than in Africa and Asia, where most health care is paid for directly by the patient. Other reasons could be more developed legal systems and higher consumer expectations in the Americas. The second limitation is that adding up the arguments used in different cases from different countries might create a false sense of statistical probability that similar arguments could work in future cases in other countries. This assumption is of course not true, since each current and future case must be judged on its individual merits and within its national legal situation. Yet cases such as the ones reported here contribute to a worldwide body of jurisprudence, which might support further developments in this area. Within these two limitations, the intended value of our analysis is to present a first overview of the situation and to generate some ideas for further analysis and study.

A successful case is defined as one that has led to new, continued, or expanded access to one or more essential medicines for an individual or group. Constitutional provisions probably contributed most to successful outcomes. All countries except Argentina and India include the right to health in their constitution. In nearly all cases, this includes a definition of State obligations with regard to health care services and social welfare. In all countries except Panama and Nigeria, one or more court rulings confirm that these constitutional rights are indeed enforceable (Table 9.1). In six countries (Argentina, Colombia, Costa Rica, Ecuador, El Salvador, and Venezuela), international treaties enjoy constitutional rank, and domestic laws should follow international treaties.

14 (24%) of 59 successful cases specifically refer to international human rights treaties to which the State is party; the other 45 successful cases refer in more general terms to the right to health, usually referring to the national constitution. When referred to, the human rights treaties are usually mentioned as a group and as a supportive argument in addition to constitutional provisions. This is probably logical when the right to health or to health care is also enshrined in the constitution. Yet there are two examples where the international human rights treaties have really made a difference. In Argentina, the right to health is not mentioned in the constitution, and could not be invoked. In an important case,[10] the Court listed all international treaties Argentina had ratified and used this as the main argument to rule that life-saving treatment of a child with a blood disease could not be interrupted. Within our series, this case features the only clear ruling in which international human rights treaties have created a state obligation towards an individual entitlement in the absence of a constitutional right to health.

In El Salvador the same point was made. Here, a slowly progressing Constitutional

Court case was accelerated by filing a parallel case before the Inter-American Commission on Human Rights, alleging the State's failure to provide the plaintiffs with antiretroviral therapy. As a provisional measure, the Commission solicited the Salvadoran State to comply with its regional obligations and to provide the needed medications. Before the regional court started its hearing procedures, the Salvadoran Constitutional Court came to its decision in support of the plaintiff.[11]

We can conclude that human rights treaties usually provide additional force to existing constitutional obligations. Additionally, national constitutions could provide that international treaties supersede domestic law. The case in Argentina further indicates that international human rights treaties can successfully be invoked in the absence of a constitutional right to health.

In 49 (83%) of 59 successful cases and in all countries, the right to health was specifically quoted as being related to the right to life. Logically, this argument was usually linked to cases of life-threatening disease in which treatment was potentially life saving. In 24 cases, this argument was for treatment for HIV/AIDS, but was also used for diseases like leukaemia, and renal and liver transplantation. In non-life-threatening conditions, more general arguments such as human dignity and physical integrity were used. Therefore, in practice, the right to health seems more linked to the right to life as such than to the quality of life.

In 11 (19%) of 59 cases, acquired rights, in the sense of non-interruption of treatment already supplied for a period of time, were quoted. In three cases (severe congenital neutropenia in a child and two cases of HIV/AIDS), this argument was used when social security rights expired after a certain period of chronic treatment—e.g., after 2 years. These cases seem to establish that in these countries the right to health cannot be limited by legal, financial, or adminis-

trative restrictions in social security coverage. Indeed, the argument could be made that the coverage of truly life-saving treatment should probably be life-long and not subject to a maximum period.

Rather surprisingly, non-discrimination, which is a cornerstone in human rights law and is included in many constitutions, was invoked in only seven (12%) of 59 cases, often together with arguments of social justice. In only two of these cases was there actual discrimination between individuals in equal circumstances: in South Africa[12] only a few HIV-infected mothers in a few hospitals could receive treatment to prevent mother-to-child-transmission, whereas large numbers in the rest of the country could not; and in Venezuela,[13] army officers were entitled to antiretrovirals whereas ordinary soldiers were not. Non-discrimination therefore seems a potentially powerful argument when certain treatments are unequally available within a country, for example only in certain types of hospitals, or only for certain categories of people.

Ten successful cases that were supported by national public health interest NGOs are among the most important and far-reaching—although to prove that NGO support was essential to the successful outcome is difficult. The first NGO-supported case took place in 1995 in Colombia.[14] Active lobbying led to a legal reform in 1997 by which antiretrovirals were included in the official medicines list. The first collective action by NGOs took place in Argentina[15] and led to a Supreme Court ruling in 2000 that confirmed that the Ministry of Health was responsible for the effective implementation of the AIDS programme; this ruling immediately benefited 15,000 people.

The South African case[12] is well known. In a joint claim against the Ministry of Health, national health advocacy NGOs and individuals challenged a government restriction on the supply of nevirapine to prevent mother-to-child transmission of HIV to 18 public hospitals undertaking a pilot study. In July, 2002, the Constitutional Court upheld earlier rulings that this restriction was unconstitutional and ordered the government to assure the general availability of this medicine. The lawsuit came after 5 years of active lobbying by civil-society organisations.

Another example is recorded in Venezuela, where a national NGO named Acción Ciudadana Contra el Sida supported a carefully constructed series of consecutive court cases between 1997 and 2001. In one case[13] on behalf of four soldiers, the organisation asked the medical services of the Venezuelan Ministry of Defence for prescription drugs for the treatment of HIV/AIDS. The Court voluntarily extended its decision to all army members in the same circumstances. A subsequent case[16] challenged the medical services of the Venezuelan Ministry of Health for its failure to ensure coverage for HIV/AIDS medications through the public health-care system for those who were not eligible under the social security scheme. This case was also awarded, but only to the plaintiff. In the next case,[17] similar to the previous one but filed by over 170 people, the collective interest was accepted by the Court. In a final case[18] of 29 people living with HIV/AIDS, a ruling in support of the regular provision of antiretrovirals and laboratory tests was extended to all people in the same circumstances.

In these cases careful litigation, supported by NGOs, has forced the government to implement its constitutional and human rights treaty obligations and has served the public-health cause of improving equitable access to essential medicines. The legal, financial, and moral support of NGOs and their effective networking have assisted plaintiffs in the presentation and defence of their case and in subsequent appeal procedures. NGOs have also mobilized public support and media interest.

All these factors seem to have contributed to the positive outcome of the case. But not all cases were successful, and lessons can be learned from the 12 cases with a negative outcome, which we have been able to identify.

Rejection of a claim for non-life-saving treatment might seem acceptable, although could leave a question about the quality of life. But what about rejected claims for potentially life-saving medicines? Six of the 12 unsuccessful cases (Table 9.3) relate to such medicines, five of them for HIV/AIDS. In one case,[19] the medicine requested was supplied in the mean time, and so could in fact be seen as a successful case. In three other HIV cases,[20–22] the court upheld the national essential medicines list and ruled that there was no medical need for the requested medicine for this patient. The fifth case[23] was dismissed because the court refused to hear the plaintiff, who was HIV-positive, fearing that her presence in the courtroom would expose the court to a risk of infection. In the sixth case, about a request for renal dialysis in a patient not eligible for transplantation in South Africa, the court specifically indicated that, in the absence of sufficient dialysis capacity in the country "it would be slow to interfere with rational decisions taken in good faith by political organs and medical authorities whose responsibility it is to deal with such matters."[24]

In two countries, negative rulings were later followed by positive outcomes. In 1992 in Costa Rica, a claim for antiretroviral treatment was rejected because the medicine was not considered to be a cure.[22] However, in 1997 the Court changed its opinion and ruled in favour of the plaintiff,[25] although the requested antiretroviral medicines were not included in the official national medicines lists. The judges based their decision on the right to life and health as enshrined in the national constitution and as endorsed by Costa Rica in international treaties. In South Africa, the negative outcome in the renal dialysis case in 1998 mentioned previously was followed in 2001 by the successful nevirapine case.[12]

18 cases from Bolivia (one case), Colombia (14), and Costa Rica (3) concluded that the right to health is not restricted by limitations in social security coverage. Some of these cases were linked to the exhaustion of time-limited coverage,[26] the non-payment of contributions by the employer,[27] or even giving the same rights to people not covered by social security at all.[28] In Colombia and Costa Rica,[25] the right to health was also defined as extending beyond the limits of the essential medicines list used to define insurance coverage. In both countries, judgments awarded life-saving treatment with antiretroviral drugs while these were not on the national list of essential medicines and were, for that reason, not made available.

From a public health point of view these judgments have both a positive and a negative side. Such judgments have led to the availability of antiretroviral treatment to patients with HIV/AIDS, which shows the value of the courts in ensuring the human rights principles of accountability and redress mechanisms. The negative side is that these cases overruled the official medicines list used for reimbursement. In the case of life-saving treatments, one could argue that this overruling is a necessary outcome if the list was not adequate or out of date. However, in another case from Costa Rica,[29] potentially life-saving treatment of leukaemia was awarded that had specifically been excluded from social security benefits because of its high cost; and in yet another case the patient won access to a branded medicine rather than the generic alternative supplied through the social security scheme.[30] Is this a positive or a negative outcome?

In some Latin-American countries, such as Colombia and Brazil, the situation is now becoming out of hand. In Colombia, most of the later successful cases in our series refer to medicines outside the national essential medicines list that is used to define the limits of social security. The first case refers to international human rights treaties, and obviously established the principle; subsequent cases only refer to the constitution and to the right to health in general. In Brazil the situation is even worse, with thousands of court cases since 1991 awarding medicines not yet approved for reimbursement, with reference to the right to health mentioned in the constitution.[31]

The solution is probably in the wording of the right to health. In Brazil, the constitution of 1988 recognizes the right to health and guarantees nearly unlimited health-care benefits to all citizens. The constitution of Venezuela of 1999 defines the responsibilities of State in more detail. However, the constitution of South Africa stands out in its simplicity and clarity. Section 27 of the constitution states that everyone has the right to have access to health-care services and social security, and that the State must take reasonable legislative and other measures, within its available resources, to achieve the progressive realisation of each of these rights.

Most public budgets are not infinite and at a certain moment choices have to be made. Progressive implementation of the right to health requires a State to choose which components should be implemented first. Under such circumstances, should courts of justice or national committees of experts decide how public funds are spent in the most equitable and cost-effective manner? The recent case of the British nurse fighting to receive a new anti-cancer medicine not yet approved for reimbursement proves that this question is also relevant in developed countries.[32] The dilemma is well described by Justice Sachs in the renal dialysis case in South Africa:

"The courts are not the proper place to resolve the agonizing personal and medical problems that underlie these choices.

Important though review functions are, there are areas where institutional incapacity and appropriate constitutional modesty require us to be especially cautious ... Unfortunately the resources are limited and I can find no reason to interfere with the allocation undertaken by those better equipped than I to deal with the agonizing choices that had to be made in this case."[24]

Many successful cases have had a substantial effect. In several countries, the court cases have led to a general availability of antiretroviral treatment for HIV/AIDS patients. In 14 cases from six countries the judgment was extended to other individuals in similar situations. In two landmark cases from Argentina and South Africa, government policies have successfully been challenged in court. Our study therefore shows that careful litigation has been one additional mechanism to promote the right to health and to encourage governments to fulfil their constitutional and international treaty obligations. In our opinion, this finding is especially relevant for countries in which social security systems are not yet fully developed.

We also conclude that constitutional guarantees on access to health care services should be well defined, for example through reference to a national list of essential medicines, to prevent abuse. Such guarantees might especially be relevant for countries with more mature social security systems. In those countries, transparent procedures should be available to define the range of goods and services covered by the social security, with the role of the judiciary focusing on general rather than on specific aspects of reimbursement.

Health policymakers in low-income and middle-income countries and the international public-health community should be aware of the increasing trend towards successful litigation. Redress mechanisms through the courts are an essential function in society, but should preferably be used as a measure of last resort. Rather, policymakers should ensure that standards for human rights guide their health policies and programmes from the outset, and should publicly be perceived as such.

REFERENCES

1. International Convention on the Elimination of All Forms of Racial Discrimination, article 5 (e) (iv), 1965.
2. Convention on the Elimination of All Forms of Discrimination against Women, article 11.1 (f) and 12, 1979.
3. Convention on the Rights of the Child, Article 24 (1989).
4. European Social Charter, Article 11 (revised) 1965.
5. African Charter on Human and People's Rights, Article 16 (1981).
6. Additional Protocol to the American Convention on Human Rights in the Area of Economic, Social and Cultural Rights, Article 10 (1988).
7. Committee on Economic, Social and Cultural Rights. The right to the highest attainable standard of health. 11/08/2000. E/.12/2000/4, CESCR General Comment 14, para 12(a).
8. WHO. The selection and use of essential medicines. Geneva: World Health Organization, 2003. Technical Report Series 920: 54.
9. United Nations High Commissioner for Human Rights, database of signed/ratified treaties.
10. Campodonico de Beviacqua, Ana Carina vs Ministerio de Salud y Acción Social. Constitutional Court, File C.823.XXXV (Oct 24, 2000; Argentina).
11. Mr Jorge Odir Miranda Cortez vs la Directora del instituto Salvadoreño del Seguro Social. Constitutional court, File no. 348–99 (April 4, 2001; El Salvador).
12. Treatment Action Campaign, Dr Haron Sallojee and Children's Rights Centre vs RSA Ministry of Health. High Court of South Africa, Transvaal Provincial Div., 12 Dec 2001.
13. Mr JRB, et al vs Ministerio de la Defensa. Supreme Court, expediente no. 14000 (Jan 20, 1998; Venezuela).
14. Mr X vs Instituto de Seguros Sociales (ISS). Constitutional Court, Judgement no. T-271 (June 23, 1995; Colombia).
15. Asociación Benghalensis et al vs Ministerio de Salud y Acción Social. Constitutional Court, File No A.186.XXXIV (June 1, 2000; Argentina).
16. Mr NA, YF, et al vs Ministerio de Sanidad y Asistencia Social. Supreme Court, expediente no. 14625 (Aug 14, 1998; Venezuela).

17. Cruz del Valle Bermúdez et al vs Ministerio de Salud y Acción Social. Supreme Court, expediente no. 15789 (July 15, 1999; Venezuela).

18. Mrs Glenda López et al vs Instituto Venezolano de Seguros Sociales. Supreme Court, expediente no. 00–1343 (April 6, 2001; Venezuela).

19. Carlos Usma Lemus, Edgar Castle Cifuentes and Mayan Polished Ramiro vs Secretariat Distrital de Salud of Bogota and the Simón Hospital Bolivar, Judgment No. T-1132/01 (Oct 25, 2001; Colombia).

20. Mr Jorge Moran vs Social Insurance Box (June 24, 1999; Panama).

21. Marina Ester Sanchez vs Ministry of Public Health and Social Assistance, case 45–2003 (Sept 14, 2004; El Salvador).

22. Mr Jacobo Schifter Sikora as President of the Association Against AIDS vs La Caja Costarricense de Seguro Social, case no. 280–92 (Feb 7, 1992; Costa Rica).

23. Ahamefule vs Imperial Medical Center & Another (Suit ID #1627/2000), Notice of Appeal, Court of Appeal (Lagos), 16 February 2001 (on file); Communication from F Mroka, Solicitor, Social and Economic Rights Action Center (SERAC), (Feb 21, 2001, and July 30, 2001; Nigeria).

24. Soobramoney vs Minister of Health, KwaZulu-Natal 1998 (1) SA 765 (CC), 1997 (12) BCLR 1696 (CC) (South Africa).

25. Mr William García Álvarez vs Caja Costarricense de Seguro Social. Constitutional Court, File 5778–V-97 (Sept 23, 1997; Costa Rica).

26. Mr Alonso Muñoz Ceballos vs Instituto de Seguros Sociales (ISS). Constitutional Court Judgment no. T-484 (Aug 11, 1992; Colombia).

27. Mr Miguel Angel Ibarguen Rivas vs Instituto de Seguros Sociales (ISS). Constitutional Court, Judgment no. T-158 (April 5, 1995; Colombia).

28. Mr X vs Secretaria de Salud Publica Municipal de Cali. Constitutional Court, Judgement no. T-177 (March 18, 1999; Colombia).

29. Ombudsman for Mrs ledi Orellana Martínez vs Caja Costarricense del Seguro Social (CCSS). Constitutional Court, File no. 02–007871 (Sept 24, 2002; Costa Rica).

30. Ms Vera Salazar Navarro vs Caja Costarricense del Seguro Social. Constitutional Court-File no. 01–009007–CO (Sept 26, 2001; Costa Rica).

31. Messeder AM, Serpa Osoria-de-Castro CG, Luiya VL. Manadados judiciais como ferramenta para garantia do acesso a medicamentos no setor publico: a experiencia de Estado do Rio de Janeiro, Brasil. Cad Saude Publica, 2005; 21: 525–34.

32. BBC Online. One woman's reaction to Herceptin. June 9, 2006.

QUESTIONS

1. The authors indicate that most court cases they reviewed invoked the right to the highest attainable standard of physical and mental health (the "Right to Health") while fewer invoked the rights to life and to non-discrimination. Where and how are these rights spelt out in the International Bill of Human Rights? What characterizes these two sets of rights from the perspective of state obligations under international human rights law? What does General Comment 14 on the Right to Health stipulate that is relevant to access to essential medicines?

2. A judge from South Africa is quoted as saying: "The courts are not the proper place to resolve the agonizing personal and medical problems that underlie these choices." What, then, could constitute a proper place, body or mechanism to determine the choice of medicines or procedures that the state would have the obligation to guarantee in fulfilment of the right to health? Who should take part or be represented in such a decision-making body or mechanism?

3. What are state obligations associated with the progressive realization of the right to health? In the context of access to essential medicines, how should the "maximum of [its] available resources" be interpreted and what implication does this have to international assistance and cooperation?

FURTHER READING

1. Report of the Special Rapporteur on the Right of Everyone to the Enjoyment of the Highest Attainable Standard of Physical and Mental Health, Expert consultation on access to medicines as a fundamental component of the right to health, Report to the Human Rights Council Seventeenth session, Agenda item 3 (2011) http://daccess-dds-ny.un.org/doc/UNDOC/GEN/G11/118/42/PDF/G1111842.pdf?OpenElement
2. Hogerzeil, Hans V., Essential Medicines and Human Rights: What Can They Learn from Each Other?' *Bulletin of the World Health Organization*, 2006; 84: 371–375.
3. Pogge, Thomas, Montréal Statement on the Human Right to Essential Medicines. *Cambridge Quarterly of Healthcare Ethics*, 2006; 15: 2.

POINT OF VIEW

The Global Commission on HIV and the Law: Building Resilient HIV Responses

Mandeep Dhaliwal

Law is a critical element of HIV, health and development responses. It can bridge the divide between vulnerability and resilience. Much in the same way that HIV has exposed health and social inequalities; it has magnified weaknesses in the rule of law that the world can no longer afford to ignore.

Human rights-based legal frameworks can be powerful tools to support countries struggling to control their epidemics. The last three decades have given rise to contentious legal debates on HIV-related issues (e.g., criminalization of HIV transmission, exposure and non-disclosure; legal restrictions on needle and syringe distribution in the US or on methadone in Russia, versus legal comprehensive harm reduction in Australia). The last few years have seen an insurgence or resurgence of punitive laws and practices related to drug use, HIV transmission and exposure, sex work, and same sex sexual relations. There is also a growing body of evidence on the relationship between HIV, violence against women and the failure of law and law enforcement to effectively protect women from violence. There is enough variation in legal responses to HIV around the world to highlight the need to rigorously examine the impact of different legal environments on HIV outcomes. This is why the Global Commission on HIV and the Law (the Commission) was created: to examine the impact of law on HIV responses and to catalyze action at

the country level, and to create legal environments, which protect and promote human rights.

Over an eighteen month period, the Commission, led by the United Nations Development Programme (UNDP) on behalf of the UNAIDS family, looked at the relationship between legal responses, human rights and HIV and developed actionable, evidence-informed recommendations for effective HIV responses. Based on an analysis of where the law could transform the AIDS response and send HIV epidemics into decline, the Commission focused on four areas: (1) laws and practices which criminalize those living with—and most vulnerable to—HIV; (2) laws and practices which sustain or mitigate violence and discrimination lived by women; (3) laws and practices which facilitate or impede access to HIV-related treatment; and (4) issues of law pertaining to children and young people in the context of HIV.

The Commission examined public health, human rights and legal scholarship, as well as evidence on the impact of legal environments on the lives of people living with and vulnerable to HIV. To inform its deliberations, the Commission received 644 submissions from 140 countries. Forty percent of the submissions were from Africa and over 70 percent of the submissions described the daily reality of stigma, discrimination, marginalization, verbal and even physical abuse experienced by people living with HIV. Sixty percent of the submissions noted human rights violations lived by women, including barriers to sexual and reproductive health and equal inheritance and property rights. Fifty percent of submissions highlighted the negative health and human rights impacts of criminal laws. Submissions highlighted issues ranging from the negative impacts of laws on age of consent which don't recognize the evolving capacity of the child and prevent young people from accessing HIV and health services to the problems posed by the current intellectual property regime and trends in intellectual property enforcement, such as free trade agreements, which impede the scale up of life-sustaining treatment.

Perhaps the most compelling evidence came from the Commission's seven regional dialogues, held from February to September 2011. The dialogues in Africa, Asia-Pacific, Caribbean, Eastern Europe and Central Asia, High Income Countries, Latin America and the Middle East created policy space for frank, constructive multi-stakeholder dialogue between those who influence, write and enforce laws, and those who experience their impacts. Through these dialogues, the Commission heard from over 700 people living with HIV, sex workers, men who have sex with men, transgender people, people who use drugs, police and prison officials, ministers of justice and health, public health officials, parliamentarians, judges and religious leaders.

The dialogues have been crucial for identifying how the law can advance health and human rights and best serve the response to HIV, for example: where police cooperation with community workers has increased condom use and reduced violence and HIV infection among sex workers; where effective legal aid has made notions of justice and equality real for people living with HIV and contributed to better health outcomes; where advocates have creatively used customary law in progressive ways to promote women's rights and health; where court and legislative actions have introduced gender-sensitive law on sexual assault and recognized the sexual autonomy of young persons; where governments have provided harm reduction and HIV infection rates among people who use drugs have dropped. The good practice and constituencies mobilized through these dialogues are vital resources for creating legal environments which support effective HIV responses.

Even before the Commission issued its final report, country level action on improving legal environments began to emerge. For instance, Fiji recently chose to not criminalize HIV transmission and lifted HIV-related travel restrictions; in Guyana, a Select Parliamentary Committee chose not to criminalize HIV transmission; the first ever judicial sensitization on HIV and the law took place in the Caribbean; national dialogues on HIV and the law have been held in Papua New Guinea, Belize, Panama and Nepal; and in Moldova and Kyrgyzstan, patent laws are being reviewed. At the Asia Pacific High-Level Intergovernmental Meeting on HIV which took place in February 2012, several governments announced their intentions to review and reform punitive legal approaches towards key populations. The Commission's work has also influenced the report of the Commonwealth Eminent Persons' Group which includes a recommendation for the removal of punitive laws blocking effective HIV responses.

The Commission's final report, *"Risks, Rights and Health"* was launched at a global dialogue in July 2012. (For more information, visit www.hivlawcommission.org.) The report emphasizes the necessity for an honest appraisal of prejudice, fear and false morality which have confounded the AIDS response for decades. The report's main messages are:

1. Bad laws are costing lives, resulting in human rights violations and fueling the spread of HIV.
2. The epidemic of bad laws is wasting money and limiting effectiveness and efficiency of HIV and health investments.
3. Good laws and practices that protect human rights and build on public health evidence already exist—they strengthen the global AIDS response, and they must be replicated.
4. We have the science and tools to end AIDS. Bio-medical tools and behavioural approaches alone will not be enough—structural drivers like the law have a vital role to play.

In 2011, at the United Nations, countries committed to reviewing laws which block effective responses. The Commission's report provides a clear blueprint for these national reviews. (United Nations. 8 July 2011. Political Declaration on HIV and AIDS: Intensifying Our Efforts to Eliminate HIV and AIDS. A/RES/65/277). The Commission's messages and recommendations must form the basis of the next generation of HIV responses, where governments and citizens approach HIV as an issue of health, development and social justice.

Mandeep Dhaliwal is Cluster Leader: Human Rights and Governance, HIV/AIDS Group, Bureau for Development Policy, United Nations Development Programme. The author is grateful for the contributions of Emilie Pradichit, Vivek Divan, Tenu Avafia, Royan Konstatinov and Jeffrey O' Malley.

CHAPTER 10

Human Rights, Health and Development

Daniel Tarantola, Andrew Byrnes, Michael Johnson, Lynn Kemp, Anthony Zwi and Sofia Gruskin

INTRODUCTION

Those who work on the implementation of human rights, improved health for all and human development have in common aspirations to improve human welfare, the relationships between people, and the environments in which we live. Each reflects shared individual and collective aspirations for a better life, and is grounded in both moral and instrumental values revolving around fundamental concepts of dignity, justice, wellbeing and progress. While all three areas have long histories of struggle, the events of the last two centuries have underlined their global significance, the need for deepening our understanding of their links and the importance of developing analytical tools to identify and manage the potential offered by a human rights approach to improving health and the process of development.

These events include the 19th century industrial revolution in Europe and the resulting expectations of an improved quality of life contrasting dramatically with the health and social inequalities increasingly visible in the streets and factories of mushrooming cities (Frank and Mustard 1994). Public health and medical advances followed, seeking through human ingenuity to apply science to address emerging problems. States that had built their industries competed with one another for economic and political influence and several states extensively exploited poorer ones through colonial domination. The atrocities of World War II led to recognition of a compelling need to set out the obligations of governments towards their populations as well as towards each other (Lauren 1998). The process of decolonisation in the 1960s, the end of the cold war in the 1990s (Tarantola 2008), and the subsequent emergence of new independent States as the process of economic globalisation rapidly escalated (Benedek et al. 2008) drew more political and public attention to global inequalities in health, disparities in wealth and the need for the realisation of human rights. The unabated spread of HIV since the early 1980s and the global response to the epidemic launched in 1987 advanced the understanding of the interdependence of health and human rights. In particular, it highlighted the fact that those subjected to discrimination and violations of other human rights—especially those living in poverty—were disproportionately affected by HIV (Mann & Tarantola 1996).

This paper explores the links between human rights concerns, improving the health of individuals and communities, and the goals and processes of develop-

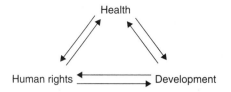

Figure 10.1 Health, human rights and development

ment that are central to improving people's living standards and life chances. It builds its analysis around a simple conceptual framework (Figure 10.1) which illustrates the interdependence of health, development and human rights. It highlights the underlying principles, values and prominent features of human rights, health and development as independent domains, and then describes their interactions. It focuses particular attention on how these linkages can be analysed and reinforced in practice. This chapter also proposes that a Health, Human Rights and Development Impact Assessment (HHRDIA) may be a practical approach that builds on the synergies between the three domains, providing structured and transparent monitoring and evaluation mechanisms to enhance accountability for progress, while revealing shortcomings in policy processes, and improve human welfare outcomes.

HUMAN RIGHTS, HEALTH AND DEVELOPMENT: ASPIRATIONS, VALUES AND DISCIPLINES

The strong causal links between human rights, health policies and programs and progressive development approaches can be demonstrated through a variety of perspectives. These include: starting with human rights (their origins and constitution being explored below); their human value (aimed at improving people's lives); social relevance (consideration of the individual as part of social constructs); normative content (standards and directions for national governance and international cooperation); instrumental application (frameworks of analysis; policy formulation, program development and evaluation); disciplinary base (exploration, documentation, research and teaching of theory and practice in separate academic institutions); and the ways in which they engage communities (building on community awareness-raising, participation and leadership). Although it risks oversimplification, for clarity of exposition we refer to health, human rights, and development below as three "domains." This section summarises the key features of each domain, in order to set out the common, cross-disciplinary information-base necessary for identifying and building upon their inter-relationships—the main objective of this contribution.

Human Rights

In the modern world human rights are often invoked to justify a variety of fundamental political, social, economic and cultural claims. The origins of rights (whether anchored in natural law, positive law, a theory of human needs, capabilities and flourishing, or some other theoretical position) and their justifications are diverse. There is nevertheless considerable international consensus about a central core of human rights claims, in particular those embodied in explicit international obligations accepted by Nation-States in the principal United Nations (UN) and regional human rights instruments adopted since World War II (see, for example, Centre for the Study of Human Rights 2005). This is so notwithstanding the challenges of cultural relativism and the need for universal human rights to be realised in the specific contexts of different communities (Baxi 2002; Steiner & Alston 2000). Challenges to dominant discourses of human rights have come in waves, with new claims to the enjoyment of universally guaranteed rights being brought by marginalised groups (racial and ethnic minorities, women, children, persons with disabilities, among others), who realise both the promise of rights and the shortfall in their practical enjoyment. Enriched by new perspectives, human rights today play an important role in shaping public policies, programs and practice aimed at improving actual and potential individual and social welfare.

Human Rights as State Obligations

Human rights constitute a set of normative principles and standards which can be traced back to antiquity although they received their particular modern imprint through the work of political philosophers and leaders of some 17th century European countries (Tomuschat 2003), and those who developed and expanded upon their ideas. The atrocities perpetrated during World War II gave rise, in 1948, to the Universal Declaration of Human Rights (UDHR) and later to a series of treaties and conventions which codified the aspirational nature of the UDHR into instruments which would be binding on States through international human rights law. Among these are the International Covenant on Civil and Political Rights (ICCPR) and the International Covenant on Economic, Social and Cultural Rights (ICE-SCR), both of which entered into force in

1976. Similar developments have also been seen at the regional level, frequently with more effective institutions for the monitoring and enforcement of those norms.

Human rights are often described as claims that individuals have on governments (and sometimes on others, including private actors such as corporations), simply by virtue of being human. In the case of the international human rights treaties and under many domestic legal systems these entitlements are embodied in legal instruments which are formally binding on States and their institutions. The formal guarantee of a right does not of itself mean that the rights-holder enjoys the right in practice and, despite their formal entitlements, people are often constrained in their ability to realise those rights fully, or indeed at all. Those most vulnerable to violations or neglect of their rights are often those with the least power to contest the denial of their rights. As a result, their well-being and health may be adversely affected (Farmer 2004).

The relationship between the individual or group who is the rights-holder and the State is central to the concept and practical enjoyment of human rights, and it is the nature and scope of the State's obligations (including in relation to the actions of private actors) which are central to the understanding of how human rights may be promoted and protected in practice (see box below).

NATURE OF HUMAN RIGHTS AND A TYPOLOGY OF STATES' OBLIGATIONS

Fundamental human rights are posited as inalienable (individuals cannot lose these rights any more than they can cease being human beings); as indivisible (individuals cannot be denied a right because it is deemed a less important right or something non-essential); and as interdependent (all human rights are part of a complementary framework, the enjoyment of one right affecting and being affected by all others) (Vienna Declaration 1993).

Currently, the most influential approach at the international level to understanding the different dimensions of human rights is a tripartite typology of the nature and extent of States' obligations: in relation to all rights, governments have obligations to respect, protect and fulfil each right (Maastricht 1997). Firstly, States must respect human rights, which requires governments to refrain from interfering directly or indirectly with the enjoyment of human rights. Secondly, States also have the obligation to protect human rights, which requires governments to take measures that prevent non-State actors from interfering with the enjoyment of human rights, and to provide legal and other appropriate forms of redress which are accessible and effective for such infringements. Finally, States have the obligation to fulfil human rights, which requires States to adopt appropriate legislative, administrative, budgetary, judicial, promotional and other measures towards the full realisation of human rights, thus creating the conditions in which persons are able to enjoy their rights fully in practice. This typology has proved particularly useful in elaborating the specific content of many economic and social rights—including the right to health.

It has been common to distinguish between civil and political rights (sometimes called "negative rights" or liberties), and economic, social and cultural rights (sometimes referred to as "positive rights"). This approach has been debunked as inaccurate and outdated (Vienna Declaration and Programme of Action 1993, art2). All rights may involve the allocation of resources (for example, the classical civil right to a fair trial is premised on the existence of a legal system resourced with judges, court buildings and legal aid). Even those rights traditionally thought of as subject only to progressive realisation have elements which require immediate action to be taken (for example, in relation to ensuring that all enjoy the right to education, carrying out a baseline analysis, the development of a plan which should be "deliberate, concrete and targeted as clearly as possible towards meeting the obligations") (UN CESCR General Comment 3), and may have justiciable elements (Eide 1995).

The Right to Health

The right of everyone to the enjoyment of the highest attainable standard of physical and mental health—or the right to health

as it is commonly referred to—appears in one form or another in many international and regional human rights documents. Furthermore, nearly every other article in these international instruments also has clear implications for health. The right to health builds on, but is not limited to, Article 12 of the ICESCR. Most of the other principal international and regional human rights treaties contain provisions relevant to health, for example, the International Convention on the Elimination of All Forms of Racial Discrimination (CERD), the Convention on the Elimination of All Forms of Discrimination against Women (CEDAW), the Convention on the Rights of the Child (CRC), and the Convention on the Rights of Persons with Disabilities (CRPD).

The right to health does not mean the right to be healthy as such, but embodies an obligation on the part of the government to create the conditions necessary for individuals to achieve their optimal health status. In 2000 the United Nations Committee on Economic, Social and Cultural Rights adopted a General Comment explicating the substance of government obligations relating to the right to health (UN CESCR General Comment No 14). In addition to clarifying governmental responsibility for policies, programs and practices influencing the conditions necessary for health, it sets out requirements for the delivery of health services, including their availability, acceptability, accessibility and quality. It lays out directions for the practical application of Article 12 and proposes a monitoring framework indicating the ways in which the State's responsibility can be implemented through national law. Currently, over 100 national Constitutions have recognised a right to health and this number continues to increase as Constitutions are rewritten or updated (Kinney 2001).

The interrelatedness of human rights, development as a process and improved health status as a measure of development can be seen clearly in the context of the right to health. Rights relating to autonomy, information, education, food and nutrition, freedom of association, reproduction, equality, sexuality, participation and non-discrimination are integral and indivisible elements of the achievement of the highest attainable standard of health. So too is the enjoyment of the right to health, inseparable from the enjoyment of most other rights, whether they are categorised as civil and political, economic, social or cultural (for example, the enjoyment of the right to work, the right to education, or the right to family life) (Leary 1994). The discourse of gender, reproductive and sexual rights also highlights the interdependency of human rights. A woman's right to health cuts across the economic, social and cultural as well as civil and political rights, affecting the individual, as well as the entire family unit (Petchesky 2003). This recognition is based on empirical observation and on a growing body of evidence which establishes the impact that lack of fulfilment of these rights has on people's health status—education, non-discrimination, food and nutrition epitomise this relationship (Gruskin & Tarantola 2001). Conversely,

ill-health may constrain the fulfilment of all rights, as the capacity of individuals to claim and enjoy all their human rights may depend on their physical, mental and social well-being. For example, when States fail to fulfil their obligations, ill-health may result in discrimination—as is commonly seen in the context of HIV, cancer or mental illness. It may cause arbitrary termination or denial of employment, housing or social security, and limit access to food or to education with the consequence that social and economic development potentials may not be achieved.

The tripartite typology of human rights obligations—to respect, to protect, and to fulfill—originally developed in the context of economic and social rights (Eide 1995) has been particularly useful in indicating what steps a government should take in relation to each dimension of its obligations. In the context of the right to health, the obligation to respect means that no health policy, practice, program or legal measure should directly violate the individual's right to health, for example, by exposing individuals to a known health hazard. Policies should ensure the provision of health services to all population groups on the basis of equality and freedom from discrimination, paying particular attention to vulnerable and marginalised groups (Hunt 2008). The obligation to protect, in relation to the right to health, means that governments must appropriately regulate such important non-State actors as the health care industry (including private health care and social services providers, pharmaceutical and health insurance companies) and, more generally, national and multinational enterprises whose contribution to market economies can also significantly affect the lifestyle, work life and health of both individuals and communities. The array of non-State actors is diverse and growing. It includes commercial enterprises whose activities have a major impact on the environment—such as energy-producing companies, manufacturers and agricultural producers—as well as the food industry and the media. Each of these actors has the capacity to promote and protect, or to neglect and violate, the right to health (and other rights) within their field of activity. Finally, the obligation to fulfil the right to health includes a duty to put into place appropriate health and health-related policies which ensure human rights promotion and protection with an immediate focus on vulnerable and marginalised groups where the value of health and other benefits to individuals and groups may be higher.

The Right to Development

In 1986 the UN General Assembly adopted the Declaration on the Right to Development, Article 1 of which states that "the right to development is an inalienable human right by virtue of which every human person and all peoples are entitled to participate in, contribute to, and enjoy economic, social, cultural and political development, in which all human rights and fundamental freedoms can be fully realized" (Declaration on the Right to Development). The human person is identified as the beneficiary of the right to development, as of all human rights. The right can be invoked both by individuals and by peoples and imposes obligations on individual States to ensure equal and adequate access to essential resources, and on the international community to promote fair development policies and effective international cooperation. The Vienna Declaration and Programme of Action adopted by the 1993 World Conference on Human Rights recognised that democracy, development, and respect for human rights and fundamental freedoms are interdependent and mutually reinforcing (Vienna 1993, art 8). The Vienna Declaration reaffirmed the right to development as a universal and inalienable

right and an integral part of fundamental human rights. It also made clear that, while development facilitates the enjoyment of all human rights, a lack of development may not be invoked to justify the abridgement of other internationally recognised human rights (Vienna 1993, art 10).

The declaration of the right to development has been controversial because some critics have seen it as having the potential for abuse by the State, which may use it to suppress concrete human rights ostensibly in order to ensure the realisation of the more amorphous right to development. Critics have also expressed concern that the State, rather than individuals or peoples, may in effect become the rights-holder, with low-income states being entitled to claim assistance from higher-income ones (see Kirchmeir 2006). Nevertheless, there is clearly a close relationship between the right to development and the right to health—enjoyment of the right to an adequate standard of health is both a goal of the exercise of the right to development, and a means of contributing to achieving development (Sengupta 2002; Marks 2005).

Health in Transition

Perspectives on health reflect the rapidly changing realities and opportunities in today's globalised world. Responding to health needs is ultimately determined by how we address the issue of rights and access to power and resources. This section seeks to identify core achievements of public health, the methods and approaches which have underpinned such achievements, and the challenges of engaging with transforming policy-making and service delivery structures.

The World Health Organization defined health in 1948, in its constitution, as "a state of complete physical, mental and social well-being and not merely the absence of disease or infirmity" (WHO 1948, 1). The definition has been modified to also include the ability to lead a "socially and economically productive life." Sen (1999) has identified health as a key determinant of the ability of an individual or group to benefit from a broader set of rights and entitlements. Public health, defined as "the art and science of preventing disease, promoting health, and prolonging life through the organised effort of society" (Acheson 1988), describes well the challenges facing the field. It also reinforces widespread recognition that promoting health requires multi-sector and "upstream" efforts to address the determinants of health, much more than simply improving access to health care (Baum 2007; Baum & Harris 2006).

Over the past two centuries, better education, improved nutrition and environmental advances, including better water and sanitation, safer working conditions and improved housing, have enhanced health outcomes (Frank & Mustard 1994; WHO 1999). Life expectancy has greatly increased in many medium and high income countries and major causes of mortality in early childhood, in particular, have been, or have the potential to be, addressed. Technologies have been developed to tackle infectious diseases, injuries and non-communicable diseases, as well as to treat and manage ill-health. Despite these significant achievements in dealing with exposures which pose a risk to life, including childbirth itself (Freedman et al. 2007), the benefits of economic advances, human security and access to health care, have not been shared equally, and significant disparities exist both within and between countries (WHO 1995). Preventable child mortality remains unacceptably high in many poor nations, in particular in Africa (Black et al. 2003). In some countries, notably those mired in conflict or under repressive regimes, population health has

deteriorated (Zwi et al. 2002) and the poorest communities are often significantly worse off.

In the past half century, the ability to control many potentially lethal infectious diseases has been achieved through better understanding of their causes, development of technologies to interrupt exposure or prevent occurrence, improved diagnosis, treatment and management, and, in the case of smallpox, the ability to eradicate an organism. Prevention and control of non-communicable diseases has been much less successful. Smoking-related diseases, obesity, cancer and injuries, are all on the increase; mental health problems, too, at a population-wide level have not been effectively addressed (Boutayeb 2006). Many countries need to simultaneously confront both communicable and non-communicable diseases (Lopez et al. 2006).

While the new public health, as enunciated in the Ottawa Charter for Health Promotion (Ottawa Charter 1986), highlighted efforts to build healthy public policy, create supportive environments, strengthen community action and reorient health services towards a health promoting perspective, the achievement in these areas has been limited (Leger 2007; Wise & Nutbeam 2007). The Charter's definition of health as being "created by caring for oneself and others, by being able to take decisions and have control over one's life circumstances, and by ensuring that the society one lives in creates conditions that allow the attainment of health by all its members" is a reality not experienced by many worldwide (Ottawa Charter 1986, art 3).

The role of the State in health services provision and in securing the basic needs required for health and development has been challenged and in many cases undermined. Increasingly, the private sector and other non-State actors have been brought into the process of providing care, often within an economic and ideological framework which positions health care as yet another commodity, without recognising the existence of significant market failures. Powerful non-State actors are increasingly involved in shaping the agenda around public health (Cohen 2006). Multilateral organisations, private foundations and the World Bank have in most cases become more influential than the World Health Organization in shaping public health policies and health care service responses in low and middle income countries (Martens 2003).

New supranational funds, such as the Global Fund to Fight AIDS, Tuberculosis and Malaria, provide substantial funds but also may end up determining how countries address major health problems (Garrett 2007). Public-private partnerships have proliferated, securing public investment to produce new technologies and programs, but also shaping what services are available and under what circumstances (Buse & Walt 2000a and 2000b; Richter 2004). Private foundations, such as the Bill and Melinda Gates Foundation, make available more funds to health development activities than any other bilateral or multilateral agency, determining priorities and shifting health and research resources with limited or no system of accountability to those often most affected by such decisions (Okie 2006). A casualty of the changed mechanisms through which development funding is made available has been the strengthening of health systems and human resource capacity not only to deliver specified programs, but to provide a comprehensive framework within which improved health, equity of access, better outcomes and greater participation can be secured. Strengthening health services has become urgent, given the gap between investments and the actual benefits that have been observed (WHO 2007).

Determinants of Health

Key health issues and challenges are increasingly presented as technical issues, requiring the engagement of "experts." This is contested by commentators and civil society organisations, such as the People's Health Movement, which draw attention to the pivotal role of communities, non-governmental organisations and the State in constructing the environment in which rights to health and broader development can be promoted and secured (People's Health Movement 2006).

While health is increasingly understood as related to a wide range of determinants, and there is recognition that health is far more than health care, strategies to secure the commitment and resources required to overcome inequities in access to these determinants of health is lacking. The ability to shape and frame how inequalities and inequities are seen, the way in which they are defined and tackled, and from where the resources to address them should come, remains crucial. Rights, politics and power are arguably moving to centre stage (Farmer 2004).

Human Development

Human development is a qualitative as well as a quantitative improvement in the level (and standards) of individual and collective welfare—welfare that includes elements contributing to self-sustenance, self-esteem and freedom and is a general goal sought by individuals, groups, Nation-States and the international community. It is also specific and can be targeted at people whose level of welfare lags below those of others and is below their potential (Thirlwall 1999). For general improvement in measures of individual and collective welfare and development to occur, factors such as the status of human rights that play a role in determining the capacity of individuals and groups to realise it must be considered.

The means adopted to achieve improvements in individual and social welfare have evolved unevenly over time as human knowledge, economic capacity and institutional sophistication have grown. It is also clearly recognised that the status of any individual or group of people is dependent for its existence on the recognition and respect exercised by others and therefore to be successful, a process of development should incorporate a "rights" perspective (Frankovits et al. 2001).

Development and Change

The process of change and development, as noted by economists from Adam Smith onwards, has never been regular, linear or distributed evenly. Indeed, it became more uneven with the advent of capitalism as social, cultural and political innovation (with an accompanying decay of traditional social, economic and political systems), capital accumulation, market development, technological change and associated nation State building accelerated in northern Europe and spread outwards. The process of development can be seen as a qualitative change in conditions and an essential prerequisite to quantitative change measured as growth. Joseph Schumpeter described this as "creative destruction," accelerating first in the most developed countries and spreading in irregular waves across the world (Schumpeter 1969, 253). Processes of change have seen the destruction and displacement of significant parts of pre-existing values (cultures) and patterns of social and economic relations, including embedded rights, in households, rural and urban settlements and nation States. New personal and social systems of rights (including property), relations, production systems and governance structures emerged to change the distribu-

tion of income and systems of social, economic and political authority (see North in Atkinson et al. 2005).

From Liberal to Neo-Liberal Model of Development

The growing differences in living standards between individuals and States that emerged with the agricultural, industrial and service revolutions in Europe almost immediately led to the study of the internal factors that contributed to the success of the first industrialised country, Britain, to see how this could be emulated in other countries and extended to the growing economic, social and political integration between countries (Cohn 2008, 8). The model of development that emerged in the 18th century, based on the early insights of John Locke and Adam Smith, focused on the importance to the emerging system of the extension of private property relations to facilitate the exercise of liberalism: the pursuit of individual economic self interest; the building of universal and secure financial systems; the establishment and extension of competitive market systems; and limits on the capacity of state policy and programs to restrict market development (Cohn 2008, 73). The objectives embedded in the dominant economic and political (liberal) policy model exercised in wealthier countries in turn were advocated in developing countries as a solution to their development problems. These objectives became part of the so-called neo-liberal approach to policy reform characterised best in relation to developing countries in the ten-point shopping list of reforms called the Washington Consensus (Stiglitz 2002; Stiglitz in Atkinson et al. 2005, 16; Williamson 1990). The goal of the Consensus through adopting policies such as reducing regulation, taxation, public expenditure (Rodrik in Atkinson 2005, 212) was to lend weight to the call to deregulate and open up to the international economy the domestic economies of developing countries, extend market exchange and achieve the most efficient allocation of resources possible and consequently maximise levels of individual welfare at any given level of financial income.

Failure of the Washington Consensus

The ideas embodied in the Washington Consensus and its predecessors have been criticised as being based on limited simplistic assumptions that reflect little consideration for what actually contributes to the development process. Claims in the Washington Consensus that the extension of property rights, the only rights mentioned there, are sufficient for development were criticised. As Sen has pointed out, the freedoms embodied in such ideas are insufficient in themselves to achieve real development which involves a process of establishing a broader set of conditions for people to develop their own capabilities for personal development (Sen 1999). In other words, the pursuit of property rights alone was not sufficient to achieve the multiple objectives of balanced multi-sectoral growth that can deepen and spread development (see Thirlwall 1999, 323). To achieve these requires the extension of a much wider range of rights than those for securing property. At a fundamental level the neo-liberal model also failed to understand the important role of institutions, defined as informal values and rules in governing behaviour (see North 1990; North in Atkinson A et al. 2005, 1) or the important role of institutions as formal organisations through which the capacity for change of individuals and communities is mediated and managed (see Jutting 2003; also Rodrik in Atkinson 2005, 209). As Sachs has summed up, the Washington Consensus is focused primarily on realising the interests (and associated ideologies) of power-ful developed countries at the expense of developing ones and has not addressed the widening gap in living standards between the developed and the developing world experiencing high levels of poverty (Sachs 2005).

Bridging the Development "Gap"

The campaigns of the last three centuries to liberate individuals and communities from formalised authoritarian systems of control such as those of feudalism and slavery have been the foundation for creating better states of psychological welfare, health, social and material welfare as well as opening up the potentials for further improvements (Grayling 2007; Ishay 2004). Development studies recognised that this process was dynamic, characterised by lags between individuals, groups and particularly nation States, in different places establishing basic human rights, improving human capacities, such as health, and building the institutions and the productive systems that create the potential for development. This perspective is also contested as revealed by the discussion of the Washington Consensus.

The problem of the development gap between the early industrial economies and other countries identified by Sachs (2005) was not new. A concern with identifying the specific development requirements necessary for the backward countries to bridge the development gap and catch-up has been recognised as important for a long time (Myrdal 1975, 65). In addition to the question of the development gap itself, longer-term questions exist as to the role of other historical factors, such as the continuing effects of colonial inheritance and the dependency of the developing world on the developed for technology, capital and markets (see, for example, Acemogolu et al., 2001, in relation to colonialism). Achieving development depends on achieving a much more complex set of goals, changes to processes and institutional system-building and it is now accepted that there could be a number of different paths to development (see, for example, Chang 2003; Rodrik in Atkinson 2005; Sengupta et al. 2005). If the choice of any specific pathway to development is subject to question, what is not in doubt is the growing recognition of the importance of development as a general goal, this being reflected also in the human rights discourse being extended to cover a broader range of rights including the right to development itself.

RECIPROCAL RELATIONSHIPS BETWEEN HEALTH, DEVELOPMENT AND HUMAN RIGHTS

A Theoretical Framework

The interactions between human rights, health and development can be illustrated by the reciprocal linkages that exist between any two of these domains. The aim is not only achieving the highest possible realisation of rights, health or development, but amplification of the synergies between them, resulting in overall benefits substantially greater than the sum of its parts. Recognising these reciprocal relationships and synergies does not imply that any policy or action in any of the three domains will positively impact the others: an untested development program may have negative effects on health or the environment; the protection of the right to health without attention to other human rights may be harmful to some individuals or communities; and disproportionate investments in a narrowly targeted health intervention may temporarily constrain progress in other health areas. The basic premise underlying our framework is that optimal policies and programs must simultaneously consider the implications for health, development or human rights, maximising overall benefit and minimising pitfalls and potential harms.

Health and Development

Health is an important prerequisite for, and desirable outcome of, human development and progress. Health is "... directly constitutive of the person's wellbeing and it enables a person to function as an agent, that is, to pursue the various goals and projects in life that she has reason to value" (Anand 2004). Health is also the most extensively measured component of well-being; it benefits from dedicated services and is often seen as a sine-qua-non for the fulfillment of all other aspirations (WHO 2002a). It can be considered to be "a marker, a way of keeping score of how well the society is doing in delivering well-being" (Marmot 2004).

Fifteen years ago, the World Bank acknowledged the reciprocal dependency between progress in health and economic development (The World Bank 1993). This acknowledgment was not an earth-shaking revelation, particularly to those who were working in health and development in Africa where the HIV pandemic was already taking a heavy toll. Yet the 1993 World Development Report marked a turning-point in the Bank's lending policy, while the nascent global movement towards poverty alleviation consistently emphasised the importance of health in the fight against poverty. It was not until 2001 that the international community, through the WHO Commission on Macroeconomics and Health, documented that poverty leads to ill-health, but also that ill-health leads to poverty (WHO 2001). The eight Millennium Development Goals (MDGs)—which set targets for 2015 to, amongst other things, halve extreme poverty, halt the spread of HIV/AIDS and improve health and education—have been agreed to by all the world's countries and leading development institutions (UNDP 2005). Arguably, all MDGs are linked to health either by their direct bearing on health outcome and the needed services (e.g., through efforts to reduce child and maternal mortality, HIV, malaria and other diseases), or by underscoring principles central to public health policy (e.g., gender equality), or else by calling for the creation of policies addressing the underlying conditions for progress in health (e.g., education, environmental sustainability, global partnerships) (Dodd & Cassels 2006).

The MDGs highlight a number of important health indicators that deserve attention, but are not in themselves sensitive to the distribution of these indicators within countries and may promote a focus on improving indicators by directing services to those easy to reach with little attention to those most marginalised or disempowered (Gwatkin 2005). Attention to process, including the provision of information, improving access, enhancing accountability and sensitivity to cultural and gender concerns may be overlooked as efforts are directed simply at increasing the number of people served or activities undertaken. Research which enhances the visibility of those least able to access services, as well as the ability of users of services to help shape them, deserve more attention, as do studies of the unanticipated impact of large-scale development initiatives on individuals, communities and systems operating within resource-poor countries.

Health and Human Rights

Viewed as a universal aspiration, the notion of health as the attainment of physical, mental and social well-being implies its dependency on, and contribution to, the realisation of all human rights. From the same perspective, the enjoyment by everyone of the highest attainable standard of physical and mental health is a human right

(UN CESCR General Comment 14). From a global normative perspective, health and human rights remain closely intertwined in many international treaties and declarations and supported by mechanisms of monitoring and accountability (the efficiency of which can be questioned) drawn from both fields.

Health and human rights individually occupy privileged places in public discourse, political debates, public policy and the media, and both are at the top of human aspirations. There is hardly a proposed political agenda that does not refer to justice, security, health, housing, education and employment opportunities. These aspirations are often not framed as human rights but the fact that they are nevertheless contained in human rights treaties and often translated into national constitutions and legislation provides policy and legal support for efforts in these areas. Incorporating the relationship of health and human rights into public health policy therefore responds to the demands of people, policy makers and political leaders for outcomes that meet public aspirations. It also creates an opportunity for helping decipher how all human rights and other determinants of well-being and social progress interact, by allowing progress to be measured towards these goals, as well as shaping policy directions and agendas for action.

Anchoring public health strategies in human rights can enrich the concepts and methods used to attain health objectives, by drawing attention to the legal and policy context within which health interventions occur, as well as bringing in rights principles such as non-discrimination and the participation of affected communities in the design, implementation, monitoring and evaluation of health programs and interventions (Gruskin et al. 2007). The introduction of human rights into public health work is about approaches and processes and their application towards maximising public health gains (Gruskin & Tarantola 2001). It does not imply that how the work is done or what its ultimate outcome will be are preordained. For example, using human rights standards with a focus on health systems requires attention to their availability, accessibility, acceptability, quality and outcomes among different population groups (UN CESCR General Comment 14). The added value of human rights for health is in systematising attention to these issues, requiring that benchmarks and targets be set and ensuring transparency and accountability for what decisions are made and their ultimate outcomes (Gruskin et al. 2007).

Development and Human Rights

Most authorities agree that achieving development implies a qualitative change in environmental, social, economic or political conditions (that may or may not generate economic growth as conventionally measured) that improves the welfare of individuals, communities and nation States (Remenyi in Kingsbury et al. 2004, 22; Sen 1999, 1; Stiglitz in Atkinson et al. 2005, 17). Welfare can be measured individually and collectively in various, potentially problematic, ways: as status (for example, measured as income or health status), capacity (for example, as human capital in the form of knowledge and skills), participation (for example, as individuals' access to employment and capacity to engage with institutions) and possibilities (for example, as the presence of pathways to future development). All these measures are intertwined with human rights, for example, for the poor to participate in the benefits of development—as is evidenced by the close relationship between the MDGs and human rights (Alston 2005). Development-specific knowledge is also required, for example, about the presence, range and roles of the different institutions, social, economic and

political, that are engaged in the development process. The specificities of different societies in terms of history, culture, technology and institutions and how these differences both can and should translate into varied "local" responses to regional or global processes, and varied strategies for development, also require attention.

BRINGING IT TOGETHER

Human rights, health and development intersect in a number of ways which, for practical purposes, can be considered on three levels: the national and international context within which policies are developed, the outcomes of these policies, and the processes through which they are developed, applied and monitored.

Context

A distinction exists between development policy affecting health (most policy does) and public health policy (often emerging from, or on the initiative of, public health governmental authorities). Development policies affecting health—for example, those related to gender, trade, intellectual property, the environment, migration, education, housing or labour—are contingent upon national laws and international treaties or agreements which often overlook—by omission or commission—their potential health consequences (Kemm 2001). Public policy is expected to aim for achieving the optimal synergy between health, development and human rights, building on the premise that the highest quality of a public health and development policy is attained when the highest possible health outcome, greatest prospects for economic and societal development and the fullest realisation of human rights are attained. This requires close interaction between public health professionals, those engaged in economic and social development work, human rights practitioners and concerned communities.

As it is generally formulated and monitored by the State, public policy operates in the context of the obligations of the State under international human rights treaties and national law. Central to these obligations are those to respect, protect and fulfil all human rights, including the rights to participate in public affairs, to equality and non-discrimination, and dignity. When a State is implementing its international obligations or international standards derived from treaties or other instruments in areas as diverse as international trade or climate change (for example, under the 2005 Kyoto Protocol, instruments adopted by the World Health Assembly, the World Trade Organization (WTO) or other international organisations), it should do so in a manner which avoids conflict between the various standards and pursues mutually supportive implementation. For example, membership in the WTO implies that members must become party to the Agreement on Trade Related Aspects of Intellectual Property Rights (TRIPS). The constraints imposed by TRIPS on developing countries with regards to intellectual property protection with respect to pharmaceuticals in particular only became known in the late 1990s as new, proven therapies for HIV/AIDS were reaching the international market. Civil society movements and some international organisations embarked on a campaign to overcome the constraints set by TRIPS to the production or importation of generic medicines by developing countries, which needed them most ('t Hoen 2002). It was not until 2002, however, that the WHO and the WTO jointly produced a document on WTO agreements and public health (WTO & WHO 2002). In most developing countries, Ministries of Health had not been consulted, were not in a position to make an assessment, or underestimated the possible health impacts of joining the WTO. Whether by oversight or through lack of capacity, States placed themselves in a situation which privileged one set of benefits while undermining others, a failure less likely to have occurred had open, transparent and participatory processes been established.

Process

The human rights to information, assembly and participation in public affairs imply, among other practical steps, the engagement of communities in decisions affecting them. As highlighted earlier, the history of health and human rights established that community representation in decision-making bodies increases the quality and impact of public health measures. Similarly, the experience, successes and failures in development have amply demonstrated that success is more likely when people are recognised as subjects and not merely objects of development (Sanoff 2000). In the last two decades, stimulated by the response to HIV in particular, nongovernmental organisations have played key roles in drawing attention to policies which were or could be detrimental to health (e.g., restrictions in access to medicines, denial of sex education to young people, lack of access to harm reduction methods among substance users) (Akukwe 1998). Civil society has also been instrumental in the development field, drawing attention, for example, to marginalised communities and low-income countries, environmental degradation, marketing of unhealthy foods and global inequities in trade, agriculture and access to technology (Howell & Pearce 2002). It is important, however, to determine who can legitimately speak on behalf of concerned communities.

The process of bringing together health, human rights and development in policy and program efforts extends beyond broad participation and transparency. It requires also verifying that decisions made and priorities set abide by human rights norms and standards, including but not limited to guarantees of non-discrimination (for example, relating to gender and vulnerable populations) and accountability.

Outcome and Impact

Human rights and health and development policies emphasise the importance of outcome and impact, crudely measured in public health terms by the reduction of mortality, morbidity and disability and in development terms by the improvement of quality of life, along with economic measurement enabling an assessment of "value for money" (Hyder & Morrow 2006). The extent to which the outcomes measured include the fulfilment of human rights is seldom factored in. For example, one would like to see the value of policies which promote sex education in school measured not only in terms of reduction of teenage pregnancy or the incidence of sexually-transmitted diseases, but how the right of the child to information is fulfilled in this way, how it affects further demands for health-related, life-saving information, and how access to this information prepares young people to benefit fully from economic and social development. Likewise, when assessing the effects of policies that prioritise childhood immunisation, one would want to know not only how immunisations make people healthier, both early and later in their childhood, but also how the right of the child to growth and development, and the right to education by improving attendance and performances at school, are factored in (Behrman 1996; Leslie & Jamison 1990).

Bringing health, development and human rights together means examining the context in which they function, seeking to identify opportunities for the elaboration of sound policy and programs, and recognising and addressing the tensions and pitfalls in their interactions. It requires ensuring that the processes of policy and program development, implementation and monitoring are informed by best knowledge and practice relevant to the three domains. Ideally, this can provide a vision of human development where policies and programs achieve the highest possible outcome and impact is measured and accounted for in health, development and human rights terms (Figure 10.2).

Context, Process and Outcome

Monitoring process and measuring outcome and impact from a combined health, development and human rights perspective implies measurement indicators which are neither fully developed nor tested. One

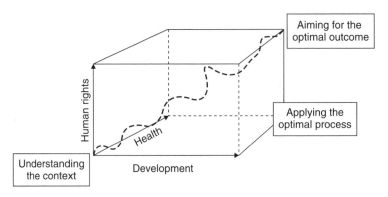

Figure 10.2 Seeking optimal synergy between health, development and human rights

of the constraints is that measurement at the national, aggregate level is not sensitive to disparities that may exist within nations, for example, as a result of discrimination. As the health and development fields are becoming more strongly rooted in robust human rights and sound public health and development principles, the concepts of a "Rights-based Approach to Development" (UNDP 1998) and "Rights-based Approach to Health" have emerged (WHO 2002b). Although these approaches will not be discussed here in great detail, they are worth mentioning as they have generated much thinking and work on how the contributions of these respective domains to strategic development, monitoring and evaluation can be brought together.

Rights-Based Approaches to Health and Development Policies and Programs

Initially conceptualised in the mid-1990s as a "human rights based approach to development programming" by the United Nations Development Programme (UNDP 1998), rights-based approaches have been applied to specific populations (e.g., children, women, migrants, refugees, Indigenous populations), basic needs (e.g., food, water, security, education, justice), health issues (e.g., sexual and reproductive health, HIV, access to medicines), sources of livelihood (e.g., land tenure, pastoral development, fisheries), and the work of diverse actors engaged in development activities (e.g., UN system, governments, NGOs, corporate sector). Even as health cuts across all of these areas and is regarded both as a prerequisite for and an important outcome of development, the understanding of what a rights-based approach actually means for public health efforts has varied across sectors, disciplines and organisations.

In order to help define the core principles of rights-based approaches (RBAs)

applicable across all sectors, a "Common Understanding" was elaborated by the UN system in 2003 (UN 2003). In short, it suggests the following: all programs should intentionally further international human rights; all development efforts, at all levels of programming, must be guided by human rights standards and principles found in international human rights law; and all development efforts must build the capacity of "duty bearers" to meet obligations and/or "rights holders" to claim rights.

This Common Understanding has clear implications for the implementation of health policies and programs as it offers a common way of thinking although, even within the health domain, what these actually mean in practice remains far from universally understood. A review of public health programs termed "rights-based" by a range of UN system actors and their partners' points to several areas relevant to what implementation of a rights-based approach to health might look like (WHO 2005). A rights-based approach to health makes explicit reference to human rights from the outset, does not invent the content of rights and does not name the relevance of rights only in retrospect; emphasises building capacity and does not use human rights norms as a way of naming violations after they have occurred but as a way of preventing violations from occurring in the first place; and is based on implementation of one or several core rights concepts including non-discrimination, participation, accountability and transparency.

In practice, bringing health, development and human rights together provides a framework within which the assessment, design, implementation, monitoring and evaluation of the progress, success or failure of a policy or program can be developed and evaluated against benchmarks relevant to all domains (Figure 10.3). Of particular interest then is to not only evaluate but also anticipate the reciprocal impacts

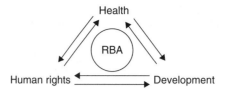

Rights-based approaches:

- Are based on international HR standards and principles
- Recognise right-holders and duty-bearers
- Focus on discriminated and marginalised groups
- Aim for the progressive achievement of all human rights
- Give equal importance to the outcome and the process of development
- Uphold principles of: *Indivisibility and interrelatedness of rights, Non-discrimination, Participation,* and *Accountability*

Figure 10.3 Rights-Based Approaches

policy and programs developed in each of these domains may have on one another through use of an assessment process.

PROJECTING THE IMPACTS OF POLICIES AND PROGRAMS: TOWARDS A HEALTH, DEVELOPMENT AND HUMAN RIGHTS IMPACT ASSESSMENT

The links between health, human rights and development described above suggest that the incorporation of human rights and development considerations into health impact assessment (HIA) may provide a structured and transparent process for incorporating understanding of the social determinants of health in the development of healthy public policy. HIA is:

A combination of procedures, methods and tools by which a policy, program or project may be judged as to its potential effects on the health of the population, and the distribution of those effects is within the population.
(European Centre for Health Policy 1999, 4)

HIA has been extensively implemented in many countries in the last two decades as a practical tool for shifting the rhetoric of healthy public policy into action (Banken

2001). During the same period, efforts have been made to develop methods and instruments for Human Rights Impact Assessment (HRIA). HRIA is:

a systematic process to ensure the integration of human rights aspects in decision making throughout the policy formulation, implementation, checking and adapting process. It includes a continuous system of monitoring and evaluation of the results of policy measures in terms of actual human rights observance.
(Radstaake & Bronkhorst 2002, 5)

HRIA has been developed predominantly as a tool for assessing macro-level policies of government, such as foreign policy, and assessment of activities of trans-national business corporations and multilateral bodies.

To date, HIA has developed primarily with an "internal" and local focus whereas HRIA has focused primarily on "external" policy and projects. While addressing different levels of institutional activity, HRIA and HIA both have at their core a systematic and transparent analysis as the basis for strategy development, policy decisions, project definition, monitoring and evaluation. The primary output in either case is "a set of evidence-based recommendations geared to informing the decision making process" (Taylor & Quigley 2002, 2).

In 1994, Gostin and Mann proposed an approach to the human rights assessment of health policy aimed at defining the optimal balance between health goals and compliance with human rights principles and standards (Gostin & Mann 1994). Yet to be explored is the reciprocal potential that adding a focus on human rights to HIA may have for enhancing assessment of internal policies, programs and projects. Other authors have suggested that human rights, including the right to health, and the related rights to education, information, privacy and decent living and working conditions, can provide a framework for the health sector to address conditions that limit achievement for optimal health in the population (Gruskin & Tarantola 2001). O'Keefe and Scott-Samuel (2002) and later Hunt and McNaughton (2006), proposed the linking of human rights with HIA. Subsequently, as the UN Special Rapporteur on the Right to Health, Hunt introduced to the United Nations General Assembly an impact assessment of the right to health as a means to strengthen national and international policies (UN 2007). The commonality of core processes, widespread support for HIA and the utility of HIA in "value adding" to decision-making processes (Wismar et al, 2006) suggests that human rights-based HIA may be successfully developed and enhance the development of healthy foreign and global policy (Scott-Samuel & O'Keefe 2007). HIA may usefully provide well accepted processes for valuing evidence, making values and assumptions explicit and assuring transparency in decision making.

Towards a Health, Human Rights and Development Impact Assessment

This chapter builds on, but extends beyond the above proposals. It suggests that the impact assessment of development policies and programs (i.e., social, economic and structural) should be carried out in view of their anticipated impacts on health and other chosen human rights. Theoretically, in most situations, greater investment in health will contribute to greater realisation of other rights, including equality, education and employment. In reality, however, choices between two or more policy options may be guided by gains anticipated in health and other sectors of development, favouring mixed investments in both health and education. Similarly, a development policy may be assessed from its isolated impact on development or health or from the broader perspective of its impacts on development, health and other human rights. This paper suggests that the latter approach is most likely to reveal possible tensions resulting from selective investments in one sector whereas a mix of investments may, together, result in advancing health along with other human rights more effectively. This fits well with HIA's recognition that the health of a population is determined by a wide range of economic, social, psychological and environmental influences, often referred to as the social determinants of health (Dahlgren & Whitehead 1991), and can lead to a Health, Human Rights and Development Impact Assessment (HHRDIA). Incorporating these considerations into a HHRDIA would thus encourage greater consideration of the impact on health of macroeconomic, political, societal and environmental structures (the macro-determinants of health).

HRIA and HIA have clear areas of overlap in both process and understanding of the causes of health. Reciprocal inclusion of one with the other offers an opportunity to greatly enhance both HRIA and HIA. At a global level HHRDIA would be enhanced by building on the widespread acceptability of HIA and of human rights to improve the development of healthy global policy. Similarly, at a local level HIA would be enhanced by the use of human rights and development as a framework for incorporating macro-level conditions in assessment to improve the development of healthy public policy. To realise this enhanced potential at both the global and local levels, however, capacity and new methods and tools will need to be developed.

IN CONCLUSION: PROGRESS THROUGH PRACTICE AND RESEARCH

Individually, the domains of health, development and human rights are currently on the forefront of political and policy debates. This is reflected in civil society movements around the world as well as in political statements heralding greater global equality, improved democratic governance and protection of public health and security, all in the context of geopolitical shifts, economic globalisation and environmental changes. These trends have emerged as knowledge and practice in each of the three domains and have advanced almost independently, along with the recognition of bridges between them. This paper is a first attempt to bring health, development and human rights together, structuring their relationship around a conceptual framework conducive to the analysis of their reciprocal interactions.

Importantly, this paper has proposed an approach incorporating health, development and human rights in the formulation and implementation of policies and programs and their monitoring. Stemming from the experience accumulated over the last decade in the application of impact assessment methods selectively to health, human rights and development programs, an approach is proposed to incorporate the three domains. To broaden and harmonise the application of impact assessment

methods raises a number of concerns. First, empirical evidence shows that impact assessments are more likely to produce quality outcomes when they are focused and able to inform decisions promptly. To overburden impact assessments by broadening their scope may affect their timeliness and quality. Second, the relationships between health, development and human rights are not yet well understood. It is our collective hope that this knowledge gap will be bridged by the experience to be gained from the practice of rights-based approaches to health and development and impact assessment, and that this will guide and monitor policies and programs towards maximising synergy into the future. Research needs in the field of health and human rights are pressing, extensive and diverse. They can be regrouped in the four main areas highlighted below.

Building the Evidence Base

This priority area focuses on advancing the research field of health, development and human rights to further build the evidence base that a human rights approach to health and development is both effective and necessary. Potential research topics may include documenting how and to what extent compliance with human rights principles enhances health, and documenting and analysing the ways and extent to which the neglect or violations of human rights impact on health and development.

Improving Governance

Good governance in regards to health, development and human rights involves public institutions providing equal distribution of services, ensuring privacy and confidentiality, permitting the right to information, promoting dignity, and creating effective mechanisms of accountability. Research in this area may focus on promoting improved governance of public institutions in relation to health, human rights and development principles. Potential research topics may include analysing political, social, cultural and other reasons for governmental lack of commitment to health, development and human rights; examining ways and the extent to which human rights have been mainstreamed or incorporated in health and development policies, strategies and actions of international, governmental, nongovernmental and private institutions; and defining health, development and human rights good practices and how they can be applied to national or institutional priority setting and resource allocation.

Focusing on Vulnerable Populations

Addressing discrimination, inequalities and inequity in access to services and systems is an important element of a human rights-based approach to health and development. These research areas may explore why, how and to what extent discrimination on the basis of gender, age, race and ethnicity, sexual orientation, health status or other civil, political, social, economic or cultural attributes such as mobility or refugee status prevails in most societies, in particular in the context of health and social services and development programs. Research is needed on how access to these entitlements can be offered in a fair and dignified manner.

Harmonising International and National Health and Development Initiatives

There are today numerous actors in international health and development initiatives labelled as "Partnerships," "Initiatives," "Funds," "Alliances" or targeted "Programs." Between 70 and 100 such initi-

atives have a health focus while the official development assistance annual funding for health has doubled from US$6 billion in 2000 to US$12 billion in 2005 (United Nations Thematic Debate: 2008 para 10). Capacity building, honouring financial commitments made by national governments and their development partners to bridge existing gaps, correcting fragmentation and inefficiencies in international efforts to achieve the MDGs and increasing the predictability of the supply of external financing to countries have been recognised at a UN General Assembly thematic debate as essential to "getting back on track to achieve the MDGs by 2015" (Ibid: para 13–18). The entry of a growing number of actors on the scene of international health assistance raises questions not only about the harmonisation of aid among these actors but also their willingness and capacity to uphold their obligations under international human rights, particularly when partnering involves international organisations mandated to uphold human rights norms and standards in their work (Hallgath & Tarantola 2008). Closer monitoring of the practices of such actors, combined with research on how to strengthen the synergy between health, development and human rights in international aid, should provide the evidence needed to guide policies and alleviate obstacles to best practice in the three domains.

Globalisation and Global Public Goods

Transnational policies and actions generated by governmental or private concerns create both risks and opportunities to advance health, development and human rights. For many populations, particularly those of low and medium income countries, the current global health trajectory is not moving towards greater equality, sustainability or even human survival.

The impact of economic globalisation on health and human rights, as well as how current global health issues are being addressed under such paradigms as social justice (Daniels 2002), bioethics (Gruskin & Daniels 2008), humanitarianism (Brauman 2000), utilitarianism (Hayry 2002), or the concept of Global Public Goods (Kaul et al. 2003) should be further explored towards ensuring greater equity in health and development. The interface between these paradigms, the value they add and the limitations they face require further research.

Meeting the above research needs will be best served by a combination of methods normally used in an array of disciplines, including those applied to policy, legal, strategic and economic analyses as well as epidemiological, behavioural, anthropological and social research.

REFERENCES

Acemogolu D, Johnson S and Robinson J (2001) 'The colonial origins of comparative development: An empirical investigation' 91 (5) *American Economic Review* pp 1369–1401

Acheson D (1988) *Committee of Inquiry into the Future Development of the Public Health Function* HMSO, London

Aggleton P and Parker R (2005) *HIV-Related Stigma, Discrimination and Human Rights Violations: Case Studies of Successful Programmes* UNAIDS Best Practice Collection, UNAIDS, Geneva pp 17–67

Akukwe C (1998) 'The growing influence of nongovernmental organisations (NGOs) in international health: Challenges and opportunities' 118 (2) *Journal of the Royal Society of Health* pp 107–115

Alston P (2005) 'Ships passing in the night: The current state of the human rights and development debate seen through the lens of the Millennium Development Goals' 27 (3) *Human Rights Quarterly* pp 755–829

Anand S (2004) 'The concerns for equity in health' in S Anand, F Peter and A Sen (eds) *Public Health and Ethics* (1st edn) Oxford University Press, Oxford pp 17–18

Atkinson A, Basu K, Bhagwati J, North D, Rodrik D, Stewart F, Stiglitz J and Williamson J (2005) *Wider Perspectives on Global Development* Palgrave Macmillan/United Nations University, Houndmills

Banken R (2001) *Strategies for Institutionalising HIA, Health Impact Assessment Discussion Papers Number 1* World Health Organization Regional Office for Europe, Copenhagen

Baum F (2007) 'Cracking the nut of health equity: top down and bottom up pressure for action on the social determinates of health' 14 (2) *Promotion and Education* pp 90–95

Baum F and Harris L (2006) 'Equity and the social determinants of health' 17 (3) *Health Promotion Journal of Australia* pp 163–165

Baxi U (2002) *The Future of Human Rights* (2nd Edn) Oxford University Press

Behrman JR (1996) 'The impact of health and nutrition on education' 11 (1) *The World Bank Research Observer* pp 23–37

Benedek W, De Feyter K and Marrella F (eds) (2008) *Economic Globalisation and Human Rights* EIUC Studies on Human Rights and Democratization, Cambridge University Press, Cambridge

Black RE, Morris SS and Bryce J (2003) 'Where and why are 10 million children dying every year?' 61 *The Lancet* pp 2226–2234

Boutayeb A (2006) 'The double burden of communicable and non-communicable diseases in developing countries' 100 (3) March *Transactions of the Royal Society of Tropical Medicine and Hygiene* pp 191–199

Buse K and Walt G (2000a) 'Global public-private partnerships: Part I—a new development in health?' 78 (4) *Bulletin of the World Health Organisation* pp 549–561

Buse K and Walt G (2000b) 'Global public-private partnerships: Part II—what are the health issues for global governance?' 78 (5) *Bulletin of the World Health Organisation* pp 699–709

Brauman R (2000) *L'action humanitaire* Flammarion

Camp Keith L (2002) Judicial independence and human rights protection around the world' 85 (4) *Judicature* pp 195–200

Centre for the Study of Human Rights (2005) *25+ Human Rights Documents* Columbia University, New York

Chang YH (ed) (2003) *Rethinking Development Economics* Anthem Press, London

Cohen J (2006) 'The new world of global health' 311.5758 *Science* pp 162–167

Cohn T (2008) *Global Political Economy* (4th edn) Pearson Longman, New York

Dahlgren G and Whitehead M (1991) *Policies and Strategies to Promote Social Equity in Health* Institute of Futures Studies, Stockholm

Daniels N (2002) 'Justice, health, and health care' in R Rhodes, MP Battin and A Silvers (eds), *Medicine and Social Justice: Essays on the Distribution of Health Care* Oxford University Press, Oxford pp 6–23

Dodd R and Cassels A (2006) 'Health, development and the Millennium Development Goals' 100 (5 and 6) *Annals of Tropical Medicine and Parasitology* pp 379–387

Eide A (1995) 'Economic, social and cultural rights as human rights' in A Eide, C Krause and E Rosas (eds) *Economic, Social and Cultural Rights: A Textbook* Martinus Nijhoff, Dordrecht pp 81–124

European Centre for Health Policy (1999) *Gothenburg Consensus Paper on Health Impact Assessment: Main Concepts and Suggested Approach* World Health Organization Regional Office for Europe, Brussels

Farmer P (2004), *Pathologies of Power: Health, Human Rights, and the New War on the Poor* California Series in Public Anthropology (4)

Frank J and Mustard J (1994) 'The determinants of health from a historical perspective' 123 (4) *Daedalus* pp 1–19

Frankovits A, Earle P and Sidoti E (2001) *The Rights Way to Development: Policy and Practice* Human Rights Council of Australia, North Sydney

Freedman LP, Graham WJ, Brazier E, Smith JM and Ensor T (2007) 'Practical lessons from global safe motherhood initiatives: Time for a new focus on implementation' 370 (9595) *The Lancet* pp 1383–1391

Garrett L (2007) 'The Challenge of Global Health' 86(1) *Foreign Affairs* pp 14–38

Gostin L and Mann J (1994) 'Towards the development of a human rights impact assessment for the formulation and evaluation of public health policies' 1 (1) *health and human rights* pp 58–80.

Grayling AJ (2007) *Towards the Light: The Story of the Struggles for Liberty and Rights that Made the Modern West* Bloomsbury, London

Gruskin S and Tarantola D (2001) 'health and human rights' in R Detels, J McEwen, R Beaglehole, and H Tanaka (eds) *The Oxford Textbook of Public Health* (4th edn) Oxford University Press, Oxford pp 311–336

Gruskin S, Mills EJ, and Tarantola D (2007) 'History, principles, and practice of health and human rights' 370 *The Lancet* pp 449–455

Gruskin S and Daniels N (2008) 'Justice and human rights: Priority setting and fair deliberative process' *American Journal of Human Rights* [in press, accepted 29 December 2007]

Gwatkin DR (2005) 'How much would poor people gain from faster progress towards the Millennium Development Goals for health?' 365 *The Lancet* pp 813–817

Hallgath L and Tarantola D, A rights-based approach to the assessment of global health initiatives. *Australian Journal of Human Rights* [in press, accepted Feb 2008].

Hayry M (2002) 'Utilitarian approaches to justice in health care' in R Rhodes, MP Battin and A Silvers (eds), *Medicine and Social Justice: Essays on the Distribution of Health Care* Oxford University Press, Oxford pp 53–64

Howell J and Pearce J (2002) *Civil Society and Development: A Critical Exploration* L. Rienner Publishers, Colorado

Hunt P and MacNaughton G (2006) *Impact Assessments, Poverty and Human Rights: A Case Study Using the Right to the Highest Attainable Standard of Health* UNESCO, Paris, pp 1–65

Hunt P (2008) *Promotion and Protection of all Human Rights, Civil, Political, Economic, Social and Cultural Rights, Report of the Special Rapporteur on the Right of Everyone to the Enjoyment of the Highest Attainable Standard of Physical and Mental Health*, Seventh Session Human Rights Council, A/HRC/7/11, 31 January

Hyder AA and Morrow RH (2006) 'Measures of health and disease in populations' in MH Merson, RE Black and AJ Mills (eds) *International Public Health: Diseases, Programs, Systems and Policies* (2nd edn) Sudbury, Massachusetts

Ishay M (2004) *The History of Human Rights: From Ancient Times to the Globalization Era* University of California Press

Jutting S (2003) *Institutions and Development: A Critical Review* OECD Development Centre, Working Paper No. 210, Paris

Kaul I, Conceicao P, Goulven KL and Mendoza RU (eds) (2003) *Providing Global Public Goods: Managing Globalization* Oxford University Press, New York

Kemm J (2001) 'Health Impact Assessment: a tool for healthy public policy' 16 (1) *Health Promotion International* pp 79–85

Kingsbury D, Remenyi J, McKay J and Hunt J (2004) *Key Issues in Development* Palgrave Macmillan, Houndmills

Kinney E (2001) 'The international human right to health: What does this mean for our nation and world?' 34 *Indiana Law Review* pp 1457–1475

Kirchmeir F (2006) 'The right to development—where do we stand? State of the debate on the right to development' 23 *Dialogue on Globalization Occasional Papers*, Friedrich-Ebert-Stiftung Geneva pp 11–14

Lauren P (1998) *The Evolution of International Human Rights: Visions Seen* University of Pennsylvania Press, Philadelphia

Leary V (1994) 'The right to health' 1 (1) *health and human rights* pp 24–56

Leger LS (2007) 'Declarations, charters and statements—Their role in health promotion' 22 (3) *Health Promotion International* pp 179–181

Leslie J and Jamison DT (1990) 'Health and nutrition considerations in education planning: 1 educational consequences of health problems among school-age children' 12 (3) *Food and Nutrition Bulletin* pp 204–214

Lopez AD, Mathers CD, Ezzati M, Jamison DT and Murry CJL (2006) 'Global and regional burden of disease and risk factors, 2001: systematic analysis of population health data' 367 *The Lancet* pp 1747–1757

'Maastricht Guidelines on Violations of Economic, Social and Cultural Rights' (1997) 20 *Human Rights Quarterly* pp 691–705

Mann J, Gostin L, Gruskin S, Brennan T, Lazzarini Z and Fineberg H (1994) 'Health and Human Rights' 1 (1) *Health and Human Rights* pp 6–23

Mann J and Tarantola D (eds) (1996) *AIDS in the World II, Global Dimensions, Social Roots and Response* Oxford University Press, Oxford and New York, pp 427–476

Marks SP (2005) 'Human rights in development: The significance for health' in S Gruskin, MA Grodin, GJ Annas and SP Marks (eds) *Perspectives on Health and Human Rights* Routledge, New York and London pp 95–116

Marmot M (2004) 'Social causes of social inequity in health' in S Anand, F Peter, and A Sen *Public Health, Ethics and Equity* (3rd edn) Oxford University Press, Oxford pp 37–62

Martens J (2003) *The Future of Multilateralism after Monterrey and Johannesburg, Dialogue on Globalization* 10 Occasional Papers, Friedrich Ebert Stiftung, Berlin

Myrdal G (1975) *Against the Stream: Critical Essays in Economics* Vintage Books, New York

North D (1990) *Institutions, Institutional Change and Economic Performance* Cambridge University Press, Cambridge

O'Keefe E and Scott-Samuel A (2002) 'Human rights and wrongs: Could Health Impact Assessment help?' 30 *Journal of Law, Medicine and Ethics* pp 734–738

Okie S (2006) 'Global health: The Gates-Buffett effect' 355 (11) *New England Journal of Medicine* pp 1084–1088

People's Health Movement (2006) *The People's Health Movement: A People's Campaign for Health for All—Now!* http://www.phmovement.org/en/node/189

Petchesky RP (2003) *Global Prescriptions: Gendering Health and Human Rights* Zed Books, London and New York

Radstaake M and Bronkhorst D (2002) *Matching Practice with Principles: Human Rights Impact Assessment: EU Opportunities* Humanist Committee on Human Rights, Utrecht

Richter J (2004) 'Public-private partnerships for health: a trend with no alternatives?' 47 (2) *Development* pp 43–48

Rodrik D, Subramanian A and Trebbi F (2002) *Institutions Rule: The Primacy of Institutions over Integration and Geography. Working Paper No. 9305* National Bureau of Economic Research, Cambridge, MA

Sachs J (2005) *The End of Poverty: How We Can Make It Happen in Our Lifetime* Penguin, London

Sanoff H (2000) *Community Participation Methods in Design and Planning* John Wiley & Sons Inc, Canada

Schumpeter J (1969) *The Theory of Economic Development* Oxford University Press, Oxford

Scott-Samuel A and O'Keefe E (2007) 'Health impact assessment, human rights and global public policy: A critical appraisal' 85 *Bulletin of the World Health Organization* pp 212–217

Sen A (1999) *Development as Freedom* Oxford University Press, Oxford

Sengupta A (2002) 'On the theory and practice of the right to development' 24 *Human Rights Quarterly* pp 837–889.

Sengupta, A Negi A and Basu M (eds) (2005) *Reflections on the Right to Development* Centre for Development and Human Rights and Sage Publications, New Delhi

Smith R, Beaglehole R, Woodward D and Drager N (eds) (2003) *Global Public Goods for Health: Health Economics and Public Health Perspective* Oxford University Press, Oxford

Steiner H and Alston P (2000) *International Human Rights in Context: Law Politics and Morals* Oxford University Press, New York

Stiglitz, J (2002) *Globalisation and Its Discontents* Allen Lane

Tarantola D (2008) 'A perspective on the history of health and human rights: From the cold war to the gold war' 29 *Journal of Public Health Policy* pp 42–53

Taylor L and Quigley R (2002) *Health Impact Assessment: A Review of Reviews* National Health Service Health Development Agency, London

The World Bank (1993) *The World Development Report: Investing in Health* The World Bank and Oxford University Press pp 156–170

Thirlwall A (1999) *Growth and Development* (6th edn) Macmillan, Houndmills

't Hoen E (2002) 'TRIPS, pharmaceuticals patents, and access to essential medicines: A long way from Seattle to Doha' 3 (1) *Chicago Journal of International Law* pp 27–46

Tomuschat C (2003) *Human Rights, Between Idealism and Realism* Oxford University Press, New York

United Nations (2003) *The Human Rights Based Approach to Development Cooperation Towards a Common Understanding Among UN Agencies.*

United Nations General Assembly Thematic Debate, "Recognizing the achievements, addressing the challenges of getting back on track to achieve the MDGs by 2015, Background Paper, Tuesday 1 April 2008, New York

United Nations General Assembly (2007) Sixty-second session, *Report of the Special Rapporteur on the right of everyone to the enjoyment of the highest attainable standard of physical and mental health* A/62/214, United Nations, New York pp 33–44

United Nation Development Program (1998) *Integrating Human Rights with Sustainable Human Development. A UNDP Policy Document* UNDP, New York

United Nations Development Programme (2005) *Investing in Development: A Practical Plan to Achieve the Millennium Development Goals* Earthscan, London

Williamson J (1990) 'What Washington means by policy reform' in J Williamson (ed) *Latin American Adjustment: How Much Has Happened* Institute for International Economics, Washington pp 5–20

Wise M and Nutbeam D (2007) 'Enabling health systems transformation: what progress has been made in re-orienting health services?' Supp 2 *Promotion & Education* pp 23–27

Wismar M, Blau J, Ernst K, Elliott E, Golby A, van Herten L, Lavin T, Stricka M, and Williams G (2006) 'Implementing and institutionalizing health impact assessment in Europe' in T Ståhl, M Wismar, E Ollila, E Lahtinen, and K Leppo (eds) Health in All Policies: *Prospects and Potentials* Ministry of Social Affairs and Health, Helsinki pp 231–252

World Health Organization (1948) *Constitution of the World Health Organization,* 7 April 1948, Amendments adopted by Res WHA26.37, WHA29.38, WHA39.6 and WHA51.23

World Health Organization (1995) *The World Health Report: Bridging the Gaps* Geneva

World Health Organization (1999) *The World Health Report: Making a Difference* Geneva

World Health Organization (2001) *Macroeconomics and Health: Investing in Health for Economic Development. Report of the Commission on Macroeconomics and Health* Geneva

World Health Organization (2002a) *Report of the WHO Commission on Macroeconomics and Health. Report by the Director-General* Fifty-fifth World Health Assembly A55/5, 23 April, Geneva

World Health Organization (2002b) *25 Questions and Answers on Health and Human Rights* Health and Human Rights Publication Series Issue No1, Geneva

World Health Organization (2003) *The World Health Report: Shaping the Future* Geneva

World Health Organization (2005) *Human Rights, Health and Poverty Reduction Strategies* Health and Human Rights No 5 WHO/ETH/HDP/05.1, Geneva

World Health Organization (2007) *Health Systems: Report by the Secretariat* 120th Session 8 January 2007, Provisional agenda item 4.7, EB120/38, Geneva

World Trade Organization and World Health Organization (2002) *WTO Agreements and Pubic Health. A joint study by the WHO and the WTO Secretariat* WTO and WHO, Geneva

Zwi AB, Garfield R and Loretti A (2002) 'Collective violence' in EG Krug, LL Dahlberg, JA Mercy, AB Zwi, R Lozano (eds) *World Report on Violence and Health* World Health Organization, Geneva, pp 215–239.

QUESTIONS

1. Using Figure 10.1 as an analytical framework, choose a public health, human rights or development issue affecting a community of your choice. Taking this entry point to the framework (i.e., one of the angles of the triangle: whether health, development or human rights), please define the issue succinctly in either public health, development or human rights terms and describe briefly who is primarily affected by it and in what ways. Following the arrows, then suggest how your chosen issue might be rooted in public health failures, lack of or inequitable development, or denial of human rights.

2. Reformulate your chosen issue in combined health, development and human rights terms.

3. Describe briefly how responding to your chosen issue through policy changes, programs or interventions may impact on health, human rights and development. Are these expected impacts positive on all accounts, or are trade-offs likely to arise? If so, what mechanism, method or process would you suggest to recognize and resolve such trade-offs?

4. Repeat the above steps 1–3, now taking gender inequality as an entry point. What important gender-related issues in human rights, health and development terms emerge from your analysis? What can be done about these issues?

FURTHER READING

1. Kirchmeir, Felix, The Right to Development: Where do we Stand? State of the Debate on the Right to Development, Dialogue on Globalization, Friedrich Ebert Stiftung, Occasional Papers, No. 23 (2006) http://library.fes.de/pdf-files/iez/global/50288.pdf
2. Kinley, David, Human Rights and the World Bank: Practice, Politics, and Law, Legal Studies Research Paper No. 07/11, Sydney Law School (2007), http://ssrn.com/abstract=962987
3. Miller, Carol & Thomson, Marilyn, *Case-studies on Rights-based Approaches to Gender Diversity*, Gender and Development Network, London, 2005. See, in particular, Case Studies 14–54.

CHAPTER 11

A Poverty of Rights: Six Ways to Fix the MDGs

Malcolm Langford

INTRODUCTION

The Millennium Development Goals (MDGs) were greeted with disbelief and praise by those focused on human rights. It was disbelief from commentators who saw the MDGs as a betrayal of more demanding and/or nuanced international human rights commitments; the 'Major Distracting Gimmicks' as one women's rights advocate labelled them (Saith 2006). It was praise from those who saw them as a bridge between the human rights and development agendas (Jahan 2003).

Between these two reactions, one can find many shades. Some like Alston (2005) and UNDP (2008) straddle the contrarian positions, arguing that the MDGs are an adequate reflection of socioeconomic rights and the real challenge is to integrate human rights into development practice. The UN Office of the High Commissioner for Human Rights (UN OHCHR 2008) has been more critical, urging States to better align the targets at the country level with human rights and then ensure integration in practice. For others, the MDGs seemed to have passed by unnoticed; possibly from ignorance, possibly from the fact that MDGs were seen as contributing little to strategies on human rights and social justice. The end result has been a mixed and fragmented engagement by human rights nongovernmental organisations (NGOs), social movements, lawyers and UN human rights bodies. One empirical survey of attitudes found that many Northern NGOs embraced the MDGs, while those in South preferred rights-based standards (Nelson 2007). From the perspective of pragmatism, it is tempting to fudge some sort of middle position on the human rights and MDGs debate. But it carries dangers. For instance, Alston (2005) seeks to largely defend the MDG design from a human rights perspective but he is simultaneously puzzled as to why human rights are almost entirely absent in MDG-related policy guidance, strategies and reporting. He does not adequately stop to ask whether the problem might be the original design. We thus need to go deeper and ask two questions. First, are the 'human rights' gaps in the MDGs architecture partly responsible for the mixed success in reaching the Targets? Second, would a critical reading from a human rights perspective alert us to the potential that the Targets could be used to avoid human rights commitments and perpetuate violations? The latter scenario has unfortunately been all too common in the history of international development policy. This is not to dismiss the sunny side of the MDGs agenda. The Goals have given a clear, communicable and quantitative focus to international and sometimes national development priorities. One can discern shifts among donors, UN agencies and the World Bank in the allocation of aid that is attributable to the Goals. Some national governments from Kenya (Government of Kenya 2005) to Indonesia (Government of Indonesia 2007), claim that the MDGs have influenced their domestic spending priorities, while political discourses and campaigns on poverty have been shaped by MDGs language. MDG 5 has seemingly inspired international campaigns on maternal mortality by the former UN Special Rapporteur on the Right to Health and now Amnesty International. Moreover, there has been some attentiveness to the MDG critiques and a target on reproductive rights was included in 2007. However, Sakiko Fukuda-Parr (2008: 1) points out that while Poverty Reduction Strategies have increased their focus on social sector investments (MDGs 2–6), other areas such as 'decent work, hunger and nutrition, the environment and access to technology tend to be neglected'.

As many development critics have discussed elsewhere, determining the impact of the MDGs in isolation from other causal factors is fraught with difficulty. Progress in some Targets such as income poverty is partly attributable to the pre-MDG efforts of China, India and Vietnam (Smith 2007). Achievements on HIV/AIDS (MDG 6) have largely occurred outside the MDG framework—for example, a slew of more precise targets on HIV were adopted in 2001 by the General Assembly but these were never integrated in the MDG monitoring system. However, less discussed in terms of impact are the negative human rights 'externalities' that have resulted from some of the MDG Targets. These are often not picked up in the monitoring. And how does one determine the human rights counter-factual—i.e., would a more human rights-friendly MDG design have done a better job?

In the emerging discussions on post-2015, it is interesting to observe the increased weight given to human rights. Calls are being made to repoliticise the MDGs, base them firmly on human rights values, return to the original rights-focused vision of the Millennium Declaration and even to frame part of the overarching development discourse in terms of rights, for example global social rights or global social citizenship. These calls are to be welcomed; indeed, one is almost tempted to hope that 2015 may be the moment when economic and social rights will come in from the global cold.

In this chapter, I want to look more at the practical consequences of bringing in human rights; both in process and substance and by looking critically backwards to 2000 and forward to 2015. The first section or 'fix' in this chapter will thus focus on the process for formulating new development mandates from a human rights perspective. It will examine what went wrong in 2001 and what could go right for 2015. The next five 'fixes' concern how the 2000/2001 MDG framework could have been better shaped by human rights, from both principled and instrumental perspectives. These latter points assume that we might continue with a target-based approach post-2015. While the target-based approach is under discussion itself, I use this framework to demonstrate the possible practical and design consequences of a human rights approach. In other words, if we accept the MDG-style targeting approach, where could human rights take us?

STOPPING AT THE PARTICIPATION SIGN

Before we begin to dream up new post-2015 roads, we need to stop at the participation sign. If we are to take human rights seriously, then the design of the MDGs cannot be simply left to a few international agencies and a group of invisible experts in New York (or Brussels) as it was in 2001. This is not to disparage the group completely. They faced the difficult task of trying to operationalise the Millennium Declaration and, to a certain degree, they were inventive in trying to fold some of the broader aspects of the Declaration, such as environment, into the Goals and push the envelope with some additional Indicators, even if they lacked Targets. At the same time, a neoliberal agenda appeared to have set in during this process, and there are many alarming omissions from the Declaration:

- Affordable water. The target for affordable water in the Declaration was dropped from the MDGs. Perhaps the target was deemed 'unmeasurable' but indexes of water affordability are available. Or was affordability dropped in order to allow space for privatisation of water utilities—a strategy very much in vogue at the time?
- Orphans from HIV/AIDS. The Declaration target of providing 'special assistance to children orphaned by HIV/AIDS', one of the world's most vulnerable groups, was likewise completely and inexplicably omitted from the MDGs.
- Equitable trade. The Declaration called for a trading system that was 'open, equitable, rule-based, predictable and non-discriminatory', but one is startled to find in MDG Target 8A that the crucial word 'equitable' was deleted.
- Gender equality and empowerment of women. The Declaration contained a general target in paragraph 20 of promoting 'gender equality and the empowerment of women as effective ways to combat poverty, hunger and disease and to stimulate development that is truly sustainable'. Instead of fashion-

ing some targets, perhaps along the lines of the Beijing Declaration, this broad Declaration target was whittled down to being the title of Goal 3 with a quantitative Target for equality in primary and secondary education. This is to be contrasted with other general targets in this paragraph where there some efforts to fashion them as (at least) qualitative Targets in Goal 8. After an initial critique, UNIFEM (2004) embarked on the task on trying to show how gender can be mainstreamed in each Target but one still wonders whether some clear Targets might have helped focus more attention on the gender gap in development: from land ownership to political representation. This omission of targets is startling on the face of the 2001 MDG list, where an additional four Indicators are added but there are no accompanying Targets.

There was also no attempt to include other key elements of the Declaration, particularly human rights, as Goals or Targets, as was done with environment. Yet, the Declaration specifically speaks of the connections between human rights and development. This orphaning of specific aspects of the Declaration is possibly the reason for the UN General Assembly's reluctance, contrary to common belief, to embrace the 2001 Goals, Targets and Indicator list. It was only in October 2005 that the General Assembly made reference to it; all earlier resolutions had focused on calling for implementation and monitoring of all the Goals and measures in the broader Millennium Declaration framework.

But not all the blame can be laid at the feet of the 2001 technocratic takeover. Some of the flaws lie in the selection of the targets in the Millennium Declaration, as will be discussed below. Broader participation and greater attention to human rights could have improved the precision and focus of the targets.

So what kind of process can take us to 2015? How can grassroots groups, Southern-based NGOs, human rights advocates, under-capacitated ministries in developing countries be properly involved this time around?

There will be great temptation to create some sort of Bruntland-style Commission of high level politicians and experts to come up with a new development vision. But the recent experience with the Commission on the Legal Empowerment of the Poor (CLEP) (led by Hernando de Soto), shows its limitations. CLEP was modelled on the Bruntland Commission but came under vociferous attack for its non-representativity and its focus on the magic bullet of formalisation, a policy which had undermined land and livelihood rights of the poor in many contexts. The outcry led to the addition of regional consultations and creation of advisory boards (see discussion of issues and process in Langford 2007). This adjustment brought in other voices but the rushed and bifurcated process led to serious splits within the Commission and a report that was balanced but fundamentally contradictory with something for everybody, as the Economist (2008) gleefully pointed out.

The key lesson from the CLEP experience is that one needs time and attention to ensure some sort of genuine bottom-up participatory process. While any final decision needs to be made within the current confines of international law, ideas for high level commissions need to be put on the backburner until a more participatory mechanism can be commenced; where those who are meant to be the 'beneficiaries' of development have a direct say in how it is conceived.

PUT THE TARGETS IN FRONT OF A HUMAN RIGHTS MIRROR

Creating a list of targets large enough to address poverty's dimensions but short enough to avoid unwieldiness is more art than science. Nonetheless, the current list of targets still begs too many questions, despite its seeming artfulness. The MDGs appear more driven by the availability of data than a concrete vision of what the global community wanted to achieve and measure. Of course it is possible to demonstrate linkages between various socioeconomic rights and existing MDG Targets, and some in the human rights community have drawn pretty tables to this effect. But it largely misses the point of a human rights approach. The key questions are whether the rights were sufficiently covered, and more importantly, whether the substance of the target actually reflects the legal standard.

If we just confine ourselves to socioeconomic rights, we would see a number of Goals, Targets and Indicators in both the 2000 and 2001 lists that are in desperate need of adjustment:

- Goal 1. First, where is the right to social security under the first Goal? Imagine if a target for building basic social protection packages had been set in 2000. The numbers of those slipping into poverty through the current global economic crises could have been palpably less. According to the International Labour Organization (ILO), the cost to Senegal, India and Vietnam of providing child grants to all households with school-age children is around 1 per cent of GDP, rising to 2 per cent in Tanzania (Gassmann and Behrendt 2006; Mizunoya et al. 2006). These estimates are close to actual costs in other developing countries which have taken the plunge. There is now a rising movement to try and insert a social protection target in 2010 but a mere glance at international human rights standards from 1948 to 2000 would have revealed a consistent and strong emphasis on this right. One might have also thought about access to land rights and inequality in distribution given the role of land for most of the rural poor in creating and sustaining livelihoods necessary to reach Goal 1.

- Goal 2. The target of universal access of primary education resonates with State obligations in the Convention on the Rights of the Child and the International Covenant on Economic, Social and Cultural Rights. However, both of these human rights treaties mandate that it must also be free, compulsory and of a certain quality. Article 14 of the International Covenant on Economic, Social and Cultural Rights (ICESCR) additionally provides that States which are not providing free primary education to all must prioritise the achievement of that commitment within a reasonable number of years (and certainly not 15 or 25!). In the MDG context, free primary education is often promoted as a good strategy—Kenya's policy shift in 2003 being promoted as the poster child. But it has been relegated to precisely that—a strategy not a right. The absence of a target for free education was evident in a recent review of a sample of MDG country reports—it was difficult to find countries measuring the affordability, quality or compulsory nature of education, which can be very important for girls' education (UN OHCHR, UNICEF and NCHR 2008)—although some countries like Malawi had recognised the importance of quality education for ensuring student attendance.

- Goal 5 is particularly impressive with its focus on a large-scale reduction of maternal mortality (75 per cent). Its inclusion of conduct-based index of birth attendants is welcome, given the problems of the maternal mortality indicators. But where are the more sophisticated and human rights-friendly targets from the 1997 UN Guidelines for Monitoring the Availability and Use of Obstetric Services? Their inclusion could have prompted countries like India to go beyond policy promises on Emergency Obstetric Services and actually measure them.

- Goal 7 is the most embarrassing of the national targets. Beyond the vacuous environmental targets, one meets the tortoise-like target of improving the lives of a mere 9 per cent of 'slum dwellers' by 2020, i.e., 100 million of 1.6 billion slum dwellers. What the target designers further failed to grasp is that the most immediate issues for many 'slum dwellers' is security of tenure, access to services and participatory planning. A cursory reading of housing rights standards, jurisprudence and practice demonstrates that these elements should be addressed first. In States where resources are few and corruption is high, these basic conditions are crucial for the poor to be able to develop their own housing solutions. Instead, the narrow focus on improving just a few lives often fuels white elephant-style slum upgrading projects (COHRE 2006). Moreover, the framing of this target has arguably helped provide justification for human rights violations (see below).

- Goal 8 looks good on first blush perspective but the developed countries have cleverly wriggled out of the types of quantitative targets that were set for developing countries. The qualitative targets are matched only with a detailed list of indicators from debt relief to development aid and trade that beg the creation of real benchmarks. This absence of quantitative targets is reflected in many donor reports, which tend to list development aid projects and programmes without a detailed assessment of how they are systematically addressing the range of issues raised in MDG 8. During 2001–08 some achievements have been made in setting such targets (e.g., on aid but not trade), but even these are far from being met and are more restrictive in practice than imagined.

- To this could be added targets on inequality—where are persons with disabilities, migrants and ethnic minorities? And where are civil and political rights, trumpeted by the Millennium Declaration and arguably crucial to long-term sustainable development? Mongolia's Goal 9 on democratic governance and human rights with time-bound targets deserves investigation.

The above critique and series of proposals is not meant to advocate an over-elasticated laundry list of goals and targets, although it is notable that Ecuador developed a list of 100 indicators to measure MDG performance. Rather it is about paying attention to whether human rights law and principles provide critical and substantive perspectives in the way in which the MDG Goals, Targets and Indicators are framed. With a little imagination, I suspect we could have ended up with ten MDGs and a few more targets.

FROM CHERRY PICKING TO EQUALITY

The Targets are problematic in being largely unfocused on the poorest of the poor or reducing inequality. These are both key requirements within human rights and the MDG approach can make it tempting for States to cherry-pick the relatively well-off among the poor and ignore long-suffering and excluded minorities. This is further accented by the fact that many marginalised groups are not recognised in the MDGs. The 2001 MDG framework did

quietly add some Indicators on the severity and depth of income poverty but there were no quantitative Targets fashioned for them.

Some countries have sought to overcome the equality problem during national tailoring and contextualisation. The MDG-plus framework in Thailand adds specific Targets for disadvantaged regions in the country. In Kenya, each region must now improve water and sanitation access by 10 per cent a year. These equality-based Targets conform with the idea proposed by Dan Seymour of UNICEF of making MDG progress conditional on meeting their Targets in all regions of a country. One could do the same with all ethnic groups, genders, etc. A second approach to such equality targeting is to provide targets for income poverty indicators such as severity and depth; something Bangladesh has done (Anderson and McKay 2008).

One additional question is whether the MDG Target framework meets the requirement that States need to immediately reach a minimum essential level of the rights unless they can demonstrably justify that resources are not available (UN CESCR 1991). For example, this could require that a very poor State devotes its limited resources to ensuring that all the hungry have improved access to food than simply halving the number of those officially classified as hungry. Should the other 50 per cent be expected to wait 15–30 years before they are addressed? In some cases, it may be highly impractical or irrelevant in attempting a modest increase in access for all. However, simple and new interventions could assist. For example, Gassmann and Behrendt (2006) econometrically model a child benefit for Tanzania and Senegal that is set at a level (35 per cent of the national food poverty line) that is not intended to take all children above the poverty line but rather move all children towards or over that line. Do we thus need to develop some targets that can be met immediately for all (particularly those affecting survival), even if it is does not fit perfectly with long-term development strategy?

FROM MDG-PLUS TO MDG-ADJUST

The MDG-plus approach of a number of countries has begun to garner favour in the development community. This is not surprising. The pitfalls of global target-setting were revealed immediately when some countries began boasting of success within a few years of the Declaration. This is particularly the case in middle-income countries which already had more ambitious targets or possessed the capacity to quickly halve or address smaller gaps. Officials at the Department of Water and Environment Affairs in South Africa recently commented that the water target is irrelevant given South Africa's earlier national commitments but that has not stopped the Government of South Africa trumpeting its success in reaching it so quickly.

Some countries and regions have taken a constructive approach to this problem and created MDG-plus Targets. The Latin American/Caribbean region amended Target 2A to include secondary education with 75 per cent of children to be accorded access by 2010, while a number of Asian countries added higher or additional targets.

This MDG-plus agenda is now centre-stage in post-2015 thinking as a way of addressing the resource imbalances between States. However, is this idea simply a band-aid to cover a flawed model? Is it the best way of dealing with a situation where Kenya is expected to halve projected income poverty of 56 per cent and Vietnam 6 per cent in the same time period? How does one have Somalia and EU member Bulgaria in the same MDG mix? There are also calls to include all States, including from the West, next time around. MDG-plus thus seems rather ad hoc without any global or normative underpinnings.

If we turn to human rights, we can find a more nuanced approach although it is only beginning to be quantified. In treaties on economic, social and cultural rights, States are only expected to progressively realise the rights within their maximum available resources. Retrogression is severely frowned upon and States are expected to set reasonable benchmarks that should be achieved over time with a reasonable set of policies. Thus, the human rights architecture allows for state particularity but has one global standard for all. It does not let middle- or high-income countries off the hook and allows some latitude to poorer states.

One obvious way to compensate for different resource levels is to adjust targets for GDP, although this ignores aid and borrowing options that may increase with lower resources. Thus we might expect greater quantitative progress in proportionately reducing gaps every five years from Vietnam compared to Kenya. A second approach would be regional targets, which would be natural considering neighbourly homogeneity and competition in much of the world. Latin American countries acknowledged as such in setting MDG-plus targets for their region. A combination of this with GDP adjustment could also work. Such approaches could be complemented by the production possibility function for economic and social rights proposed by Fukuda-Parr et al. (2008) or country-based econometric methods for determining available resources (Anderson 2008). Of course such approaches should not distract attention from countries which require greater assistance in reducing large poverty gaps but they would at least keep in check middle and higher income countries.

When it comes to income poverty, a way must also be found to bring existing national poverty lines into the method for calculating the currently flawed international poverty line (Pogge 2005). For example, in Senegal the $1-a-day measurement is substantially below the national poverty line, while it is the reverse in Tanzania (Gassmann and Behrendt 2006). In August 2008, the World Bank further confirmed these suspicions around the $1-a-day measurement by releasing new poverty figures based on 2005 (instead of 1993) cost-of-living data which showed that a further 400 million people lived below an adjusted poverty measure of $1.25/day. In Anderson and McKay's (2008) review of a sample of MDG reports, they found many countries measuring with national poverty lines, as opposed to the international poverty line.

TRADE-OFFS WITH RIGHTS

The divorce of the MDGs from the Millennium Declaration has arguably led to a value-free policy space for the MDGs. It seems that anything goes in the quest to meet the MDGs. If massive human rights violations are the method, no one is the wiser as the figures show 'progress'. Take, for example, Target 7D where Vietnam reports slum clearance as part of their efforts in achieving the MDGs (Government of Vietnam 2005: 12). This is pronounced despite countless international standards inveighing against forced evictions (e.g., see UN Commission on Human Rights 1993). Marie Huchzermeyer (2008) argues that a provincial slum clearance law in South Africa and moves to replicate it country-wide are based on a 'fundamentally flawed' interpretation by governments of MDG Target 7D and its accompanying slogan of 'Cities without Slums'. The sloppiness of the MDG target formulation has allowed states to use it as a pretext for violations of the housing rights of those who were intended to benefit from the Target.

Likewise, the MDGs have coincided with renewed interest in dams and a continuing focus on promoting large-scale commercial agriculture, although the World Bank is now sending out markedly contradictory signs on the latter. Such projects are regularly justified on the basis of addressing income poverty or providing clean energy and water resources, arguments that resonate with MDGs 1 and 7. However, development-based displacement continues apace (UN-Habitat 2007) and the MDGs risk being added as another 'public interest' criterion to justify gross violations of human rights. This is not to rule out relocation per se but most States do not have proper mechanisms in place to ensure individuals and communities are only evicted in accordance with human rights standards, i.e., there is substantive justification, due process and remedies.

Therefore, human rights need to be integrated into the MDG policy process. Red lines need to be drawn under what policies are permissible and under what normative framework trade-offs and choice making will occur (Seymour and Pincus 2008). The principle of do no harm needs real teeth and must be foregrounded in the development package. The policy choice spectrum also needs to be proactively influenced by human rights. Some policy options are more likely to both fulfil development goals and tick off human rights objectives. Thus, future MDGs need to better encourage economic trade-offs which favour human rights. For example, if the research shows that smaller farmers are more, or as, efficient as larger farmers (Brink et al. 2006), why has large-scale agriculture been pushed so hard? Likewise, space needs to be opened for different ways of economic development, particularly for indigenous peoples. There needs to be an emphasis on more bottom-up participation in deciding trade-offs, as has been very strongly recognised in the 2007 UN General Assembly Declaration on the Rights of Indigenous Peoples.

FROM WORDS TO ENFORCEMENT

For a bunch of words with a simple monitoring system, the MDGs have had considerable success. Not radical but enough to influence global development discourse and the practice of some countries. Even still, the MDGs often seem to be a game of Forrest Gump's box of chocolates. Donors and governments pick and choose according to their own tastes despite the attempts at harmonisation à la Paris Declaration. MDG targets on sanitation, maternal mortality and slums are virtually invisible in many donor platforms let alone national policy.

Other forms of accountability are needed to complement the political rewards of MDG attainment. In Targeting Development, Black and White (2004: 17), acknowledge that a major weakness of the MDGs is the lack of rights-based accountability even though it has a rights-based flavour in setting a political form of accountability. In relation to the international actors they concede:

> What is missing from discussion of targets for international development agencies is any theory of accountability. For real accountability, at the very least there needs to be more transparency as to who is responsible for what, and more ownership of goals by those expected to meet them. In this sense, scale is also important. Individuals and agencies need to be held accountable for targets that are realistic and achievable at the level at which they are working.

One approach is to look to the international human rights system with its engine of periodic reviews, complaint systems and expert mandates. It could play a larger role in development policy but is limited by design and suffers from some of the same weaknesses as the MDG monitoring system (see a general discussion in Alston 2005).

We thus need to be more imaginative and there follows a few suggestions:

- First, articulate specific development targets that require States to ensure that domestic accountability systems are in place. One could draw from the UN Committee on Economic, Social and Cultural Rights (CESCR) General Comment No. 9 on domestic provision of enforceable remedies. Judicial enforcement of socioeconomic rights has been particularly important in Latin American and South Asian countries and increasingly elsewhere (Langford 2008).
- A second and similar road to take is to ensure that domestic space for political mobilisation and participation around poverty issues is encouraged and even targeted. The experience of Porto Alegre demonstrated that direct participation in discretionary budge allocations led to a remarkable and speedy closure of large gaps in access to basic services such as water and sanitation.
- Third, can we imagine a stronger international monitoring system? Can 2015 be a date to bring together development and human rights systems and create something more powerful? Does 2015 present a window of opportunity for some sort of big bang reform that cements global social citizenship at the core of international processes? And the creation of a stronger and broader human rights monitoring and enforcement system?
- And lastly, can one introduce some carrots? The EU accession process has been remarkably successful in spurring on domestic reform. Could improvement on domestic targets be rewarded with automatic progress on MDG 8 Targets (aid, trade, debt relief and, critically, labour mobility) in the future?

CONCLUSION

Starting to dream up a post-2015 approach to international development obviously carries dangers as it could distract those genuinely seeking to reach the 2015 Goals in an appropriate manner. At the same time, it provides a useful forum to unpick some of the key faultlines in the MDGs and start to address the key weaknesses now rather than later. As the Office of the United Nations High Commissioner for Human Rights (UN OHCHR 2008), there is already much that can be done to align current targets at the national level with human rights and possibly some targets such as inequality, climate change and social protection could be added in 2010.

But a full-scale integration of human rights into international development policy is an idea whose time has not yet come and is still not desired in some quarters. The point of this chapter, however, was to show that a human rights approach not only provides the poetry for new development visions or the complication of introducing civil and political rights, but that it also provides a framework for operationalising development in ways that have not yet been properly explored. Post-2015 provides a new opportunity for human rights to be taken seriously in international development. We need to be begin with a commitment to participatory process and attention to contributions that international and national human rights jurisprudence and practice can bring to the table, whether in the selection and framing of targets, the setting of state obligations or the creation of accountability frameworks that can ensure development, is not only achieved but sustained.

REFERENCES

Alston, Philip (2005) 'Ships Passing in the Night: The Current State of the Human Rights and Development Debate Seen Through the Lens of the Millennium Development Goals', *Human Rights Quarterly* 27.3: 755–829

Anderson, Edward (2008) *Using Quantitative Methods to Monitor Government Obligations in Terms of the Rights to Health and Education*, New York: Center for Economic and Social Rights

Anderson, Edward and McKay, Andy (2008) *Human Rights, the MDG Income Poverty Target and Economic Growth*, Background Paper for UN OHCHR Africa and Asia Regional MDGs and Human Rights Dialogues for Action, Geneva: UN Office of the United Nations High Commissioner for Human Rights

Black, R. and White, H. (2004) Targeting *Development: Critical Perspectives on the Millennium Development*, London: Routledge

Brink, R.; Thomas, G.; Binswanger, H.; Bruce, J. and Byamugisha, F. (2006) *Consensus, Confusion and Controversy. Selected Land Reform Issues in Sub-Saharan Africa*, Washington DC: World Bank

COHRE (2006) *Listening to the Poor: Housing Rights in Nairobi, Kenya*, Geneva: Centre on Housing Rights and Evictions

Economist (2008) 'Legal Titles for the Poor', 5 June

Fukuda-Parr, Sakiko (2008) *Are The MDGs Priority in Development Strategies and Aid Programmes? Only Few Are!*, International Poverty Centre Working Paper 48, Brasilia

Fukuda-Parr, S.; Lawson-Remer, T. and Randolph, S. (2008) *Measuring the Progressive Realization of Human Rights Obligations*, Economic Rights Working Paper Series, University of Connecticut, Storrs

Gassmann, Franziska and Behrendt, Clarissa (2006) *Cash Benefits in Low-income Countries: Simulating the Effects on Poverty Reduction for Senegal and Tanzania*, Issues in Social Protection, Discussion Paper 15, Geneva: Social Security Department, International Labour Organization

Government of Indonesia (2007) *Let's Speak Out for the MDGS: Achieving the Millennium Development Goals in Indonesia*, Jakarta: Government of Indonesia and United Nations Development Programme

Government of Kenya (2005) *MDG Status Report for Kenya*, Nairobi: UNDP, Government of Kenya and Government of Finland

Government of Vietnam (2005) *Vietnam Achieving the Millennium Development Goals*, Fourth MDG Report, Hanoi: Government of Vietnam

Huchzermeyer, Marie (2008) 'Slums Law Based on Flawed Interpretation of UN Goals', *Business Day*, 19 May

Jahan, Selim (2003) 'Millennium Development Goals and Human Rights', in *Human Rights in Developing Countries: How can Development Cooperation Contribute to Furthering their Advancement*, Berlin: InWent

Langford, Malcolm (ed.) (2008) *Social Rights Jurisprudence: Emerging Trends in International and*

Comparative Law, New York: Cambridge University Press

Langford, Malcolm (2007) 'Beyond Formalisation: The Role of Civil Society in Reclaiming the Legal Empowerment Agenda', Norwegian Ministry of Foreign Affairs, *Legal Empowerment—A Way Out Of Poverty* 4: 41–66

Mizunoya, S.; Behrendt, C.; Pal, K. and Léger, F. (2006) *Can Low Income Countries Afford Basic Social Protection? First Results of a Modelling Exercise for Five Asian Countries,* Issues in Social Protection Discussion Paper 17, Geneva: Social Security Department, International Labour Organization

Nelson, P. (2007) 'Human Rights, the Millennium Development Goals, and the Future of Development Cooperation', *World Development* 35.12: 2041–55

Pogge, Thomas (2005), 'The First UN Millennium Development Goal: A Cause for Celebration?', in A. Føllesdal and T. Pogge (eds), *Real World Justice: Grounds, Principles, Human Rights, and Social Institutions,* Berlin: Springer: 317–38

Saith, A. (2006), 'From Universal Values to Millennium Development Goals: Lost in Translation', *Development and Change* 37.6: 1167–99

Seymour, Dan and Pincus, Jonathan (2008) 'Human Rights and Economics: The Conceptual Basis for their Complementarity', *Development Policy Review* 26.4: 387

Smith, Stephen (2007) 'The Millennium Development Goals and the Struggle Against Poverty Traps', presentation at the United Nations Economic and Social Council meeting on 'Eradicating Poverty and Hunger—Joining Forces to Make it Happen', 2 April

UN CESCR (1991) *General Comment No. 3, The Nature of States Parties' Obligations* (Fifth Session 1990), UN Doc. E/1991/23, annex III at 86, UN Committee on Economic, Social and Cultural Rights

UN Commission on Human Rights (1993) *Resolution 1993/77 on Forced Evictions,* Geneva

UNDP (2008) *Human Rights and the Millennium Development Goals Making the Link,* Oslo: United Nations Development Programme Oslo Governance Centre

UNIFEM (2004) *Pathway to Gender Equality: CEDAW, Beijing and the MDGs,* New York: United Nations Development Fund for Women

UN-Habitat (2007) *Forced Evictions—Towards Solutions? Second Report of the Advisory Group on Forced Evictions to the Executive Director,* Nairobi: UN-Habitat

UN OHCHR (2008) *Claiming the MDGs: A Human Rights Approach,* Geneva: Office of the United Nations High Commissioner for Human Rights

UN OHCHR, UNICEF and NCHR (2008) *Human Rights and MDGs in Practice: A Review of Country Strategies and Reporting,* Geneva: Office of the United Nations High Commissioner for Human Rights

QUESTIONS

1. Refer to the United Nations Millennium Declaration (UN General Assembly Resolution 55/2, 18 September 2000) http://www.un.org/millennium/declaration/ares552e.htm and to the MDG formulation, targets and monitoring indicators http://mdgs.un.org/unsd/mdg/. How does health relate to each of the eight MDGs? Which particular human rights resonate with each of the MDGs? How explicit or implicit are references to human rights in the formulated MDGs, their targets and monitoring indicators? What are possible reasons for the emphasis being placed explicitly on human rights in the MDG Declaration and their implicit or absent mention in the formulation of the MDGs and their targets and monitoring indicators?

2. Review the 2010 (or later) progress report on the MDGs: http://www.un.org/millenniumgoals/pdf/MDG%20Report%202010%20En%20r15%20–low%20res%2020100615%20–.pdf. Towards which of the MDGs is progress on track? Towards which of the MDGs is progress notably lagging behind? To what extent and how can these different trends be explained by lack of state unwillingness, state incapacity, or what the author describes as "genuine

bottom-up participatory process"? How should this impact the participation of state actors in the formulation of goals, targets and indicators?

3. In the 2010 (or later) progress report on the MDGs cited above, examine facts, figures and narratives reporting in particular on Goals 4, 5 and 6. Do these reports provide evidence supporting the author's assertion, echoing the OHCHR, that "there is already much that can be done to align current targets at the national level with human rights." Can you suggest one or two examples of what could be achieved in this direction and through what process?

FURTHER READING

1. Human Rights and Poverty Reduction: Realities, Controversies and Strategies, Human Rights and the Millennium Development Goals: Contradictory Frameworks?, Speakers: Simon Maxwell, Overseas Development Institute, and Robert Archer, International Council on Human Rights Policy, (1999), http://webcache.googleusercontent.com/search?q=cache:ze8J7i4tFaEJ:www.sarpn.org/documents/d0002022/3–ODI_Human-Rights_Mar2006.pdf+&hl=en
2. Tomasevski, Katarina, Girls' Education Through a Human Rights Lens: What Can be Done Differently, What Can be Made Better? Rights in Action, ODI, 2005.
3. Alston, P., Ships Passing in the Night: The Current State of the Human Rights and Development Debate Seen through the Lens of the Millennium Development Goals. *Human Rights Quarterly*, 2005; 27: 755–829.

POINT OF VIEW

A Failure to Act: Human Rights and the Social Determinants of Health

Jeffrey O'Malley

Even in wealthy countries with relatively widespread access to the latest medical technologies, only a small fraction of premature death is due to lack of access to quality health care. One review estimates that in the United States, about 10% of premature death is primarily related to lack of access to quality health care and about 30% is primarily related to genetic predisposition. The balance, about 60%, is attributable in one way or the other to social determinants of health.[1] Social determinants have an even greater impact on health outcomes in developing and middle income countries.

In 1946, stating what was already obvious, the Constitution of the World Health Organization noted that "Governments have a responsibility for the health of their peoples which can be fulfilled only by the provision of adequate health *and social* measures" (my emphasis). Over thirty years later, in September 1978, WHO appeared to rediscover this truth in the Declaration of Alma-Ata, which argued that economic and social development is a pre-requisite to the attainment of health for all, while also noting the inverse contribution of good health to peace and development. After another thirty year gap, WHO's "Commission on Social Determinants of Health" (CSDH) issued its final report in 2008. The CSDH's report, *Closing the Gap*, provided compelling evidence that both "the circumstances in which people are born, grow, live, work, and age" and "the inequitable distribution of power, money and resources" dramatically drive health outcomes, concluding

that "social injustice is killing people on a grand scale."

These advances within the global public health architecture had a parallel in the human rights world. The 1946 World Health Organization's constitution itself asserted that "the enjoyment of the highest attainable standard of health is one of the fundamental rights of every human being without distinction of race, religion, political belief, economic or social condition." Two years later, in 1948, Article 25 of the Universal Declaration of Human Rights referred not only to "the right to a standard of living adequate for the health and well-being of himself and of his family" but to a specific list of social determinants of that right, including "food, clothing, housing.. necessary social services, and the right to security in the event of unemployment, sickness, disability, widowhood, old age or other lack of livelihood in circumstances beyond his control." In 1966, the International Covenant on Economic, Social and Cultural Rights (ICESCR) reasserted the right to the highest attainable standard of health, which was then described in far more detail in General Comment 14 in 2000, including attention not just to medical services but to "*underlying determinants of health,*" linked to other rights entrenched in the ICESCR such as food, nutrition, housing, employment and a healthy environment, as well as to determinants of health "*such as resource distribution and gender differences.*" In 2009, Paul Hunt, having recently ended his term as UN Special Rapporteur on the Right to the Highest Attainable Standard of Health, concluded "there can be no doubt that the right to the highest attainable standard of health encompasses social determinants. This fundamental human right places legal obligations on governments to tackle social determinants where they harm health."[2]

There is a large and constantly growing body of evidence that social determinants of health, collectively, may well be responsible for a majority of morbidity and mortality globally. A large number of foundational documents of international public health governance reflect this insight, from the Constitution of the World Health Organization, to the Declaration of Alma-Ata to the final report of the CSDH. Accordingly, through numerous declarations, resolutions and binding conventions, States have committed to individual and collective action. In particular, International human rights instruments establish state obligations for action on social determinants of health: both directly and through the principal that human rights are interdependent and indivisible.

So why has so little been done? There is a wide range of barriers and obstacles hindering action, including limitations in the evidence base, complexity of program design, limitations to national and international health governance, disconnects between the worlds of health and human rights, and of course power and politics.

Social epidemiology has repeatedly provided powerful evidence of associations between social determinants and health outcomes but the evidence base that tests action and demonstrates results has been much weaker until recently. Beginning with a pioneering evaluation in Mexico, there is now robust evidence that cash transfer programmes can improve access to health services, especially for children and pregnant women.[3] The quasi-experimental IMAGE trial in South Africa and the Zomba trial in Malawi both showed how development interventions can influence risk for HIV acquisition, including a 50% reduction in intimate partner violence in South Africa and a 60% reduction in HIV risk in Malawi within 18 months.[4] Unfortunately, even these more recent and relatively robust studies have had difficulty demonstrating actual impact on health outcomes. Just as important, multi-dimensional interventions with multiple potential health and development benefits are not prone to cost-effectiveness analysis, which in turn limits the extent to which they will beconsidered by policy makers, and ultimately therefore their value in driving widespread policy change.

Health governance structures pose other major barriers. At a global level, the World Health Organization on its website describes itself as the "directing and coordinating authority for health within the United Nations system," yet WHO has no formal convening or coordinating structure with UN actors dedicated to development or human rights issues, let alone any potential for enforcement. At a national level, health ministries rarely have the authority or the systems to coordinate, encourage or leverage non-health ministries to care about and act on social determinants, with rare exceptions such as Finland's "Health in All" initiative.

Those most involved in either social determinants of health or health and human rights would seem to be natural allies in designing and advocating for increased action and accountability, but they more often seem like "two ships passing in the night," as described by Audrey Chapman, citing an analogy originally drawn by Philip Alston about the disconnect between the human rights and development communities. Chapman goes on to describe both the scant attention to human rights instruments and methodologies in the work of the Commission on Social Determinants of Health and the limited scope of attention to social determinants by those working on health and human rights. As one example, Chapman notes that "of the 65 paragraphs in the Committee on Economic, Social And Cultural Rights' General Comment 14 interpreting the 'right to health', only five mention the underlying determinants of health" while most of the rest address "obligations of the state related to the health systems and health services."[5]

Finally, it is essential to note that evidence related to social determinants of health increasingly underlines the profound limitations of liberal, individualistic approaches to either economic development or human rights. Non-discrimination, equal access to health services, participation and focus on the poor are important but inadequate on their own: relative equality of social and economic outcomes, not just of opportunities, is the most powerful action against health inequity.

Each of the obstacles described above can be addressed to some degree and must be addressed if the world is going to break through the current reality of atrocious health outcomes for the poor and marginalized. The evidence base can be increased and political leaders and policy makers can be educated to understand that social policy does not always require or generate evidence to the same level of precision as biomedical interventions. Policy and programme experimentation must increasingly focus on relatively simple and scalable approaches, accompanied by robust evaluation to ensure course corrections as needed and to sustain political will. International and national health structures, as well as civil society movements, must see health, development and human rights actors as partners rather than rivals, and demonstrate that vision through action. The last challenge is of course the most difficult: recognizing that the highest attainable standard of health ultimately requires a more just, equitable and sustainable world.

REFERENCES

1. Schroeder. We Can Do Better—Improving the Health of the American People. *New England Journal of Medicine.* 2007; 357;12.
2. Hunt. Missed Opportunities: Human Rights and the Commission on Social Determinants of Health. *Global Health Promotion* 1757–9759, Supp (1) (2008).
3. DFID 2011. Cash Transfers Evidence Paper.
4. UNDP 2012, Understanding and Acting on Critical Enablers and Development Synergies.
5. Chapman 2010. The Social Determinants of Health, Health Equity and Human Rights *Health and Human Rights*, 2010; 12.

Jeffrey O'Malley is Director, Division of Policy & Strategy, UNICEF.

CHAPTER 12

Child Rights and Child Poverty: Can the International Framework of Children's Rights Be Used to Improve Child Survival Rates?

Simon Pemberton, David Gordon, Shailen Nandy, Christina Pantazis and Peter Townsend

THE CONSEQUENCES OF CHILD POVERTY

It is estimated that over 10 million children in developing countries die each year, mainly from preventable causes. In approximately half of these deaths, malnutrition is a contributory cause.[1, 2] However, the World Health Organization has argued that seven out of ten childhood deaths in such countries can be attributed to just five main causes, or their combination. In addition to malnutrition,[3] these causes are pneumonia, diarrhoea, measles, and malaria. Around the world, three of every four children seen by health services are suffering from at least one of these conditions. Many of these deaths could be prevented using readily available medical technologies at comparatively little cost. In 1997, the United Nations Development Programme estimated that the cost of providing basic health and nutrition for every person on the planet was $13 billion per year for ten years.[4] To place this sum in perspective, in 2002, the United States population spent $30 billion on pizza and Europeans spent $12 billion on dog and cat food. While medical interventions can, in principle, prevent most young children from dying early, they cannot remove the underlying causes of poor health,

which are linked directly to the severely deprived or absolutely poor living conditions suffered by 30% of the world's children.[5, 6] For example, almost a third of the world's children live in squalid housing conditions, with more than five people per room or with mud flooring. Over half a billion children (27%) have no toilet facilities whatsoever and over 400 million children (19%) are drinking from unsafe open water sources (e.g., rivers, lakes, ponds) or have to walk so far to fetch water that they cannot carry enough to meet minimum health requirements.[6] The World Health Organization has argued that: "The world's biggest killer and the greatest cause of ill health and suffering across the globe is listed almost at the end of the International Classification of Diseases. It is given code Z59.5—extreme poverty."[7] Eliminating extreme poverty is the key to improving global child survival rates, particularly over the long term.

CHILD SURVIVAL AND CHILD RIGHTS

In recent years, the importance of the link between child rights and child survival has been contested. In 2004, an editorial in The Lancet[8] argued that UNICEF's focus on child rights had been detrimental to international campaigns to improve child survival. In particular, the article claimed that the outgoing UNICEF Director (Carol Bellamy) had focused on "girl's education, early childhood development, immunisation, HIV/AIDS, and protecting children from violence, abuse, exploitation, and discrimination," and that in doing this she had "failed to address the essential health needs of children." The current Director of UNICEF (Ann Veneman) has so far given much less prominence to child rights, making "child mortality public enemy number one for the agency."[9]

We argue that a rights-based strategy will increase child survival, in part by reducing child poverty, but only if some rights are prioritised over others. UNICEF, under Bellamy, adopted a position in which all the rights in the UN Convention on the Rights of the Child (UNCRC) were regarded as of equal importance, and both developed and developing countries were urged to realise these rights progressively (i.e., one after the other).[5, 10] This position has become hard to defend, since some rights are clearly more important than others and/or contingent on others. For example, whilst UNICEF recognises that children living in poverty are more likely to experience non-fulfilment of other rights,[5] the right to vote is little use to a child who has died in infancy as a result of a lack of medical care due to poverty.

There is a clear need to prioritise the realisation of rights in policy so that action can be divided into successive stages according to degree of severity of transgression and available resources. Ensuring child survival provides a good basis for this prioritisation, but to be effective, actions need to tackle both the symptoms and the underlying causes. The UNCRC (see Box 12.1) established a strong ideological, moral, and political tool for challenging these structural causes and its utility should not be undervalued.

Article 24 (1) of the UNCRC states that:

States Parties recognize the right of the child to the enjoyment of the highest attainable standard of health and to facilities for the treatment of illness and rehabilitation of health. States Parties shall strive to ensure that no child is deprived of his or her right of access to such health care services.

Similarly, Article 24 (2) of the UNCRC continues:

States Parties shall pursue full implementation of this right and, in particular, shall take appropriate measures:

a. *To diminish infant and child mortality;*
b. *To ensure the provision of necessary medical assistance and health care to all children with emphasis on the development of primary health care;*
c. *To combat disease and malnutrition, including within the framework of primary health care, through, inter alia, the application of readily available technology and through the provision of adequate nutritious foods and clean drinking-water, taking into consideration the dangers and risks of environmental pollution;*
d. *To ensure appropriate pre-natal and post-natal health care for mothers;*
e. *To ensure that all segments of society, in particular parents and children, are informed, have access to education and are supported in the use of basic knowledge of child health and nutrition, the advantages of breastfeeding, hygiene and environmental sanitation and the prevention of accidents;*
f. *To develop preventive health care, guidance for parents and family planning education and services.*

If these rights were to be fulfilled, child survival rates would rapidly improve.

BOX 12.1 THE FIVE CORE PRINCIPLES OF THE UN CONVENTION ON THE RIGHTS OF THE CHILD

- The right to life, survival, and development
- Non-discrimination
- Devotion to the best interests of the child
- Respect for the views of the child
- The right to an adequate standard of living and social security.

THE POTENTIAL OF A HUMAN RIGHTS APPROACH

A human rights approach offers the possibility for progressive interventions into child poverty and child survival in three ways. First, conventions like the UNCRC have been signed by most countries in the world and thus can be considered to embody universal values and aspirations. Second, human rights conventions place a legal obligation upon states, a view endorsed by Mary Robinson (former UN High Commissioner for Human Rights) in her speech to the 2002 World Summit on Sustainable Development in Johannesburg, South Africa: ". . . a human rights approach adds value because it provides a normative framework of obligations that has the legal power to render governments accountable."[11]

Any comprehensive understanding of the root causes of poverty and the 10 million annual premature child deaths cannot ignore the legal and institutional structures that create and perpetuate income and wealth imbalances within society. Thus, human rights provide a challenge to these structures.[12]

Third, rights-based language can help to direct policy. It shifts the focus of debate from the personal failures of the "poor" to the failure of macro-economic structures and policies implemented by nation states and international bodies (World Trade Organization, World Bank, International Monetary Fund, etc.) to eradicate poverty. Hence, child poverty in this context is no longer described as a "social problem" but a "violation of rights."[13]

HUMAN RIGHTS AS A TOOL FOR POVERTY REDUCTION: SOME PRACTICAL ISSUES

There are objections to the human rights approach. One question is whether human rights, as formally expressed in human rights conventions, are genuinely universal.[14] Critiques based on cultural relativism and Asian values have suggested that human rights are "western" in orientation and content and, consequently, promote liberal/individualist social preferences over more "collective" forms of organisation.[15, 16] However, it is a fact that every country in the world (the 193 UN Member States) has signed the UNCRC—implying that negotiated moves towards the realisation of the agreed goals are feasible. There is a near-unanimous consensus on objectives and values. Only two countries have to date failed to ratify the UNCRC—Somalia and the US.

A second question is whether economic, social, and cultural rights (including child health and survival) have been subjugated to civil and political rights, despite the insistence of human rights advocates on the "indivisibility" of these rights (see Box 12.2 for definitions of different categories of rights).[17] Following the Universal Declaration of Human Rights in 1948, civil and political rights have tended to be promoted over economic, social, and cultural rights.[18] Two specific international covenants were agreed upon: the International Covenant on Civil and Political Rights and the International Covenant on Economic, Social and Cultural Rights, and signatories are committed to the realisation of all these rights.[18, 19] Ironically, the act of creating two covenants has served to provide contradictory messages about the "indivisibility" of rights. This distinction has become entrenched in the legal systems of nation states, which sometimes place civil and political rights in the "justiciable" section of their constitution, while relegating economic, social, and cultural rights to the realm of directive principles.[20] Civil and political rights have entered into law ahead of economic, social, and cultural rights, which are crucial for poverty eradication and health improvements.

A third question about human rights is whether the "non-justiciability" and non-enforcement of certain economic, social, and cultural rights makes the development of anti-poverty policies difficult. It is often argued that "rights," as they have been defined in human rights conventions, are imprecise or are moral claims that are not legally enforceable.[20] Many "rights" have so far been largely ignored by national courts, and the realisation of economic, social, and cultural rights is particularly difficult. Domestic courts have been adept at arriving at complex decisions in cases relating to civil and political rights, but they have tended to dodge issues of poverty, access to health care, and non-fulfilment of other economic and social rights. They cite the non-justiciability of such rights and have not been aided by international jurisprudence, which is currently lacking in this area.

However, both domestic and international judiciaries could follow the inventive and progressive approach of treaty committees and special rapporteurs who scrutinize and regularly report on nation states' adherence to the conventions.[20] For instance, the Committee on the Rights of the Child has, on a number of occasions, refused to accept the "non-affordability" claims made in the progress reports of states. For instance, in the light of the funding of their defence budgets, Indonesia and Egypt were invited to justify their failure to make significant progress in implementing the UNCRC.[20]

There are notable examples where economic and social rights have been written into nation states' constitutions. Rights thus removed from the political sphere into the legal sphere are less contested. The advantage of this shift is that the courts can help to set minimum welfare stand-

---

BOX 12.2 DEFINITIONS OF CATEGORIES OF RIGHTS

Social and economic rights relate to guaranteeing individuals a minimum standard of living, such as a minimum income, housing, health care, and education.

Cultural rights relate to the recognition and safeguarding of ethnic/religious groups' practices and beliefs.

Civil rights relate to personal freedoms, such as the right to privacy, freedom of movement, and right to a fair trial.

Political rights relate to political participation, such as the right to vote and the right to peaceful assembly.

ards—through reviewing government budgets, vetoing legislation that is likely to increase rather than reduce poverty, and so on. Examples of such an approach can be found in India, the Republic of South Africa, and Finland.[21]

THE RELATIONSHIP BETWEEN THE RIGHTS OF THE CHILD AND CHILD POVERTY

The UNCRC does not contain an explicit human right to freedom from poverty. Hence, to measure poverty in terms of rights, a selection process is required to match these rights to the severe deprivations of basic human need that characterise poverty and cause ill health. Giving greater priority to selected groups of rights does not imply that rights are divisible in any ultimate or "perfect" sense. It allows planned actions to be taken, progressively by stages, to achieve agreed ends. Human rights are interrelated, so the fulfilment of some rights is reliant on the prior realisation of others.[15]

Many of the rights, as expressed in the relevant charters and conventions, are ambiguous or imprecise. This is often the case with social and economic rights where access to some rights is easier to define and measure than others. The right to survival—preventing early deaths—is less difficult to measure than access to adequate health or educational services. Many phenomena (such as "health") can be considered to be on a continuum ranging from "good health" to "poor health/death."[22] Similarly, fulfilment of rights can be considered to be on a continuum ranging from complete fulfilment to extreme violation. Courts can make judgments on individual cases on the correct threshold level at which rights are found to have been violated or fulfilled (see Figure 12.1).

Regrettably, there is little international case law at present that identifies the location of this "judicial" threshold with respect to many social, economic, and cultural rights, such as the right to health care. Social scientists therefore have a responsibility to help identify such "judicial" thresholds—a methodological issue we have sought to address in previous research.[23]

CONCLUSION

The international framework of child rights is a useful theoretical and political tool in taking action to reduce child poverty and improve child health.[24-29] A rights-based strategy is necessary to the development not only of international and national jurisprudence but to a global civil society that challenges the structures of global poverty, so that child rights may move from the realms of rhetoric to those of tangible reality. However, in order to provide clear guidance for policy, we need to move away from an approach that gives all rights equal weight, to a strategy of choosing clear implementation priorities. We suggest that the rights contained in the UNCRC relating to child survival and non-discrimination be prioritised, i.e., these rights should be

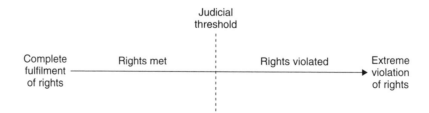

Figure 12.1 Continuum of Rights

implemented first in situations where child rights cannot be implemented all at once. An emphasis on both survival and non-discrimination is vital to prevent unequal health provision from developing—for example, privileging the survival of boys over girls or one ethnic group over another. If such priorities are not set, then governments may decide to implement those rights first that are least expensive and easiest to fulfil and only implement more expensive rights, which would improve child survival, at a later date.

Child rights fulfilment by states can only be properly assessed within the global context of poverty and an equal appraisal of developed and developing countries. Thus, the guidance given by the Committee on the Rights of the Child (General Comment No. 5),[30] which specifies that the realization of child rights is the responsibility of all nation states, be it within their jurisdiction or through international cooperation and action, requires widespread reinforcement and support. This places special obligations upon those who operate in the interests of the powerful nation states at the supranational level to ensure that child survival rates are improved by the fulfilment of children's human rights, particularly their economic and social rights. Solely concentrating on medical interventions that increase child survival, while ignoring other violations of children's human rights, is unlikely to ensure the health and well being of children in the long term.

REFERENCES

1. UNICEF (2002) State of the world's children 2002: Leadership: The rate of progress. New York: UNICEF.
2. Black RE, Morris SS, Bryce J (2003) Where and why are 10 million children dying every year? Lancet 361: 2226–2234.
3. World Health Organization (2002) The world health report 2002: Reducing risks, promoting healthy life..
4. United Nations Development Programme (1998) Human development report 1998: Consumption for human development.
5. UNICEF (2004) State of the world's children 2005: Childhood under threat.
6. Gordon D, Nandy S, Pantazis C, Pemberton SA, Townsend P (2003) Child poverty in the developing world. Bristol: The Policy Press.
7. World Health Organization (1995) World health report 1995: Bridging the gaps.
8. Horton RJ (2004) UNICEF leadership 2005–2015: A call for strategic change. Lancet 364: 9451.
9. Kapp C (2006) Ann Veneman: getting UNICEF back to basics. Lancet 368: 1061.
10. UNICEF (1999) Human rights for children and women: How UNICEF helps make them a reality.
11. Robinson M (2002) Statement by Mary Robinson, United Nations High Commissioner for Human Rights, at the World Summit on Sustainable Development plenary session.
12. Williams LA (2003) Introduction. In: Williams LA, Kjonstad WA, Robson P, editors. Law and poverty: The legal system and poverty reduction. London: Zed.
13. Chinkin C (2001) The United Nations decade for the elimination of poverty: What role for international law? Current Legal Problems 54: 553–589.
14. Kallen E (2004) Social inequality and social injustice: A human rights perspective. New York: Palgrave.
15. Doyal L, Gough I (1991) A theory of human need. London: Macmillan.
16. Sen A (1991) Development as freedom. Oxford: Oxford University Press.
17. Commonwealth Human Rights Initiative (2001) Human rights and poverty eradication: A talisman for the commonwealth. New Delhi: Commonwealth Human Rights Initiative.
18. Perez-Bustillo C (2003). Poverty as a violation of human rights: The Pinochet case and the emergence of a new paradigm. In: Williams LA, Kjonstad A, and Robson P, editors. Law and poverty: The legal system and poverty reduction. London: Zed.
19. Aoeud A (2003) the right to development as a basic human right. In: Williams LA, Kjonstad A, Robson P, editors. Law and poverty: The legal system and poverty reduction. London: Zed.
20. Van Bueren C (1999) Combating child poverty— Human rights approaches. Human Rights Quarterly 21: 680–706.
21. Campbell T (2003) Poverty is a violation of human rights: Inhumanity or injustice? Ethical and human right dimensions of poverty: Towards a new paradigm in the fight against poverty. Sao Paolo: UNESCO.
22. United Nations Development Programme (2000)

Human development report 2000: Human rights and development.

23. Gordon D (2002) The international measurement of poverty and anti-poverty policies. In: Townsend P, Gordon D, editors. World poverty: New policies to defeat an old enemy. Bristol: Policy Press.

24. Pemberton S, Gordon D, Nandy S, Pantazis C, Townsend P (2005) The relationship between child poverty and child rights: The role of indicators. In: Minujin A, Delamonica E, Komarecki M, editors. Human rights and social policies for children and women: The MICS in practice. New York: UNICEF/New School University.

25. MacDonald R (2007) An inspirational defence of the right to health. Lancet 370: 379–380.

26. MacDonald TH (2007) The global human right to health: Dream or possibility? Oxford: Radcliffe Publishing.

27. Gruskin S, Mills EJ, Tarantola D (2007) History, principles and practice of health and human rights. Lancet 370: 9585.

28. Singh JA, Govender M, Mills EJ (2007) Do human rights matter to health? Lancet 370: 9586.

29. Veit-Wilson J (2007) Some social policy implications of a right to social security. In: Van Langendonc J, editor. The right to social security. Antwerp: Intersentia. pp 57–83.

30. United Nations Committee on the Rights of the Child (2003) General comment no. 5: General measures of implementation for the Convention on the Rights of the Child 03/10/2003. CRC/GC/2003/5.

QUESTIONS

1. Children's rights are human rights, so why is a special convention needed for children? How is the child defined? What is the age cutoff? Should this cutoff be extended or reduced, and if so for what reasons? Do governmental policies impact adults and children equally?

2. The CRC insists that each child should be able to develop to the fullest. Does "developing to the fullest" have the same definition everywhere? Does a young girl in a community that limits the education a woman can receive have the same rights as a young girl with full access to any level of education she desires?

3. The author mentions that only Somalia and the US have failed to ratify the United Nations Convention on the Rights of the Child. What US administration was in power when the CRC was first proposed? What objections did the US raise? Why does this continue to be a problem despite a number of changes in the US administration? Do you believe that the US should ratify the CRC? Why or why not?

4. Pemberton suggests that social scientists have a responsibility to help identify "judicial thresholds" with respect to social, economic and cultural rights. Propose some appropriate judicial thresholds that could be used as functional indicators in the oversight of universal social, economic or cultural rights for children. You may wish to consult the previous research of the authors.

FURTHER READING

1. Office of the United Nations High Commissioner on Human Rights (OHCHR) The Convention on the Rights of the Child, OHCHR (1989). See also General Comments on the Rights of the Child. http://www2.ohchr.org/english/law/crc.htm

2. Lewis, S., Promoting Child Health and the Convention on the Rights of the Child. *Health and Human Rights*, 1997: 2: 77–82

3. World Health Organization, Tobacco and the Rights of the Child, WHO, Geneva, (2001) http://whqlibdoc.who.int/hq/2001/WHO_NMH_TFI_01.3_Rev.1.pdf
4. Price Cohen, Cynthia, The Role of the United States in Drafting the Convention on the Rights of the Child. *Emory International Law Review,* Vol. 20: 185–198, 2006.
5. Tarantola, D., & Gruskin, S., Children Confronting HIV/AIDS: Charting the Confluence of Rights and Health. *Health Human Rights,* 1998; 3: 60–86.

CHAPTER 13

Using Indicators to Determine the Contribution of Human Rights to Public Health Efforts

Sofia Gruskin and Laura Ferguson

INTRODUCTION

Despite increasing attention paid to the apparent integration of human rights into public health policies and programs, it is difficult to find concrete examples of the benefits that have been derived from linking human rights norms and standards to public health imperatives. There is a need to identify existing approaches that link human rights and health concerns and then to determine the best ways to assess their impact on the effectiveness and outcomes of health policies and programs. As basic as it sounds, this approach requires clarity, not only in defining human rights, but also in recognizing what incorporation of identified norms and standards should look like in practice.

In the interests of validity and comparability, from a public health perspective, assessment requires appropriate quantitative indicators. Implicit in the use of such indicators is a sense that they are both impartial and objective. Yet a human rights perspective suggests querying the assumed neutrality of an indicator: we should think about who uses it, for what purposes and in what ways. What occurs before, during and after the measurement process itself is equally important as what is being measured. Thus, the purpose of this paper is to begin to disentangle the diversity of approaches to health and human rights indicators and to suggest issues to consider in determining the value of existing approaches.

HUMAN RIGHTS AND PUBLIC HEALTH PRACTICE

Human rights bring into focus the relationship between the government, which is the first-line provider and protector of human rights, and individuals (who hold these rights as human beings).[1] Every country in the world is party to at least one human rights treaty and all have made rights-related commitments relevant to health.[2] While for many years it was unclear what the incorporation of human rights principles meant for public health practice, certain actions are increasingly considered part of a human rights-based approach to health (Box 13.1).

Although generally not incorporated so systematically, many of the interventions implied by the actions named in Box 1 are familiar to people involved in public health. Those that are not so familiar, such as ensuring transparency for how decisions are made, are unique contributions that the human rights field offers to public health. A difficulty lies in determining whether, by drawing attention to the human rights aspects of those actions traditionally in the domain of public health, the nature of the indicator appropriate for their measurement should remain the same or change. Additionally, the fact that institutions may engage differently with the same concepts and even the same indicators has implications for assessing the ways in which monitoring and evaluation are done across the fields of health and human rights.

INDICATORS

A wide range of actors use indicators to capture human rights concerns relating to health including international and national human rights mechanisms, governments, health and development organizations and civil society.

In general terms, an indicator is "a variable with characteristics of quality, quantity and time used to measure, directly or indirectly, changes in a situation and to appreciate the progress made in addressing it."[4] Table 13.1 lays out definitions and examples of the two types of indicators used to capture health and human rights concerns.

It is immediately apparent that many of the human rights indicators constitute measures that fall outside the traditional definition of a health indicator. To assess the degree to which human rights are respected, protected and fulfilled in the area of health is to expand the notion of what constitutes an indicator in this field. Inevitably this brings with it complications, some of which are explored in this paper.

Human Rights Indicators to Measure Health

For those involved in monitoring the human rights compliance of States, indicators are primarily used to enhance the practice of accountability for health-related rights issues. In this context, interest in health arises primarily from its relevance to a range of rights, in particular when nonfulfilment of health-related rights is thought to impede fulfilment of a range of human rights. For example, human rights organizations may quantify violations in specific areas to highlight governmental failure to protect human rights relevant to health, e.g., sexual violence in conflict situations.[8] Further, some treaty monitoring bodies ask governments to show the kind of legislation that exists to protect population groups from discrimination in their access to health care,[9] while others ask for such information as disaggregation by ethnicity of the reported number of births attended by skilled health personnel.[10]

BOX 13.1 ACTIONS SUGGESTED TO CONSTITUTE A RIGHTS-BASED APPROACH TO HEALTH

- Considering the legal and policy context within which interventions occur.
- Supporting the participation of affected groups, especially vulnerable groups, in all efforts that concern them.
- Working to ensure discrimination does not occur in the delivery of services nor in the health outcomes experienced among different population groups.
- Using human rights standards to deliver services in particular with respect to ensuring their availability, accessibility, acceptability and quality.
- Ensuring transparency and accountability both for how relevant decisions are made and their ultimate impact.[3]

Attention to the use of such human rights indicators by actors in the health arena is rapidly increasing. To ensure a shared understanding of why and how they are being used, as well as transparency, it is important to make explicit the justification for the assumption that these indicators are grounded in international human rights law and they are linked to the field of health. Highlighting the legal bases from which such indicators are derived can also help to minimize bias in how they are used.

Health Indicators to Measure Human Rights

Within the human rights field, compliance with human rights norms and standards and assessment of government accountability is often done through use of "traditional" health indicators. An example is infant mortality rates, which are used as a measure of State Party compliance with their obligation to respect the child's right to life, survival and development, even though they were created as an indicator of population health.[10]

For those involved in health, the fact that health indicators draw attention to rights issues is generally a by-product of efforts to determine the appropriateness and effectiveness of policies and programs. As one example, disaggregation of data on the basis of sex and age may be used to gauge usage of available health services,[11] but may also draw attention to larger underlying concerns related to inequities in access. In other instances, attention to human rights may be driven by a genuine, but nebulous, desire to "do good" and thus give insufficient attention to why a particular health indicator, or set of indicators, is assumed to measure human rights.

Even as indicators are frequently used for purposes beyond those for which they were originally intended, it is useful to consider whether health indicators ostensibly used to measure human rights would have been constructed differently if human rights considerations had formed part of their design, and also to consider the criteria that are or should be used to determine how health indicators are linked to specific human rights for valid inferences to be made.

Indicators of Health and Human Rights

With regard to the capture of information at the intersection of health and human rights, increasingly a third category of indicators exists—those created in the health field to capture information specifically relating to human rights issues in the design and delivery of health policies and programs.[12-15]

This can most plainly be seen in relation to the components noted previously as key aspects of a human rights approach. Some examples follow.

Assessment of laws that may present obstacles to effective HIV prevention and care for vulnerable populations provide a useful example of an indicator that brings to light issues equally of interest to both fields.[16] Laws that criminalize injecting drug use, sex work or consensual sex between men may deter people who engage in these behaviours from seeking HIV-related services even if they are available. Knowledge of the existence of such laws provides context within which the public health community can plan and implement programmatic activities, and can help the human rights community to inform advocacy and push for any legal reform necessary. These indicators could be improved by capturing not simply the existence of a law but also its quality, as well as the degree to which it is implemented.

Indicators relating to the participation of vulnerable groups bring several concerns relevant for both health and rights. For example, the Greater Involvement of People Living with or Affected by HIV/AIDS (GIPA) principle draws its strength and legal grounding in the right to participation and has also been recognized as critical to effective HIV programming.[17] It is crucial that appropriate participation be sought from affected communities to ensure the acceptability of interventions to the population for whom they are intended. Additional thought is required on the way to determine in each instance which populations are considered vulnerable. This determines not only whose participation is solicited and measured, but also which populations are acknowledged to exist.

LINGUISTIC CHALLENGES

Semantics pose challenges as there are differences in understanding across the fields even when using the same terminology. For example, stigma and discrimination have precise definitions such that, in relation to health, "stigma" means being devalued by individuals or communities on the basis of real or perceived health status. "Discrimination" refers to the legal, institutional and procedural ways that people are denied access to their rights because of their real or perceived health status.[18,19] In public health, these terms are increasingly used but often without distinction. For example, several instruments ostensibly assess both stigma and discrimination within the context of HIV/AIDS.[20–23] While presumably excellent for their own purposes, most mix the definitions and concepts of stigma and discrimination, thereby detracting from the ultimate utility of the data from a human rights perspective for both advocacy and accountability purposes.

Along similar lines, in 2003 the United Nations Special Rapporteur on the Right to Health suggested that the categories of structural, process and outcome indicators be introduced into the monitoring of health-related human rights,[24] and the validity of this approach for a wide range

Table 13.1 The two types of indicators used to capture health and human rights concerns

	Definition	*Examples*
Health indicator	A health indicator has been defined as a "variable that helps to measure changes in a health situation directly or indirectly and to assess the extent to the objectives and targets which of a program are being attained."[5]	The number of maternal deaths is a raw statistic that takes on greater meaning when converted into an indicator of number of maternal deaths/live births/year, which can be tracked over time alongside programmatic activities. Other examples include: the percentage of the population that has sustained access to improved drinking water sources, the percentage of children aged less than 5 who sleep under insecticide-treated bed-nets, and total expenditure on health as a percentage of gross domestic product.
Human rights indicator	A human rights indicator has been defined as a measure that provides information on the extent to which human rights norms and standards are addressed in a given situation.[6]	Indicators of fulfilment of human rights would include, for example, the extent to which international human rights obligations are incorporated into national laws and policies relevant to maternal health. Human rights indicators also include indicators of violations such as quantitative summaries of human rights violations, legal audits and determination as to the existence and use of mechanisms for challenge and redress if violations are alleged to occur.[7]

of rights is increasingly under discussion in the human rights community.[6] While, to those working in the health field, this would seem to be a familiar delineation of indicators and an important step in bringing together the human rights and health fields, the differences in how these categories are defined is worthy of note. In human rights terms, "structural indicators" capture the existence of laws, policies and regulations considered key to the functioning of health systems [24] as opposed to variables reflecting the system in which care is delivered.[25] "Process indicators" are defined as measuring "programs, activities and interventions,"[24] which is different from the traditional public health definition of measuring the mechanisms through which interventions have an impact.[25] The fields more or less come together in their definition of "outcome indicators," which aim to capture the impact of programs, activities and interventions on health.[24, 25]

Thus even when the same terminology is used, unless recognized and addressed, definitional differences between the health and human rights fields can lead to confusion and limitations in the presentation and use of the information collected.

USING EXISTING INDICATORS

It is clearly preferable to first determine the concept that is to be assessed and then find an appropriate measure. However, given the veritable plethora of indicators already in existence, one should look at how existing indicators can be better understood and used to capture issues relevant to both health and human rights before giving consideration to the creation of any new indicators. For an indicator to be valid from both a health and human rights perspective, irrespective of why it was initially constructed, it is essential to determine the extent of its human rights sensitivity and its validity in public health terms. We propose a series of questions to help guide determination of the health and human rights appropriateness of any given indicator.

Why Was It Designed?

The design of every indicator is influenced by the priorities shaping its use. An indicator will look quite different if its intended purpose is to inform strategy and program development as opposed to monitoring targets and holding specific actors accountable. While in the end the issues of concern may be similar, decisions relating to such issues as specificity, comparability and cost will, to a large extent, be determined by the intended purpose of the indicator as well the interests of the entity funding its construction. Careful consideration and due attention to transparency are obviously required as to whose values are incorporated and the extent to which the indicator was designed with both health and human rights concerns in mind.

Who Is Using It?

Beyond the question of whether an organization's primary area of focus is health, human rights or both, the use of an indicator is likely to look different in the hands of a nongovernmental organization, a donor, a national government institution or an international organization. If the indicator is designed by one actor but used by others, it is unclear the extent to which all actors need to be aware of its original purpose in order for their efforts, including the interpretation and use of any data, to be valid.

What Kind of Indicator?

Within the public health community, statistical significance achieved through use of quantitative indicators has long been seen as the gold standard for research and evaluation.[26] Attention to human rights concerns sheds light on the inadequacy of quantitative indicators alone for fully understanding and addressing a situation. Likewise, surveys of client perceptions of the availability, accessibility, acceptability and quality of health services (key aspects of the right to health) are useful for raising human rights concerns, but they too are inadequate in painting a full picture. In an ideal world, not only would indicators be constructed to take into account both health and human rights considerations, but quantitative and qualitative indicators would be considered together to allow for interventions shaped by a more complete picture of the issues at hand.

Does It Provide Information on Vulnerable Populations?

Disaggregation of information to reflect where the needs are most acute is undisputed. The question ultimately boils down to what disaggregation criteria are applied and in response to whose demand. In light of the acknowledged importance of non-discrimination and the recognized need for appropriately targeted interventions, at first glance it is problematic that most indicators do not capture information about specific population subgroups. An inherent tension between public health and human rights concerns surfaces here. Statistical validity requires carefully planned sampling strategies, which become increasingly costly, time-consuming and complicated as categories of disaggregation are added. Conversely, attention to human rights concerns would seem to suggest that disaggregation needs to go beyond sex and geographical location to include such factors as race, language, sexual orientation, and civil, political, social or other status.[27] Determining the appropriate level of disaggregation for any given setting requires conscious attention to both public health and human rights considerations to ensure the situation of vulnerable populations with respect to specific health issues is appropriately addressed without inadvertent exacerbation of discrimination.

How Are Data Collected?

The public health community's interest in the process of collecting data is to a large extent centred around determining ways to ensure reported results are valid,[28] whereas a human rights perspective is concerned with the processes of why and how data are collected. Egregious examples within the public health field, such as Nazi human experimentation[29] and the Tuskegee Syphilis Study,[30] have drawn attention to ethical concerns but a human rights perspective highlights the responsibility of the researcher, policy-maker and health programer to know the source of data in all instances. This helps to ensure not only that efforts are appropriately informed but also, if necessary, that data collection efforts be amended to ensure human rights violations do not inadvertently occur in the process.

HOW ARE DATA USED?

Once data are collected, there are issues to consider with respect to whether the information is made publicly available, released to the affected community with proper education or only known to a small subset of actors; concerns may exist in each of these scenarios. Transparency in how this decision is reached will help ensure legitimacy and accountability for any problems that may occur from subsequent use of the data. Attention to human rights considerations can also make an important contribution to the use of purportedly neutral health data and help to ensure these data do not end up unintentionally fostering stigma, discrimination or further violations of human rights. Table 13.2 draws on examples from HIV to

Table 13.2 Using HIV to highlight the issues raised by questioning indicators

Question	Example
Why was this indicator designed?	Tracking the total number of people on antiretroviral therapy (ART) might suffice for monitoring governmental accountability and progress towards achieving universal access targets. However, to inform the provision of ART, a detailed breakdown of which populations are (and are not) accessing ART would be more useful.
Who is using the indicator?	Designed by international organizations, early indicators of the number of people on ART included women who were given prophylaxis to prevent vertical transmission of HIV to their infants. These numbers were initially used by other organizations who were unaware that data which appeared to show some degree of gender equity in access to ART were in fact masking the low numbers of women accessing ART outside the context of preventing vertical HIV transmission.
What kind of indicator is it?	The number of people who have been tested for HIV is a quantitative indicator often used in the field of HIV. However, this does not capture the quality of the HIV testing process such as the type of counselling, ensured confidentiality and appropriate referral, all of which are critical to people's ability to process the information presented both for behaviour change and to promote long-term connection with HIV-related services. Bringing together qualitative and quantitative indicators can not only improve use of services but provide a more accurate picture of the long-term impact of HIV testing on communities and more broadly.
Does the indicator provide appropriate information with regard to vulnerable populations?	Access to services for the prevention of mother-to-child transmission of HIV is often used as an indicator of coverage of HIV services. However, an aggregate figure can hide under-served populations: disaggregation by age, for example, might highlight adolescents as an under-recognized population; or disaggregation by locality might draw attention to the need to improve these services for remote rural populations.
How are data collected?	Estimates of prevalence of HIV infection among sex workers and intravenous drug users are sometimes presented as evidence of commitment to vulnerable populations. These estimates could be modeled from data collected from sex workers or drug users who voluntarily came forward for HIV counselling and testing, but the information equally could be collected at centres for rehabilitation where people are pulled off the streets, detained, tested without their consent and given no access either to their test results or to adequate care.
How are data used?	The withholding of information by government officials in the context of HIV, for example when governments refuse(d) to report accurately the numbers of people estimated to be living with HIV in their borders, is well known. Equally troubling have been documented instances of the inappropriate use of data fuelling stigma, discrimination and human rights violations such as occurred for people from communities identified in government statistical reports as having high rates of HIV infection including immigrants, sex workers and drug users.[31]

highlight the sorts of issues raised by previous questions.

CONCLUSION

Different types of indicators capture different sorts of data through diverse mechanisms. Consequently, effective assessment of health and human rights concerns may require innovative application of proven monitoring and evaluation methodologies, such as triangulation across different data sources. Such an approach would promote pioneering use of existing indicators thereby maximizing the potential use of existing data without further burdening monitoring and evaluation systems with new indicators.

The value of what can genuinely be called health and human rights indicators is not only to show progress, disparities and gaps within countries and globally: the process of measurement matters as much as the data themselves. Health and human rights indicators can show the extent to which governments and other entities are meeting their health-related human rights obligations, highlight areas where further efforts might lead to increased fulfilment of these obligations and, by extension, improve health outcomes. Drawing attention to all elements of a rights-based approach, indicators which genuinely capture both sets of concerns will ultimately help to determine whether policies and programs that are the most effective in health terms are also those that have achieved the greatest level of compliance with human rights principles. Even as clarifying these links is important, all of this will remain purely academic unless the data are used to improve support for affected communities. Although still young and fairly amorphous, the potential of health and human rights indicators for informing evidence-based policies and programs underscores the need for their further development.

REFERENCES

1. Clapham A. *Human rights: a very short introduction.* Oxford: Oxford University Press; 2007.
2. United Nations Treaty Collection [Internet site]. Geneva: United Nations; 2009.
3. Gruskin S, Tarantola D. Universal access to HIV prevention, treatment and care: assessing the inclusion of human rights in international and national strategic plans. *AIDS* 2008; 22 Suppl 2; S123–32.
4. Management effectiveness program. In: *Health systems: concepts, design & performance.* Cairo: World Health Organization Regional Office for the Eastern Mediterranean; 2004.
5. *Health systems performance glossary.* Geneva: World Health Organization; 2000.
6. Malhotra R, Fasel N. Quantitative Human Rights Indicators: a survey of major initiatives. In: *Expert Meeting on Human Rights Indicators, Abo Akedemi University, Turku, Finland, 10–13 March 2005.*
7. Landman T. Measuring human rights: principle, practice and policy. *Hum Rights Q* 2004; 26: 906–31.
8. *Five years on: no justice for sexual violence in Darfur.* New York, NY: Human Rights Watch; 2008.
9. International Convention on the Elimination of All Forms of Racial Discrimination, Article 5 paragraph e (iv). Geneva: Office of the United Nations High Commissioner for Human Rights.
10. Committee on the Rights of the Child. *General guidelines regarding the form and content of initial reports to be submitted by States Parties under article 44, paragraph 1(a), of the Convention [CRC/C/5].* Geneva: Office of the United Nations High Commissioner for Human Rights; 1991.
11. *Reproductive health indicators for global monitoring* [Report of the second inter-agency meeting, WHO/RHR/01.19]. Geneva: World Health Organization; 2000.
12. Hunt P. Human right to the highest attainable standard of health: new opportunities and challenges. *Trans R Soc Trop Med Hyg* 2006; 100: 603–7.
13. Green M. What we talk about when we talk about indicators: current approaches to human rights measurement. *Hum Rights Q* 2001; 23:1063–97.
14. Report of Turku expert meeting on human rights indicators. In: *Expert Meeting on Human Rights Indicators, Abo Akedemi University, Turku, Finland, 10–13 March 2005.* Available from: web.abo.fi/instut/imr/research/seminars/indicators/Report.doc [accessed on 3 July 2009].

15. Raworth K. Measuring human rights. In: Gruskin S, Grodin MA, Annas GJ, Marks

16. *Monitoring the Declaration of Commitment on HIV/AIDS: guidelines on construction of core indicators reporting.* Geneva: Joint United Nations Program on HIV/AIDS (UNAIDS); 2008.

17. The Paris Declaration. In: *Paris AIDS Summit, Paris, 1 December 1994.*

18. Definition of "stigma", no. 2. *The Oxford English Dictionary.* 2nd edition. Oxford: Oxford University Press; 1989.

19. Definition of "discrimination", no. 1. *The Oxford English Dictionary.* 2nd edition. Oxford: Oxford University Press; 1989.

20. UNAIDS General Population Survey. Geneva: UNAIDS; 2000.

21. Demographic and Health Survey AIDS Module. Calverton, MD: ORC Macro; 2000.

22. Behavioral Surveillance Surveys. Adult and youth modules. Research Triangle Park, NC: Family Health International; 2009.

23. Multiple Indicator Cluster Survey (MICS). New York, NY: UNICEF; 2009.

24. Right of everyone to enjoy the highest attainable standard of physical and mental health [Interim report of the Special Rapporteur of the Commission on Human Rights, agenda item 117 (c)]. In: *United Nations 58th session of the General Assembly, Geneva, 2003.*

25. Donabedian A. Evaluating the quality of medical care. *Milbank Mem Fund Q* 1966; 44: 166–206.

26. Baum F. Researching public health: behind the qualitative-quantitative methodological debate. *Soc Sci Med* 1995; 40: 459–68.

27. General comment 14 on the right to the highest attainable standard of health [E/C.12/2000/4]. In: *United Nations Committee on Economic, Social and Cultural Rights, Geneva, 20 May 2000.*

28. Shadish WR, Cook TD, Campbell DT. *Experimental and quasi-experimental designs for generalized causal inference.* Boston, MA: Houghton Mifflin; 2002.

29. Annas GJ, Grodin MA. *The Nazi doctors and the Nuremberg Code.* New York, NY: University Press; 1992.

30. Brandt AM. Racism and research: the case of the Tuskegee syphilis study. *Hastings Cent Rep* 1978; 8: 21–9.

31. De Lay P, Manda V. Politics of monitoring and evaluation: lessons from the AIDS epidemic. *N Dir Eval* 2004: 13–31.

QUESTIONS

1. What are the commonalities and differences between health indicators and human rights indicators? With reference to Table 13.1, how would you define an indicator relevant to human-rights based approaches to health? Could you provide an example?

2. What influence on policies, program and actions can be exerted by the formulation and choice of health and human rights indicators? If anyone, who should take part in formulating and choosing such indicators and through what process?

3. Could you formulate a single health and human rights indicator for the monitoring of a national program aimed at combating gender-based violence? What events or trends is this indicator likely to reveal? What may not be captured by the use of this single indicator? What additional means of monitoring could be suggested to bridge this gap?

FURTHER READING

1. WHO: Consultation on Indicators for the Right to Health, Meeting Report, Health and Human Rights, Department of Ethics, Trade, Human Rights and

Health Law, Sustainable Development and Healthy Environments, World Health Organization, Geneva (2004).

2. McInerney-Lankford, S., & Sano, H.O., Human Rights Indicators in Development: An Introduction, The World Bank Studies (2010) http://webcache.googleusercontent.com/search?q=cache:1K1C-BC6EYcJ:siteresources.worldbank.org/EXTLAWJUSTICE/Resources/HumanRightsWP10_Final.pdf%3F%26resourceurlname%3DHumanRightsWP10_Final.pdf+&cd=10&hl=en&ct=clnk

3. Rosga, A. & Satterthwaite, M.L., The Trust in Indicators: Measuring Human Rights, *Berkeley Journal of International Law* (2009) http://www.boalt.org/bjil/docs/BJIL27.2_Satterthwaite_Rosga.pdf

4. *Reproductive Health Indicators for Global Monitoring* [Report of the second inter-agency meeting, WHO/RHR/01.19]. Geneva: World Health Organization (2000). http://who.int/reproductive-health/publications/rhr_01_19/index.htm

CHAPTER 14

Mainstreaming Wellbeing: An Impact Assessment for the Right to Health

Rebekah Gay

The World Health Organization has written that 'without health, other rights have little meaning' (Jamar 1994). Over the past decade, the full ramifications of this statement have become clearer, as the health and human rights movement has endeavoured to establish conceptual and analytical bridges between the two disciplines of health and human rights, to create a field of discourse that goes to the very essence of human wellbeing.

That discourse now faces the challenge of evolving itself from the conceptual to the operational, so that the linkages between health and human rights are explicitly recognised and incorporated in decision-making processes. There is therefore a rising call for new methodologies that can advance this ongoing evolution. A right-to-health impact assessment has been suggested as one such methodology, on the basis that it might provide decision makers across sectors with an evidence-based mechanism for analysing and anticipating the effects of their decisions.

This chapter seeks to explore that possibility by examining the experiences of health impact assessment and human rights impact assessment and considering whether a right-to-health impact assessment offers anything more than these existing methodologies. These considerations belie complex conceptual and methodological issues, and the chapter offers some preliminary thoughts on the issues with which the health and human rights movement will need to grapple as it continues its struggle to mainstream human wellbeing.

HEALTH AS A HUMAN RIGHT

Written in 1946, the Constitution of the World Health Organization (WHO) contains in its preamble one of the most enduring statements of health as 'a state of complete physical, mental and social wellbeing' and its conception as a fundamental human right (Toebes 1999, 36). While this definition catapulted health into the human rights framework, there has been a degree of inconsistency in the articulation of the right to health and the more delimited right to the 'highest attainable standard of health' in the human rights documents that have emerged since that time (Leary 1994). Such inconsistency can be partly attributed to the lack of conceptual clarity that has been associated with the normative content and scope of the right to health. As one of the bundle of economic, social and cultural rights, it was long overlooked on the basis that it was too vague and predominantly aspirational (Alston and Quinn 1987, 159; Meier 2006,

733; Chapman 1998, 390). However, in more recent times, the health and human rights movement has sought to revolutionise the linkages between health and human rights, and to give much-needed substance to the right to health as enshrined in international human rights law (Mann 1994; Gruskin and Tarantola 2005).

Through this process, there is now an understanding that the right to health is an inclusive one, and is inextricably related to and dependent on the realisation of other rights, which are also essential determinants of human wellbeing (CESCR 2000, para 3; Toebes 2001, 175). There is also a growing consensus that, notwithstanding the qualifying principles of progressive realisation and resource availability, the right to health has a core content that imposes immediate obligations upon states. That core content mandates state adherence to the fundamental principles of non-discrimination and participation (CESCR 2000, paras 11, 18 and 19) and compels states to provide minimum essential levels of primary health care, food, housing, sanitation and essential drugs, and to adopt and implement a national public health strategy (CESCR 2000, para 43). At the same time, the interrelated and essential elements of availability, accessibility, acceptability and quality provide a concrete standard against which state conduct can be measured (CESCR 2000, para 12; Toebes 2001, 177; Asher 2004, 37).

The right to health has therefore been invested with a substantive meaning that is capable of being operationalised. Such an evolution, from conceptual to operational, is essential if the right to health is to move beyond a slogan to something that has meaningful and useful application in the real world. This task presents a series of significant challenges, and the United Nations Special Rapporteur for Health has articulated the need for new techniques that are capable of engaging with rele-

vant players, including policy makers and health practitioners, so as to mainstream the right to health (Hunt 2007a, paras 9 and 26; Farmer and Gastineau 2002, 663; Roth 2004). Impact assessment, particularly a right-to-health impact assessment, has been suggested as one such technique (Hunt 2007b, para 44; Gruskin et al. 2007, 453).

HEALTH IMPACT ASSESSMENT

The past decade has seen the emergence of health impact assessment (HIA), which has been defined as:

> . . . a combination of procedures, methods and tools by which a policy, program or project may be judged as to its potential effects on the health of a population, and the distribution of those effects within the population.
>
> (ECHP 1999)

While HIA traces its origins to earlier methodologies of impact assessment, such as environmental impact assessment and social impact assessment, it also owes much of its existence to public health practitioners who perceived the potential of HIA as a means of promoting 'healthy public policy' (Kemm and Parry 2004, 16; Mahoney and Durham 2002; Mittelmark 2000). Through the influence of these practitioners, HIA has embraced a broad definition of health and has developed a clear understanding that the wellbeing of people is dependent on a spectrum of factors (ECHP 1999). These determinants of health have been illustrated as layers of influence, as depicted in Figure 14.1 (Dahlgren and Whitehead 1991).

By adopting this multidimensional model of health, HIA recognises that most policies or programs, including those in non-health sectors, have the potential to impact significantly through these layers of

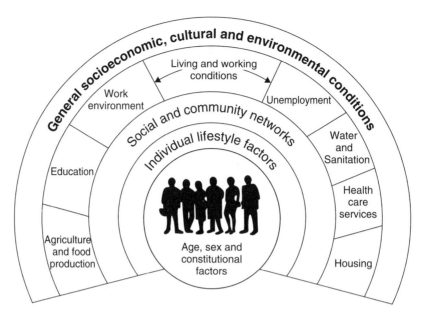

Figure 14.1 Layers of Infference

influence (Lock 2006, 11). In doing so, HIA advocates for a multidisciplinary approach to health, so that the responsibility for health is necessarily expanded to a range of sectors that would not otherwise give explicit consideration to health-related issues.

At the same time, this model of health enables HIA to provide a practical means of assessing potential health impacts. The links between health outcomes and health determinants are complex and multifactorial, so that it is often impossible to identify clear causal relationships. HIA offers a mechanism for overcoming that complexity by considering impacts in terms of health determinants rather than health outcomes, and by examining those determinants as categories and subcategories which correspond to the layers of influence depicted in Figure 14.1 (Lock 2006, 11). An assessment of the likely impact of a proposal on the various categories of determinants then provides a basis for drawing conclusions as to antici-

pated effects on the health of a community (Birley 2002).

Another significant dimension of HIA is health equity, and its recognition that the impacts of a policy or program will rarely be uniform throughout a population. HIA is therefore concerned to identify both the potential impacts of a proposal on the health of a population and the distribution of those impacts within the population. To that end, HIA has developed its capacity to ascertain how a proposal will impact on different population groups, including whether it might compound the distribution of existing health inequalities or impose new health burdens on specific groups (Taylor et al., 2003; Harris-Roxas et al. 2004).

One of the key methodologies for identifying such health inequalities is the use of a participatory approach to HIA, which allows those most likely to be affected by an intervention to identify the anticipated impacts on their state of wellbeing (ECHP 1999; Douglas et al. 2001, 152; Elliot et al.

2004, 81). It also democratises both the process of HIA and the decisions that HIA seeks to influence, by emphasising community participation in a transparent process for the formulation, implementation and evaluation of policies that affect the community (Kemm 2005; ECHP 1999). In this way, the process of HIA becomes as important as its outcomes, as it provides an empowering and consensus-building experience for community participants (Taylor et al. 2003; Kemm 2005; Mahoney and Durham 2002; Mahoney and Potter 2005, 19; Gillis 1999; O'Mullane 2007).

As HIA enters its second decade of experience, while many of the underlying principles of HIA have gained general acceptance, HIA practitioners have identified that if HIA is to achieve its ultimate goal of promoting healthy public policy, a vital challenge will be its ability to become entrenched within the decision-making process (Kemm 2005; Banken 2003; Davenport et al. 2006). Assuming HIA is up to this challenge, HIA has the potential to facilitate an awareness and understanding of health and its determinants across policy spheres and, in doing so, to introduce the core values of equity and democracy into decision-making processes. Expressed in these terms, it is not difficult to recognise that in bringing health into the consciousness of decision makers, HIA is also emphasising many of the core values that underpin the right to health. However, the concept of health as a human right has received little explicit consideration within HIA methodologies. In terms of impact assessment, that discussion has been left to the relatively embryonic field of human rights impact assessment.

HUMAN RIGHTS IMPACT ASSESSMENT

Much of the activity around human rights impact assessment (HRIA) has been in the field of business and human rights, as a result of the recent calls for businesses to take active steps to avoid human rights violations within their spheres of influence. HRIA has been perceived as one means of operationalising this call to action, with a number of different HRIA tools being developed to assist businesses in assessing the human rights impacts of their activities.

For example, the International Business Leaders Forum and the International Finance Corporation (IBLF/IFC) have collaborated in developing a self-assessment tool for businesses (IBLF/IFC 2007; Ersmaker 2007). The tool emphasises consultation with stakeholders, and encompasses eight steps sequencing from knowledge building to impact assessment, to final monitoring and evaluation (IBLF/IFC 2007, 40). In its summary of the human rights issues that may require assessment, IBLF/IFC categorises rights by those of workers, communities and customers (IBLF/IFC 2007, Appendix 4). Within each of these categories, the right to health is addressed in terms of the entitlement of workers to protection from risks to their health and safety in the workplace; the right of communities to be protected from adverse impacts on their health and safety arising from a company's operations; and the obligation on companies to ensure that their products are not detrimental to the health of customers.

The human rights concerns associated with corporate involvement in foreign investment projects have also prompted Rights and Democracy to propose the use of HRIA for such projects (Rights and Democracy 2005; 2007; Brodeur 2007). The methodology developed by Rights and Democracy is intended as a community-led impact assessment of existing investment projects, and has been the subject of five reported case studies (Rights and Democracy 2007, 35). With respect to the right to health, the results of the case studies usefully illustrate how dependent the outcome of the assessment process is on the substantive meaning given to the underlying right. While Rights and Democracy cites the WHO definition of health, the main focus of its right-to-health questions is the impact of a project on health care and health services, as assessed using the criteria of accessibility, availability, acceptability and quality (Rights and Democracy 2005, 53). As a result, the consideration given to the right to health in the reports of the case studies is limited and in two of the five case studies an impact on the right to health is not identified at all as a concern.

The Halifax Initiative Coalition has also proposed the use of HRIA to develop a rights-based approach to trade and finance (Halifax Initiative Coalition 2004). The Coalition has outlined an impact assessment process that applies a human rights framework to existing impact assessment methodologies, such that the values of accountability, participation, equity and sustainability are placed at the core of the assessment process (Halifax Initiative Coalition 2004, 17). This approach is intended to produce an integrated impact assessment that identifies potential cultural, economic, social, civil and political rights impacts of a proposed project (Halifax Initiative Coalition 2004, 14).

There has also been consideration given to the use of HRIA to inform government decision-making processes. One of the earliest proposals was expounded by Larry Gostin and Jonathan Mann, who envisaged the use of HRIA in the formulation and assessment of public health policies (Gostin and Mann 1994). Their proposed tool was designed to provide policy makers with a systematic approach to exploring the human rights dimensions of such policies, and to assist them in balancing the public health benefits of a policy against its human rights burdens on individuals. In doing so, the tool recognised that human rights and public health may have competing priorities, and required assessors to explore how those priorities could be counterpoised (Watchirs 2002, 723).

More recent HRIA activity has focused on the application of HRIA as a means of mainstreaming human rights in policies or programs with international application. For example, the Norwegian Agency for Development Corporation (NORAD) has developed a handbook aimed at integrating human rights into development programs (NORAD 2001), while the Netherlands Humanist Committee on Human Rights (HOM) has similarly proposed the application of HRIA to policy measures of the European Union with an external effect (Radstaake and Bronkhurst 2002). In an early case study undertaken by HOM, the criteria used to assess the right to health, such as mortality rates and access to health-care facilities, suggest that within the overall HRIA process health is given a narrower meaning, with the broader determinants of health left to be considered in the context of other rights (Radstaake and de Vries 2004).

HOM has also developed a 'Health Rights of Women Assessment Instrument' (HeRWAI) as an advocacy tool for non-government organisations seeking to influence government policies that affect women's health (Bakker 2006). The impact of a policy is assessed by considering a set of questions, which are accompanied by a checklist of qualitative indicators. These questions and indicators are derived from a right-to-health framework which recognises that the right to health requires the availability, accessibility, acceptability and quality of health care and other determinants of health; people have the right to participate in decisions that affect their health; and violence against women is a violation of women's right to health.

In addition to these initiatives, the Commission of the European Communities

(CEC) has outlined a methodology for ensuring that legislative proposals are scrutinised for compatibility with the Charter of Fundamental Rights of the European Union (CEC 2005a). The CEC's methodology integrates the assessment of human rights impacts into its existing impact assessment framework by including a series of additional questions into the CEC's impact checklist. That checklist is divided into economic, environmental and social impacts, with questions directed towards the assessment of fundamental rights being incorporated within those categories, although such questions are not explicitly framed in terms of human rights (CEC 2005a, paras 18–19; CEC 2005b).

HRIA AND THE RIGHT TO HEALTH

A clear indication to emerge from a brief review of existing HRIA methodologies is that the consideration expressly given to the right to health within HRIA is relatively limited where the HRIA process is intended to assess the full spectrum of rights enshrined in international human rights law. In these circumstances, despite the interconnectedness and indivisibility of human rights, as a practical matter, HRIA is forced to consider individual human rights in a relatively piecemeal fashion. That is, the most common approach is to identify a given right and attribute to it a series of questions that act as indicators as to the likely impact of the relevant intervention on that right. In ascribing those indicators, to avoid duplication within the HRIA methodology, the questions for each right will generally have a relatively specific focus. Accordingly, in relation to the right to health, questions tend to focus on health in a more biomedical sense. As a consequence, the assessment procedure may not identify that the right to health is likely to be impacted, even though impacts on a number of rights which are themselves determinants of health are predicted.

Of course, given that HRIA needs to be undertaken in the real world, HRIA cannot be all things to all rights, and it is likely that HRIA will tend to focus on certain human rights depending on the circumstances in which it is being applied (Hunt and MacNaughton 2006, 30). The HeRWAI developed by HOM demonstrates how different the assessment procedure looks where the focus of HRIA is specifically trained on health. However, this leads us back to HIA. HIA has developed increasingly well-established methodologies for examining health impacts; it is not distracted by the need to conceptualise impacts in terms of a range of different rights; and there are a number of clear synergies between HRIA and HIA. Indeed, in many ways, HIA is already implicitly operating in relation to a human rights discourse (O'Keefe and Scott-Samuel 2002, 737). These characteristics of HIA might therefore suggest that it is just as able as, and in many circumstances better able than, HRIA to operationalise the right to health.

THE SYNERGIES BETWEEN HIA AND HRIA

There are four features of HIA and HRIA that usefully elucidate the synergies between these two forms of impact assessment. First, both HIA and HRIA are generally democratic processes that emphasise the importance of participation. Engagement with relevant stakeholders as part of the assessment process is seen as both an empowering experience for affected communities and a means of gathering evidence about the likely impacts on the community (IBLF/IFC 2007, 6; Rights and Democracy 2007, 18; Halifax Initiative Coalition 2004, 19). In relation to HRIA, in particular, participation is an enabling mechanism, which allows communities to actively assert their human rights (Rights and Democracy 2007, 18). At other levels, it is a key aspect of both HIA and HRIA that people are able to participate in the preparation, implementation and evaluation of the relevant program or policy. Such emphasis on participation means that in both HIA and HRIA, the assessment process is as important as its outcomes.

Second, HIA and HRIA are equally concerned to identify the differential impacts of a proposed intervention. HRIA endeavours to do this through its consideration of the right to non-discrimination. It asks assessors to consider whether an intervention is likely to have a discriminatory effect on a group within a population, either at a general level or in relation to the exercise of specific rights by that group. HIA asks assessors to consider the same issues when it speaks to them in the analogous language of health equity, and seeks to ensure both that existing inequalities are not deepened and that new inequalities are not created by a particular intervention (Braveman and Gruskin 2004).

Third, there is a concurrence between HIA and HRIA in terms of their ability to assess how a policy or program is likely to impact on the broader determinants of health. That is, given the interconnections between health and human rights, when HIA sets out to assess likely impacts on the determinants of health, it is inevitably giving consideration to a similar set of questions as HRIA when it assesses the impact of an intervention on a bundle of identified human rights. Conversely, even though HRIA tends to focus its assessment on a biomedical model of health, it nevertheless implicitly addresses each of the determinants of health by reason of its consideration of those additional rights that are necessary to the full enjoyment of the right to health. Indeed, in many ways, the practice in HIA of categorising and assessing the determinants of health in order to facilitate a systematic method of impact assessment is akin to the methodologies of HRIA, which segregate individual human rights and consider the likely impact on each of those rights.

Finally, both HIA and HRIA advocate for a multidisciplinary approach to impact assessment. While HRIA, in practice, has not developed its methodologies to the same stage as HIA, it is nevertheless clear that HRIA is seeking to assess impacts on rights that span a spectrum of sectors. To do this most effectively, it is necessary to involve practitioners from those other sectors in the assessment process. Similarly, HIA, in its endeavour to assess the impact of a policy or program on the determinants of health, seeks to engage with a broad audience both inside and outside public health. In adopting this intersectoral approach, both HRIA and HIA are concerned not only to call on the technical assistance of experts in a range of disciplines but, even more importantly, also to enhance recognition among decision makers across sectors of the human rights or health implications of their decisions.

These synergies demonstrate that there is considerable affinity between the core values and principles of HIA and HRIA. Yet, it is also clear that, despite this affinity, the focus of HIA remains embedded in the public health space rather than in the human rights paradigm. This, therefore, raises for consideration the question of whether a focus on the right to health rather than health itself offers anything over and above what HIA already provides.

WHY AN IMPACT ASSESSMENT FOR THE RIGHT TO HEALTH?

Accountability

International human rights law is a formal body of law which imposes legal obligations on states. Accordingly, to speak of the right to health is to speak of a legal norm which is embedded in a framework that imposes clear and enforceable duties on states as duty-bearers. A failure to comply with those duties represents a violation of a state's legal obligation and gives rise to enforceable claims by rights-holders.

Health, as understood from the public health perspective, is not invested with the same legal authority. Public health is quintessentially a social movement, and HIA is therefore a methodology that is founded on notions of social democracy (Mann 1997). This is reflected in the language of public health practitioners who describe HIA as deriving from 'a belief that governments are benevolent in purpose and have the capacity to play an active role in developing a society based on principles of social justice' (Mahoney and Durham 2002, 18). Within this paradigm, the failure of a government to act in the interests of good public health may give rise to moral culpability, but does not give rise to any form of legal accountability (Scott-Samuel and O'Keefe 2007, 213).

A method of impact assessment that focuses on the right to health therefore offers a legal framework of accountability that is not available through HIA. Where an assessment is made that a proposed intervention is likely to result in a violation of a government's legal obligations, government decision makers are legally bound to take action in response to that assessment. This represents a significant advantage over HIA, which is ultimately reliant on the largesse of the decision maker to respond to a negative assessment in an appropriate way. In this regard, the accountability framework provided by a right-to-health impact assessment also has the potential to equip HIA with at least one mechanism for attempting to overcome the difficulties that it has experienced to date with respect to successfully influencing the decision-making process (Hunt and MacNaughton 2006, 13).

International Legal Standards

The legal nature of human rights obligations also means that an impact assessment for the right to health emphasises standards that are established by international law, and focuses on measuring the gap between those standards and the experience created by an intervention (Rights and Democracy 2007, 16). This may be contrasted to HIA, which lacks a clear conceptual framework for identifying the conditions required for public health, and so tends to use an existing situation as a baseline from which all else is measured. Further, even once an assessment has been made that an intervention is likely to have a health impact, there may be a lack of clarity in relation to the nature and extent of any changes that are required in response to that assessment (Mann 1997). For example, an HIA conducted on proposed changes to Slovenia's agricultural and food policies identified a number of key determinants of health that were likely to be affected by the changes. One of the predicted effects was increased rural unemployment and a consequent increase in ill-health in a region that already had high rates of alcohol-related deaths and suicides. To address these anticipated problems, the HIA recommended that steps be taken to maintain small farms, so as to avoid farm intensification and greater unemployment (Lock and Gabrijelcic-Blenkus 2004; Lock et al. 2003). While this prediction and recommendation are clearly useful, it essentially begins with the premise that the existing situation was bad, and ends by concluding that steps need to be taken to ensure things do not get any worse as a result of the proposed policy.

A right-to-health impact assessment has the potential to begin and end in a different position. It begins by considering the pre-existing conditions in light of the international legal standards by which the state is bound, and almost certainly reaches the conclusion that violations of the state's core obligations, such as with respect to non-discrimination, are already occurring. From that starting point, a right-to-health impact assessment may then predict the same impacts as HIA, but its end point differs. It will recommend not only that steps be taken to avoid a deterioration of pre-existing conditions, but also that pro-active and concrete steps be taken to improve upon the conditions of rural communities, with a view to moving towards the full realisation of their right to health.

This example emphasises a further aspect of a method of impact assessment that sees health as a human right—namely, its recognition that governments have positive obligations with respect to the right to health. Of course, HIA also has the goal of achieving healthy public policy, which inherently requires governments to take positive steps towards the creation of optimal conditions for people's wellbeing. However, entrenched as it is in more traditional forms of impact assessment, HIA has a tendency to nevertheless focus on the negative or unintended impacts of a particular intervention, with a view to ultimately minimising or mitigating those impacts. A right-to-health impact assessment therefore advocates an expansion of the assessment process to a consideration of whether a government has taken, or needs to take, positive action in order to comply with its legal obligations with respect to the right to health (Evans 2005, 692).

Consensus

Given its emphasis on an intersectoral approach to health, it is an important element of HIA that it seeks to assimilate a wide variety of perspectives from different disciplines. This is a difficult task under any circumstances, and HIA suffers particularly from its inability to speak to different disciplines in a consensual language (Mann 1997). So long as HIA speaks of health, a term that lacks a degree of conceptual clarity even within the health sector, it will always be at risk of being misunderstood by those outside the health sector. Further, health is likely to be seen as something that competes with, and is to be traded off against, the foci of other sectors, such as employment, housing or transport (Lee et al. 2007).

A right-to-health impact assessment offers a potential solution to this problem, by providing a consensual language that is capable of engaging across sectors (Gostin et al. 2003). Predicated as it is on an internationally sanctioned legal framework, a right-to-health approach to impact assessment compels every sector to consider whether its policies or programs are likely to impact on that right. Further, in speaking the language of law and human rights, a right-to-health impact assessment is able to engage with powerful and political vested interests to mainstream health concerns, and give them the same priority as matters such as economic prosperity and national security. It also provides all sectors with a clear statement that the right to health is interconnected with other human rights and extends to the enabling conditions required for a complete state of wellbeing. In this way, a right-to-health impact assessment not only advocates for an intersectoral approach, but goes a step further by providing a framework that facilitates a coherent and consistent application of the right to health across sectors.

The Determinants of the Determinants of Health

There is no question that HIA is concerned to explore the impact of an intervention on the broader determinants of health. However, the ability of HIA to explore the determinants of health is nevertheless constrained by its public health origins, which have historically been concerned with disease prevention and the promotion of physical health at a community level (Gostin 2001). While public health has evolved to embrace broader notions of social wellbeing, public health practitioners have recognised the problem with adopting an overly expansive view of public health, such that its scope becomes limitless. The reach of public health is therefore constrained by both its traditional role and its need to contain itself so as to maintain a meaningful function and agenda (Gostin 2001). In addition, the primary research and analytical tool of public health is epidemiology, in which researchers seek to understand the causal relationships between risk factors and public health (Freedman 1999). This is very much a scientific inquiry, which is limited by the need to be able to analyse and understand the pathways that connect health and its underlying determinants.

Against this background, if we envisage the determinants of health as the layers of influence depicted in Figure 14.1, then it becomes apparent that HIA is inherently limited in its ability to reach all of those layers. Certainly, it is able to extend to a consideration of individual lifestyle factors, social and community networks, and living and working conditions. However, despite its rhetoric, it is less clear that it is truly able to extend as far as a robust assessment of the general socioeconomic, cultural and environmental conditions that are the outermost layer of the spheres of influence, or the determinants of the determinants of health. These layers would seem to be beyond the causal reach of HIA.

Modern human rights, on the other hand, are fundamentally concerned with articulating the societal conditions for wellbeing (Mann 1996–97), with an object of the human rights discourse being to define the individual rights that are necessary for the achievement of those conditions. It follows that by reason of its grounding in the human rights framework, a right-to-health impact assessment promises a methodology that is capable of considering the impact of an intervention on the so-called determinants of the determinants of health. Indeed, it is the examination of those outer spheres of influence that, on one view, ought to be the primary concern of a model of impact assessment that is grounded in the human rights paradigm. This represents an opportunity to radically transform HIA, which presently trains its focus on health, and then moves outwards through the spheres of influence to explore the full impact of an intervention. A right-to-health impact assessment could begin its inquiry by considering the state of general socioeconomic, cultural and environmental conditions and then narrow its focus until it understands how those conditions impact on the enjoyment of the right to health.

Individual Rights and Public Health

From the above discussion it is apparent that, theoretically, a right-to-health impact assessment promises to provide a number of normative and conceptual advantages over HIA. However, the above discussion is predicated on an assumption that a right-to-health impact assessment conceptualises the right to health in the same broad terms advocated by the modern health and human rights movement. It is essential to recognise that an expansive vision of the right to health is not explicitly reflected in the language of international human rights instruments, which express the right to health as a positivist individual right that may be asserted by individuals against state actors. Further, despite endeavours to reconceptualise the right to health in broad terms, at an operational level the right to health has, to date, most often focused on individual access to health services (Meier 2006).

This is very much reflected in many of the existing HRIA methodologies in which the consideration of the right to health has generally been confined to a clinical and individualistic model of health and an assessment of access to, and availability of, health-care services. While it is possible to understand this approach as being the result of HRIA's methodological need to compartmentalise its assessment of a bundle of interconnected rights, it nevertheless demonstrates the tendency of human rights discourse to discuss the right to health in narrow terms. By comparison, public health and, as a consequence, HIA have evolved to embrace an expansive conception of health and a clear understanding of its location within personal, social, cultural and environmental structures.

If a right-to-health impact assessment is intended as a tool for operationalising the right to health, it is essential that the right be understood in a broader sense—that is, it must not be limited to the atomised version that comes from a narrow, strictly textual interpretation of the right to health as enshrined in international human rights instruments. General Comment 14 of the CESCR goes a long way towards providing an authoritative exposition of a new conceptual framework for the right to health, as do the efforts of the Special Rapporteur on Health (Meier 2006; Gostin and Gable 2004, 109; Hunt 2003a). This framework, although not explicitly, moves the right to health away from its individualistic origins towards a social or public health interpretation. In this evolutionary, or perhaps revolutionary, process, properly applied, a right-to-health impact assessment in fact offers a mechanism for operationalising the synergies between public health and the right to health, by providing what might be described as a public health approach to the right to health. To the extent that this is seen as advancing a collectivised form of the right to health, then,

notwithstanding the controversy that surrounds the notion of collective rights, it is submitted that this approach is necessary if the full spectrum of right-to-health concerns within society are to be addressed (Meier 2006, 748–52).

In adopting this approach, a right-to-health impact assessment can, and should, draw on the practical experiences of HIA, which has its foundations in the public health paradigm. HIA has already been through the experience of attempting to put into practice methodologies that seek to operationalise a broad conception of health and are underpinned by core values of equity and democracy. Accordingly, while it is possible to anticipate the advantages that a right-to-health impact assessment ultimately offers over HIA, a right-to-health impact assessment should nevertheless draw on the lessons learned by HIA as it seeks to embed a broad understanding of the right to health in decision-making processes (Krieger et al. 2003).

DEVELOPING A RIGHT-TO-HEALTH IMPACT ASSESSMENT

The idea of developing a form of impact assessment that is intended to focus on the right to health has begun to be explored by a small number of practitioners (Bakker 2006; People's Health Movement 2006; Center for Economic and Social Rights—Latin Program 1999; Hilber 2007; Nhelko 2007). Paul Hunt and Gillian Mac-Naughton have also proposed an approach to HRIA using the right to health as a case study (Hunt and MacNaughton 2006). Their rights-based approach to impact assessment requires that the methodology be explicitly grounded in a human rights normative framework, and be based on the fundamental principles of progressive realisation; equality and non-discrimination; participation; provision of information to stakeholders; accountability; and the interdependence of rights (Hunt and MacNaughton 2006, 32).

In the case study of a right to health, the normative framework for an impact assessment is drawn from General Comment 14, while the fundamental principles identified by Hunt and MacNaughton are consistent with approaches proposed in existing HRIA methodologies. There therefore appears to be an emerging consensus as to the principles that ought to underpin both HRIA and a right-to-health impact assessment. However, a number of difficult questions remain unresolved. These include whether integration of a right-to-health impact assessment into other forms of impact assessment is desirable and necessary for the mainstreaming of the right to health; how and whether existing methodological variations should be resolved; what type of evidence a right-to-health impact assessment should rely upon; and how it should deal with indicators.

Integration and Mainstreaming the Right to Health

With the impact assessment space becoming ever more crowded, a key consideration for a right-to-health impact assessment is whether it is realistic to expect policy makers to undertake yet another form of impact assessment. Hunt and MacNaughton have suggested that such an expectation is not realistic, and have therefore proposed that any right-to-health impact assessment, along with HIA, be integrated into existing assessment processes (Hunt and MacNaughton 2006, 31). This is proposed both on the basis that policy makers are more likely to integrate right-to-health considerations into an impact assessment that they are already required to undertake, and because such an approach is consistent with the desire to mainstream human rights into all government processes.

However, attempts to integrate health into other forms of impact assessment do not bode well for the integration of a right-to-health impact assessment. While advocates of integration have claimed that impact assessment methodologies such as environmental impact assessment are sufficiently flexible to tackle health concerns, experience suggests there is a considerable risk this theoretical flexibility will not translate into practice. Indeed, practical experience clearly demonstrates the difficulties associated with effectively integrating health concerns into a broader impact assessment, where the agencies controlling the assessment process have no direct stake in the health of a population, and their interests in fact lie elsewhere (Lock 2006; Birley 2003; Bond et al. 2001).

The approach taken in the EU with respect to the development of an integrated impact assessment also raises concerns as to the efficacy of integrating human rights into an all-encompassing impact assessment process. Where decision makers, who do not speak a language of human rights in the first place, are being asked to consider a number of different impacts and then balance and trade those off against each other, it is difficult to see how that process is likely to instil a genuine commitment to human rights. Far from mainstreaming human rights, the assessment process seems to be at real risk of becoming an administrative compliance check, undertaken by people with little or no understanding of human rights (Toner 2006, 319; de Schutter 2005, 37).

So what is the future of a right-to-health impact assessment, if a standalone model is likely to be seen by decision makers as just another procedural headache, while integration risks diluting right-to-health concerns beyond any substantive meaning? One answer is that, given the synergies between HIA and HRIA, there may be a possibility of effectively integrating a right-to-health impact assessment into HIA. Unlike attempts to integrate health or human rights within an integrated impact assessment model, integration of a right-to-health impact assessment within HIA would not require assessors to consider a number of different impact categories. Instead, because both health and human rights are concerned with the promotion and protection of human wellbeing, there is substantial concurrence between the considerations that are given to health and its underlying determinants within both HIA and a right-to-health impact assessment. Further, while a right-to-health impact assessment is based on a normative framework that derives from international human rights law, many of those underlying norms are consistent with the values that underpin HIA. Integrating a right-to-health impact assessment within HIA does not therefore require a radical value shift, but instead is more a change in emphasis and language that has the potential to be revolutionary.

The integration of a right-to-health impact assessment within HIA can also be seen as offering a better solution for mainstreaming the right to health than a consideration of the right to health within HRIA, which seeks to consider a bundle of human rights. Within the human rights matrix, an assessment of the right to health will generally need to be contained in order to give meaning to the assessment of other rights. Accordingly, regardless of how interconnected or indivisible those rights may be to the right to health, from a practical perspective, health is almost inevitably conceptualised and disserted in a narrower sense.

Of course, this is not to say that the proposal for the integration of a right-to-health impact assessment within HIA is a perfect solution. Even before the right to health is plunged headlong into HIA, HIA still has much work to do in order to institutional-ise itself in decision-making circles. There is also a growing trend towards integrated impact assessment methodologies, which means the present proposal runs counter to that trend (Birley 2003). Nevertheless, if the object of a right-to-health impact assessment is to mainstream the right to health in decision-making processes, then subjugating it within an all-encompassing integrated impact assessment seems unlikely to be a solution. On the other hand, embedding an impact assessment of the right to health within HIA offers the right to health the opportunity to take advantage of the work already done by HIA practitioners, both methodologically and with respect to the mainstreaming of health concerns. In this regard, HIA may be capable of incorporating right-to-health impact assessment in a way that recognises its connection with the suite of rights enshrined in international human rights law and, at the same time, sees those rights as essential preconditions to the enjoyment of the right to health. In doing so, HIA offers a practical impact assessment methodology that locates the right to health within the human rights matrix, without seeing it being subsumed by it. At the same time, this approach also presents the possibility of providing HIA with some solutions to the challenges that it is presently facing, so that it can ensure its long-term effectiveness in promoting healthy public policy.

Different Methodologies

The methodological variation that presently exists between HRIA tools raises the further question of whether it is desirable to strive towards an agreed form of right-to-health impact assessment. The lessons of HIA suggest that, in the practical world, it will be essential for right-to-health impact assessment to establish some consistency so that it provides an easy-to-use and transparent screening tool (Cole et al.

2005; Douglas et al. 2001; Mindell 2001). However, methodological variation also enures right-to-health impact assessment with a degree of flexibility that enables it to adapt to different settings and uses.

For example, where impact assessment is to be undertaken by governments, its methods will need to adapt to the political and administrative reality of the decision-making environment. In particular, a key requisite will be its ability to provide decision makers with a way of navigating the right to health, such that it is properly balanced and prioritised among competing objectives. On the other hand, where the right-to-health impact assessment is intended for use by non-government organisations, its priority will be to provide conclusions that are sufficiently justifiable and robust to be worthy advocacy tools. The methodologies may also need to be varied depending on the type and stage of the intervention under consideration. The challenge for right-to-health impact assessment will therefore be to develop itself to a point of methodological maturity and consistency that gives it traction with decision makers, while still maintaining enough flexibility to adapt to the variety of circumstances in which it may be applied.

In addition to this balancing act, the experience with HRIA anticipates that a right-to-health impact assessment will need to achieve a balance between developing comprehensive tools, which tend to be complex and time consuming, and limited tools, which may be more user-friendly but which may not achieve the desired right-to-health outcomes. The three levels at which HIA has been undertaken may provide a right-to-health impact assessment with some guidance in this respect. HIA has been undertaken as a desk-based audit, an intermediate HIA and a comprehensive HIA (Simpson et al. 2004, 164; Harris 2005, 108). Accordingly, consideration might be given to whether it is either feasible or desirable to develop right-to-health impact assessment methodologies that mirror some or all of these approaches. Certainly, to date, none of the right-to-health methodologies proposed have envisaged anything like a desk-based audit, and the dangers of reducing right-to-health impact assessment to an administrative function have already been discussed. Nevertheless, as right-to-health impact assessment seeks to find its place in the decision-making world, the experience of these various levels of HIA will be invaluable indicators of how the methodologies of a right-to-health impact assessment should best position themselves.

A further issue that arises from both a methodological and a conceptual perspective is the extent to which a right-to-health impact assessment differs from a rights-based approach to health impact assessment. In many ways, HOM's Health Rights of Women Assessment Instrument looks more like a rights-based approach to health impact assessment. This appears to be reflected in at least one experience with its practical application, which has identified HeRWAI as a useful tool for 'highlighting the links between women's rights violations and their poor health' (Nahar 2007)—that is, it begins with women's health, and then applies a rights-based lens in its analysis of the contributors to the state of women's health in a given population. This mirrors the rights-based approaches taken in the development space (Ruggie 2007, para 27; Human Rights Council of Australia 1995; Boesen and Martin 2007) and the approach proposed by the Halifax Initiative Coalition for its HRIA methodology (Halifax Initiative Coalition 2004, 17). A potential differentiator for a right-to-health impact assessment is that it begins with a series of inputs that are themselves human rights, and then considers how those inputs affect a population's enjoyment of the right to health. In this way, both the input and the outcome of the assessment process are driven by human rights norms and principles. The extent to which these conceptual differences correspond to methodological differences, and the relative merits of a rights-based approach to HIA versus a right-to-health impact assessment, will require further explication as this field of impact assessment develops and matures.

Evidence and Indicators

Closely related to the methodological issues surrounding a right-to-health impact assessment are questions as to the type of evidence that should be relied upon, and the use of indicators. A right-to-health impact assessment, like other forms of impact assessment, is intended as an evidence-based tool for informing the decision-making process. Accordingly, both its methods and the evidence it relies upon must be capable of withstanding close scrutiny and challenge. Within HIA circles, the same need for robust evidence has given rise to considerable debate as to whether quantitative or qualitative evidence ought to be used, with the use of quantitative evidence being preferred by some practitioners on the basis that it provides HIA with a robust scientific base and is likely to be more influential on decision makers (Cole et al. 2005; Mindell 2001). However, in the context of a right-to-health impact assessment, even more so than in HIA, it seems highly improbable that the multidimensional causal pathways through which an intervention may impact on a population's right to health can be properly explored and predicted through quantitative evidence.

At the same time, express recognition should be given to the inherent limitations associated with making predictions and fully elucidating causal connections. Regardless of the type of evidence used, a right-to-health impact assessment is unlikely to ever offer a mechanism by which scientifically accurate predictions can be made. Accordingly, a right-to-health impact assessment should not be concerned to identify an objective truth, but rather to fully examine the range of pathways through which a proposed intervention may influence the enjoyment of the right to health of a population The essential aspect of a right-to-health impact assessment should therefore be its systematic nature and its use of a range of appropriate quantitative and qualitative evidence to create a better understanding of, and better outcomes with respect to, the right to health in the decision-making process.

Further, notwithstanding the problems associated with undertaking accurate impact analysis in relation to the right to health, it is still possible to develop better analytical tools through the development and use of appropriate indicators (Andreassen and Sano 2007). Buoyed by the success of indicators in development analysis, human rights indicators, both qualitative and quantitative, have been proposed as valuable tools in the struggle for human rights, as they can be used to monitor human rights, build accountability and capture the attention of policy makers (Chapman 2000; Raworth 2001; UNDP 2000, chapter 5). In relation to economic, social and cultural rights, in particular, human rights indicators have been perceived as being especially helpful, as they offer the possibility of measuring the somewhat elusive concepts of progressive realisation and resource availability (Hunt 1998; Chapman 2000, 4).

With respect to health, the use of indicators is also well known. For example, a number of key indicators have long been used as part of the reporting requirements under ICESCR in relation to the right to the highest attainable standard of health (CESCR 1991). These indicators are derived from health indicators developed by the WHO, which makes extensive use of indicators in its endeavour to promote global public health (WHO 2007, 7). More recently, the Millennium Development Goals (MDGs) have also given much prominence to health indicators (Hunt 2003a, para 47).

In the context of a right-to-health impact assessment, it will be important to distinguish between health indicators and right-to-health indicators. In this regard, the Special Rapporteur for Health has identified that while the substance of health indicators and right-to-health indicators may often not differ, the essential distinguishing feature of a right-to-health indicator is that it is derived from and is designed to monitor the realisation of specific right-to-health norms (Hunt 2003b). Accordingly, as the concepts and methods of right-to-health impact assessment continue to be developed, greater clarity will be required in relation to the indicators that are being used, in terms of both what is being assessed and how it will be measured. It will be also be necessary to consider how indicators with respect to the underlying determinants of the right to health can be developed and incorporated into the assessment process. This will be a complex task, given the range of factors that are preconditions to human wellbeing and the concurrent need to contain the scope of the assessment process, so that it does not become too chaotic or onerous. It will also be necessary to ensure that indicators be selected according to their appropriateness for effective monitoring of the right to health in the specific circumstances (WHO 2004).

In developing right-to-health indicators, it is also important that the limitations of indicators be expressly recognised. Indicators alone will never give a complete picture of the multiple dimensions of a government's performance with respect to the right to health (Hunt 2006, para 30; de Beco 2007, 271). This is particularly the case where indicators are being used within an assessment process that is seeking to predict a likely impact (Anderson and Sano 2006, 21). Indicators are therefore one piece of the assessment puzzle, and must be used together with benchmarks, which provide an essential means of measuring performance over time, and other forms of quantitative and qualitative evidence. It is the combination of this evidence that is best able to inform both the predictions made by a right-to-health impact assessment and the decision makers that it is seeking to influence.

CONCLUSION

A right-to-health impact assessment has the potential to be a powerful tool in the struggle to ensure that the right to health is embedded within the decision-making processes that affect our wellbeing. While it is clear that, at a practical level, right-to-health impact assessment still has much work to do in resolving the methodological challenges that it presently faces, the challenges that lie ahead should not discourage efforts to further explore its potential and develop its methodologies. One of the most important lessons to be learnt from earlier forms of impact assessment is that it is possible to move beyond rhetoric and shift entrenched practices and attitudes through the use of these tools. A right-to-health impact assessment therefore holds the promise of taking the health and human rights message to the decision-making corridors, where it might ultimately be heard and heeded by the decision makers who are responsible for shaping the societies in which we live.

REFERENCES

International legal materials

Commission of the European Communities (CEC) (2005a) *Compliance with the Charter of Fundamental Rights in Commission Legislative Proposals*

—*Methodology for Systematic and Rigorous Monitoring*, COM (2005) 172 (27 April 2005)

Commission of the European Communities (CEC) (2005b) *Impact Assessment Guidelines*, SEC (2005) 791 (15 June 2005)

Committee on Economic, Social and Cultural Rights (CESCR) (2000) *The Right to the Highest Attainable Standard of Health, General Comment No 14*, UN Doc E/C/2000/4 (11 August 2000)

Committee on Economic, Social and Cultural Rights (CESCR) (1991) *Revised General Guidelines Regarding the Form and Contents of Reports to Be Submitted by States Parties Under Articles 16 and 17 of the International Covenant on Economic, Social and Cultural Rights*, UN Doc E/C.12/1991/1 (17 June 1991)

Hunt P (2007a) *Report of the Special Rapporteur on the Right of Everyone to the Highest Attainable Standard of Physical and Mental Health*, UN Doc A/HRC/4/28 (17 January 2007)

Hunt P (2007b) *Report of the Special Rapporteur on the Right of Everyone to the Highest Attainable Standard of Physical and Mental Health*, UN Doc A/62/214 (8 August 2007)

Hunt P (2006) *Report of the Special Rapporteur on the Right of Everyone to the Highest Attainable Standard of Physical and Mental Health*, UN Doc E/CN.4/2006/48 (3 March 2006)

Hunt P (2003a) *Preliminary Report of the Special Rapporteur on the Right of Everyone to Enjoyment of the Highest Attainable Standard of Physical and Mental Health*, UN Doc A/CN.4/2004/58 (13 February 2003)

Hunt P (2003b) *Report of the Special Rapporteur on the Right of Everyone to the Highest Attainable Standard of Physical and Mental Health*, UN Doc A/58/427 (10 October 2003)

Hunt P (1998) *State Obligations, Indicators, Benchmarks and the Right to Education*, UN Doc E/C.12/1998/11 (16 July 1998)

International Convention on the Elimination of All Forms of Racial Discrimination, 21 December 1965

International Covenant on Economic, Social and Cultural Rights, 16 December 1966

Ruggie J (2007) *Human Rights Impact Assessments—Resolving Key Methodological Concerns*, report of the United Nations Special Representative of the Secretary-General on the issue of human rights and transnational corporations and other business enterprises to the Human Rights Council, UN Doc A/HRC/4/74 (5 February 2007)

Books, articles and reports

Alston P and Quinn G (1987) 'The nature and scope of states parties' obligations under the International Covenant on Economic, Social and Cultural Rights' 9(2) *Human Rights Quarterly* p. 156

Anderson E A and Sano H (2006) *Human Rights Indicators at Program and Project Level—Guidelines for Defining Indicators, Monitoring and Evaluation* Danish Institute for Human Rights, Copenhagen

Andreassen B and Sano H (2007) 'What's the goal? What's the purpose? Observations on human rights impact assessment' 11 *International Journal of Human Rights* p. 275

Asher J (2004) *The Right to Health: A Resource Manual for NGOs* Commonwealth Medical Trust, London

Bakker S (2006) *Health Rights for Women Assessment Instrument* Humanist Committee on Human Rights, Utrecht

Banken R (2003) 'Health impact assessment—how to start the process and make it last' 81(6) *Bulletin of the World Health Organization* p. 389

Birley M (2003) 'Health impact assessment, integration and critical appraisal' 21(4) *Impact Assessment and Project Appraisal* p. 313

Birley M (2002) 'A review of trends in health-impact assessment and the nature of the evidence used' 13(1) *Environmental Management and Health* p. 21

Boesen J K and Martin T (2007) *Applying a Rights-Based Approach: An Inspirational Guide for Civil Society* Danish Institute for Human Rights, Copenhagen

Bond R, Curran J, Kirkpatrick C and Lee N (2001) 'Integrated impact assessment for sustainable development: a case study approach' 29 *World Development* p. 1011

Braveman P and Gruskin S (2004) 'Health equity and human rights: what's the connection?' in D Fox and A Scott-Samuel (eds) *Human Rights, Equity and Health* Nuffield Trust, London

Brodeur C (2007) 'Rights & democracy's initiative on human rights impact assessment' in Netherlands Humanist Committee on Human Rights (HOM) *Human Rights Impact Assessment in Practice—Conference Report* HOM, Utrecht

Center for Economic and Social Rights—Latin Program (1999) *From Needs to Rights: Recognizing the Right to Health in Ecuador* CESR, New York

Chapman A (2000) *Indicators and Standards for Monitoring Economic, Social and Cultural Rights*, paper given to the American Association for the Advancement of Science

Chapman A R (1998) 'Reconceptualising the right to health: a violations approach' 65 *Tennessee Law Review* p. 389

Cole B L, Shimkhada R, Fielding K E, Kominski G and Morgenstern H (2005) 'Methodologies for realizing the potential for health impact assessment' 28(4) *American Journal of Preventive Medicine* p. 382

Dahlgren G and Whitehead M (1991) *Policies and Strategies to Promote Social Equity in Health* Institute of Future Studies, Stockholm

Davenport C, Mathers J and Parry J (2006) 'Use of health impact assessment in incorporating health considerations in decision making' 60 *Journal of Epidemiology and Community Health* p. 196

de Beco G (2007) 'Measuring human rights: underlying approaches' 3 *European Human Rights Law Review* p. 266

de Schutter O (2005) 'Mainstreaming human rights in the European Union' in P Alston and O de Schutter *Monitoring Fundamental Rights in the EU: The Contribution of the Fundamental Rights Agency* Hart Publishing, Oxford

Douglas M, Conway L, Gorman D, Gavin S and Hanlon P (2001) 'Developing principles for health impact assessment' 23 *Journal of Public Health Medicine* p. 148

Elliot E, Williams G and Rolfe B (2004) 'The role of lay evidence in HIA' in J Kemm, J Parry and S Palmer (eds) *Health Impact Assessment* Oxford University Press, Oxford

Ersmaker E (2007) 'A guide to human rights impact assessment—IBLF/IFC/UNCG' in Netherlands Humanist Committee on Human Rights (HOM) *Human Rights Impact Assessment in Practice—Conference Report* HOM, Utrecht

European Centre for Health Policy (ECHP) (1999) *Health Impact Assessment—Main Concepts and Suggested Approach* WHO Regional Office for Europe, Brussels

Evans S (2005) 'Improving human rights analysis in the legislative and policy processes' 29 *Melbourne University Law Review* p. 665

Farmer P and Gastineau N (2002) 'Rethinking health and human rights: time for a paradigm shift' (2002) 30 *Journal of Law, Medicine & Ethics* p. 655

Freedman L (1999) 'Reflections on emerging frameworks of health and human rights' in J Mann, S Gruskin, M A Grodin and G J Annas *Health and Human Rights: A Reader* Routledge, London

Gillis D (1999) 'The "People Assessing Their Health" (PATH) Project: tools for community health impact assessment' 90 *Canadian Journal of Public Health* p. S53

Gostin L (2001) 'Public health, ethics and human rights: a tribute to the late Jonathan Mann' 29 *Journal of Law, Medicine & Ethics* p. 121

Gostin L and Gable L (2004) 'The human rights of persons with mental disabilities: a global perspective on the application of human rights principles to mental health' 63 *Maryland Law Review* p. 20

Gostin L, Hodge J G, Valentine N and Nygren-Krug H (2003) *The Domains of Health Responsiveness—A Human Rights Analysis*, WHO Health and Human Rights Working Paper Series No 2, World Health Organization, Geneva

Gostin L and Mann J (1994) 'Toward the development of a human rights impact assessment for the formulation and evaluation of public health policies' 1 *Health and Human Rights: An International Journal* p. 58

Gruskin S, Mills E J and Tarantola D (2007) 'History, principles, and practice of health and human rights' 370 *The Lancet* p. 449

Gruskin S and Tarantola D (2005) 'Health and human rights' in S Gruskin (ed) *Perspectives on Health and Human Rights*, Taylor & Francis Group, New York

Halifax Initiative Coalition (2004) *Risk, Responsibility and Human Rights: Taking a Rights-based Approach to Trade and Project Finance* NGO Working Group on EDC, A Working Group of the Halifax Initiative Coalition, Ottawa

Harris E (2005) 'Contemporary debates in health impact assessment: what? why? when?' 16 *NSW Public Health Bulletin* p. 107

Harris-Roxas B, Simpson S and Harris E (2004) *Equity-focused Health Impact Assessment—A Literature Review* Centre for Health Equity Training Research and Evaluation on Behalf of the Australasian Collaboration for Health Equity Impact Assessment, Sydney

Hart D (2004) 'Health impact assessment: where does the law come in?' 24 *Environmental Impact Assessment Review* p. 161

Hilber A M (2007) 'Maternal and neonatal health: using a human rights approach' in Netherlands Humanist Committee on Human Rights (HOM), *Human Rights Impact Assessment in Practice—Conference Report*, HOM, Utrecht

Human Rights Council of Australia Inc (1995) *The Rights Way to Development—A Human Rights Approach to Development Assistance: Policy and Practice* Human Rights Council of Australia, Maroubra

Hunt P and MacNaughton G (2006) *Impact Assessments, Poverty and Human Rights: A Case Study Using the Right to the Highest Attainable Standard of Health* UNESCO

Ingram A (2006) 'Health impact assessment of foreign and security policy: a critical analysis' in K Lee, A Ingram and K Lock (eds) *The Role of Health Impact Assessment* Nuffield Trust, London

International Business Leaders Forum and International Finance Corporation in Consultation with the United Nations Global Compact Office (IBLF/IFC) (2007) *Guide to Human Rights Impact Assessment and Management: Road-testing Draft* International Business Leaders Forum and International Finance Corporation

Jamar S (1994) 'The international human right to health' 22 *Southern University Law Review* p. 1, citing UN Document A/CONF.32/8

Jobin W (2003) 'Health and equity impacts of a large oil project in Africa' 81(6) *Bulletin of the World Health Organization* p. 461

Kemm J (2005) 'The future challenges of HIA' 25 *Environmental Impact Assessment Review* p. 799

Kemm J and Parry J (2004) 'The development of HIA' in J Kemm, J Parry and S Palmer (eds) *Health Impact Assessment* Oxford University Press, Oxford

Krieger N, Northridge M, Gruskin S, Quinn M, Kriebel D, Davey Smith G, Bassett M, Rehkopf D H and Miller C (2003) 'Assessing health impact assessment: multidisciplinary and international perspectives' 57 *Journal of Epidemiology and Community Health* p. 659

Leary V (1994) 'The right to health in international human rights law' 1 *Health and Human Rights* p. 24

Lee K, Ingram A, Lock K and McInnes C (2007) 'Bridging health and foreign policy: the role of health impact assessments' 85(3) *Bulletin of the World Health Organization* p. 207

Lock K (2006) 'Health impact assessment of foreign and security policy: background paper' in K Lee, A Ingram and K Lock (eds) *The Role of Health Impact Assessment* Nuffield Trust, London

Lock K and Gabrijelcic-Blenkus M (2004) 'HIA of agricultural and food policies' in J Kemm, J Parry and S Palmer (eds) *Health Impact Assessment* Oxford University Press, Oxford

Lock K, Gabrijelcic-Blenkus M, Martuzzi M, Otorepec P, Wallace P, Dora C, Robertson A and Zakotnic J M (2003) 'Health impact assessment of agriculture and food policies: lessons learnt from Slovenia' 81 *Bulletin of the World Health Organization* p. 391

Mahoney M and Durham G (2002) *Health Impact Assessment: A Tool for Policy Development in Australia* Report for the Commonwealth Department for Health and Ageing, Deakin University, Melbourne

Mahoney M and Potter J (2005) *Taking It to the Streets: Health Impact Assessment as a Health Promoting Activity to Reduce Inequalities within the Community* Deakin University, Melbourne

Mann J (1997) 'Medicine and public health, ethics and human rights' 27 *Hastings Center Report* p. 6

Mann J (1996–97) 'Human rights and AIDS: the future of the pandemic' 30 *John Marshall Law Review* p. 195

Mann J (1994) 'Health and human rights' (1994) 1 *Health and Human Rights: An International Journal* p. 6

Marks S P (2002) 'The evolving field of health and human rights: issues and methods' 30 *Journal of Law, Medicine & Ethics* p. 739

Meier B (2006) 'Employing health rights for global justice: the promise of public health in response to the insalubrious ramifications of globalization' 39 *Cornell International Law Journal* p. 711

Mercier J (2003) 'Health impact assessment in international development assistance: the World Bank experience' 81(6) *Bulletin of the World Health Organization* p. 461

Mindell J (2001) 'What do we need for robust, quantitative health impact assessment?' 23 *Journal of Public Health Medicine* p. 173

Mittelmark M B (2000) *Promoting Social Responsibility for Health: Health Impact Assessment and Healthy Public Policy,* paper presented at the Fifth Global Conference on Health Promotion, Mexico City (5–9 June 2000)

Nahar N (2007) 'Working with HeRWAI: interrogating the maternal health conditions in Bangladesh' in Netherlands Humanist Committee on Human Rights (HOM) *Human Rights Impact Assessment in Practice—Conference Report* HOM, Utrecht

Nhelko P A (2007) 'Positive women monitoring change' in Netherlands Humanist Committee on Human Rights (HOM) *Human Rights Impact Assessment in Practice—Conference Report* HOM, Utrecht

Norwegian Agency for Development Corporation (NORAD) (2001) *Handbook in Human Rights Assessment: State Obligations, Awareness & Empowerment* Norwegian Agency for Development Corporation, Oslo

O'Keefe E and Scott-Samuel A (2002) 'Human rights and wrongs: could health impact assessment help?' 30 *Journal of Law, Medicine & Ethics* p. 734

O'Mullane M (2007) *Utilisation of Health Impact Assessment (HIA) Evidence in Decision-making: An Exploratory Study of Policy Formulation in Ireland,* paper presented at the Political Studies Association of Ireland Postgraduate Conference, Trinity College, Dublin (27–28 April 2007)

Parry J and Stevens A (2001) 'Prospective health impact assessment: pitfalls, problems, and possible ways forward' 323 *British Medical Journal* p. 1177

People's Health Movement (2006) *The Assessment of the Right to Health and Health Care at the Country Level—A People's Health Movement Guide* People's Health Movement

Radstaake M and Bronkhurst D (2002) *Matching Practice with Principles—Human Rights Impact Assessment: EU Opportunities* Humanist Committee on Human Rights, Utrecht

Radstaake M and de Vries J (2004) *Reinvigorating Human Rights in the Barcelona Process: Using Human Rights Impact Assessment to Enhance Mainstreaming of Human Rights* Humanist Committee on Human Rights, Florence

Raworth K (2001) 'Measuring human rights' 15 *Ethics and International Affairs* p. 111

Rights and Democracy (2007) *Human Rights Impact Assessments for Foreign Investment Projects—*

Learning from Community Experiences in the Philippines, Tibet, the Democratic Republic of Congo, Argentina and Peru International Centre for Human Rights and Democratic Development, Montreal

Rights and Democracy (2005) *Human Rights Impact Assessment for International Investment—A Research Guide for Civil Society Groups* International Centre for Human Rights and Democratic Development, Montreal

Roth K (2004) 'Defending economic, social and cultural rights: practical issues faced by an international rights organization' 26 *Human Rights Quarterly* p. 63

Scott-Samuel A and O'Keefe E (2007) 'Health impact assessment, human rights and global public policy: a critical appraisal' 85(3) *Bulletin of the World Health Organization* p. 212

Simpson S, Harris E and Harris-Roxas B (2004) 'Health impact assessment: an introduction to the what, why and how' 15(2) *Health Promotion Journal of Australia* p. 162

Taylor L, Gowman N and Quigley R (2003) *Addressing Inequalities Through Health Impact Assessment* Health Development Agency, Yorkshire

Toebes B (2001) 'The right to health' in A Eide, C Krause and A Rosas (eds) *Economic, Social and Cultural Rights* Kluwer Law International, The Hague

Toebes B (1999) *The Right to Health as a Human Right in International Law* Intersentia, Antwerpen

Toner H (2006) 'Impact assessments and fundamental rights protection in EU law' 31 *European Law Review* p. 316

United Nations Development Program (UNDP) (2000) *Human Development Report 2000* UNDP, Geneva

Watchirs H (2002) 'Review of methodologies measuring human rights implementation' 30 *Journal of Law, Medicine & Ethics* p. 716

World Health Organization (2007) *World Health Statistics 2007* World Health Organization, Geneva

World Health Organization (2004) *Consultation on Indicators for the Right to Health*, meeting report

QUESTIONS

1. The author distinguishes two ways to integrate human rights and health in Impact Assessment: a Human Rights Impact Assessment, inclusive of the right to health (HRIA) and a Health Impact Assessment (HIA) focusing on the right to health. What are the respective attributes, potential usefulness and pitfalls of these two approaches and their commonalities? Could you, in a context of your choice, formulate two sets of Impact Assessment objectives for which each of the proposed approaches would, respectively, be best suited?

2. Assuming a Health Impact Assessment (HIA) focused on the right to health is envisaged to project the impacts of a proposed cervical cancer screening scheme, who should participate or be represented in the consensus building process and what respective contribution would they be expected to bring to it?

3. With reference to Figure 14.1, and specifically to the layer of social determinants of health labeled as "living and working conditions," which human rights are particularly relevant to the determinants of health figuring in this layer? What potential benefits and shortcomings would there be in explicitly linking these determinants to specific human rights?

FURTHER READING

1. Pock, Karen, Health Impact Assessment, *BMJ*, 2000; 320: 1395–1398. http://www.ncbi.nlm.nih.gov/pmc/articles/PMC1118057/

2. Gostin, Lawrence, & Mann, Jonathan M., Towards the Development of a Human Rights Impact Assessment for the Formulation and Evaluation of Public Health Policies. *Health and Human Rights*, 1994; 1: 58–80.

3. Hunt, Paul, & MacNaughton, Gillian, Impact Assessments, Poverty and Human Rights: A Case Study Using the Right to the Highest Attainable Standard of Health. *Health and Human Rights Working Paper Series* No 6, World Health Organization (2006) http://www.who.int/hhr/Series_6_Impact%20Assessments_Hunt_MacNaughton1.pdf

Pillars for Progress on the Right to Health: Harnessing the Potential of Human Rights through a Framework Convention on Global Health

Eric A. Friedman and Lawrence O. Gostin

INTRODUCTION

Each year, nearly 20 million people die—one in three global deaths—as a result of inequities between richer countries and the rest of the world and within low- and mid-income countries.[1] A child entering the world today in sub-Saharan Africa has a life expectancy more than a quarter century shorter than a child born in a wealthy country.[2] Women in the poorest quintile in Southern Asia are five times less likely to be attended by a skilled birth attendant than those in the wealthiest quintile.[3] The comparable disparity between wealthier and poorer women in West and Central Africa is three-and-a-half times.[4]

These persisting inequalities live alongside a far more promising reality for global health. The past several decades have demonstrated that great progress is possible. Child mortality has fallen from 16 million in 1970 to 7.6 million in 2010.[5] Maternal mortality has fallen from more than 500,000 maternal deaths every year to approximately 287,000 in 2010.[6] The number of people with HIV/AIDS in sub-Saharan Africa on antiretroviral medication increased from about 50,000 in 2000 to 5,064,000 by the end of 2010.[7] In Brazil, the inequalities between rich and poor women in their access to skilled birth attendants

that mark so much of the world have been close to eliminated, with near universal coverage of skilled birth attendants.[8]

How can the international community bring the first tragic reality in line with the second, far more hopeful, reality? We believe the right to the highest attainable standard of physical and mental health can be a force to enable even the world's poorest people to benefit from the immense health improvements that we know to be possible—interventions that are proven and affordable.[9] Increasingly, civil society and communities, courts and constitutional assemblies, are turning to the right to health as tool for developing a more just society. The six new national constitutions adopted in 2010 all codified the right to health.[10] Court decisions based on the right to health are burgeoning. Social movements are turning to the right to health in their advocacy. The UN General Assembly has recognized the right to clean drinking water and sanitation—two of the underlying determinants of health.[11] The days when a government could argue that the right to health was simply aspirational and unenforceable seem distant.

Yet none of this progress has fundamentally changed the gaping inequalities between rich and poor and other marginalized and disadvantaged populations.

How, then, is it possible to accelerate and consolidate the progress already made in improving health and closing health inequalities? Here we propose a four-part approach to accelerating progress towards fulfilling the right to health and reducing both global and domestic health inequities: 1) incorporating right-to-health obligations and principles into national laws and policies; 2) using creative strategies to increase the impact of national right-to-health litigation; 3) empowering communities to claim their right to health and building civil society's health and human rights advocacy capacity, and; 4) bringing the right to health to the center of global governance for health.

These facets will be mutually reinforcing. Empowered communities are more likely to take advantage of the potential for litigation to enforce national policies, while global governance structures could bolster support for public right-to-health education and establish policy standards. A global health agreement—a Framework Convention on Global Health (FCGH)—could help construct these pillars.[12] A civil society-led international coalition, the Joint Action and Learning Initiative on National and Global Responsibilities for Health (JALI), is steering a process to develop just such a treaty.[13] The FCGH would aim to dramatically reduce health inequities and establish a post-Millennium Development Goals (MDGs) global health agenda rooted in the right to health, placing such right-to-health principles as equality, accountability, and empowerment—as well as clearly defined responsibilities—at the center of this agenda in ways that the MDGs did not. The treaty would further elaborate on the right to health, from clarifying and codifying the interpretation of this right by the Committee on Economic, Social, and Cultural Rights to setting clearer standards for the progressive realization and maximum of available resource obligations in the International Covenant on Economic, Social, and Cultural Rights. The FCGH would also establish norms, targets, mechanisms, processes, and specific obligations that would give further life to central principles, such as accountability, participation, non-discrimination, and equality, while incorporating approaches to ensure proper prioritization of health, and of the right to health in other sectors such as trade, investment, and the environment.

In the spirit of the principles that comprise the right to health itself, JALI intends the FCGH to be developed through an inclusive and consultative process that amplifies the voices of the people who suffer most from national and global health inequities. To help inform this dialogue, we explore this four-pronged framework to better realize the right to health and offer ideas on how an FCGH could advance each pillar.

INCORPORATING THE RIGHT TO HEALTH INTO NATIONAL LAW AND POLICY

National legal and policy reform should begin at the top, incorporating the right to health into the constitution. A constitutional right to health does not guarantee that the government will respect the right or that health outcomes will improve. However, it does provide a foundation for action, whether catalyzing legal and policy reforms or unlocking the potential for litigation to enforce this right where other routes (e.g., constitutional right to life, judicially enforceable international treaties, and legislation) are unavailable or insufficient.

Incorporating the right to health does not require wholesale constitutional reform, but rather can be incorporated as a separate constitutional amendment. Civil society campaigns could valuably direct national attention to this and other socioeconomic rights. Right-to-health provisions in other constitutions and information on their implementation should be readily available to assist advocates in determining the specific amendment language that they seek, and to build public and political understanding of what such a right would entail and its possible benefits. This is not presently the case.[14]

The World Health Organization (WHO), civil society, and academics could establish an online, dynamic, regularly updated list of all right-to-health constitutional provisions, and analysis of how these provisions have been interpreted and implemented. This could help expand the scope of the possible, as advocates see how constitutions like Kenya's incorporate rights to such fundamental human needs as sufficient food, water, sanitation, and adequate housing; how Brazil's constitution demands universal and equal access to health care and establishes a formula for minimum government health spending on public health activities and services; and how Bolivia's constitution guarantees participation of the population in the decision-making processes of the public health system.[15]

An FCGH could aid in these efforts, requiring that states make the right to health justiciable. In countries that already have the right to health in their constitutions, or in which the FCGH (or other treaties with the right to health to which they are party) is self-executing, the right to health would already be justiciable. Elsewhere, states might meet this obligation by passing legislation to domesticate the FCGH—or by enacting a constitutional amendment. This requirement would be comparable to provisions in the International Covenant on Civil and Political Rights obliging parties to develop the possibility of a judicial remedy, and to enforce that remedy for violations of treaty rights.[16]

Laws, regulations, and policies should incorporate principles of equity, participation, and accountability. Comprehensive approaches to health equity will include non-discrimination legislation with effective sanctions, disaggregated health data and equity targets for poor and marginalized populations with accompanying strategies and time-bound benchmarks; and equitably distributed funding, health workers, and facilities. Legislation should require that all processes involving health-related decision making engage civil society and community members with standards to ensure that members of marginalized groups are able to fully participate.

Countries could commit through an FCGH to disaggregate health data by sex, rural or urban residence, and other dimensions, and through periodic surveys or other means assess health disparities that may be harming other populations. Health information systems could also be strengthened to capture how health funds are disbursed, both to monitor funding across regions (for example, whether indigenous areas are receiving disproportionately few funds) and to compare actual disbursements with committed funds, which could reveal corruption or other malfeasance. Perhaps within prescribed minimum benchmarks, equity-related targets could be among the targets in an FCGH, or those that the FCGH commits countries to set for themselves. The treaty could commit countries to a multi-faceted approach—addressing a patient bill of rights, pre- and in-service health worker training, structural measures (e.g., infection control and prevention), and effective complaint mechanisms—to reduce health sector stigma and discrimination. It could also establish guidelines for inclusive health decision making at sub-national, national, and international levels.

The FCGH could encourage wealthier countries to fund these measures. It might even establish a right-to-health capacity-building fund to which FCGH parties would contribute, possibly under an agreed formula to ensure that the fund contains at least minimum necessary resources for the full gamut of right to health related capacity-building activities under the FCGH. This could represent a distinct channel of funding within a larger global health funding mechanism.

Accountability requires that people have the opportunity to understand and question government policies and actions, get answers, challenge responses, and obtain redress for rights violations. Transparency is critical for accountability: India's Right to Information Act of 2005 has proven one of civil society's most important recent new tools to advance human rights.[17] Transparency will also help tackle corruption and protect rights, as will powerful, independent anti-corruption bodies.

Improving domestic accountability would be one of the chief goals of an FCGH. It could require countries to develop, implement, monitor and evaluate, and report back on a strategy to improve health accountability at the community level, such as through functioning village health committees, community scorecards, or community monitoring. The treaty could require and support capacity-building for maternal, newborn, and child mortality audits.[18] It could ensure and provide standards for implementing the right to information, akin to India's law, at the least for health and related sectors. The treaty could also prescribe a multitude of measures to improve transparency in health and related sectors, such as publishing (including on the Internet) all health plans and strategies, including in minority languages; discouraging corruption by requiring health ministry officials to publish their private assets online; in general, using open, transparent, competitive bidding processes for contracts of the ministry of health (and of related ministries, such as water); and informing communities of health funds that they are supposed to receive for local health services.

A right-to-health approach requires adequate funding. Laws could establish minimum funding levels for health, as in Brazil. Governments should use all policy levers to increase funding for health and its determinants. One analysis identified five such levers: 1) the proportion of government expenditure that is health-related; 2) overall government revenue; 3) official development assistance; 4) borrowing (deficit financing); and 5) monetary policy and financial regulation.[19] We would add a sixth: ensuring the efficient use of resources. The WHO conservatively estimates that fully 20–40% of the world's health "spending is consumed in ways that do little to improve people's health."[20] Changed incentive structures for health providers, strategic health sector purchasing, reduced fragmentation of health financing, and greater focus on health equity are just some of the ways to improve efficiency and meaningfully channel available resources to health.[21]

Countries should explore innovative approaches to raising revenue, such as taxing unhealthy foods and imposing special levies on large, profitable companies.[22] An FCGH might commit countries to implement a minimum number of such approaches, which the treaty could delineate. Beyond establishing domestic and international assistance funding benchmarks, the treaty could state circumstances under which countries are obliged to seek international assistance, owing to domestic resources that are inadequate to meeting their populations' right to health.

The rights approach to health also demands respect for the central, but often violated, public health principles of developing policies based on evidence and adopting an all-of-government approach in advancing the public's health.

Countries could develop institutions specifically charged with advocating for and coordinating government efforts to incorporate health and human rights into all policies. For instance, Uganda established a right-to-health desk in the health ministry, charged with building capacity among health professionals on the right to health, mainstreaming the right to health in the health sector, and advocating for incorporating right-to-health-based policies in other sectors.[23] Parliamentary committees responsible for health or human rights oversight should hold hearings on health and human rights. An FCGH could commit governments to establishing a right-to-health office to coordinate a health—and right to health—in all policies approach, as well as to educate the public on their right to health, promote health worker education on human rights, motivate support for the right to health within the government, and provide or ensure legal assistance for people when their right to health has been violated.[24] The treaty could require a comprehensive public health strategy encompassing social determinants of health, and its funding benchmarks could extend beyond health care to address underlying determinants of health.

Codifying the right to health and developing accountability mechanisms will transform sound health policy into enforceable legal requirements. Policies on particular health issues must also integrate human rights standards, such as funding clean needle exchange to reduce HIV transmission among drug users, domesticating the Convention on the Rights of People with Disabilities, and conducting right-to-health assessments.

Health and right-to-health assessments are seeing growing use across a great variety of contexts, from assessing health and health-related policies—such as a gender action plan in Pakistan and maternal health policy in Bangladesh—to projects that might at first glance seem to have little relation to health, such as replacing a bridge.[25] They can lead to critical recommendations. The maternal health policy assessment in Bangladesh, using the Health Rights of Women Impact Assessment Instrument, led to recommendations to strengthen sub-district health advisory committees and have health facilities accommodate social and religious practices. The health impact assessment of the bridge included recommendations to minimize risk of injury to pedestrians and bicyclists and to reduce air pollution and other negative health effects of construction.

An FCGH could set minimum standards on when countries should conduct right-to-health assessments of policies outside the health sector that could impact health, and require a right-to-health assessment of the health system itself as a foundation for revising a national health strategy, as well as to assess the impact of health policy changes on the right to health. The treaty could require that countries follow the policy that would most positively affect health or the right to health or, if they do not, to publicly justify the chosen approach and establish processes for affected populations or civil society organizations to challenge the decisions. Beyond right-to-health assessments, an FCGH might even direct countries to implement specific policies, such as permitting syringe exchange.

Beyond the FCGH itself, how to give life to this ambitious agenda? As a foundation, government officials need to understand the right to health. Civil society, academics, and international civil servants all have a role in educating government officials, including parliamentarians, on health and human rights. To enable health in all policies, this education should cover all officials, not only those with an explicit health mandate.

BUILDING RIGHT TO HEALTH CAPACITY

A right-to-health capacity-building fund in an FCGH could support these efforts. WHO could train and designate a human rights point person in each of its country offices. Such point people will need to closely collaborate with partners to ensure that their impact extends beyond the health ministry.

Policymakers will need to be convinced of the link between the right to health and improved health outcomes. For example, they need to be convinced that public participation in health decision making and community-based accountability structures indeed impacts health services and health outcomes. More research is needed, but evidence is emerging.[26]

Organizations supporting these types of mechanisms should carefully monitor and evaluate their impact, and explore possibilities for linking with researchers to develop rigorous evidence of success. Foundations should fund this research and the community monitoring efforts themselves. The health impacts of these empowering community mechanisms can be every bit as great as many of the most powerful biological medicines.

Whether established through an FCGH or an independent effort, a global database collecting information on these initiatives could both help countries and communities design the most effective mechanisms and convince policymakers of their importance. If linked to the treaty, it could encourage states to submit examples of such approaches to the FCGH Secretariat to feed into the database. This should increase uptake of these practices, strengthening accountability to the right to health and thus improving compliance with the FCGH. As part of an FCGH monitoring and evaluation process, states might even be required to report on measures that they are taking—including by making use of the best available evidence, including through the database—to adopt measures that will enhance accountability to the right to health from the community to national levels.

Leadership is essential. Right-to-health proponents can identify and nurture respected officials in government to chart the way. And they can advocate for government positions that are mandated to pursue the right to health, like Uganda's right-to-health desk, and for dynamic individuals to fill such positions.

Motivated policymakers will need the means to effectively implement the right to health. A growing set of health and human rights tools can support this capacity (see Table 15.1), and assure policymakers that FCGH mandates, such as right-to-health assessments, are feasible. The human rights community can create more advanced tools, such as further practical guidance to policymakers in specific health areas and right-to-health issues.

USING CREATIVE STRATEGIES TO ENHANCE NATIONAL RIGHT-TO-HEALTH LITIGATION

From increasing access to food and medicine to supporting tobacco prevention and control, constitutional provisions and court cases are contributing to healthier populations. AIDS advocates from South Africa and India to Latin America took to the courts to argue that human rights obligate government to provide AIDS medications—and they won.[37] In India, the right to food has resulted in cooked meals for millions of school children.[38] A regional human rights commission catalyzed the transformation of Paraguay's mental health system from institutionalization to community care.[39] In Colombia, where unsafe abortions are a leading cause of maternal death, the

Table 15.1 Health and human rights tools

Tool	Description	FCGH Implementation
Health, human rights, and impact assessments		
Human Rights Impact Assessment for the Formation and Evaluation of Public Health Policies (Lawrence O. Gostin and Jonathan M. Mann, 1994)[27]	Provides questions to guide public health policies that may burden human rights	These tools will help implement an FCGH mandate on health and human rights assessments, including to incorporate the right to health in health strategies and interventions, and to ensure that policies and projects beyond the health sector that impact health are consistent with the right to health. Some of these tools address specific areas that health strategies should address, including the health work force and reducing health sector discrimination. Many can be used proactively to design health strategies and polices and activities in other sectors that protect and promote the right to health. Civil society can use them to evaluate government implementation of the right to health. The first tool is slightly different, aimed at minimizing the possible burden of public health strategies on other human rights.
Health Rights of Women Assessment Instrument (Aim for Human Rights, 2010)[28]	Instrument to assess impact of policies on women's health rights and develop action plans to better realize women's health rights	
The Assessment of the Right to Health and Health Care at the Country Level: A People's Health Movement Guide (People's Health Movement, 2006)[29]	Guide to assess government implementation of right to health obligations and develop recommendations to address violations	
Health Impact Assessment (World Health Organization)[30]	Tools and guidance documents to determine how policies in different sectors will affect the public's health and the health of vulnerable groups	
Human Rights Impact Assessment Tools and Instruments (Human Rights Impact Resource Center)[31]	Various tools to assess the impact of policies on human rights, including rights to health, food, and housing	
Incorporating the Right to Health into Health Workforce Plans: Key Considerations (Health Workforce Advocacy Initiative, 2009)[32]	Questions to guide policymakers and civil society on incorporating the right to health into health workforce plans and policies	
Ensuring Equality: A Guide to Addressing and Eliminating Stigma and Discrimination in the Health Sector (Physicians for Human Rights, 2011)[33]	Guide to a comprehensive approach to reduce stigma and discrimination in the health sector	
Enforcing the right to health		
Global Health and Human Rights Database (O'Neill Institute for National and Global Health Law at Georgetown University Law Center, World Health Organization, and Lawyers Collective, launching summer 2012)[34]	Database of more than 350 health and human rights cases from around the world and international instruments and national constitutions from around the world that	An FCGH could encourage or require countries to contribute to this or a similar database, which could assist civil society and legal professionals in using litigation to enforce the right to health,

		and aid the judiciary in using the effective approaches to adjudicate health rights claims, including by prescribing innovative remedies.
Monitoring the right to health		
Health Systems and the Right to Health: An Assessment of 194 Countries (Gunilla Backman, Paul Hunt, Rajat Khosla et al., 2008)[35]	Preliminary set of 72 health and human rights indicators	These indicators, including as they may be further refined, could inform countries in developing right to health-based health strategies, as an FCGH would require; contribute to monitoring implementation of the right to health; and assist in monitoring FCGH compliance.
Maternal Death Audit as a Tool Reducing Maternal Mortality (World Bank, 2011)[36]	Provides guidance on and a sample form for maternal death audits	This tool could assist countries in implementing a possible FCGH mandate to conduct maternal death audits.

highest court demanded abortion legalization to protect women's health.[40] And an Indian court prohibited smoking in public places to safeguard the right to life.[41]

Yet even constitutional rights and successful litigation do not always lead to better health. Enforcing anrogrammes individual's right to health without regard to the cumulative impact of individual cases risks unintended negative effects on equity. Courts may feel institutionally constrained from issuing bold orders, and without a watchful eye upon them, states may fail to implement court directives.

Three steps could take right-to-health litigation to the next level. First, courts could adapt and build upon the most progressive approaches. Where constitutions do not expressly guarantee the underlying determinants of health, courts can read them into the right to health or life. Courts could be open to claims of immediate enforceability of minimum core obligations.

They should constantly interrogate the policy and equity implications of their judgments and of government policies. As South Africa's Constitutional Court insisted in the landmark right-to-housing case Government of the Republic of South Africa v. Grootboom, to meet the constitutional standard of reasonableness, the government's housing plan would have to "provide relief for people who have no access to land, no roof over their heads, and who are living in intolerable conditions or crisis situations."[42] Courts could institute a comparable test in all areas connected to health and its underlying determinants.

Pushing the boundaries of the right to health requires engaging some of the most doctrinally difficult challenges: What precisely are the minimum core obligations? What are the proper benchmarks for maximum available resources? What pace of progress does progressive realization require? With respect to the minimum core obligations requirement to ensure "essential primary care," courts could require a government strategy to achieve universal primary care.[43] Courts could assess whether the strategy is fully funded and adequately prioritizes reaching poor and other marginalized groups. Going a step further, courts could directly require countries to establish and define a benefit package to which everyone would be entitled.

Courts' role in establishing and passing judgment on minimum core obligations has been challenged from several directions. In Grootboom, the court doubted its own competence to establish such obligations. The South African Court has also sought a level of deference to the elected branches of government in evaluating the government's implementation of socioeconomic rights.[44] Meanwhile, experience elsewhere suggests that case-by-case challenges of often expensive health services not included in national health benefit packages risk diverting funds from other services that could better meet the needs of the whole population, including its poorer members. This is particularly true when limited access to courts means that the poorest members of the population are unlikely to be the litigants. However, new evidence from Brazil, challenging earlier findings, suggests that this case-to-case approach can be an important way for even very low-income individuals to secure needed medicines.[45]

Courts might take a lesson from the Constitutional Court of Colombia in combining the clarity, accountability, and equity of a defined set of minimum health services for all with the inclusive, participatory processes that ensure democratic legitimacy, competence, and equity. In 2008, the Colombian court required the government to unify two health insurance schemes and to achieve the government's stated goal of universal insurance coverage by 2010. The unification process had "to be participatory, transparent, and evidence-based, and to include relevant indicators and benchmarks."[46] Rather than determining the benefits of the unified scheme itself, the court ordered the relevant health authority "to immediately and on an annual basis comprehensively update the benefits included . . . through a process that included 'direct and effective participation of the medical community and the users of the health system,' in particular those who would be most affected by policy changes."[47] Such benefits would be immediately enforceable, as would other health services needed to address threats to a person's minimum level of subsistence that the person could not afford.[48] The court recognized resource limitations: the benefits "need not be infinite but can be circumscribed to cover the health needs and priorities determined by the competent authorities in light of the efficient use of scarce resources."[49] The benefits plan had to be "designed to protect the right to health according to the needs of the population," with limitations being "reasonable and proportionate."[50]

Universal health coverage could extend to underlying determinants of health. Courts could be deferential if these guaranteed minimums have been developed through an inclusive, participatory process, adhere to requirements of equity, are consistent with maximum resource availability requirements, are regularly reviewed and updated, and are well implemented.

Courts could demand specific, time-bound action, with experts and community members themselves developing the remedy, much as the Colombian court sought to put the nature of universal coverage in the democratic domain. The approach adopted by the Inter-American Court of Human Rights in Xákmok Kásek Indigenous Community could similarly serve as a model. The court held that the Paraguayan government had a duty to guarantee the right to life to community members who lacked basic services as they sought to reclaim traditional lands. The court required Paraguay to prepare a study, involving specialists and community perspectives, on obstacles to health care and other basic needs, including food, water, and sanitation. Paraguay was then obliged to adapt its services to the study's conclusions.[51] A participatory approach could be linked to substantive parameters encompassing areas including equity and resources to ensure a robust outcome.

Courts are most likely to adopt these approaches if judges and lawyers are well-versed in the right to health. Therefore, a second step to better realize the right to health through litigation is training for legal professionals on health and human rights, courts' approaches in other jurisdictions, and the real-world impact of their decisions (including on equity and implementation). A new health and human rights database opens up new possibilities for cross-border learning.[52] Judges and lawyers could be exposed to innovative applications of socioeconomic rights, such as the South Africa Constitutional Court finding that these rights required an independent anti-corruption body.[53]

The FCGH might require countries to periodically submit relevant cases to the treaty Secretariat to ensure that the database is comprehensive and current, maximizing its potential to aid litigants in protecting their rights and courts in adjudicating and offering the most effective remedies for violations. There is precedent for such a data-sharing requirement. The WHO Global Code of Practice on the International Recruitment of Health Personnel, for example, encourages countries to establish and maintain a database of laws and regulations relevant to health worker migration and recruitment, as well as their implementation. Countries are supposed to provide this information to WHO every three years.[54]

An FCGH could establish one or several lead agencies, such as the WHO or the UN Office of the High Commissioner for Human Rights (OHCHR), or another process (involving such partners as the International Commission of Jurists), to establish a plan for this training. If such direct support for legal capacity-building within the judicial system stands out among human rights treaties, it builds upon other legal capacity-building stipulations in international law. The other health framework convention, the Framework Convention on Tobacco Control, stands as an important precedent, with its support for technical assistance to develop "a strong legislative foundation" for tobacco control measures.[55] Further afield, with the centrality of law enforcement to the treaty—though looking towards prosecutions by the state, rather than potentially against the state—the Convention against Corruption requires that countries, "to the extent necessary, initiate, develop or improve specific training programs for its personnel responsible for preventing and combating corruption." This is much as an FCGH might require training personnel responsible for enforcing the right to health. The Convention against Corruption encourages international technical assistance for this capacity-building, including training through international institutions.[56] In the realm of human rights itself, a resolution of the Pan American Health Organization calls for educating legislative and judicial personnel on human rights standards.[57]

Third, lawyers and civil society organizations need to view court victories as only part of a continuum of change. Compliance is a pervasive problem. In Grootboom, seen as a landmark victory for socioeconomic rights, the seemingly victorious plaintiff, Irene Grootboom, died eight years after the judgment, "still homeless and penniless."[58] Advocates for victorious parties in right-to-health cases must follow through to see that policies—and lives—really change.

Change is most likely if advocates combine litigation with a broader strategy. For example, in 2011 Ugandan health and human rights advocates initiated a case against the government to force action to reduce maternal mortality, asserting violations of the rights to life and health, and the rights of women. Civil society organizations have coordinated the litigation with a comprehensive advocacy strategy including petitions, civil society and public mobilization, and media pressure. Since the Centre for Health, Human Rights and Development initiated the case, more than 35 civil society organizations in Uganda have come together to form a coalition advocating for maternal health.[59]

EMPOWERING CIVIL SOCIETY AND COMMUNITIES TO CLAIM THEIR RIGHT TO HEALTH

Pressure from civil society and the broader public can generate the political imperative to secure the right to health. Empowering communities to understand and claim their rights represents the third pillar of a health and human rights strategy. This pillar is constructed of public understanding, participation, accountability, and advocacy. It recognizes that more than a set of legal doctrines, human rights demand a fundamental redistribution of power from states to individuals, especially those who have traditionally held the least power.

Incorporating the right to health into laws, regulations, policies, and practices begins with establishing participatory and inclusive policy development processes that provide a privileged place for poor and marginalized communities. Public input and civil society organizations should inform health-related policies and identify areas where policy reform is required. Community involvement in implementing, that reforms are carried out effectively, respond to local priorities and

realities, and reach those in greatest need. Mechanisms range from the national (e.g., national health assemblies and multi-sector health committees) to the local (e.g., village health committees), and from open processes that engage many people (e.g., regulatory notice comments procedures) to those engaging selected community and civil society representatives (e.g., community health boards).

In addressing community level accountability and offering health decision-making guidelines, an FCGH should insist that countries incorporate ways to ensure meaningful participation of marginalized and vulnerable populations and to emphasize their needs. A central aspect of an FCGH would be to establish standards of universal health coverage, for both health care and the underlying determinants of health. Countries could be required to follow inclusive, participatory approaches to translating these global guidelines into specific national standards and policies, and not rely solely on a technocratic approach (e.g., by setting the standards simply by determining most cost-effective interventions that would comply with the global guidelines; such evidence should have a role, but not an exclusive one).

People will be best equipped to pursue the right to health if they understand their rights. Civil society and the media can educate the populace. Journalists will themselves often need to be educated on, and sensitized to, health and human rights. Government institutions have an educational role. The Uganda Human Rights Commission's health rights unit seeks to help "people realise what they are entitled to in the health units and empower them to demand . . . the services," and offers legal aid to people whose health rights are violated.[60] Health workers can be a powerful force for the right to health, respecting it in their own practices, educating patients, and advocating locally and nationally.

Their educational curricula should incorporate human rights, including the right to health. An FCGH could commit countries to incorporating human rights into training for all health workers and to establishing an agency—perhaps a governmental entity within the health ministry, or perhaps an empowered independent institution, such as a strong human rights commission—charged with facilitating implementing the right to health. This should encompass assisting people in claiming this right, including through education on the right to health, and ensuring that people can access legal recourse to remedy violations. Such a requirement would be similar to, if more specific than, the duty in the Convention on the Rights of People with Disabilities to "maintain, strengthen, designate or establish . . . a framework, including one or more independent mechanisms . . . to promote, protect and monitor implementation of the present Convention."[61]

Knowledge of the right to health alone, even combined with access to the legal system, is not enough. Civil society capacity-building is needed, including core and programmatic funding; fundraising, budgeting, management, and information technology skills; strategic planning; and training in advocacy strategies and tactics (e.g., budget monitoring and community scorecards). Capacity-building should be supplemented by capacity sharing, that is, facilitating connections among civil society organizations: developing health and human rights networks within countries and regions to share skills, experiences, and lessons, and to join forces in advocacy campaigns. The PAHO human rights resolution incorporates some of these capacity-building measures, namely human rights training for health workers and promoting dissemination of human rights information among civil society organizations.[62]

It is critical that an FCGH support often beleaguered civil society organizations that seek to advance health and other human rights, but find their time consumed by fundraising as much as change-making. This support could be part of the proffered right-to-health capacity-building fund, or a distinct mechanism, and should encompass less formally organized community groups and networks, whether geographically centered or sharing other common characteristics (e.g., disease status, gender, or disability). Such a fund could overcome the potential ineffectiveness of good intentions not backed by resources, such as the pledge in the Rio Political Declaration on Social Determinants of Health to "empower the role of communities and strengthen civil society contribution to policy-making and implementation by adopting measures to enable their effective participation for the public interest in decision-making."[63]

With increased funding and support should also come measures to augment the accountability of civil society organizations, particularly to the people on whose behalf they work. This accountability could come through their constituents' direct involvement and decision-making authority within the organizations, NGOs effectively and transparently evaluating their own activities, and regular channels of communication, input, and feedback. Meanwhile, when one or several civil society organizations represent broader civil society, those organizations need to accurately portray the positions and ideas of broader coalitions, report back on results, and gather feedback to contribute to a cycle of meaningful representation.

Health and human rights advocacy cannot be viewed apart from the broader human rights environment that will impact this advocacy, such as freedom of expression and assembly, the right to information, and the free operation of civil society organizations. Feeling their power and control over society threatened, a growing number of regimes have restricted NGOs' ability to register and raise money, especially from foreign sources, and have limited the activities of internationally supported NGOs, including human rights advocacy.[64]

The FCGH might require countries to review, rescind, and avoid future laws that could obstruct civil society right-to-health advocacy through the type of laws described above. An internationally financed civil society fund might help give some solace to—or more likely, remove a propaganda point from—governments that are skittish about the foreign influence of NGOs. It will provide funds that are clearly not linked to an agenda of any particular country—only to advancing the human rights and well-being of their people.

BRINGING THE RIGHT TO HEALTH TO THE CENTER OF GLOBAL GOVERNANCE FOR HEALTH

Much of this chapter is devoted to showing how an FCGH could help bring the right to health to the center of global governance for health. Here we expand on this concept to show how the international community could support effective health and human rights policies, progressive litigation, and empowered civil society and communities. These international efforts comprise the fourth pillar and build on ideas enunciated earlier, such as increasing funding for health and human rights organizations; providing technical support to build their capacity; and sharing lessons, facilitating international connections, and developing health and human rights tools and indicators that can be adapted locally.

Beyond this, countries must meet their own right-to-health obligations in the global arena. These include sustained, sufficient, and predictable development assistance, and protecting and advancing health and human rights in trade, investment, environment, and other spheres of international law.

An FCGH could codify and expand upon the foregoing responsibilities. It could establish an international financing framework that delineates funding obligations for each country, addressing both domestic and international responsibilities. It could establish new financing mechanisms, and unambiguously specify the priority to be given to health and human rights in other international legal regimes. An FCGH could go further by delineating what such priority would entail in these other areas, from affirmative requirements to address the health impact of climate change when developing adaptation measures, to protecting bilateral and regional trade agreements from provisions that could reduce access to medicine. It could require countries to assess the impact of macroeconomic policies on the right to health and avoid any that could undermine the right. The treaty could codify public health and human rights approaches to illicit drug use, which recognize addiction as a health condition requiring treatment and demand respect for the human rights of drug users. A treaty might also establish formal mechanisms of coordination among the WHO, the OHCHR, and key actors in other regimes, such as the World Trade Organization, World Bank, International Monetary Fund, International Labour Organization, UN Office on Drugs and Crime, and UN Environment Program. Civil society and communities, as well as governments, would need to be assured of formative roles in any such mechanism. The WHO and OHCHR, with their health and human rights mandates, would be well-placed to lead such an entity.

The WHO should strengthen its own human rights capacity in line with its constitutional mandate.[65] The WHO should assume this leadership role, mainstreaming human rights throughout its programming, increasing its own human rights capacity in terms of staffing, funding, and organizational knowledge, and elevating the priority it gives human rights. It should lead and help coordinate international support for local health and human rights activities and advocate for other international legal regimes to incorporate health and human rights concerns.

Academia and think tanks can make human rights law itself more effective. By analyzing the fast-growing body of right-to-health law, examining how the right is being implemented, and offering new ideas, they can contribute to greater clarity of health and human rights law and to its progressive development. And they can increase understanding on the real-life impact of this law, factors that facilitate and impede its impact, and mechanisms to improve enforcement.

AN FCGH AND THE FOUR PILLARS OF HEALTH AND HUMAN RIGHTS

These four pillars—incorporating the right to health into national laws, using creative strategies to increase the impact of national right to health litigation, empowering communities to claim their rights, and bringing the right to health to the center of global governance for health—are integrally intertwined. Social movements spur legal and policy reform. Legal and policy change creates new opportunities for litigation. Elevating human rights in and integrating it throughout global governance for health will facilitate national progress, even as national processes, priorities, and experiences should inform global action.

An FCGH could help to simultaneously erect all four pillars. A successful FCGH will need to incorporate strong compliance mechanisms. These would begin with regular, public country reports on how they are implementing the treaty. Whether by requiring an inclusive process in developing these state reports, explicitly considering parallel civil society reports in evaluating state compliance, or both, the treaty should ensure that evaluation of compliance is not based simply on states' say-so.

Reporting cannot be the end of compliance strategies, however. While countries have considerable self-interest in improving the health of their own and the world's population, the treaty should also include creative incentives for compliance and sanctions for non-compliance.[66] For example, certain forms of international funding might be available or ensured only for countries that are meeting their own funding obligations. Non-compliance might open up the possibility of suspension from the possibility of serving on the WHO Executive Board or UN Human Rights Council. Given the lives on the line, targeted sanctions of the sort usually reserved for traditional national security concerns, such as freezing assets and travel bans on individuals, could be options in severe cases. Any sanctions must themselves adhere to the highest human rights standards and not degrade the health and undermine the rights of the very people they are meant to help. Populations of countries whose governments are failing to meet their FCGH obligations should have a central role in determining what sanctions, if any, would be most appropriate and effective.

Critical to a successful FCGH will be a social movement that supports the treaty and the right to health more broadly. A powerful social movement, one that includes labor, environmental, and other broader concerns, can ensure that pressure for compliance comes from domestic as well as international sources. Indeed, a widely supported FCGH with clear standards could be a powerful tool for civil society advocacy in both the global South and North, even in countries that have not ratified the Convention themselves.

A comprehensive approach to advancing the right to health, backed by a global treaty, could prove a commanding counterweight to competing interests and political forces, advance effective policies and mechanisms for implementing the right to health, further clarify human rights law and attendant obligations, and enhance accountability and enforcement through community, national, and international actions.

Due regard to each pillar, drawing on and adding to innovative right-to-health approaches and capturing the synergies among the pillars, holds much promise for global health. With bold, systematic, and innovative actions, human rights stand to have a transformative impact in making global health better tomorrow than it is today.

We believe an FCGH could powerfully advance the right to health and close national and global health inequities. JALI envisions a treaty developed through a broadly inclusive "bottom-up" process. While hoping that our ideas contribute, we know that ultimately the most important input into an FCGH will come from the people whose health realities are worlds away from our own. The treaty must speak to the realities of slum dwellers who live near centers of power yet lack the most basic services, to farmers who find themselves and their children without proper nourishment, and to the orphans and widows, indigenous populations, sexual minorities, women, people with disabilities, and others who often suffer the ugliest discrimination and most extreme poverty. It is their voices that JALI most hopes to hear and incorporate in guiding a process to develop an FCGH.[67]

REFERENCES

1. J. Garay, "Global health (GH)=GH equity=GH Justice=Global social justice: The opportunities of joining EU and US forces together," Newsletter of the European Union of Excellence at the University of California, Berkeley (Winter 2012). The figure derives from the difference in death rates between high-income countries and other regions of the world.

2. United Nations Development Program, *Human development report 2011* (New York: UNDP, 2011), p. 130.

3. UNICEF, *State of the world's children 2009* (New York: UNICEF, 2008), p. 38.

4. UNICEF, *Progress for children: A report card on maternal mortality, number 7* (New York: UNICEF, 2008), p. 16.

5. J. K. Rajaratnam, J. R. Marcus, A. Flaxman et al., "Neonatal, postneonatal, childhood, and under-5 mortality for 187 countries, 1970–2010: A systematic analysis of progress towards Millennium Development Goal 4," *Lancet* 375/9730 (2010), pp. 1988–2004; UNICEF, World Health Organization, World Bank, and United Nations DESA/Population Division, *Levels and trends in child mortality, Report 2011, Estimates developed by the UN Inter-agency Group for Child Mortality Estimation* (New York: UNICEF, 2011), p. 1.

6. World Health Organization, UNICEF, UNFPA, and World Bank, *Trends in maternal mortality: 1990 to 2010* (Geneva: WHO, 2012), p. 19.

7. World Health Organization, UNAIDS, and UNICEF, *Global HIV/AIDS response: Epidemic update and health sector progress towards universal access, progress report 2011* (Geneva: WHO, 2011), p. 89.

8. Z. A. Bhutta, M. Chopra, H. Axelson et al., "Countdown to 2015 decade report (2000–10): Taking stock of maternal, newborn, and child survival," *Lancet* 375/9370 (2010), pp. 2032–2044.

9. We will use "right to health" as shorthand for "the right of everyone to the enjoyment of the highest attainable standard of physical and mental health." International Covenant on Economic, Social, and Cultural Rights (ICESCR), G.A. Res. 2200A (XXI), Art. 12. (1966).

10. These are the constitutions for Angola, Dominican Republic, Kenya, the Kyrgyz Republic, Madagascar, and Niger. Note that the international community did not recognize the government of Madagascar, which came to power in a 2009 coup d'état led by Andry Rajoelina; "Madagascar approves new constitution," *Voice of America* (November 22, 2010). Available at

http://www.voanews.com/english/news/afrca/Madagascar-Approves-New-Constitution-109912629.html; A. Iloniaina, "Madagascar's gov't hopes for recognition after poll," *Reuters Africa* (December 6, 2010). Four of the listed countries had previously recognized the right to health. This recognition is new for Kenya and the Dominican Republic, though the latter had previously addressed health in its constitution; E. D. Kinney and B. A. Clark, "Provisions for health and health care in the constitutions of the countries of the world," *Cornell International Law Journal* 37/2 (2004), pp. 285–355.

11. The Human Right to Water and Sanitation, G.A. Res. 64/292 (July 28, 2010).

12. L. O. Gostin, "Meeting basic survival needs of the world's least healthy people: Toward a framework convention on global health," *Georgetown Law Journal* 96/2 (2008), pp. 331–392.

13. L. O. Gostin, E. A. Friedman, G. Ooms et al., "The Joint Action and Learning Initiative: Towards a global agreement on national and global responsibilities for health," *PLoS Medicine* 8/5 (2011).

14. To the best of our knowledge, the most recent comprehensive listing of right to health and other health-related constitutional provisions dates back to 2004. See Kinney and Clark (note 10).

15. Constitution of Kenya (2010), Art. 43. Constitution of the Federative Republic of Brazil (1988), Arts. 196,198. Constitution of the Republic of Bolivia (2009), Art. 40.

16. International Covenant on Civil and Political Rights (ICCPR), G.A. Res. 2200A (XXI), Art. 3 (1966). An FCGH could, for at least one right, remedy the distinction among categories of rights with respect to their justiciability; the ICESCR does not contain a comparable provision on ensuring a judicial remedy for rights violations.

17. India Together, *Right to information in India*. Available at http://indiatogether.org/rti/.

18. South Africa Every Death Counts Writing Group, "Every death counts: Use of mortality audit data for decision making to save the lives of mothers, babies, and children in South Africa," *Lancet* 371/9620 (2008), pp. 1294–1304.

19. R. Balakrishnan, D. Elson, J. Heintz, and N. Lusiani, *Maximum available resources and human rights: Analytical report* (New Brunswick, NJ: Center for Women's Global Leadership, Rutgers, State University of New Jersey, 2010), p. 5.

20. World Health Organization, *The world health report—Health systems financing: The path to universal coverage* (Geneva: WHO, 2010), pp. 71–72 (2010).

21. Ibid., pp. 72–79.

22. Ibid., p. 29.

23. Information regarding the right-to-health desk in Uganda is from a July 28, 2009, interview between Physicians for Human Rights and Dr. Faustine Maiso, who was a Right to Health Officer with the Ugandan Ministry of Health and the World Health Organization.

24. In Uganda, a separate unit in the Human Rights Commission engages in several of these functions. C. Businge, "Health rights unit launched," *New Vision* (September 30, 2008).

25. R. Zahid, *Gender reform action plan—A breakthrough for Pakistani women? A policy research using Health Rights of Women Assessment Instrument* (HeRWAI) (Seattle, United States: University of Washington, 2007). Naripokkho, *HeRWAI Study of the Bangladesh national strategy for maternal health* (Dhaka, Bangladesh: Naripokkho, 2006). M. Bhat and E. Clapp, *The Sellwood Bridge: A health impact assessment* (Multnomah County, OR: Multnomah County Health Department, 2011).

26. In a study involving villages in Uganda, researchers found that community scorecards led to a 33% reduction in child mortality. M. Björkman and J. Svensson, "Power to the people: Evidence from a randomized field experiment on community-based monitoring in Uganda," *Quarterly Journal of Economics* 124/2 (2009), pp. 735–769. Citizen monitoring of health services has also had an impact; H. Potts, *Accountability and the right to the highest attainable standard of health* (Essex, United Kingdom: Human Rights Centre, University of Essex, 2008), pp. 35–36.

27. L. Gostin and J. M. Mann, "Human Rights Impact Assessment for the Formation and Evaluation of Public Health Policies," *Health and Human Rights: An International Journal* 1/1 (2004), pp. 58–80.

28. S. Bakker, H. Plagman, and M. Nederveen, *Health rights of women assessment instrument* (Utrecht, The Netherlands: Aim for Human Rights, 2010).

29. People's Health Movement, *The assessment of the right to health and health care at the country level: A people's health movement guide* (People's Health Movement, 2006) Human Rights Impact Resource Center, *Human Rights Impact Assessment (HRIA) tools and instruments*.

30. World Health Organization, Health Impact Assessment (HIA): HIA related sites. Available at http://www.who.int/hia/network/related/en/index.html.

31. Human Rights Impact Resource Center, Human Rights Impact Assessment (HRIA) Tools and Instruments. Available at www.humanrights

impact.org/resources-database/toolsets/

32. Health Workforce Advocacy Initiative, *Incorporating the right to health into health workforce plans: Key considerations* (Health Workforce Advocacy Initiative, 2009).

33. L. Peugh and E. A. Friedman, *Ensuring Equality: A Guide to Addressing and Eliminating Stigma and Discrimination in the Health Sector* (Cambridge, MA and Washington, DC: Physicians for Human Rights, 2011).

34. O'Neill Institute for National and Global Health Law (Georgetown University Law Center), World Health Organization and Lawyers Collective, Global Health and Human Rights Database.

35. G. Backman, P. Hunt, R. Khosla et al., "Health systems and the right to health: an assessment of 194 countries," *Lancet* 372/9655 (2008), pp. 2047–2085.

36. S. Mills, Maternal Death Audit as a Tool Reducing Maternal Mortality (Washington, DC: World Bank, 2011).

37. See, for example, *Minister of Health & Others v. Treatment Action Campaign & Others* (July 5, 2002), CCT 8/02 (Constitutional Court of South Africa). *Cruz del Valle Bermúdez & Others. v. Ministerio de Sanidad y Asistencia Social* (Supreme Court of Justice of Venezuela, Case No. 15.789, Decision No. 916, July 15, 1999). *Asociación Benghalensis v. Ministerio de Salud y Accion Social-Estado Nacional* (National Supreme Court of Justice of Argentina, A. 186, XXXIV, June 1, 2000); O. Conroy, "Free second-line medication for HIV/ AIDS to be available in non-metro Indian cities from March," *TopNews* (January 12, 2011).

38. See, for example, *People's Union of Civil Liberties v. Union of India & Others* (November 28, 2001), Writ Petition (Civil) No. 196 of 2001, Supreme Court Order (Supreme Court of India). Available at http

39. The Inter-American Commission issued precautionary measures to protect against life-threatening conditions in a psychiatric institution in Paraguay, and facilitated negotiations that led to an accord requiring the country to create community-based mental health services. A. Hillman, "Protecting mental disability rights: A success story in the Inter-American Human Rights System," *Human Rights Briefs* 12/3 (2005), pp. 25–28.

40. *Roa López v. Colombia* (Constitutional Court of Colombia, C-355/06, May 10, 2006).

41. K. *Ramakrishnan & Another v. State of Kerala & Others* (July 12, 1999), AIR 1999 Ker 385 (Kerala High Court, India). Available at http://

indiankanoon.org/doc/1480636/.

42. *Government of the Republic of South Africa v. Grootboom* (October 4, 2000), CCT 11/00 (Constitutional Court of South Africa), para. 99. Available at http://www. saflii.org/za/cases/ZACC/2000/19.html.

43. Committee on Economic, Social, and Cultural Rights, General Comment No. 14, The Right to the Highest Attainable Standard of Health, UN Doc. No. E/C.12/2000/4 (2000), at para. 43.

44. See, for example, *Lindiwe Mazibuko & Others. v. City of Johannesburg & Others* (October 8, 2009), CCT 39/09 (Constitutional Court of South Africa), para.161.

45. O. L. M. Ferraz, "The right to health in the courts of Brazil: Worsening health inequities?" *Health and Human Rights: An International Journal* 11/2 (2009), p. 40. Biehl, J.J. Amon, M.P. Socal, and A. Petryna, "Between the court and the clinic: Lawsuits for medicines and the right to health in Brazil," *Health and Human Rights: An International Journal* 14/1 (2012).

46. A. E. Yamin and O. Parra-Vera, "Judicial protection of the right to health in Colombia: From social demands to individual claims to public debates," *Hastings International and Comparative Law Review* 33/2 (2010), pp. 101–129.

47. Ibid., pp. 116–117.

48. Judgment T-760/08 (Constitutional Court of Colombia, July 31, 2008), at para. 4.4.3.; Yamin and Parra-Vera (see note 46), pp. 116–117.

49. Judgment T-760/08 (see note 48), para. 3.5.1.

50. Ibid., para. 6.1.1.2.2.

51. *Xákmok Kásek Indigenous Community v. Paraguay* (Inter-American Court of Human Rights, Series C, No. 214, August 24, 2010), paras. 300–306.

52. The Global Health and Human Rights Database is a collaborative effort of the O'Neill Institute for National and Global Health Law at the Georgetown University Law Center, the World Health Organization, and the Lawyers Collective in India. It will become available in summer 2012 at http://www.ghhrdb.org.

53. *Hugh Glenister v. President of the Republic of South Africa & Others* (March 17, 2011), CCT 48/10 (Constitutional Court of South Africa).

54. WHO Global Code of Practice on the International Recruitment of Health Personnel, World Health Assembly Res. 63.16 (2010).

55. WHO Framework Convention on Tobacco Control, World Health Assembly Res. 56.1 (2003), Art. 22(1)(b)(i).

56. UN Convention against Corruption, G.A. Res. 58/4 (2003), Art. 60.

57. Health and Human Rights, Pan American Health

Organization (PAHO) Directing Council 50.R8 (2010).

58. P. Joubert, "Grootboom dies homeless and penniless," *Mail and Guardian* (August 8, 2008).

59. M. Mulumba, D. Kabanda, and N. Hafsa, "Holding the Ugandan government to account for maternal mortality," *Equinet Newsletter* (December 1, 2011).

60. Businge (see note 24).

61. International Convention on the Protection and Promotion of the Rights and Dignity of Persons with Disabilities, G.A. Res. 61/106 (2006), Art. 33(2).

62. PAHO (see note 57).

63. Rio Political Declaration on Social Determinants of Health, World Conference on Social Determinants of Health, Rio de Janeiro, Brazil (2011), Para. 12(2) (ii).

64. International Center for Not-for-Profit Law, "Recent laws and legislative proposals to restrict civil society and civil society organizations," *International Journal of Not-for-Profit Law* 8/4 (2006), pp. 76–85; International Center for Not-for-Profit Law, "Barred from the debate: Restrictions on NGO public policy activities— Letter from the editor," *Global Trends in NGO Law* 1/3 (2009), pp. 1–12.

65. "The enjoyment of the highest attainable standard of health is one of the fundamental rights of every human being without distinction of race, religion, political belief, economic or social condition." Preamble to the Constitution of the World Health Organization (1948).

66. For a brief explanation of benefits that countries in both the Global South and North would receive, see Gostin, Friedman, Ooms et al. (see note 13).

67. To learn more about JALI, and to offer your own perspectives on an FCGH, we encourage you to visit http://www.jalihealth.org.

QUESTIONS

1. What are commonalities and differences between a Convention and a Framework Convention? Could you provide one or two examples fitting each category? According to the authors, what would a Framework Convention on Global Health critically add to the existing "Right to Health" entrenched in the International Covenant on Economic, Social and Cultural Rights?

2. Refer to the WHO Constitution and its governance http://www.who.int/governance/eb/constitution/en/index.html and summarize what the Framework Convention on Global Health proposed by the authors would add to global health governance in terms of shared responsibility, transparent accountability and harmonization across funding entities, technical agencies, states and civil society. Is there any apparent tension between the Framework Convention and the mandate and mission of WHO? If so, what mechanisms or safeguards could be considered to minimize or eliminate this tension? What are potential pitfalls associated with the formulation, implementation and monitoring of the proposed Framework Convention? How could these be prevented or mitigated?

3. What is the usual process that should be gone through for an International Framework Convention to enter into force? Who are the key actors and in what ways do they contribute to this process? Judging, for example, by the experience of the Tobacco Framework Convention, what timelines could be considered reasonable for a framework convention to come into force if the process were to start now?

FURTHER READING

1. WHO Framework Convention on Tobacco Control, World Health Organization (2003) http://whqlibdoc.who.int/publications/2003/9241591013.pdf
2. Hathaway, O.A., Do Human Rights Treaties Make a Difference? *Faculty Scholarship Series.* Yale Law School Legal Scholarship Repository, Paper 839 (2002). http://digitalcommons.law.yale.edu/fss_papers/839
3. Gennarini, Stefano, Human Rights Roulette: What it Means to Ratify a New Treaty, Turtle Bay and Beyond: International Law, Policy and Beyond, August 3, 2012, Blog accessed on 4 August, 2012 to hear the voice of those who have dissenting views. http://www.turtlebayandbeyond.org/2012/abortion/playing-human-rights-roulette-the-un-treaty-on-disabilities/
4. Wolff, Jonathan, *The Human Right to Health.* New York: Norton, 2012.

PART III

*H*eightened Vulnerability and the Need for Special Protection

Introduction

In the context of health and human rights, vulnerability is understood as limited control over one's life and decision-making as a result of lack of power or oppression or violence, intense discrimination, or social exclusion. Vulnerability can be mitigated or redressed through greater human rights protection. In situations of heightened vulnerability, however, such as extreme violence and threats to individuals and communities, special measures may be needed. Special protection should also be considered when the state is the perpetrator or when state actions to respect, protect and fulfill human rights are insufficient to prevent severe violations of human rights to defined populations. This part develops a theme: when advocacy for special populations is framed within a rights based approach, a more effective force is created that can enable increased protection of vulnerable populations. In policy and practice, populations with heightened vulnerability largely remain separate; they have not been recognized as groups entitled to equal human rights protection. As the concept of special protection continues to evolve, so too will a deeper understanding of populations in need of such protection, as well as the extent to which this new contextualization can synergistically support human rights.

This part addresses issues of health and human rights in extremis, and the resultant heightened vulnerability. The readings begin with a discussion of war and its consequences. In the first chapter, Annas and Geiger remark "War is always and everywhere a public health disaster." War may be associated with massive relocation of populations, environmental destruction, loss of livelihood, high levels of civilian insecurity, and wide spread human rights abuses. War also leads to a breakdown of social fabric, increased chaos with civilian-combatants, disruption of families, and increased risk to women and to children. On an individual level, the direct consequences of armed conflict include morbidity and mortality due to violence in combat, long-term disability, and the sequalae of psychological trauma. Indirect consequences of armed conflict range from malnutrition resulting from loss of agriculture, to infectious disease and the collapse of social and medical infrastructure.

International Humanitarian Law has developed under the four treaties of the Geneva Convention and its three additional protocols for the humanitarian treatment of victims of wars, including civilian populations and non-combatant military prisoners. While International Humanitarian Law has helped limit abuses perpetrated during inter-state conflicts, it has limited relevance to intra-state conflicts, particularly when one or more of the belligerents do not have state status. In such situations, there is a lack of an enforcement system (arrest, detention and adjudication) to hold perpetrators accountable. For this reason, Annas and Geiger call for increased support of the International Criminal Court and increased focus of the Court on such actors. Another reason that International Humanitarian Law has fallen short of addressing the wartime needs of vulnerable populations in the 21st century is that, as discussed by Bruderlein and Leaning, the nature of warfare has changed significantly. For example, today it is a practice of some armies to deliberately target civilian populations. This is not only contrary to the Geneva Conventions, but also gravely undermines humanitarian relief efforts. To this end, Bruderlein and Leaning consider strategies to "re-establish civilian protection and provide neutral space where medical and aid workers can deliver relief." They further suggest that physicians have a duty as key actors to provide humanitarian relief.

In the chapter on "Torture and Public Health," Piwowarczyk, Crosby, Kerr and Grodin provide an introduction to the history and epidemiology of torture as a public health problem. They also address the treatment and rehabilitation of survivors of torture and refugee trauma. This provides background for Taylor's chapter that follows. It discusses health policy in the context of health and human rights issues faced by refugees and asylum seekers. Taylor concludes that, "in almost all indices of physical, mental, and social well being, asylum seekers and refugees suffer a disproportionate burden of morbidity."

The study of male sexual violence against women in Botswana and Swaziland by Tsai, Leiter and Heisler provides a compelling example of the value of collecting empirical data to support redress for human rights violations, and to help inform policy. They also address a significant area of health amd human rights, as sexual violence is associated with health and psychological sequalae which contribute to power differentials that further limit women's rights. Their identification of risk factors, such as heavy drinking is vital to developing preventative strategies and policies. This is followed by a Point of View by Calma, which provides evidence of the link between indigenous health and human rights. Many indigenous populations face similar challenges as refugees, and other vulnerable populations.

The part ends with a discussion of the heightened vulnerability of prisoners and their need for special protections. Metzner and Fellner begin with a discussion of the human rights abuses associated with the solitary confinement of mentally ill prisoners in the US. London's Point of View addresses the subordination of clinical independence in the interest of the state where the physician is an employee of the state. He uses the rubric of "divided loyalty." Annas believes a more accurate description is "dual use." This piece highlights many of the themes present in the work that follows, American Vertigo, in which Annas examines the role of physicians in prisons with special attention to how the state can (and does) use physicians to further national security and research interest of the state. The war on terror has permitted governments, especially the US government, to use physicians for national security reasons in ways that directly violate medical ethics, Guantánamo Bay prison and the use of physicians in torture and interrogation are the most spectacular examples. To protect the human rights (and health) of their patients, with special attention to patients who are prisoners, he argues, "physicians must refuse to comply with any order . . . that is inconsistent with medical ethics," such as the forced feeding campaigns, and suggests that physicians have a special ethical responsibility to act as leaders in upholding health and human rights standards.

Collectively, these chapters frame questions regarding the nature of responsibility, and the need for international accountability for providing special protection to vulnerable populations. These chapters emphasize the need to define key players (allies and detractors) in human rights abuses. In times of war, it is necessary for the international community to immediately recognize and respond when combatants transgress international humanitarian law. In the health area, physicians have a responsibility to become key actors in upholding human rights.

TOPICS FOR DISCUSSION

1. Are human rights abuses more egregious in contemporary warfare than in interstate armed conflicts? How does contemporary warfare challenge the health, international humanitarian protection and human rights of populations that are today most exposed to violence, injury, ill-health and premature death? Who is ultimately responsible for protecting the health and rights of populations discussed in this part?

2. What other populations are in need of special protection? If human rights are universal, why should certain groups be viewed as requiring special protection? Whose obligation is it to protect them?

3. What roles can civil society organizations and academia play in helping to protect populations with heightened vulnerability?

CHAPTER 16

War and Human Rights

George J. Annas and H. Jack Geiger

War is always and everywhere a public health disaster. Because of war's inherent cruelty and savagery, as historian John Keegan has observed, "It is scarcely possible anywhere in the world today to raise a body of reasoned support for the opinion that war is a justifiable activity."[1]

There is a bloody paradox in the world's political and social history. There has never been such universal recognition of human dignity, including the claim that everyone—regardless of race, nationality, religion, gender, sexual orientation, or political belief—is entitled to rights, especially what have been aptly called "life integrity rights."[2] These human rights include the right to life; the right to personal inviolability; not to be hurt; the right to be free of arbitrary seizure, detention, and punishment; the freedom to own one's body and labor; the right to free movement without discrimination; and the right to create and cohabit with family. Life integrity rights embrace, but transcend, the conventional classes of human rights, which include political and civil rights (aspects of freedom or democracy), and social and economic rights (aspects of social justice). They are embodied in a remarkable variety of international human rights and humanitarian laws, conventions, and declarations, including:

- The Charter of the United Nations
- The Universal Declaration of Human Rights
- The International Covenant on Civil and Political Rights
- The Convention on the Prevention and Punishment of the Crime of Genocide
- The Convention against Torture and Other Cruel, Inhuman or Degrading Treatment
- The Convention on the Elimination of All Forms of Discrimination against Women
- The International Convention on the Elimination of All Forms of Racial Discrimination
- The Convention on the Rights of the Child.

These, in turn, are supplemented by specific agreements concerning the conduct of armed conflict (humanitarian law): The Geneva Conventions of 1949 and the Additional Protocols of 1977.

The paradox is that while today's recognition of human rights is unprecedented, with the exception of slavery, human rights have never been violated on so massive a scale, nor with such efficacy and savagery, and the chief instrument of violation is war. The evolution and varieties of warfare over the past century, aided by the technological sophistication, destructive power, and accessibility of new weapons, has all but obliterated the distinction between warfare and mass terrorism. In the early years of the 21st century, with this paradox unresolved, and accompanied by a poorly defined "global war on terror," the fledgling post-World War II commitment to effective and vigorous protection of human rights is under siege.

"War" is no longer the phenomenon simplistically defined as "a contest between armed forces carried on in a campaign or series of campaigns."[2] The diverse forms of armed conflict now include declared and undeclared wars between nations; full-scale civil wars, including many with genocidal motivations; so-called low-intensity conflicts between competing national political groups (which are often highly intense); and a wide variety of "dirty wars" of repression mounted by governments against their own citizens. The defining characteristic of most of these types of war is a calculated and deliberate assault on civilians in contravention of international humanitarian law. All wars put civilian populations at risk of trauma, illness, or death, and threaten to create humanitarian crises.[3]

Violations of international humanitarian and human rights law can be categorized into five areas, as described in the following sections.

DIRECT ASSAULTS ON CIVILIANS BY "CONVENTIONAL" MEANS

The wanton killing of civilians in war was defined as a crime by the Hague Convention of 1907. Nonetheless, millions of civilians have been killed in war since then. In the 1930s, the bombing of Ethiopian civilians by Italian planes and of Spanish civilians at Guernica by German planes drew international condemnation as frightening examples of the criminal use of powerful military technology to harm innocent noncombatants, as did Japanese assaults on cit-

ies in China. World War II saw the abandonment of scruples by all parties. Examples of assaults on essentially nonmilitary and civilian targets included rocket and bomb attacks on London and Coventry and fire-bombings of Dresden, Hamburg, and Tokyo. Tens of thousands of civilians died, mostly elderly people, women, and children.

The wanton killing of civilians was reaffirmed as a war crime by the Geneva Conventions of 1949—again with little effect. Although the regional and surrogate conflicts of the Cold War replaced massive international confrontations, they were almost uniformly characterized by the indiscriminate bombing and fire-bombing of cities and villages, typified by the armed conflicts in Vietnam and Afghanistan. But the almost automatic assumption that civilians were legitimate and inevitable targets of war was reinforced most during the Cold War by the targeting of cities with intercontinental ballistic missiles and the elaboration of absurd, but massive, "civil defense" plans in both the United States and the Soviet Union.

The end of the Cold War did not change this pattern except, perhaps, to emphasize artillery shelling over bombing as the instrument of choice for attacks on noncombatants and the outright destruction of urban life. The conflict in the former Yugoslavia was marked by the sustained and systematic shelling of many cities.[4, 5] These attacks were exceeded in intensity by the Russian assault on Grozny in Chechnya. The highest level of recorded attacks reached was 3,500 shells per day in Sarajevo, and 4,000 per hour in Grozny. The first 3 months of conflict in Chechnya killed an estimated 15,000 civilians and made hundreds of thousands of people refugees.[6, 7]

ETHNIC CLEANSING AND EXTRAJUDICIAL KILLINGS

During the 1980s and 1990s, an old and ugly variant of human rights abuse reappeared: conflicts in which the central purpose of military action was the forced removal of civilian populations from their homes and land on the basis of religion, nationality, or ethnic identity. Such actions constitute a crime against humanity under international law. Many of the episodes involved mass killing; although they did not approach the methodical slaughter of the Holocaust—industrialized mass murder with the goal of extermination of victimized populations—they were genocidal in spirit. The same was true of the systematic mass murders, forced deportations, detention camps, and enslavement carried out by the Khmer Rouge regime in Cambodia under Pol Pot, a bizarre variant in which victims were characterized not by ethnicity but by urban residence and education.

Other notorious examples of ethnic cleansing are the wars in the former Yugoslavia and in Rwanda. In both conflicts, the instruments of ethnic cleansing were massive assaults on noncombatants: the torture and murder of men, women, and children: the widespread and systematic use of rape to terrorize whole communities; the destruction, by explosives and arson, of homes, farms, industries, and basic infrastructures that provided water, electrical power, food, fuel, sanitation, and other necessities; denial of medical care and other violations of medical neutrality; and siege, blockade, and interference with humanitarian relief. Soldiers and noncombatants alike were starved, tortured, or killed in prison camps, to many of which the International Committee of the Red Cross was denied access.[8] Thousands were victims of arbitrary and extrajudicial execution and were buried in mass graves. Refugees and internally displaced persons were denied protection and deliberately attacked: subjected to beatings, rape, and extortion; forced to walk through minefields: and slaughtered in churches, hospitals, and other sanctuaries (Figure 16.1).

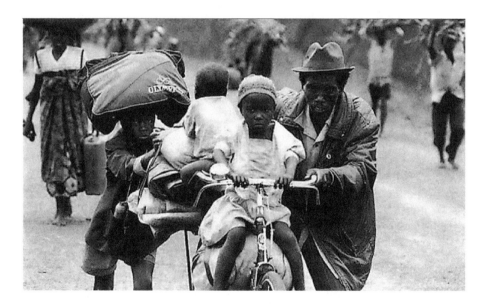

Figure 16.1 A family of Rwandan refugees, their bicycle loaded, make their way along the road to the Benaco Camp in the remote Ngara district, a day's walk from the river where they crossed from Rwanda into Zaire.

(Source/photographer: UNICEF/94/0065/Howard Davies.)

Ethnic cleansing in Yugoslavia and Rwanda are the best-known cases of massive human rights abuses, but attention focused on them has tended to obscure many others, such as those in Sri Lanka, East Timor, Armenia and Azerbaijan, Ossetia and Georgia, China and Tibet, and Iraq and Kurdistan.

In 1988, Iraq destroyed thousands of Kurdish villages. A report on the fate of one such village[9] described murder, forcible disappearance, involuntary relocation, and the refusal to provide minimal conditions of life to detainees. Blatant human rights violations represented by ethnic cleansing will likely continue for decades to come, because dozens of nations have minorities at risk of such onslaughts.[10]

The history of warfare during the past 100 years is replete with smaller-scale, more singular examples of civilian massacres and the punitive destruction of "enemy" villages. The cumulative suffering and loss of life has been enormous. In addition, incidents on the smallest scale, the one-by-one murders by death squads in the so-called dirty wars of repression in El Salvador,[11, 12] Nicaragua, Guatemala,[13] Chile,[14] Argentina, Brazil,[15] Haiti,[16] Colombia, Ethiopia, the Philippines, Kashmir,[17] and South Africa over the past six decades, have resulted in hundreds of thousands of dead and "disappeared" civilians.

DIRECT ASSAULTS ON CIVILIANS CAUSED BY INDISCRIMINATE WEAPONS

Indiscriminate weapons are those which, by their effects and defining characteristics, are almost certain (and are usually intended) to harm military combatants and civilians alike and therefore by definition violate the humanitarian law prohibition of wanton killing. They include, but are not limited to, weapons of mass destruction as usually defined: nuclear, chemical, and biological weapons, as well as landmines.

The nuclear bombings of Hiroshima and Nagasaki were transforming events of 20th-century warfare. That more than 200,000 civilians died from blast, incineration, and radiation is widely recognized; that such mass killing is a violation of human rights is not widely recognized, despite the multiple specific provisions in international law that (1) prohibit attacks that cause unnecessary suffering, (2) require implementation of the principle of proportionality, and (3) affirm the basic immunity of civilian populations and civilians from being objects of attack during armed conflict.

INDIRECT ASSAULTS ON CIVILIAN POPULATIONS

Modern military technology, especially the use of high-precision bombs, rockets, and missile warheads, has now made it possible to attack civilian populations in industrialized societies indirectly—but with devastating results—by targeting the facilities on which life depends, while avoiding the stigma of direct attack on the bodies and habitats of noncombatants. The technique has been termed "bomb now, die later."[18]

U.S. military action against Iraq in the 1991 Persian Gulf War and in the Iraq War has included the specific and selective destruction of key aspects of the infrastructure necessary to maintain civilian life and health. During the bombing phase of the Persian Gulf War, this deliberate effort almost totally destroyed Iraq's electrical-power generation and transmission capacity and its civilian communications networks. In combination with the prolonged application of economic sanctions and the disruption of highways, bridges, and facilities for refining and distributing fuel by conventional bombing, these actions had severely damaging effects on the health and survival of the civilian population, especially infants and children. Without electrical power, water purification and pumping ceased immediately in all major urban areas, as did sewage pumping and treatment. The appearance and epidemic spread of infectious diarrheal disease in infants and of waterborne diseases, such as typhoid fever and cholera, were rapid. At the same time, medical care and public health measures were totally disrupted. Modern multistory hospitals were left without clean water, sewage disposal, or any electricity beyond what could be supplied by emergency generators designed to operate only a few hours per day. Operating rooms, X-ray equipment, and other vital facilities were crippled. Supplies of anesthetics, antibiotics, and other essential medications were rapidly depleted. Vaccines and medications requiring refrigeration were destroyed, and all immunization programs ceased. Because almost no civilian telephones, computers, or transmission lines were operable, the Ministry of Health was effectively immobilized. Fuel shortages and the disruption of transportation limited civilian access to medical care.[19–21]

Many reports provide clear and quantitative evidence of violations of the requirements of immunity for civilian populations, proportionality, and the prevention of unnecessary suffering. They mock the concept of "life integrity rights." In contrast to the chaos and social disruption that routinely accompany armed conflicts, these deaths have been the consequence of an explicit military policy, with clearly foreseeable consequences to the human rights of civilians. The U.S. military has never conceded that its policies violated human rights under the Geneva Conventions or the guidelines under which U.S. military personnel operate. Yet the ongoing development of military technology suggests that—absent the use of weapons of mass destruction—violations of civilians' human rights will be the preferred method of warfare in the future.

VIOLATIONS OF MEDICAL NEUTRALITY

The Geneva Conventions, customary international law, and medical ethics all mandate

- Medical neutrality
- Protection of medical facilities, personnel, and patients from military attack or interference
- Humane treatment of civilians
- The right of access to care
- Nondiscriminatory treatment of the ill and wounded in time of war.

In the wide range of human rights concerns, medical neutrality is of particular concern to health workers. This is more than a matter of narrow self-interest. Concern for the rights of individual patients and the health of populations is at the core of mandates for health professionals.

Yet in almost every recent armed conflict violations of medical neutrality have been widespread, systematic, and almost routine. All seven major hospitals in Grozny were destroyed.[6] In the conflict in the former Yugoslavia, hospitals were routinely shelled—in some cases, reduced to rubble—and physicians were special targets of sniper attacks. In Haiti, Kuwait, the West Bank and Gaza Strip, Somalia, and Sudan, hospitals, clinics, and first-aid stations were invaded and patients, medical personnel, and relief workers were assaulted, abducted, tortured, and murdered. In El Salvador, where civil conflict was marked by almost every conceivable violation of medical neutrality, health and relief workers were beaten, imprisoned, or murdered for activities as innocent as the vaccination of children. In many conflicts, ambulances are routinely attacked, seized, or blocked. In some civil wars and in so-called "low-intensity conflicts" (somewhat of a misnomer), the destruction of civilian health services has been defended as a legitimate tactic to punish populations suspected of supporting dissident armed forces. In some wars, physicians have been arrested, tortured, or executed for fulfilling their ethical obligation to provide medical care regardless of the patient's political or military affiliation; in others, physicians have actively participated in the torture of dissidents.[22]

Contemporary warfare, focused increasingly on assaulting civilian populations and their support structures, is replacing medical neutrality—in practice, if not in law—with strategies in which no civilian systems and no human rights are immune.

WAR AND INTELLECTUAL CORRUPTION: JUSTIFYING VIOLATIONS

The Geneva Conventions and other embodiments of human rights protection are undermined by the corrupt view that victory in war is its own justification, so virtually any abuse or atrocity can be rationalized. It is a position most frequently articulated as a self-evident necessity by the military, the very institution that is supposed to be constrained by human rights in wartime, and it is strikingly uniform in its expression by soldiers from nations with widely varied political systems.

Is it possible that the existence of laws of war that seek to limit death, pain, and suffering of civilians can actually make war appear more benign than it is, encouraging brutal wars that would not have otherwise been contemplated? Can it ever make sense to go to war to protect civilians from human rights abuses, as has recently been attempted in Kosovo, Bosnia, East Timor, Liberia, and Haiti? These questions are complex and require much more attention than they have received, because war, even when waged for "good" purposes, always terrorizes civilians.

INTERNATIONAL LAWS TO PROTECT HUMAN RIGHTS DURING WAR

World War I, with its horrors of trench warfare and chemical weapons, was meant to be the war to end all wars. The failure of the League of Nations to prevent World War II—a global disaster—led to what was hoped were much stronger instruments to prevent war, including the United Nations and specific international human rights laws. The most important human rights documents, including the Universal Declaration of Human Rights, the International Covenant on Civil and Political Rights, and the International Covenant on Economic, Social and Cultural Rights, were all direct products of World War II. The same can be said about the most important humanitarian treaty, the Geneva Conventions of 1949, and the Nuremberg Principles, which were established in the major war crimes trial of Nazi leaders after World War II. The Nuremberg Principles, which must be distinguished from the Nuremberg Code on human experimentation developed during the Nuremberg Doctors' Trial, are the following:[23]

- There are war crimes and crimes against humanity (including murder, torture, and slavery).
- Individuals—not just states—can be held criminally responsible for committing them.
- It is no defense that an individual was "just obeying orders" or following the law of one's country.

The rapid growth of international human rights laws in reaction to the horrors of World War II has been so profound that we need to have some familiarity with what preceded their development before discussing these instruments and their contemporary application and efficacy.

HUMANITARIAN LAW

"Humanitarian law" is the unlikely term for the law of war, especially that part of the law of war devoted to rules designed to restrain the actions of the warring parties. The law of war is generally divided into two parts: (1) the law relating to primary prevention by discouraging going to war in the first place (*jus ad bellum*); and (2) the law relating to what may be thought of as secondary prevention, rules for the conduct of war—especially as related to the protection of civilians (*jus in bello*).[24]

Because war is so terrible, it has, at least since Roman times, required justification, usually set forth in various versions of the "just war" doctrine. This doctrine requires that the war be waged under a public authority, be instigated either for self-defense or to punish a grievous injury, and be pursued only to achieve the just ends—not for vengeance. What constitutes self-defense is open to some interpretation, but the current position of the United States that permits "preemptive" war when a future threat, even one involving weapons of mass destruction, is thought to exist has no "just war" pedigree. Nations need not wait to defend themselves until they are actually attacked, but an attack must be imminent and unstoppable by other means to justify a self-defense war response. Public health principles, which focus on prevention as a means of protecting the health of the public, demand that all reasonable steps be taken to prevent war, including support of international treaties designed to limit the development and use of weapons of mass destruction and support of the United Nations, which was founded primarily to keep the peace.

Secondary prevention or damage control is the goal of *jus in bello*—the attempt to produce rules that limit the destructiveness of an inherently destructive activity. It is strange, and even macabre, to try to develop rules of conduct for mass killings. It is even possible that such rules could make it easier to justify going to war in the first place. Nonetheless, the wholesale slaughter of civilians has been unacceptable since the Thirty Years War (1618–1648) and the work of Dutch jurist Hugo Grotius. Before then, humanitarian rules simply did not exist. Shakespeare's rendition of Henry V's threat to the mayor of a French city, from whom he demanded unconditional surrender or else he would let loose his troops to murder, rape, and pillage, reflects the practice of the Middle Ages:[25]

> Take pity of your town and of your people
> Whiles yet my soldiers are in my
>   command. . . .
> If not, why, in a moment look to see
> The blind and bloody soldier with foul hand
> Defile the locks of your shrill-shrieking
>   daughters;
> Your fathers taken by the silver beards,
> And their most reverend heads dashed to
>   the walls;
> Your naked infants spitted upon pikes,
> Whiles the mad mothers with their howls
>   confus'd
> Do break the clouds, as did the wives of
>   Jewry
> At Herod's bloody-hunting slaughtermen.
> What say you? Will you yield, and this avoid?
> Or, guilty in defence, be thus destroy'd?

The Hague Conventions, established before World War I, specifically apply to land warfare and prohibit, among other things, "the attack or bombardment of towns, villages, habitations or buildings which are not defended," as well as "the pillage of a town or place, even when taken by assault." The League of Nations was singularly ineffective in preventing World War II. The Hague rules designed to protect civilians were systemically ignored, not only by Germany and the Soviet Union, but also by Britain in its fire-bombing of German cities (especially Dresden and Hamburg) and by the United States in 1945 in its fire-bombing of more than two dozen Japanese cities and its use of atomic weapons on Hiroshima and Nagasaki.

The basic justification for dropping the atomic bombs was that the laws of warfare applied only to the "civilized nations," and uncivilized peoples could be killed with impunity.[26] As President Harry Truman said 3 days after the bomb was dropped on Hiroshima, "I know that Japan is a terribly cruel and uncivilized nation in warfare. . . ."[27] His position had a long pedigree, including the Crusades, the conquest of the New World, and colonization. A second rationale—that use of atomic weapons on civilian Japanese populations would shorten the war—is simply a restatement of a proposition highlighted earlier in this chapter: War has its own logic, and almost any tactic, regardless of its impact on civilian populations, can be, and often is, justified as militarily necessary.

World War II was followed by the first international war crimes trial in history, conducted at Nuremberg. In his opening statement to the international tribunal, composed of judges from the United States, England, France, and the Soviet Union, Justice Robert Jackson made it clear to all that he understood the critique that the tribunal was designed to render a "victor's justice" based on vengeance "which arises from the anguish of war," rather than justice based on international law. The final judgment not only labeled the waging of aggressive war as a crime against humanity but also catalogued specific acts, including murder, torture, and slavery, as war crimes and crimes against humanity. It was hoped that holding individuals accountable for committing such crimes would help prevent them in the future. It was also hoped, at least by the prosecution team, that the world would establish a "permanent Nuremberg" to be on hand to hold individuals

in the future accountable for war crimes and crimes against humanity. In 2000, the International Criminal Court was finally established, based on this model. However, the major military powers, including the United States, have refused to agree to its jurisdiction, primarily because they fear being judged unfairly and arbitrarily by the community of nations for waging aggressive warfare and for using a disproportionate amount of force in so doing.

In short, the legacy of Nuremberg is mixed—perhaps inherently so, since the primary sponsor of Nuremberg, the United States, continues to oppose a "permanent Nuremberg" court; has never publicly acknowledged any doubts about the justice of using atomic weapons on civilian targets; and opposes treaties that would explicitly make first use of nuclear weapons a war crime and a crime against humanity.

The killing of millions of civilians during World War II, as well as the deaths of millions of prisoners of war, led to an expansion of the Geneva Conventions, first with the Geneva Conventions of 1949 (especially Convention IV regarding the protection of civilians), and the two protocols of 1977 (especially Protocol 1 related to the protection of victims of international armed conflicts). Under Protocol 1, "civilian objects" include all things that are not "military objects"—that is, not "objects which by their nature, location, purpose or use make an effective contribution to military action and whose total or partial destruction, capture or neutralization, in the circumstances ruling at the time, offers definite military advantage." An occupying power is also responsible under Geneva Convention IV and Protocol 1 to ensure that the civilian population is provided with food and medical supplies and, "to the fullest extent of the means available to it," with "clothing, bedding, means of shelter, [and] other supplies essential to the survival of the civilian population."

HUMAN RIGHTS LAW

The development of international human rights law based on the horrors of World War II has been more promising. The Charter of the United Nations, signed by the 50 original member nations in 1945, spells out the goals of the United Nations. The first two are "to save succeeding generations from the scourge of war . . .; and to reaffirm faith in fundamental human rights, in the dignity and worth of the human person, in the equal rights of men and women and of nations large and small." After the Charter was signed, the adoption of an international bill of rights with legal authority proceeded in three steps: a declaration, two treaties, and implementation measures.

The Universal Declaration of Human Rights was adopted by the United Nations General Assembly in 1948 without dissent as "a common standard for all peoples and nations." Its precepts apply in war and peace and provide, among other things, that "Everyone has the right to life, liberty and security of person"; "No one shall be subjected to torture or to cruel, inhuman or degrading treatment or punishment"; "No one shall be subjected to arbitrary arrest, detention or exile"; and "Everyone has the right to freedom of thought, conscience and religion . . . [and to] freedom of opinion and expression." Of special interest to public health is Article 25:

1. Everyone has the right to a standard of living adequate for the health and well-being of himself and his family, including food, clothing, housing and medical care and necessary social services . . .
2. Motherhood and childhood are entitled to special care and assistance.

This was a declaration of principles and thus aspirational. It took a treaty process to make these provisions an obligatory part of international law. Because of another

war, the Cold War, two separate treaties were developed, both of which were opened for signature in 1966: the International Covenant on Civil and Political Rights (ICCPA), which the United States supported and which is most directly applicable to war, and the International Covenant on Economic, Social and Cultural Rights, which the United States did not and does not support. The latter contains a more specific right to health, "the right of everyone to the enjoyment of the highest attainable standard of physical and mental health." Given the horrors of poverty, disease, and armed conflicts since World War II, it is easy to dismiss as empty gestures the rights enunciated in these documents.[28] But our disappointments with human rights reflect more our own failures than the failure of the human rights framework. We need not be naïve to continue to believe that the best hope of humankind lies in the protection and promotion of human rights.

How do human rights work in war? Article 4 of the ICCPR provides that, "In time of public emergency which threatens the life of the nation and the existence of which is officially proclaimed," a state may derogate from its obligations under the treaty if contrary measures are "strictly required" for its survival and they are not "inconsistent with their other obligations under international law and do not involve discrimination solely on the ground of race, colour, sex, language, religion or social origin." Even in emergencies, some human rights cannot be compromised by the state, including the right to life; the right not to be tortured or subjected to cruel, inhuman, or degrading treatment or punishment; the right not to be held in slavery; and the right not to be subject to arbitrary arrest or imprisonment. Finally, rights to freedom of thought, conscience, and religion are also protected absolutely. Standards, known as the Siracusa Principles, explain how to apply the emergency derogation provision. They require that when a derogation of the other rights in the ICCPR is made for public emergency, including a public health emergency, the aim must be legitimate and the measure "proportionate to that aim," and "a state shall use no more restrictive means than are required for the achievement of the purpose of the limitation." The principle of proportionality applies directly to warfare; a parallel principle of requiring the use of the "least destructive means necessary" to achieve the military mission has not yet been articulated.

War puts all human rights at risk by its brutal nature. Humanitarian law applies only to armed conflicts and cannot be suspended during hostilities. People around the world continue to suffer, at least in part, because of the lack of effective enforcement mechanisms for human rights and humanitarian law violations. While not a complete solution, the newly established International Criminal Court deserves the support of everyone who believes that human rights and humanitarian law should be taken seriously, and that those who commit war crimes and crimes against humanity should be held accountable for their actions.[29]

REFERENCES

1. Keegan J. A History of Warfare. New York: Vintage Books, 1993, pp. 56–57.
2. The Shorter Oxford English Dictionary, 3rd ed. London: Oxford University Press, 1964.
3. Geiger HJ, Cook-Degan RM. The role of physicians in conflicts and humanitarian crises. JAMA 1993; 270: 616–620.
4. Reiff D. On your knees with the dying. In Rabia A, Lifswchultz L (eds.). Why Bosnia? Writings on the Balkan War. Stony Creek, CT: The Pamphleteer's Press, 1993.
5. Magas B. The Destruction of Yugoslavia. London: Verso Press, 1993.
6. Cuny F. Killing Chechnya. New York Review of Books, April 6, 1995, pp. 15–17.
7. Human Rights Watch/Helsinki. Russia: Three months of war in Chechnya. New York: Human Rights Watch/Helsinki Newsletter, February 1995; 7(6).
8. Gutman R. A Witness to Genocide. New York: Macmillan, 1993.
9. The Anfal campaign in Iraqi Kurdistan: The destruction of Koreme. New York and Boston: Middle East Watch and Physicians for Human Rights, 1993.
10. Gurr TR, Scaritt JR. Minorities' rights at risk: A global survey. Human Rights Quarterly 1989; 11: 379–405.
11. El Salvador: Health Care Under Siege. Boston: Physicians for Human Rights, 1990.
12. Geiger HJ, Eisenberg C, Gloyd S, et al. Special report: A new medical mission to El Salvador. N Engl J Med 1989; 321: 113–114.
13. Getting Away with Murder. Boston: Physicians for Human Rights, 1991.
14. Sowing Fear: The Uses of Torture and Psychological Abuse in Chile. Somerville, MA: Physicians for Human Rights, 1988.
15. The Search for Brazil's Disappeared: The Mass Grave at Dom Bosco Cemetery. Washington, DC, and Somerville, MA: Amnesty International, Physicians for Human Rights, and American Association for the Advancement of Science, 1991.
16. Return to the Darkest Days: Human Rights in Haiti Since the Coup. Boston: Physicians for Human Rights, 1992.
17. The Crackdown in Kashmir: Torture of Detainees and Assaults on the Medical Community. Boston and New York: Physicians for Human Rights and Asia Watch, 1993.
18. Geiger HJ, quoted in Kandela P. Iraq: Bomb now, die later. The Lancet 1991; 337: 967.
19. Report to the Secretary-General on Humanitarian Needs in Kuwait and Iraq in the Immediate Post-Crisis Environment by a Mission to the Area Led by Mr. Martti Ahtisaari, Under-Secretary for Administration and Management. United Nations, March 10, 1991.
20. Report of the WHO/UNICEF Special Mission to Iraq. New York: United Nations Children's Fund, February, 1991.
21. Iraq's Food and Agricultural Situation during the Embargo and the War. Congressional Research Service Report for Congress, February 26, 1991. Washington, DC: The Library of Congress.
22. Medicine Betrayed: The Participation of Doctors in Human Rights Abuses. London: Zed Books and the British Medical Association, 1992.
23. Drinan RF. The Nuremberg Principles in international law. In Annas GJ, Grodin MA (eds.). The Nazi Doctors and the Nuremberg Code. New York: Oxford University Press, 1992, pp. 174–230.

24. O'Brien WV, Arend AC. Just war doctrine and the international law of war. In Bean TE, Sparacino LA (eds.). Military Medical Ethics, Vol. I. Falls Church, VA: Office of The Surgeon General, United States Army; Washington, DC: Borden Institute, Walter Reed Army Medical Center; and Bethesda, MD: Uniformed Services University of the Health Sciences, 2003, pp. 221–240.

25. Shakespeare W. Henry V, III, ii.

26. Lindqvist S.A History of Bombing. New York: New Press, 2000.

27. McCullough D. Truman. New York: Simon & Schuster, 1992, p. 458.

28. Annas GJ. Human rights and health: The Universal Declaration of Human Rights at 50.N Engl J Med 1998; 339: 1778–1781.

29. Annas GJ. Human rights outlaws: Nuremberg, Geneva, and the global war on terror. Boston U. Law Rev. 2007; 87: 427–466.

QUESTIONS

1. What is the difference between international humanitarian law and international human rights law? What is the difference between *jus ad bellum* and *jus in bello*?

2. The authors ask, "can it ever make sense to go to war to protect civilians from human rights abuses, as has recently been attempted in Kosovo, Bosnia, East Timor, Liberia and Haiti?" Respond to the authors' question. Consider broadly, what is a "just" war? Also, using the examples above, consider whether any of these contemporary armed human rights interventions have been "successful."

3. Why is there the need for rules of war? What do you believe are appropriate rules of war? Feel free to use outside resources to formulate your answer, such as the Geneva and Hague Conventions and the Nuremberg Trials.

FURTHER READING

1. Schabas, William, *An Introduction to the International Criminal Court.* Cambridge, UK: Cambridge University Press, 2004.

2. Barnett, Michael, *Empire of Humanity: A History of Humanitarianism.* Ithaca NY: Cornell University Press, 2011.

3. Byron, Christine, *War Crimes and Crimes Against Humanity in the Rome Statute of the International Criminal Court,* Manchester: Manchester University Press, 2009.

4. Lifton, Robert Jay & Mitchell, Greg, *Hiroshima in America: A Half Century of Denial.* New York: Avon, 1995.

CHAPTER 17

New Challenges for Humanitarian Protection

Claude Bruderlein and Jennifer Leaning

INTRODUCTION

The fourth Geneva Convention, adopted 50 years ago, on 12 August 1949, describes the actions that warring parties must take to protect civilian populations from the worst excesses of war. Building on the concept developed in the previous three conventions—that certain activities and people, especially civilians, can be seen as hors de combat—the fourth Geneva Convention defines in detail the many ways in which civilians must be dealt with to shield them from the direct and indirect effects of conflict between combatant forces.

Among the responsibilities that this convention sets for the warring parties are explicit actions that would grant medical personnel, and all aspects of the medical enterprise, complete protection from interference or harm. This neutral status for medical relief (and, by extension, all humanitarian aid) rests on the reciprocal assumption that those who deliver this relief are practising in accord with their professional ethics and will take specified steps to maintain their neutral posture vis à vis the warring parties.

The moral impetus for this addition to the Geneva Conventions derived from international reaction to the great civilian death toll of the second world war. In virtu-ally all wars of the subsequent 50 years the fourth Geneva Convention has been variously observed and routinely violated—and there has been no calling to account. Moreover, and this is what prompts new attention to the issue of humanitarian protection in war, in recent wars the warring parties have shown an increasing tendency to flout the fourth convention entirely. The problem is no longer a failure to abide by the rules but a failure to acknowledge that the rules even exist.[1]

This failure is particularly relevant for the medical community. Without the guarantees of protection defined in the fourth convention, civilians can be slaughtered with impunity and physicians and other relief workers swept up in the ensuing carnage. Once the notion of civilian protection is abandoned, the terrain of war is changed utterly. At the very moment we celebrate the 50th anniversary of the Geneva Conventions, we find that effective respect for humanitarian protection has reached its nadir.

TRADITIONAL APPROACH TO HUMANITARIAN PROTECTION

The traditional legal effort to protect civilians in war has long centred on distinguishing between civilian persons or objects and military targets. This approach was based on two key assumptions: that attacking civilian targets would provide little military advantage; and that, quite apart from their legal or moral obligations, parties to a conflict would thus seek to optimise their resources by targeting military assets. Therefore the most effective approach to protect civilians in international legal treaties on the conduct of war would be to build on this assumed basic military preference and promote the concept of civilian distinctiveness. This approach has inspired the development of international humanitarian law since its inception.

A corollary of this approach is to designate the armed forces of the warring parties as the principal implementing agents of the protection. International humanitarian law states that those who seek to be protected cannot engage in any hostile activities without losing their protected status. If the armies confirm that the civilians are abiding by these constraints then the armies are obliged to ensure that the civilians are indeed protected. An essential element of this legal regime therefore is the commitment of the parties to the conflict to abide by the rules.

INTENSIFIED THREATS TO PROTECTION OF CIVILIANS

The traditional approach taken by international humanitarian law thus rests on a particular and rational view of military interests and behaviour. However, military strategies from the second world war onwards have departed significantly from this classic perception of the non-military worth of civilian assets. The bombardments of London, Rotterdam, Dresden, Hamburg, Hiroshima, and Nagasaki in the second world war were only the precursors of military tactics aimed at obtaining significant military advantage from the destruction, terror, flight, and chaos caused by attacks on civilians. In the 54 years since 1945, civilians have constituted the overwhelming majority of war casualties.[2] What has evolved now, with the waning of the cold war, is a pattern of deliberate war against civilians, waged by relatively untrained forces wielding relatively light arms.[3] Civilian populations have come to acquire a strategic importance, including:

- As a cover for the operations of rebel movements
- As a target of reprisals
- As a shield against air or artillery attacks
- As a lever for exerting pressure on the adverse party, by terrorising and displacing populations, or even
- As a principal target of ethnic cleansing operations and genocide.

In internal conflicts civilian populations are caught in the crossfire between insurgents and state forces and bear most of the casualties. In extreme situations (Rwanda 1994; Bosnia-Herzegovina 1992–4; and Kosovo 1998–9) entire segments of the civilian population have been perceived as a primary military target. Civilian deaths in just these three wars amount to over 1 million people—far greater than the estimated military casualties.

Death is not the only outcome of a war strategy that targets civilians. In the past decade armed conflict has turned over 40 million people into refugees or internally displaced people. The consequences of such displacement are severe and include:

- Breakdown of the social fabric and disintegration of communities
- Production of chaotic situations, where the mixture of civilians and combatants puts civilians at risk and endangers medical and humanitarian relief workers

- Disruption of family groupings, exposing women and girls to sexual violence, prostitution, and sex trafficking
- Forced military recruitment of children, sending those as young as 7 years old into battle.

In addition, warring factions have increasingly denied civilian populations access to humanitarian relief. They defend their actions by appealing to the principle of national sovereignty. Within their national boundaries these warring parties block relief convoys, obstruct ambulances, invade hospitals, destroy clinics, and harass and terrorise national and international medical and other humanitarian relief workers.[4–8] In these circumstances the assumption in international humanitarian law that civilians would be protected simply by establishing their distinct nonmilitary character seems outdistanced by recent changes in warfare and thus fundamentally flawed. In the absence of alternative credible and effective enforcement mechanisms, it would seem that the international community can offer little help to civilian populations targeted in today's wars.

POSSIBLE NEW STRATEGIES

The international community has thus been compelled to reconsider its approach towards protecting civilians. When states or parties to conflicts are unable or unwilling to protect civilians during armed conflict, the international community must develop specific mechanisms to ensure that protection. To that end, new strategies are being developed to expand the concept of humanitarian protection and to consider new alliances with other potential enforcement agents, including the United Nations Security Council and regional organisations and their military outfits.

Accordingly, human rights and humanitarian organisations are pursuing three distinct strategies to bolster the protection given to civilians: reasserting the role and validity of international humanitarian law, and developing new judicial implementation mechanisms; expanding the scope of humanitarian protection; and diversifying the implementation strategies of humanitarian protection, involving the use of various diplomatic and coercive measures, including the use of force under chapter VII of the UN Charter.

Reasserting the Role of International Humanitarian Law

The first strategy has been to recall the objectives of international humanitarian law and promote further efforts nationally and internationally for enforcing these rules. International humanitarian law is seen as essential in determining the illegal character of violence perpetrated against civilians in war. It should therefore be at the centre of any strategy to protect them and to restore the integrity of international law. The proponents of this approach, particularly the International Committee of the Red Cross, acknowledge that war has changed and that civilians have increasingly become the objects of attacks. In their view, however, violations of law do not necessarily signify its obsolescence. On the contrary, international humanitarian law remains highly relevant in contemporary conflicts (such as instances of ethnic cleansing and failed states) and serves to mobilise considerable efforts to further its application.

The key focus of these efforts has been to strengthen international judicial institutions. The culture of impunity that shelters individuals responsible for violent assaults against civilians is one of the biggest obstacles to protecting civilians in most conflicts. The unwillingness or inability of states to bring these people to justice undermines the effectiveness of the entire legal framework. An international remedy for such situations has been identified in the establishment of an International Criminal Court and the creation of the two ad hoc tribunals for the former Yugoslavia and for Rwanda by the UN Security Council.

Action from Professional Groups

Professional groups, including lawyers, doctors, and journalists, have also played a part in reinforcing traditional mechanisms of protection by recalling the legal obligations of parties to armed conflicts under humanitarian law. The successes of "sans-frontières" nongovernmental organisations, such as Médecins Sans Frontières, International Commission of Jurists, or Reporter Sans Frontières, is a demonstration of this mobilisation of professionals. The medical and public health communities, through international societies, human rights groups, or relief agencies, played a pioneering role here, taking a strong interest in upholding established international principles of human rights in relation to medical ethics and international humanitarian law and in documenting violations. Beginning with the founding of the World Medical Association in 1947, the world's national medical societies have tried to uphold professional norms in the face of potential or actual confrontation with developments in peace and war. An early leader was the British Medical Association, which in the 1980s spurred organised medicine to combat the participation of physicians in torture.[9, 10]

Physician based human rights organisations have sought to provide governments and judicial bodies with evidence of major violations of the Geneva Conventions during conflict or civil war in the West Bank and Gaza in 1988–90,[11] Somalia in 1992,[12] Bosnia-Herzegovina in 1992–5,[13] Rwanda-Eastern Congo in 1994–7,[14] and Kosovo in 1998–9.[15] A major effort is now underway among several such organisations to provide documentary and forensic evidence to the international criminal tribunals of Yugoslavia and Rwanda.

Relief organisations, under increasing public scrutiny and subject to ever more frequent danger in the field, have also realised that they must educate their staff in the principles of human rights and international humanitarian law.[16] Their staff will thus operate within internationally respected norms and know what should be expected from warring parties and the international community in terms of humanitarian protection.

Expanding the Scope of Humanitarian Protection

The need to expand the scope of humanitarian protection arises directly from the changing nature of war. Were civilians not terrorised into fleeing from their homes, issues relating to internally displaced people would be less acute. Were regular forces fighting according to standard rules of weaponry, the proliferation of unmarked antipersonnel landmines would be less of a problem. Were children not being forcibly inducted into irregular armies and then forced to commit unspeakably brutal acts, the minimum age and its enforcement would not attract such attention.

The increasing involvement, over the past decades, of UN agencies and nongovernmental organisations in humanitarian operations has increased the number of humanitarian actors in conflict situations.[17] This in turn has affected the perceived scope of humanitarian protection from one that is basically driven by international humanitarian law to one that is driven by the many needs of specific groups of victims in specific circumstances. Children need caring adults; terrified refugees need to be able to feel safe; people from diverse cultures seek respectful space for religious practice; women in camps should not be forced into prostitution.

The humanitarian community has sought legal confirmation of this needs based expansion by referring to several key human rights documents that it regards as relevant in conflict settings. These include the 1951 Convention Relating to the Status of Refugees, the 1979 Convention on the Elimination of all Forms of Discrimination against Women, the 1984 Convention against Torture, and the 1989 Convention on the Rights of the Child. The insistence that key provisions of these documents do, indeed, apply in a state of conflict[18] has produced a growing recognition that just because people are trapped in war, they do not in any moral sense, and thus should not legally, lose the protection that they could claim if they were living in a country at peace. International humanitarian law remains the primary legal reference in conflicts. Nevertheless, these developments in humanitarian practice and policy, and the new guidelines on internally displaced peoples (which combine elements of human rights law with international humanitarian law) show an encouraging convergence between these two basic ways of defining protections for civilians in war.

The concept of humanitarian protection is also being extended in terms of time frame. International humanitarian law traditionally applies during the actual conduct of hostilities. From a public health and human rights perspective, however, the phases that lead up to a conflict and the extended reconstruction period afterwards are of equal concern. Issues such as the repatriation of refugees[19] or the status of vulnerable groups, such as women and girls in Afghanistan,[20] become central concerns of those engaged in humanitarian and human rights action in war.

This expansion arises out of a decade of work in which these humanitarian concerns were slowly shaped by bitter experience. The humanitarian community has provided the data that has forced the international legal and political community to develop an expanded scope of protection. As early witnesses to and occasional victims of child soldiers, as surgeons in field hospitals overwhelmed by landmine injuries, or as the only source of help in a region suddenly flooded by internally displaced people, medical relief workers had first to act without the benefit of guidelines and were then compelled to become more systematic. Internal critiques and published reviews of this experience[21] have accelerated our understanding of the complexity of the issues facing those who try to provide relief when established norms of protection are violated and when new forms of attacks on civilians take place in the absence of consensus on what the international community should do next.

International Initiatives

To establish this expanded scope of humanitarian protection in the legal and operational sphere is a complex challenge. Three recent initiatives, undertaken at international legal levels and pursued by many humanitarian and human rights organisations, have focused on protecting civilians against the use of antipersonnel landmines, protecting internally displaced persons, and prohibiting the military recruitment of children.

The 1997 Ottawa Landmines Treaty (entered in force in March 1999) bans the use, production, stockpiling, and transfer of antipersonnel landmines. Groups such as the International Campaign to Ban Landmines (comprising many humanitarian and human rights groups) were critical in mobilising states. This grass roots coalition, and others associated with it, has now embarked on monitoring compliance with the treaty and running local landmine awareness campaigns throughout the world.

The forced displacement of people within the borders of their own countries by armed conflicts has become a central feature of the post cold war era. In its classic form international humanitarian law does not protect internally displaced people since they remain primarily under the protection of their own state. Yet some of the worst assaults on civilians in war have taken place against internally displaced people (Srebrenica),[22] and some of the more intractable humanitarian dilemmas relate to supporting those forced to survive away from home but within the borders of their state (Sudan).[23] As a result the United Nations presented "Guiding Principles for the Protection of Internally Displaced Persons" to the Commission on Human Rights in 1998. These combine elements of humanitarian law and human rights law, which recognise, among other rights, a right not to be unlawfully displaced, the right of access to assistance and protection during displacement, and the right to a secure return and reintegration.

Finally, the use of children in armed conflicts has been another dramatic feature of post cold war hostilities. An estimated 300,000 child soldiers are actively involved in armed conflicts around the world.[24] According to both international human rights and humanitarian law, the current minimum age for participation in armed conflict is 15 years. Although the recruitment of children as young as 7 already falls far below this international standard, Unicef and other humanitarian organisations have tried to raise awareness and affect realities on the ground by crafting the Optional Protocol to the Convention of the Rights of the Child. This sets a minimum age of 18 years. This campaign has also highlighted the many difficulties presented by child soldiers: demobilisation, re-entry into society, and education.

Diversifying Implementation Strategies of Humanitarian Protection

The expansion of the concept of humanitarian protection has resulted in a more sophisticated understanding of the rights of civilians in times of war. Such protection still relies primarily, however, on the ability and willingness of implementing agents (states, the UN Security Council, and regional organisations such as NATO) to enforce this protection. When warring parties fail to abide by the rules of international humanitarian law, it falls to the international community to enforce them.

The practical importance of this responsibility remains unclear. Proponents of more assertive regimes of civilian protection believe that new political and security strategies are required, to provide more tactical options along a continuum within the current legal framework of the UN Charter's chapter VI (entry with the permission of the sovereign state) and chapter VII ("non-permissive" entry). Such protection strategies need to involve political and military actors, such as the UN Security Council, regional organisations, and specialised agencies (such as the UN Department of Peacekeeping Operations) and would constitute the next generation of international security response to humanitarian crises. The current rationale for international political and military intervention is based on threats to international peace and security; in the next generation this would also include threats to civilian protection.

Throughout this decade we have been in the midst of that transition. In the former Yugoslavia and Rwanda, the international security regime failed to act decisively to end wars that caused great civilian suffering. Humanitarian and human rights organisations decried the role that international relief organisations were forced to play, filling a power vacuum, assuaging the conscience of the international community.[25] In northern Iraq, in Somalia, and again in Kosovo, various sets of international political and military actors took more aggressive action, in each case different, and in each case with mixed and disputed results.

Discussion and Force

As we continue through this transition the humanitarian community, including those in medical relief organisations, must participate in the discussion and develop strategies that would maximise the humanitarian resources available under a given set of political and security constraints. In settings where the consent of warring parties can be obtained such options include establishing humanitarian corridors, delivering targeted relief, planning the safe exit of a population from an emergency, and creating protected areas.

If the warring parties do not consent and civilians continue to be at risk, the international community must consider using force to uphold international humanitarian law. The UN Security Council might consider intervening under chapter VII to re-establish the necessary conditions for providing humanitarian assistance and protecting civilians. These conditions might include creating and enforcing security corridors and areas, protecting humanitarian convoys, disarming populations or groups, and deploying forces to protect civilians. These measures might be particularly relevant in situations that have generated, as a consequence of grave violations of international humanitarian law, major displacements of population and widening social chaos, further contributing to regional and international instability. As in Kosovo, the use of force, in association with diplomatic negotiation, could help to restore a minimal political and security environment, thus permitting delivery of humanitarian assistance and restoration of minimum levels of civilian protection.

Whenever any of these strategies have been attempted during this decade, some humanitarian analysts and practitioners have raised concerns about the mixture of humanitarian and political goals.[26, 27] The use of force mandated by the Security Council or regional organisations entails political agendas that may jeopardise the neutrality of protective humanitarian arrangements.[28] Furthermore, the use of force against warring parties may put civilians at even more at risk, as their status and safety become central issues in resolving the conflict. Finally, the extent to which UN Security Council members consider internal conflicts of the magnitude of the Kosovo crisis or the Rwanda genocide to be within the competence of the council remains to be ascertained. The question then arises as to which regional organisation, when, and on what grounds, can be permitted to intervene?

A Role for the Humanitarian Community

Yet many humanitarian organisations, including many engaged in medical relief, have already begun to accumulate experience in humanitarian interventions that involve a mixture of players—civilian, security, and military.[29] The future success of these strategies of humanitarian intervention will depend to a large extent on the ability of humanitarian organisations to engage the interest of political and security authorities in the task of developing clear, adequate, and practical options for protecting civilians.[30] It is also possible that, having participated in and witnessed a series of failures and partial small gains, having played a bit part in a drama determined by others, the humanitarian community could in future decide to play a significant role in mobilising political authorities around specific preferred strategic options.[31] It comes back to the aim of creating in times of war a distinct and neutral place for civilians, where medical and relief workers can reach the population and build a system of adequate supports, sustainable for as long as is necessary. The end is the same as that described in the fourth Geneva Convention of 1949, but the means no longer obtain. The world and its wars have changed, so other means to secure that same high purpose have to be developed and deployed.

REFERENCES

1. Russbach R, Fink D. Humanitarian action in current armed conflicts: Opportunities and obstacles. *Med Global Survival* 1994; 1: 188–99.
2. Sivard RL. *World military and social expenditures 1996.* Washington, DC: World Priorities, 1996.
3. Kaldor M, Vashee B, eds. *Restructuring the global military sector.* Vol 1. *New wars.* London: Pinter, 1997.
4. Leaning J. When the system doesn't work: Somalia 1992. In: Cahill KM, ed. *A framework for survival: health, human rights, and humanitarian assistance in conflicts and disasters.* New York: Basic Books, Council on Foreign Relations, 1993:103–20.
5. Ramsbotham O, Woodhouse T. *Humanitarian intervention in contemporary conflict.* Cambridge: Polity Press, 1996: 167–92.
6. Jean F. The problems of medical relief in the Chechen war zone. *Central Asian Survey* 1996; 15: 255–8.
7. Hansen G. Aid in war-ravaged Chechnya: a severe test for humanitarians. *Christian Science Monitor* 1997 Dec 31: 19.
8. Physicians for Human Rights. *Medical group documents systematic and pervasive abuses by Serbs against Albanian Kosovar health professionals and Albanian Kosovar patients.* Boston: PHR, 1998. (Preliminary report 23 December.)
9. British Medical Association. *Torture report.* London: BMA, 1986.
10. British Medical Association. *Medicine betrayed.* London: Zed Books, 1992.
11. Geiger HJ, Leaning J, Shapiro LA, Simon B. *The casualties of conflict: medical care and human rights in the West Bank and Gaza Strip.* Boston: Physicians for Human Rights, 1988.
12. De Waal A, Leaning J. *No mercy in Mogadishu:* *the human cost of the conflict and the struggle for relief.* Boston, New York: Physicians for Human Rights, Africa Watch, 1992.
13. Physicians for Human Rights. *Medicine under siege in the former Yugoslavia 1991–1995.* Boston: PHR, 1996.
14. Africa Rights. *Genocide in Rwanda.* London: Africa Rights, 1994.
15. Physicians for Human Rights. *War crimes in Kosovo 1998–1999.* Boston: PHR, 1999.
16. Porter K. Human rights medicine. 1. An introduction. *Student BMJ* 1996; 4: 146–7.
17. US Mission to the UN. *Global humanitarian emergencies, 1998.* New York: United Nations, 1998.
18. O'Donnell D. Trends in the application of international humanitarian law by United Nations human rights mechanisms. *Int Rev Red Cross* 1998; 324: 481–503.
19. Boutroue J. *Missed opportunities: the role of the international community in the return of the Rwandan refugees from eastern Zaire July 1994–December 1996.* Cambridge: Massachusetts Institute of Technology, 1998.
20. Iacopino V, Rasekh Z, Yamin AE, Freedman L, Burkhalter H, Atkinson H, et al. *The Taliban's war on women: a health and human rights crisis in Afghanistan.* Boston: Physicians for Human Rights, 1998.
21. Joint Evaluation of Emergency Assistance to Rwanda. *The International response to conflict and genocide: Lessons from the Rwanda experience.* Copenhagen: Steering Committee of the Joint Evaluation of Emergency Assistance to Rwanda, 1996.
22. Ignatieff M. *The warrior's honor: ethnic war and the modern conscience.* New York: Henry Holt, 1997.
23. Hart M, van Praet S. The Sudan: dying a slow death. In: *World in crisis: The politics of survival at the end of the 20th century.* London, New York: Médecins Sans Frontières, 1997: 181–203.
24. Brett R, McCallin M. *Children: the invisible soldiers.* Stockholm: Swedish Save the Children, 1998.
25. Martin I. Hard choices after genocide: human rights and political failures in Rwanda. In: Moore JM, ed. *Hard choices: moral dilemmas in humanitarian intervention.* Lanham, MD: Rowman and Littlefield, 1998: 157–75.
26. De Waal A. Humanitarianism unbound? *Current dilemmas facing multimandate relief operations in political emergencies.* London: African Rights, 1994.
27. Perrin P. The risks of military participation. In: Leaning J, Briggs SM, Chen LC, eds.

Humanitarian crises: the medical and public health response. Cambridge: Harvard University Press, 1999: 309–23.

28. Sandoz, Y. The establishment of safety zones for persons displaced within their country of origin. In: Al-Nauimi NN, Meese R, eds. *International legal issues arising under the United Nations Decade of International Law.* Dordrecht: Kluwer Law International, 1995: 899–927.

29. Minear L, Weiss TG. *Humanitarian action in times of war: a handbook for practitioners.* London: Lynne Rienner, 1993.

30. Stremlau J. *People in peril: human rights, humanitarian action, and preventing deadly conflict.* New York: Carnegie Corporation, 1998.

31. Weiss TG. *Military-civilian interactions: intervening in humanitarian crises.* Lanham, MD: Rowman and Littlefield, 1999.

QUESTIONS

1. In the last line of the chapter, the authors remark, "The world and its wars have changed, so other means to secure that same high purpose have to be developed and deployed." How have the "world and its wars" changed and why? In general, how do the authors suggest that the means to secure the fourth Geneva Convention must change? Whose responsibility is it to instigate this change? Do you expect the "world and its wars" to continue to change and, if so, how?

2. Consider the fourth Geneva Convention and rules of war in general. Why is there an ever-increasing blur between combatants and noncombatants? What is meant by the US-invented term "enemy combatant," and how does the term relate to international humanitarian law?

3. How has the US "war on terror" changed the global understanding of the rules of war? Can this war ever end?

FURTHER READING

1. Solis, Gary D., *The Law of Armed Conflict: International Humanitarian Law in War.* Cambridge: Cambridge University Press, 2010.

2. Weissman, Fabrice, *In the Shadow of 'Just Wars': Violence, Politics and Humanitarian Action.* London: Hurst, 2004.

3. Byers, Michael, *War Law: Understanding International Law and Armed Conflicts.* New York: Grove Press, 2006.

4. Polman, Linda, *The Crisis Caravan: What's Wrong with Humanitarian Aid?* New York: Metropolitan Books, 2010.

CHAPTER 18

Torture and Public Health

Linda Piwowarczyk, Sondra Crosby, Denali Kerr and Michael A. Grodin

INTRODUCTION

Historically, the practice of torture focused on the dyad of the torturer and his or her victim in the quest to obtain information. In the past few decades it has become clear that the impact of torture is far beyond the individual and includes society as a whole. The practice of torture is an attempt to instill fear in the community, not merely to oppress a single individual, and as such, the public health impact of torture is far reaching. In response to increasing recognition of torture as a public health problem, a field of research is evolving which seeks how best to help survivors. International law has also provided mechanisms to hold perpetrators accountable. However, the ultimate human rights and public health goal is to prevent torture from occurring at all.

DEFINING TORTURE

Torture has been practiced over the centuries, at times in public view and often with social and government sanction. But it was only in the wake of the atrocities of World War II that torture was publicly condemned as an abuse of human rights. Article 5 of the Universal Declaration of Human Rights (1948), proclaimed that "No one shall be subjected to torture or cruel, inhuman or degrading treatment or punishment" The World Medical Association's Declaration of Tokyo (1975) provided the first explicit definition of torture, declaring that it was the "deliberate, systematic or wanton infliction of physical or mental suffering by one or more persons acting alone or on the orders of any authority, to force another person to yield information, to make a confession, or for any other reason." Ten years later, governments united to denounce state-sponsored torture when they ratified the Convention Against Torture and Other Cruel Inhuman or Degrading Treatment or Punishment (1984) which defines torture as:

any act by which severe pain or suffering, whether physical or mental is intentionally inflicted on a person for such purposes as obtaining from him or her or a third person information or a confession, punishing him for an act he or a third person has committed, or intimidating or coercing him or a third person, or for any reason based on discrimination of any kind, when such suffering is inflicted by or at the instigation of or with the consent or acquiescence of a public official or other person acting in an official capacity. It does not include pain or suffering arising from, inherent in or incidental to lawful sanctions.

Today there are many international and regional instruments prohibiting torture and ill-treatment, which are listed in Table 18.1 Some of those declarations and treaties have helped develop mechanisms by which torture can be monitored and perpetrators held accountable, which is discussed further on.

Table 18.1 International instruments on the absolute prohibition of torture and ill treatment

Universal texts on torture

The United Nations Charter
International Covenant on Civil and Political Rights
Optional Protocol to the International Covenant on Civil and Political Rights
International Covenant on Economic, Social and Cultural Rights
Convention against Torture and Other Cruel, Inhuman or Degrading Treatment or
 Punishment
Convention on the Rights of the Child
International Convention on the Elimination of All Forms of Racial Discrimination
Convention on the Elimination of All Forms of Discrimination Against Women
Optional Protocol to the Convention on the Elimination of Discrimination against Women
Convention on the Prevention and Punishment of the Crime of Genocide
International Convention on the Suppression and Punishment of the Crime of Apartheid

Nonbinding texts adopted by the UN

Universal Declaration of Human Rights
Declaration on the Protection of All Persons from Being Subjected to Torture and Other Cruel,
 Inhuman or Degrading Treatment or Punishment
Vienna Declaration and Programme of Action
Declaration on the Elimination of Violence Against Women
Declaration on the Protection of Women and Children in Emergency and Armed Conflict
United Nations Standard Minimum Rules for the Administration of Juvenile Justice
United Nations Rules for the Protection of Juveniles Deprived of Liberty
Body of Principles for the Protection of All Persons under Any Form of Detention or
 Imprisonment
Basic Principles for the Treatment of Prisoners
Standard Minimum Rules for the Treatment of Prisoners Principles of Medical Ethics relevant to
 the Role of Health Personnel, particularly Physicians, in the Protection of Prisoners and
 Detainees against Torture and Other Cruel, Inhuman or Degrading Treatment or Punishment
Basic Code of Conduct for Law Enforcement Officials
Basic Principles on the Use of Force and Firearms by Law Enforcement Officials
Guidelines on the Role of Prosecutors
Declaration of Basic Principles of Justice for Victims of Crime and Abuse of Power
Declaration on the Human Rights of Individuals who are not Nationals of the Country in which
 They Live
Declaration on the Protection of all Persons from Enforced Disappearance
United Nations Declaration on the Elimination of All Forms of Racial Discrimination
Declaration on the Right and Responsibility of Individuals, Groups, and Organs of Society to
 Promote and Protect
Universally Recognized Human Rights and Fundamental Freedoms

Prohibition of torture in humanitarian law

Common Article 3 of the Geneva Conventions
Geneva Convention for the Amelioration of the Condition of the Wounded and Sick in Armed
 Forces in the Field
Geneva Conventions for the Amelioration of the Condition of Wounded, Sick, and Shipwrecked
 Members of Armed Forces at Sea

Table 18.1 (Continued)

Geneva Convention relative to the Treatment of Prisoners of War
Geneva Convention relative to the Protection of Civilian Persons in Time of War
Protocol I Additional to the Geneva Conventions of 12 August 1949, and relating to the Protection of Victims of International Armed Conflicts
Protocol II Additional to the Geneva Conventions of 12 August 1949, and relating to the Protection of Victims of Non-International Armed Conflicts

Prohibition of torture in the international criminal court and the ad hoc tribunals

Statute of the International Criminal Tribunal for the Former Yugoslavia
Statute of the International Criminal Tribunal for the Rwanda
Rome Statue of the International Criminal Court

Regional texts concerning torture

African Charter on Human and Peoples' Rights
African Charter on the Right and Welfare of the Child
American Convention on Human Rights
Inter-American Convention to Prevent and Punish Torture
Inter-American Convention on the Prevention, Punishment and Eradication of Violence Against Women
Inter-American Convention on the Forced Disappearance of Persons
European Convention for the Protection of Human Rights and Fundamental Freedoms
European Convention for the Prevention of Torture and Inhuman or Degrading Treatment or Punishment
Resolution 690(1979) on the Declaration on the Police
Recommendation No. R(87) 3 of the Committee of Ministers to Member States on the European Prison Rules
Recommendation No. R(98) 7 of the Committee of Ministers to Member States concerning Ethical and Organizational Aspects of Health Care in Prisons
Recommendation No. R(99) 3 of the Committee of Ministers to Member States on the Harmonization of Medico-Legal Autopsy Rules
Concluding Document of the Third Follow-up Meeting (OSCE/CSCE)
Document of the Copenhagen Meeting of the Conference on Human Dimension and the OSCE
Document of the Moscow Meeting of the Conference on the Human Dimension of the OSCE
Charter for Human Security
Charter of the Fundamental Rights of the European Union
Guidelines to EU policy towards third countries on torture and other cruel, inhuman or degrading treatment or punishment
The Cairo Declaration on Human Rights in Islam
Arab Charter on Human Rights

Compiled by L. Piwowarczyk from International Rehabilitation Council for Torture Victims (2006) International Instruments and Mechanisms for the Fight Against Torture: A Compilation of Legal Instruments and Standards on Torture. Copenhagen: IRCT. http://www.irct.org/Default.aspx?lD=159&M=News&PID=5&NewsID=39

EPIDEMIOLOGY

As the global community has turned its attention to torture, reporting of torture has increased. The Amnesty International (AI) Annual Report (2006) showed that torture and ill-treatment currently occur in 150 countries. However, torture still goes underreported. Survivors often choose not to disclose their experiences because of fear of putting themselves and their families in further danger, impairment of memory resulting from torture, cultural sanctions, or simply as a coping strategy (Mollicia and Caspi-Yavin, 1991). Therefore, it is difficult to determine the true prevalence of torture.

Complex humanitarian disasters, characterized by massive population dislocation, are often accompanied by an erosion of international humanitarian law and a breakdown of security which put individuals at greater risk of being subject to torture. Torture is frequently an element of war, conflict, ethnic and religious persecution, and ethnic cleansing, although it can also be an isolated event. Today, there are 9.2 million refugees and approximately 10 million people of concern (asylum seekers, returned refugees, internally displaced persons, stateless persons, and others) who are at high risk for human rights abuses (UN High Commission for Refugees, 2006). Torture can be found in 5–30% of the world's refugees, and in even higher percentages in certain ethnic groups (Baker, 1992; Jaranson *et al.*, 2004). Efforts have been made in a variety of settings to document the prevalence and incidence of torture in community and clinic samples, and across specific cultural groups and ethnicities; the results are summarized in Table 18.2.

TORTURE AS A PUBLIC HEALTH PROBLEM

Impact

Torture is highly destructive toward individuals and can have long-term physical

Table 18.2 Prevalence of torture

Type of sample	Author[a]	Sample Size	Location	Prevalence
National	De Jong *et al.*, 2001		Algeria	8%
			Cambodia	9%
			Gaza	15%
			Ethiopia	26%
	Modvig, 2001		1033 East Timor households in 13 districts	39%
Prison detainees	Paker *et al.*, 1992	246	Turkish prisons	85%
Refugees	Shresta *et al.*, 1998	85078	Bhutanese refugees in a UNHCR camp in Nepal	2.74%
	Iacopino *et al.*, 2001	1180	Kosovar refugees in Albanian and Macedonian camps	3%
	Tang and Fox, 2001	242	Senegalese in two refugee camps in Gambia	16%
General ambulatory clinics	Crosby *et al.*, 2006	142	Foreign-born- Boston hospital, USA	11%
	Eisenman *et al.*, 2000	638	Three primary care Latino clinics in Los Angeles, USA	8%
	Eisenman and Keller, 2000	121	Foreign-born- New York hospital, USA	6.6%
Selective ethnic	Lie, 2002	426	Resettled refugees in 20 municipalities in Norway (5/04–9/05)	6%
groups	Montgomery and Foldspang	74	Middle Eastern asylum seekers	30%
		218	Airline list of accepted refugees arriving in Sweden	51%
	Elkblad *et al.*, 2002	622	Somalis resettled in Minneapolis St. Paul, Minn, USA	36%
	Jaranson *et al.*, 2004	512	Oromos (of Ethiopia)	55%
	Marshall *et al.*, 2005	586	Cambodians in Long Beach, California	54%

a Cited in Quiroga and Jaranson (2005).

and psychological effects on survivors, which are summarized in Table 18.3 and Table 18.4. There is international discourse about the potential psychological sequelae in torture survivors, and at one time, questions were raised as to the presence of a torture syndrome. This idea was replaced by Western phenomenology using diagnostic criteria such as 'post-traumatic stress disorder' and 'depression.' Globally questions have been raised about the possibility of different cultural expressions of traumatic stress, which require more cross-cultural research to be resolved.

Table 18.3 Physical findings in torture survivors

Skin	Scars from lesions inflicted by torture, such as abrasions, contusions, lacerations, puncture wounds, cutting wounds, gunshot wounds; burns from cigarettes or heated instruments; electrical injuries; injuries to nail beds
Face	Evidence of fracture, crepitation, swelling or pain
Eyes	Conjunctival hemorrhage, lens dislocation, subhyeloid hemorrhage, retrobullar hemorrhage, retinal hemorrhage, and visual loss
Ears	Rupture of the tympanic membrane; hearing loss; otorrhea, vestibular dysfunction
Nose	Misalignment, crepitation, and deviation of the nasal septum
Jaw, neck, oropharynx	Mandibular fractures and/or dislocations, temporomandibular joint syndrome, crepitation of the hyoid bone or laryngeal cartilages, lesions in the oropharynx, injury to parotid gland or ducts
Oral cavity/ teeth	Tooth avulsions, fractures of the teeth, dislocated fillings and broken prostheses
Chest and abdomen	Lesions of the skin; pain; tenderness and discomfort related to injuries of the musculature, ribs (including rib fractures), or abdominal organs; retroperitoneal, intramuscular, and intra-abdominal hematomas
Musculoskeletal system	Musculoskeletal aches and pains including changes in mobility of joints, contractures, compartment syndrome (acutely), fractures with or without deformity, and dislocations, amputations
Genitourinary system	In females: bruises, lacerations, tears, bleeding, or vaginal discharge, ecchymoses, sexually transmitted diseases (including human immunodeficiency virus), scarring, and deformity. In males: pain and sensitivity, hydrocele and hematocele, testicular torsion, erectile dysfunction, injuries to the penile ligaments, strictures, atrophy of the testes, and scarring anal region: fissures, rectal tears, disruption of the rugal pattern/scarring, skin tags, and purulent drainage
Central nervous system	Cognitive and mental status changes; motor and sensory neuropathies related to trauma (including painful peripheral neuropathies); brachial plexopathy; radiculopathies; cranial nerve deficits; hyperalgesia; parathesias; hyperesthesia; change in position and temperature sensation, motor function; gait and coordination disturbances

Adapted from Plwowarczyk LA, Moreno A, and Grodin M (2000) Health care of torture survivors. *Journal of the American Medical Association* 284(5): 539–541. Copyright© 2000 American Medical Association.

Table 18.4 Common psychological responses to torture

Posttraumatic stress disorder
Somatic complaints such as pain and headaches
Depressive disorders
Substance abuse
Neuropsychological impairment
Psychosis
Enduring personality change
Generalized anxiety disorder
Panic disorder
Acute stress disorder
Somatoform disorders
Bipolar disorder
Phobias

Adapted from Piwowarczyk LA, Moreno A, and Grodin M (2000) Health care of torture survivors. *Journal of the American Medical Association* 284(5): 539–541. Copyright © 2000 American Medical Association. All rights reserved.

Torture can take many different forms, some of which are quite common and others that are specific to certain geographic regions. Examples of different forms of torture are listed in Table 18.5. As a response to the increase in human rights monitoring over the past few decades, torture methods are now often devised so that they leave no physical signs or evidence of torture after the fact (Forrest, 1996).

Although torture victims are sometimes killed, the true aim of torture is not murder, but to send a message of fear to the community through the returning

Table 18.5 Examples of the forms of torture

Beating
   with hands or fists
   with batons, rods, sticks, canes, whips on the soles of the feet (falanga) resulting in head trauma
Kicking, pushing, being jumped on
Being suspended or restrained
Being forced to hold certain body positions
Forced to walk on one's knees
Electric shocks
Asphyxiation
   choking, submersion, with chemicals
   dry asphyxiation: covering of head with plastic bag, use of ligature
Burned
   with cigarette butts, rubber, wax, hot oil, or battery acid
Excessive noise, cold, heat, isolation
Sexual violence
   rape, attempted rape
   nudity or humiliation
   instrumentation
   direct sexual trauma
Waterboarding
Threats to self or family
Mock executions
Forced to sign fake confessions or denounce others
Witness the torture of others
Forced to participate in the torture of others

victim. The traumatic effects of torture can be transmitted intergenerationally to the family, thus spreading the impact beyond the individual (Danieli, 1998). Torture also has impacts on the broader community by sowing widespread mistrust of the government and social structures. When military and police officials commit acts of torture, they undermine the relationship between peoples and their government. Sadly, health professionals also sometimes participate in torture; physicians and psychiatrists can be employed to monitor torture, approve its continuation, and write fraudulent documentation, including death certificates and medical records of injuries sustained by torture victims (Miles, 2006). These acts of complicity by medical professionals validate the culture of torture. The impacts of torture on a community which must live in constant fear of reprisals affect the ability of citizens to challenge the status quo or speak in favor of human rights.

Prevention

The end goal of human rights advocates and health professionals is the complete eradication of torture. However, there are many levels to the prevention of torture. Primary prevention focuses on high-risk groups which may be recruited for involvement in torture, including medical professionals and law enforcement officials, and uses training to help these individuals prevent acts of torture. Secondary prevention can include human rights monitoring in areas of social unrest or political instability. Tertiary prevention encompasses the institution of legal frameworks which allow survivors of torture to seek justice and restitution.

Public involvement in the prevention of torture is helpful in bringing pressure on governments and also important because civilians are frequently targeted for torture.

When a spotlight is placed on any known acts of torture, perpetrators are more likely to be held accountable for their actions, and society engages in broad discussions about the inalienability of certain human rights. Increased public awareness of the prevalence of torture and its impacts on society makes it more difficult for perpetrators to attempt to justify their actions as necessary for the defense or stability of society.

Health professionals, especially, can engage in the prevention of torture on many levels. Not only can physicians provide direct care to survivors and provide expert testimony for individuals seeking asylum, but also public health professionals in general can act on the front lines of torture prevention through identification of possible victims and perpetrators, research on torture, and education. It is critical for professional organizations around the world to speak out against torture, to support members working on behalf of survivors, and to hold accountable any health professionals involved in or complicit with acts of torture. There are specialized organizations for health and legal professionals, including Amnesty International, Physicians for Human Rights, Global Lawyers and Physicians, and Human Rights First. However, to reach a broader base of support it is important that broader national or international professional organizations, such as the American Medical Association and the World Medical Association, take on torture as a health problem. Clear ethical statements and guidelines by professional organizations about involvement in torture are important aids to prevention, as is offering continuing education to members. Advocacy for not just an end to torture itself but also for strong international humanitarian law and legal frameworks of accountability is critical for solving the problem.

Legal Frameworks for Reporting and Responding to Torture

The first campaign against torture launched by Amnesty International (AI) in December 1972 was meant to educate the public and engage governments in ending torture. In 1984, AI's second campaign developed a 12-point program for the prevention of torture (Amnesty International, 1983). This campaign added weight to the Convention Against Tormre and Other Criminal, Inhuman, or Degrading Treatment or Punishment, which was adopted by the United Nations (UN) in that same year, although it didn't come into force until 1987. This convention requires state parties to outlaw and prevent torture within their borders, and speaks to the complete indefensibility of torture as well as the need for accountability. It also established a monitoring body, the Committee against Torture, which in certain jurisdictions conducts investigations, hears complaints against torture, and receives state reports on states' compliance with the Convention.

Since the Convention against Torture went into effect, several other monitoring bodies have been created. The Special Rapporteur on Torture reports to the UN High Commission on Human Rights, which investigates complaints. In addition, the Optional Protocol to the UN Convention against Torture (United Nations General Assembly, 2002) put in place a subcommittee to the UN Committee against Torture, international visiting bodies, and a national visiting body which go to detention centers to monitor for torture. The work of the Committee for the Prevention of Torture has shown that monitoring can (1) provide opportunities to make recommendations about conditions and procedures; (2) facilitate ongoing communication between authorities and detention personnel; (3) provide support to detainees; and (4) encourage detention personnel to improve conditions (United Nations, 2002).

The European Convention for the Prevention of Torture (1989) established a further commitment to monitor special populations, including persons institutionalized in psychiatric hospitals and prisons. The terms of this convention allow monitors unlimited access to any persons "deprived of their liberty by a public authority." The visiting committee can then make private recommendations to the government, which will be made public if the recommendations go unheeded. This regional commitment to preventing torture provides support for international efforts to go further with monitoring for human rights abuses.

One area of the Convention against Torture that still needs much support to be put into effect is that addressing the issue of reparations. Article 14 of the Convention against Torture states that victims of torture "shall obtain redress, compensation, and rehabilitation from the state." As of 2003, there still existed large discrepancies between this law and its implementation, and a study concluded that perpetrator impunity is currently the single largest obstacle both to the prevention of torture and to obtaining equitable reparations (Redress Trust, 2003). In *most* cases, torture survivors and their families do not have legal recourse or receive reparations of any kind. Although some survivors have received monetary compensation, there are no legal guarantees that torture will not recur, and survivors are not provided with rehabilitation. The paucity of data makes it difficult to quantify the number of complaints and determine whether reparation has been awarded. This is further aggravated by the fact that in many countries, torture is not an offense within domestic law, which limits the incentive to pursue and prosecute torturers.

Treatment and Rehabilitation of Survivors

In December 1972, Amnesty International engaged health professionals to document torture as part of their effort to abolish it (Eitinger and Weisaeth, 1980). A medical group affiliated with AI established the first Rehabilitation and Research Centre for Torture Victims (RCT) in Denmark in an effort to help survivors. Their initial publication in the *Danish Medical Bulletin* of the characteristics of 200 survivors from many countries shed light on torture and its effects and the potential role for health providers in healing and recovery, but it also heightened awareness of the role of health professionals in torture itself (Rasmussen and Lunde, 1980). The next major step forward in torture treatment came in 1999, when an ad hoc committee presented to the UN the *Manual on Effective Investigation and Documentation of Torture and Other Cruel, Inhuman or Degrading Treatment or Punishment*, now known as the Istanbul Protocol (Iacopino *et al.*, 1999). The Istanbul Protocol is a set of international guidelines on how to assess torture survivors, document and investigate torture, and present findings to judiciaries. It has been promoted by the UN and various nongovernmental organizations (NGOs), such as Physicians for Human Rights, Global Lawyers and Physicians, and Amnesty International, with the goal of global implementation.

There are now 119 programs in the International Rehabilitation Council for Torture Survivors (IRCT) network (International Rehabilitation Council for Torture Victims, 2006). The treatment movement overall contributes to the advance of human rights by (1) increasing knowledge that torture can have long-term effects contrary to what is postulated by torturers; (2) increasing awareness that torture and trauma can have intergenerational effects; (3) engaging the community in the recovery of survivors, leading to broader human rights-related activity; and (4) educating policymakers at treatment centers(Johnson, 1998).

Controversy exists as to whether the care of torture survivors should be mainstreamed or whether specialized centers should continue to operate and teach other providers and sectors of society (Gurr and Quiroga, 2001). Closing down the specialized centers would result in the loss of multidisciplinary services with expertise in engaging with the community and working with multicultural patients. However, the specialized centers cannot reach everyone in need of their services, so it is important torture treatment centers collaborate with local hospitals and networks of general health practitioners. Through cooperation between mainstream and specialized health centers, knowledge about the identification and rehabilitation of torture survivors can be disseminated, and survivors will be more likely to receive the care they need.

RESEARCH ON TORTURE

There are many challenges to researching torture. Although there are universal guidelines defining torture, individuals may define their experiences otherwise; for example, in some places, beatings are *so* commonplace that survivors of such brutality might not consider it torture. This can make it difficult to identify survivors. In addition, ethical issues arise when doing international or multicultural research. There may be limited understanding of informed consent in cultures unaccustomed to legal expectations of privacy or rights of refusal.

When research on torture occurs in a country where torture is taking place, there can be risks for both the researchers and the participants. Government operatives in some countries have harassed health professionals known to treat torture survivors (Physicians for Human Rights, 1996). If information from the study is released or leaked, the torture survivors may be exposed to risk of further abuses. Other ethical issues include the paucity of resources as an incentive for participation in studies, the power dynamics between the researcher and the participant, how the results will be used, and whether communities interviewed are benefited by their participation in research.

Research can also occur in receiving countries to which torture survivors flee for asylum. In these countries there can be additional stressors for the survivor such as persecution, loss, bereavement, and the challenges of acculturation, all of which confound the effects of torture. In addition, when research or treatment involves extensive questioning that may simulate interrogation, there *is* a risk of retraumatizing the survivor.

A great deal of research is needed on the effects of torture. Quantitative studies could elicit the psychobiological mechanisms of torture, the neuropsychological effects of head injury, the coping mechanisms of survivors, and the influences of culture and gender on the response to trauma. In addition, outcomes research to develop standardized assessment instruments and analyze the efficacy and cost-effectiveness of treatment approaches could aid in the development of highly responsive and effective treatment for torture survivors (Quiroga and Jaranson, 2005).

CONCLUSION

Torture is a global public health problem and an abuse of human rights that requires a multiperspective approach to its prevention. Public health professionals and human rights advocates must unite. Lawyers, doctors, researchers, educators, and politicians must come together to work on every angle of this issue. Health professionals in particular are in a unique position to work for the eradication of torture and the promotion of human rights. Whether through research, education, or advocacy, public health workers have the power to provide a far-reaching response to the problem of torture.

REFERENCES

Amnesty International (1983); (revised 2000 and 2005). *Amnesty international 12-Point Program for the Prevention of Torture by Agents of the State.*

Amnesty International (2006) *Annual Report 2006: The State of the World's Human Rights.* London: Amnesty International.

Baker R (1992) Psychological consequences for tortured refugees seeking asylum and refugee status in Europe. In: Basoglu M (ed.) *Torture and Its Consequences: Current Treatment Approaches,* 1st edn., pp. 83–106. Cambridge, UK: Cambridge University Press. .

Danieli Y (1998) *International Handbook of Multigenerational Legacies of Trauma.* New York: Plenum Press.

Eitinger Land Weisaeth L (1980) The Stockholm syndrome. *Tidsskrift for Den Norske Laegeforening* 100(5): 307–309.

Forrest D (1996) *A Glimpse of Hell: Reports on Torture Worldwide.* New York: New York University Press.

Gurr Rand Quiroga J (2001) Approaches to torture rehabilitation: A desk study covering effects, cost-effectiveness, participation, and sustainability. *Torture* 11 (Suppl 1): 1–35.

Iacopino V, Özkalipci Ö, and Schlar C (1999} *Manual on Effective Investigation and Documentation of Torture and Other Cruel, Inhuman or Degrading Treatment or Punishment* ("The Istanbul Protocol"). Geneva, Switzerland: United Nations Publications.

International Rehabilitation Council for Torture Victims (2006) *International Instruments and Mechanisms for the Right Against Torture: A Compilation of Legal Instruments and Standards on Torture.* Copenhagen, Denmark

Jaranson JM, Butcher J, Halcon L, *et al.* (2004) Somali and Oromo refugees: Correlates of torture and trauma history. *American Journal of Public Health* 94(4): 591–598.

Johnson D (1998) Healing torture survivors as a strategic advancement of human rights. *Torture* 8: 128–129.

Miles S (2006) *Oath Betrayed: Torture, Medical*

Complicity, and the War on Terror. New York. Random House.

Mollica RF and Caspi-Yavin Y (1991) Measuring torture and torture-related symptoms. *Psychological Assessment* 3(2): 1–7.

Physicians for Human Rights (1996) *Torture in Turkey and Its Unwilling Accomplices.* Cambridge, MA: Physicians for Human Rights.

Piwowarczyk LA, Moreno A, and Grodin M (2000) Health care of torture survivors. *Journal of the American Medical Association* 284(5): 538–541.

Quiroga J and Jaranson J (2005) Politically-motivated torture and its survivors: A desk-study review of the literature. *Torture* 15(2–3): 1–111.

Rasmussen OV and Lunde I (1980) Evaluation of investigation of 200 torture victims. *Danish Medical Bulletin* 27: 241–243.

Redress Trust (2003) *Reparation for Torture: A Survey of Law and Practice in Thirty Selected Countries.* London: Redress Trust. United Nations General Assembly (2002) *Optional Protocol to the Convention Against Torture or Other Cruel, Inhuman, or Degrading Treatment or Punishment.* New York: United Nations.

United Nations High Commissioner for Refugees (2006) *The State of the World's Refugees: Human Displacement in the New Millennium.* New York: Oxford University Press.

QUESTIONS

1. The authors states "in the past few decades it has become clear that the impact of torture goes far beyond the individual, and includes society as a whole." How does torture impact the "society as a whole"? What are the implications of this broad impact for human rights campaigning? What is the difference between primary, secondary and tertiary prevention of torture?

2. What is the definition of torture, and what are its goals? In what context might you find an alternate definition of torture? Why does this matter? Why is it difficult to collect epidemiologic data regarding torture?

3. Amnesty International's 12 point program to prevent torture includes: condemn torture, prosecute, and provide reparation. Which of these do you think is the most effective and why? The full 12 points are on Amnesty's website.

FURTHER READING

1. United Nations, *Istanbul Protocol Manual on the Effective Investigation and Documentation of Torture and Other Cruel, Inhuman or Degrading Treatment or Punishment.* New York: United Nations, 2004. http://search.ebscohost.com/login.aspx?direct=true&scope=site&db=nlebk&db=nlabk&AN=131338.

2. Wilson, John P., & Droek, Boris, *Broken Spirits: The Treatment of Traumatized Asylum Seekers, Refugees, War, and Torture Victims.* New York: Brunner-Routledge, 2004.

3. Baolu, Metin, *Torture and Its Consequences: Current Treatment Approaches.* Cambridge: Cambridge University Press, 1992.

4. Siems, Larry, *The Torture Report: What the Documents Say About America's Post-9/11 Torture Program.* New York: OR Books, 2011.

5. Joshua Phillips, *None of Us Were Like This Before: American Soldiers and Torture.* New York: Verso, 2010.

CHAPTER 19

Asylum Seekers, Refugees, and the Politics of Access to Health Care: A UK Perspective

Keith Taylor

We must remember that the NHS is a national institution and not an international one . . . The aim of these proposals is to ensure that the NHS is first and foremost for the benefit of residents of this country.

John Hutton (former Minister for Health, 2004)[1]

It is the duty of a doctor . . . to be dedicated to providing competent medical service in full professional and moral independence, with compassion and respect for human dignity.

World Medical Association, Geneva Declaration 1948[2]

INTRODUCTION

The UK government has recently consulted on proposals to exclude some 'overseas visitors', including asylum seekers, from NHS care.[1] A judicial review took place at the high court in April 2008 regarding the rights of a failed asylum seeker to receive free hospital treatment in the UK.[3] In this case the government's policy of selectively prohibiting access to care was initially overturned although the government was successful in its appeal against this verdict.[4] This chapter will examine the wider ethical, moral, and political issues that are raised by this debate.

Studies suggest that in almost all indices of physical, mental, and social wellbeing, asylum seekers and refugees suffer a disproportionate burden of morbidity.[5–8] This population is already disempowered and restricted in access to services, and any further policy moves to limit access may therefore be unjust and exacerbate existing inequalities.

Many of the tensions at the heart of this debate provoke wider questions regarding the ethics of population health. How should we fund our healthcare system? Who should be entitled to care? Where and when should rationing be applied? How does society conduct this debate? These are some of the defining questions in the health inequalities arena. This paper will argue that this debate also raises far-reaching questions about the relationship between the NHS, society, government, and international governance.

SOME DEFINITIONS

The term 'refugee' covers immigrants at all stages in the asylum process. Under the Geneva Convention, this includes any individual fearing persecution for reasons of race, religion, nationality, social, or political group, and who is consequently unwilling or unable to return to their home country.[9] The UK categorises refugees according to the definitions outlined in Box 19.1.[10]

The UK is a signatory to the European Convention on Human Rights, the United

---

BOX 19.1 DEFINITIONS OF REFUGEE STATUS (ADAPTED FROM BUR-NETT AND PEEL, 2001) [10]

- Asylum seeker: claim submitted (awaiting verdict).
- Refugee status: given leave to remain for 4 years and can then apply for indefinite leave. Restricted entitlement to family reunion.
- Indefinite leave to remain: indefinite residence. Restricted entitlement to family reunion.
- Exceptional leave to remain: right to remain for up to 4 years but expected to return to home country.
- Refusal: person has right of appeal within strict time limits and criteria.

Nations Convention Against Torture, and the International Covenant on Economic, Social and Cultural Rights. These treaties oblige host countries to protect the most vulnerable people, offer 'the highest attainable standard of health', and specify not to limit equal access to health care.[11]

In some ways the Home Office application process is an attempt to homogenise an extremely diverse cohort. The demographic mix of the migrant population varies hugely, depending on the current geopolitical climate.[12] Consequently, refugees' health needs are diverse and they may differ as much from each other as they do from the domestic population. Nevertheless, there are several unifying themes that affect all migrant groups in terms of their physical, psychological, and social wellbeing.

THE UK ASYLUM PROCESS

Ultimately, decisions on immigration lie with the UK Home Office. By definition, demographic data for this population are difficult to collect. Numbers are possibly underestimated, as only those living in the country who have lodged an official application or appeal are included.[13, 14]

Pressure on migration is multifactorial and dependent on numerous host and recipient sociopolitical factors (including war, famine, and poverty).[12] Recently, the most common nationalities seeking asylum have included Eritrean, Afghan, Iranian, Chinese, and Somali (countries where torture, war, anarchy, and other human rights abuses are commonplace). There is little evidence that migrants are specifically attracted by access to a higher standard of living or the welfare system.[11, 15] Nevertheless, this remains a dominant perspective in some aspects of public debate.[16]

Asylum applications in the UK were at a peak of over 80,000 in 2002. Since then, this has reduced and remained at approximately 25,000 per year. The majority of applications tend to be unsuccessful. For example, of all applications lodged in 2006 only 10% were granted refugee status. Of those who were able to launch an appeal against this decision, 73% were dismissed.[13]

'Failed' asylum seekers are not necessarily 'bogus' asylum seekers, but have been unable to establish 'to a reasonable degree of likelihood' that they would suffer persecution if they were to return to their home nation. It is estimated that there may be as many as 450,000 failed asylum seekers remaining in the UK.[17, 18]

For individuals the process can be lengthy, bureaucratic, and confusing. At any one time an individual may be lodging an application, awaiting a decision, awaiting an appeal, or have been refused asylum. For some this can take several years.[19] The length and complexity of this process has been criticised by the United Nations (UN), the House of Commons Home Affairs Committee, and several campaign groups.[20] In comparison with its neighbours, the UK currently ranks 12th for number of asylum seekers per head of population.[11]

HEALTH ISSUES AFFECTING ASYLUM SEEKERS

Health needs assessment data for UK asylum seekers are scarce.[21] Evidence suggests that asylum seekers fare worse than the UK population on almost all measures of health and wellbeing. The health effects of the immigration process may be considered in terms of the past and present consequences of forced migration (Figure 19.1).

For this group, there is an unequal distribution not only of ill-health but also of the social determinants of ill-health (including poverty, social isolation, literacy, self-efficacy, and so on). It is generally agreed that there is a reciprocal relationship between ill-health and these wider determinants.[22] This is a crucial point in considering how

to reduce health inequalities, as it may not simply be a question of providing 'more or better' health care.[23]

Physical Health

Physical health needs of migrants tend to reflect the endemic spectrum of disease in their home country. Thus, infectious disease including HIV, tuberculosis, malaria, and other parasitic diseases are often more prevalent among immigrants from sub-Saharan Africa.[5, 6] In many refugees from eastern Europe, higher rates of chronic disease, including diabetes and cardiovascular disease, have been reported.[7]

Other problems include poor dentition, malnutrition, and incomplete immunisation. In addition, health behaviour may be affected by forced migration. Several studies have reported a high prevalence of non-specific or somatising presentations as a result of psychosocial distress.[8]

Psychological Health

It is unsurprising that symptoms of depression, anxiety, and agoraphobia have been reported among refugees and asylum seekers.[5] These symptoms may result from

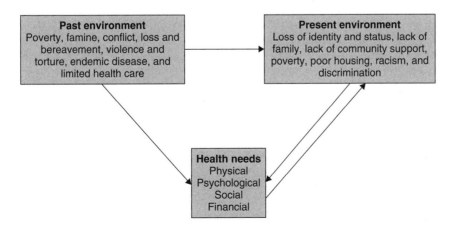

Figure 19.1 Model of health effects of forced migration and refugee status.

stressors including bereavement, displacement, or torture. Many of these symptoms are further exacerbated by conditions in the host country, including compulsory detention, poverty, unemployment, housing, and social isolation. Different cultures have different models for conceptualising mental health and seeking help, which may complicate the provision of services such as counselling.[24]

Although high rates of post-traumatic stress disorder (PTSD) have been reported,[25] much of the burden of illness may be beneath the level of formal psychiatric diagnosis.[26] It is paradoxical, however, that those affected may only be able to seek help through a medical system that may stigmatise or label them. A diagnosis of PTSD may be sought in support of an asylum application. Some argue that the solutions to most psychological distress among refugees require social rather than medical intervention.[8, 24]

Financial Issues

Most asylum seekers and refugees are impoverished on arrival. Many may have specific skills and training that they are prevented from using in the UK, thus fostering a culture of dependence.[27]

Those who apply for asylum are subsequently entitled to benefits equivalent to approximately 70% of normal income support. This is dependent on remaining at a particular allocated accommodation. If an individual moves (which could be for reasons of seeking a social support network or because of racist abuse) or if their claim is refused, their benefits cease immediately, often leading to destitution.

Under the Immigration and Asylum Act 1999, most asylum seekers are not entitled to additional welfare benefits. As well as these theoretical restrictions, there are significant practical ones. For example, applicants on a low income can claim exemption from prescription charges if they complete an AG2 form. However, this is 16 pages long and available only in English. Therefore, there is a potential gap between entitlement to and provision of support.[11]

Social Issues

Social isolation is common among migrants as they may be separated from their family, friends, and functional role in society. The effects of this can be powerful. One study of Iraqi refugees in the UK suggested that depression was more strongly associated with social isolation than with a past history of torture.[28] Many immigrants are deprived of the principles of respect, autonomy, and self-efficacy, which are increasingly thought of as contributing to positive health.[29]

Geographical Issues

Under the Immigration and Asylum Act 1999, many asylum seekers are relocated in areas with little experience of the needs of refugees. Some suggest that this may have worsened the problem of social isolation by actively discouraging integration.[17, 21]

Accommodation for asylum seekers is often in areas of existing deprivation, and they therefore inherit the same social determinants of ill-health as the native population, yet with additional barriers to care.

Detention is a particularly controversial topic, as there is increasing evidence that it leads to adverse mental health outcomes.[30, 31] As well as prompting humanitarian concern, there is no evidence that this functions as a 'deterrent' to immigration. This might suggest that this policy is being pursued more as a political gesture.[32]

Women and Children

The UN Convention on the Rights of the Child recognises that children often suffer disproportionately as a result of government policy.[33] Children face a double burden of lack of provision of current basic needs and future loss of opportunity through lack of education, socialisation, and normal development.[34, 35]

For women, there is the additional burden of child care and having to adapt to new roles and responsibilities. Women are more likely to report poor health and depression, yet in some cultures may be dependent on a man to disclose this. Women are often neglected in training and employment programmes. They are also more likely to suffer domestic violence and separation during periods of stress.[36] Refugee women are also less likely to engage in screening, health promotion, family planning, and maternity services.[7]

There is a clear burden of need among this diverse population. At present the NHS barely meets these needs. Even if the government were to improve access and provision of services, many individuals would encounter other barriers that may be institutionally discriminatory. These include difficulties with literacy, cultural sensitivity, interpretation, confidentiality, and racism.[37] For healthcare workers too, there is evidence of inadequate training, time, and resources to meet the needs of this group.[38]

ACCESS TO CARE

At present, government policy differentiates between access to primary and secondary care and between entitlement to 'routine' and 'emergency' treatment. The government also differentiates between failed asylum seekers and those who are applying for asylum. Current Department of Health guidance is summarised in Table 19.1.[39]

Table 19.1 Current entitlement of 'overseas visitors' to NHS treatment.

Status	*Primary Care*	*Secondary Care*
• Asylum seeker (application under under consideration) • Asylum seeker appealing refusal • Asylum seeker denied financial support but still claiming asylum • Given refugee status • Discretionary leave to remain • Given humanitarian protection[a]	Entitled to NHS treatment without charge (except prescription charges where exempt). Can register with GP. Exempt from charges for NHS hospital treatment.	
• Failed asylum seekers (including those awaiting departure)[b]	• GP practices have discretion to register under the NHS • Emergency treatment free of charge	• Not eligible for NHS treatment • Life-saving treatment should not be withheld but charge should be pursued in the event of recovery • If receiving treatment while under appeal this should be continued but discretion applied as to when treatment is 'completed' • Any further treatment is chargeable • Some exemptions apply (for example, tuberculosis)

a Humanitarian protection: technically this is not the same as asylum. The criteria for humanitarian protection are defined by the European Convention on Human Rights. The criteria for asylum are influenced by the United Nations Convention Relating to the Status of Refugees.

b The government's policy of selectively prohibiting access to care was initially overturned although the government was successful in its appeal against this verdict.[4, 39]

This two-tier system gives rise to several situations in which care may be deliberately withheld. For example, in the case of HIV, failed asylum seekers are entitled to testing and counselling but not to treatment of HIV with antiretroviral drugs. In the case of diabetes, patients may complete a course of treatment for complications but would not be entitled to ongoing care if their asylum appeal was subsequently unsuccessful.

Prior to the recent high court ruling, the government has advised that 'best practice is to ensure that overseas visitors are aware of the expectation to pay charges . . . before they start treatment, so they can consider alternatives like a return home, if they are well enough to travel'.[40] Most undocumented and failed asylum seekers will, of course, be unable to pay and in effect will be refused treatment.

A further implication of this policy is that the onus is placed on healthcare staff to discern a patient's immigration status. Some argue that this places doctors in the impossible position of either breaking the law by maintaining the principles of 'Good Medical Practice' and providing care on the basis of need, or complying with the current political imperative by applying a discriminatory policy.[41, 42]

Perhaps the fundamental issue here is the extent to which an individual doctor practising within the NHS is governed by a moral versus a political obligation. At present there is an uneasy tension between the NHS as a monopoly provider of health care on one hand, and on the other, the duty of the medical professional as an advocate for the care of the sick irrespective of issues of citizenship.

The Case of HIV

The case of HIV exemplifies some of the implications of recent policy. People of 'uncertain immigration status' are currently entitled to treatment for sexually transmitted infection and illnesses that may be a threat to public health. However, despite meeting these criteria, HIV is explicitly excluded from this list. There are a number of practical, ethical, and moral problems with this position.

First, there is a clear clinical case that treatment early in the disease may prevent long-term death, disease, and disability. Harm can therefore either be avoided in the present or at some point in the future (when there is a 'life-threatening situation' as defined by the Department of Health). There is no clear ethical argument for withholding intervention in the present, while permitting action in the future.[43]

Second, the concept of 'duty of easy rescue' holds, whereby minimal cost to an individual (the tax payer) should not prevent significant benefit to another (that is, to provide life-saving treatment).[44] In the context of the NHS as a whole, the cost of treating refused asylum seekers with antiretroviral therapy is minimal compared to the cost of not acting and treating the eventual consequences.[45]

Third, current 'loopholes' in the system lead to discrepancies that may be inconsistent and arbitrary. For example, HIV treatment may be available through genitourinary departments where residential status may be withheld, but not in obstetric departments where the full cost of care would payable. Treatment is allowed for 'life-threatening' or 'immediately necessary' situations and it could be argued this should include antiretroviral treatment for all women of childbearing age.

THE ETHICS OF POPULATION HEALTH

It may be argued that the inverse care law applies to refugees in the UK, whereby disproportionate needs are met by insufficient access, empowerment, and provision.[46, 47] The government proposes to restrict entitlement to care further. The ethical implications of this approach to provision of health care may be far reaching. In particular, it challenges us to define the basic rights that all patients may be entitled to as opposed to those rights that may be regarded as discretionary. In many ways this debate highlights the modern tension between a libertarian and egalitarian perspective of health care.[48]

The NHS was founded on the principle of universal care with equal access to all on the basis of need, and no charge at the point of care. For a number of reasons this value is being challenged.[49, 50] In particular, there is uncertainty over what services should be funded by the NHS and whose rights should take precedence.[51]

Proponents of restricted access on the basis of citizenship argue that allowing treatment of those of uncertain or illegal status would lead to further pressure on migration and 'health tourism'. There is little evidence for this proposition.[11] Most immigration is driven by much wider sociopolitical considerations than simply access to treatment.[15, 17, 52]

A further concern that has been raised is that the treasury should not fund highly expensive treatment to non-UK tax payers. There are three counter-arguments to this. First, in terms of cost–benefit analysis there is evidence that primary or secondary prevention (for example, antiretroviral therapy) may greatly curtail future spending on complications.[45] Second, the NHS does not currently differentiate between UK resident citizens on the basis of means. This is an extension of the libertarian view that all citizens have equal basic rights.[53] Third, the government covertly prohibits asylum seekers from skilled employment, and hence integration and contribution to tax revenue.

It could be argued then that the government is confusing two difficult yet distinct decision-making processes: the decision on immigration status and the decision on access to treatment for those who are already resident in the UK. Furthermore, by linking asylum application to the provision of health care, the government may be forcing health professionals to collude in applying the sharp end of immigration policy.[11]

TACKLING SOCIAL INJUSTICE

If we accept then that current treatment of refugees in the UK is unjust, how should we move to reduce inequalities? As with many health inequalities, it is not simply a case of providing 'more or better' health care. Experience has shown that many inequalities persist over time.[54] We must then also attend to their root causes. In doing so we should be cautious about medicalising what may be largely social problems.

It is likely that many of the strategies for reducing health inequalities in this population may also empower other marginalised groups to achieve their potential. Such potential benefits ought to be considered in any broad economic analysis. A vast improvement in data collection and needs assessment is an obvious precursor to planning service provision.[55]

Practical Solutions

Health screening should be made routinely available on entry to the UK. Tuberculosis screening is already supposed to occur, although coverage is variable.[6] The World Health Organization (WHO) strongly advises against compulsory testing for HIV due to fears it may be used to discriminate. Instead, immigrants should be offered voluntary testing and counselling.

One of the fundamental improvements in healthcare provision would be to overcome the information barrier. A coordinated interpretation and translation service may help interactions with healthcare staff. At present, this tends to vary significantly from area to area. The temptation to rely on family members should be avoided due to the potential for conflict of interest, although this should be challenged sensitively.[56, 57] Similarly, healthcare workers need prompt access to patients' records where available. Many asylum seekers tend to be registered as temporary residents, and a coordinated unified record may make this easier.

Many doctors mention time as a limiting factor in encounters with this group of patients.[38] Some argue that unless care of this population is incentivised, it will succumb to the pressure of competing demands.[58] Others suggest that continuity of care and an open narrative approach may help to address complex presentations progressively.[8] If so, then sophisticated communication skills may be required.[56, 57]

Advocacy may be essential for vulnerable patients who are not sure of what they can and cannot expect from the health service. This may also offer a stepping stone between the health service and voluntary sectors. Some authors suggest that investment in advocacy workers may be more efficient than providing more healthcare staff.[58] Specific steps to improve the health of women and children may be undertaken by the extended role of the health visitor, and liaison with the voluntary sector and support networks where they exist.

There is a need for further training throughout the health sector in areas of cultural, religious, and gender sensitivity.[19] Again, the benefits of this may apply to many other areas. Many of these strategies need multi-agency coordination, depending on the specific needs of the community.

Social Solutions

There is convincing evidence that social integration improves health outcomes for refugees.[30, 31] Education, employment, and social networks are the three main routes. As well as reducing isolation and dependency, integration may also improve future opportunities and provide financial gain and a sense of self-worth. For children, successful integration into schools can be enormously therapeutic.

In many areas of deprivation there is a need to improve the basic minimum standard of housing available.[59] Compulsory detention should be avoided on health and humanitarian grounds.[31]

Efforts to build social networks and support groups are necessary if a dispersal policy is to be successfully implemented.[19] This would avoid the inevitable process of asylum seekers moving to bigger cities for support. Where possible, support groups should be led by asylum seekers themselves and encouraged to identify their own needs. A growing body of evidence demonstrates the positive health impact of promoting social inclusion.[60]

The role of the voluntary sector is critical. It is uniquely flexible and responsive to local needs. There is potential, however, for the unintended consequence of excusing mainstream NHS services from responsibility. In the provision of primary care, for example, this may lead to a fragmented and uncoordinated approach whereby 'core services' are increasingly provided outside the NHS.[61]

Political Solutions: Advocacy and the Medical Profession

The care of refugees may bring the medical profession into direct conflict with the government.[62] The duty of a doctor as described by the General Medical Council is 'not to discriminate on the basis of race or background'.[63] The Geneva Declaration of the World Medical Association specifically exhorts doctors not to allow '... considerations of age, disease or disability, creed, ethnic origin, gender, nationality, political affiliation, race, sexual orientation, social standing or any other factor to intervene between my duty and my patient'.[2]

Some have criticised the British Medical Association (BMA) for being ready to condemn human rights abuses in other countries while being reluctant to criticise the UK government's approach to domestic health rights;[64] however, the BMA have responded to this criticism.[65]

One possible strategy for those who care for refugees is for doctors to offer voluntary or charitable care outside of the NHS. This may be difficult given the virtual monopoly that the NHS has on health care. The danger of this approach is that it may give rise to a piecemeal and unintegrated service that does not significantly reduce inequalities.

An alternative then is for the NHS as an employer to acknowledge that doctors may at times have a moral duty of care to patients that transcends their duty to the NHS itself. This is recognised to some extent in other contentious areas; for example, the right of doctors to object conscientiously to certain practices or, conversely, to exceed the norms of expected care.

Perhaps this argument is symptomatic of a greater contemporary tension within primary care between the utilitarian 'gatekeeper' and libertarian 'consumer–provider' roles. If primary care drifts further towards a consumerist model, then health inequalities may well widen. Moreover, there may be even less will or coordination among the profession to speak out and advocate against government policy.

International Perspective

This debate is not confined to the UK, as similar moral and political arguments may confront all developed countries. The UK is a signatory to the International Covenant on Economic, Social and Cultural Rights, the International Covenant on Civil and Political Rights, and the Universal Declaration of Human Rights. Together these form the International Bill of Human Rights, ratified by the UK in 1976.

The fact that these agreements are not justiceable raises questions about the nature of international governance itself. Worldwide, there are at least 20 million refugees. Most of the burden for care of refugees is currently placed on neighbouring countries that are themselves often greatly under-resourced.

A further implication of international agreements is that while they necessitate shared responsibility, they also permit limited responsibility. Thus the UK need do no more than any other state. The counter-argument is that the UK is one of the wealthiest countries in the world, and as such may have a moral responsibility to care for its inhabitants accordingly, that is to say it should be 'leading rather than following'.

Others would claim that the UK presently targets significant debt relief overseas, and that this may be a more sustainable way of reducing forced migration at its source. In a sense this may be a false dichotomy, as the issue ought to be whether or not care is offered rather than where that care is delivered. The two options are not mutually exclusive, however. Developed countries could still attempt to tackle the root causes of forced migration while offering equal care to those individuals who are resident within their borders.

CONCLUSION

Ultimately, government policy is directed by political will, legislature, and public debate. This discussion raises questions of how this debate is conducted. Many support groups point to the relentlessly negative portrayal of refugees in the press.[17, 19] Political parties ought to resist the temptation to endorse these views for popular support alone. It could be argued that the medical profession is uniquely poised to advocate for the needs of patients, irrespective of issues of citizenship.

There is a wider debate taking placed in many liberal democracies about provision of universal health care. At present we may not possess the ethical framework and language to conduct this debate explicitly.[51] A first step would be to separate healthcare policy from immigration policy. The government should then be more explicit about what healthcare services are available to all of its inhabitants.

An inevitable consequence of democratic decision making is that some people may differ and vote accordingly. Yet we should acknowledge that the decision-making process may be influenced by moral as well as political argument, and the medical profession has a responsibility to engage in this debate.

Loewy specifies three preconditions for a nation to achieve political democracy in a 'decent society'.[66] First we should understand democracy as a moral value: this implies an individual respect for one another. Second, we should strive for economic democracy to minimise the gap between rich and poor. Third, educational democracy should offer the opportunity for all to achieve their potential. In the absence of these conditions, refugees might well ask themselves 'what is the state of democracy in the UK?'

Migratory pressures are likely to increase significantly this century as a result of factors such as population growth, climate change, and political instability. On an international level we should attend to the route causes of migration. As individuals we may find ourselves considering who we wish to regard as a patient and who we do not. I would argue that as many refugees are already disadvantaged by the determinants and effects of migration, we should be cautious in implementing further barriers to care.

REFERENCES

1. Department of Health. Proposals to exclude overseas visitors from eligibility to free NHS primary medical services. A consultation. London: Department of Health, 2004.
2. World Medical Association. World Medical Association International Code of Medical Ethics. Ferney-Voltaire, France: World Medical Association.
3. Dyer O. News: Health department's denial of free health care to asylum seekers was unlawful, judge says. BMJ 2008; 336(7649): 849.
4. Flory D. Failed asylum seekers and ordinary/lawful residence; and when to provide treatment for those who are chargeable. Dear colleague letter, Department of Health, 2 April 2009.
5. Walker PF, Jaranson J. Refugee and immigrant health care. Med Clin North Am 1999; 83(4): 1103–1120.
6. Dick B. Diseases of refugees—causes, effects and controls. Trans R Soc Trop Med Hyg 1984; 78(6): 734–741.
7. Burnett A, Peel M. Health needs of asylum seekers and refugees. BMJ 2001; 322(7285): 544–547.
8. Burnett A, Peel M. Asylum seekers and refugees in Britain. The health of survivors of torture and organised violence. BMJ 2001; 322(7286): 606–609.
9. United Nations. Convention relating to the status of refugees. Geneva: United Nations, 1951.
10. Burnett A, Peel M. Asylum seekers and refugees in Britain. What brings asylum seekers to the United Kingdom? BMJ 2001; 322(7284): 485–488.
11. Hall P. Failed asylum seekers and health care. BMJ 2006; 333(7559): 109–110.
12. UNHCR: UN Refugee Agency. 2008 global trends: refugees, asylum-seekers, returnees, internally displaced and stateless persons. UNHCR: UN Refugee Agency.
13. Bennett K, Heath T, Jeffries R. Asylum statistics United Kingdom 2006. Home Office Statistical Bulletin. 3rd ed. London: Home Office, 2007.
14. Bilsborrow RE, Hugo G, Oberai S, Zlotnik H. International migrations statistics: guidelines for improving data collection systems. Geneva: International Labour Office, 1997.
15. Glover S, Gott C, Loizillon A, et al. Migration: an economic and social analysis. RDS Occasional Paper No 67. London: The Home Office, 2001.
16. Raymond M. Tabloids blame asylum seekers for GP shortages. BMJ 2003; 326: 290.
17. The Refugee Council. Basics on asylum.
18. Stevenson R, Grant H. Land of no return. The Guardian, 13 June 2008.
19. Barclay A, Bowes A, Ferguson I, et al. Asylum seekers in Scotland. Edinburgh, Scottish Executive Social Research, 2003

20. Amnesty International. Get it right: how Home Office decision making fails refugees. London: Amnesty International, 2004.

21. Audit Commission. Another country. Implementing dispersal under the Immigration and Asylum Act 1999. Abingdon: Audit Commission Publications, 2000.

22. Evans RG, Barer ML, Marmor TR, editors. Why are some people healthy and others not? The determinants of health of populations. New York: Aldine de Gruyter, 1994.

23. Evans RG, Stoddart, GL. Producing health, consuming health care. Soc Sci Med 1990; 31(12): 1347–1363.

24. Bracken P, Giller J, Summerfeld D. Psychological responses to war and atrocity: the limitations of current concepts. Soc Sci Med 1995; 40(8): 1073–1082.

25. Bison J. Post-traumatic stress disorder. BMJ 2007; 334: 789–793.

26. American Psychiatric Association. Diagnostic and statistical manual of mental disorders. 4th ed. Washington: American Psychiatric Association, 2000.

27. Pile H. The asylum trap: the labour market experiences of refugees with professional qualifications. London: Low Pay Unit, 1997.

28. Gorst-Unsworth C, Goldenberg E. Psychological sequelae of torture and organized violence suffered by refugees from Iraq. Trauma related factors compared to social factors in exile. Br J Psychiatry 1998; 172: 90–94.

29. Sennett R. Respect: the formation of character in an age of inequality. London: Penguin, 2004.

30. Porter M, Haslam N. Pre-displacement and post-displacement factors associated with mental health of refugees and internally displaced persons: a meta-analysis. JAMA 2005; 294(5): 602–612.

31. Arnold F. Detained asylum seekers may be being re-traumatised. BMJ 2007; 334(7600): 916–917.

32. Fazel M, Silove D. Detention of refugees. BMJ 2006; 332(7536): 251–252.

33. UNICEF. Convention on the Rights of the Child.

34. Noglik A, Bassi Z. Eligibility of non-residents for NHS treatment: children of asylum seekers are special case. BMJ 2004; 329(7467): 683.

35. Fazel M, Stein A. UK immigration law disregards the best interests of children. Lancet 2004; 363(9423): 1749–1750.

36. Wallace T. Refugee women: their perspectives and our responses. Oxford: Oxfam, 1990.

37. Williams P. Why failed asylum seekers must not be denied access to the NHS. BMJ 2004; 329: 298.

38. Ramsey R, Turner S. Refugees health needs. Br J Gen Pract 1993; 43(376): 480–481.

39. Department of Health. Asylum seekers and refugees: entitlement to NHS treatment. London: Department of Health, 2008.

40. Department of Health. Proposed amendments to the National Health Services (Charges to Overseas Visitors) Regulations 1989: a consultation. London: Department of Health, 2003.

41. Harding-Pink D. Humanitarian medicine: up the garden path and down the slippery slope. BMJ 2004; 329(7462): 398–399.

42. Forrest D, Barrett J. Ethical pitfalls can be hard to avoid. BMJ 2004; 329(7462): 399–400.

43. Rawls J. A theory of justice. Oxford: Oxford University Press, 1972.

44. Singer P. Practical ethics. Cambridge: Cambridge University Press, 1993.

45. Fowler A, Collins L, Larbalestier N, et al. HIV, HAART and overseas visitors. Sex Transm Infect 2006; 82(6): 516.

46. Watt G. The inverse care law today. Lancet 2002; 360(9328): 252–254.

47. Stirling AM, Wilson P, McConnachie A. Deprivation, psychological distress and consultation length in general practice. Br J Gen Pract 2001; 51(467): 456–460.

48. Berwick DM. A transatlantic review of the NHS at 60. BMJ 2008; 337: a838.

49. Klein R. What does the future hold for the NHS at 60? BMJ 2008; 337: a549.

50. Coombes R. NHS anniversary: the NHS debate. BMJ 2008; 337: 628.

51. Roberts M, Reich M. Ethical analysis in public health. Lancet 2002; 359(9311): 1055–1059.

52. Romero-Ortuno R. Eligibility of non-residents for NHS treatment: failed asylum seekers should not be denied access to free NHS care. BMJ 2004; 329(7476): 683.

53. Kant I. The critique of practical reason. New York: Liberal Arts Press, 1956.

54. Acheson ED. Independent enquiry into inequalities in health. London: HMSO, 1998.

55. Scottish Needs Assessment Programme. A rough guide to needs assessment in primary care. Glasgow: Scottish Needs Assessment Programme, 1997.

56. Bischoff A, Perneger T, Bovier P, et al. Improving communication between physicians and patients who speak a foreign language. Br J Gen Pract 2003; 53(541): 546.

57. Phelan M, Parkman S. How to do it; work with an interpreter. BMJ 1995; 311(7004): 555–557.

58. Jones D, Gill P. Refugees and primary care: tackling the inequalities. BMJ 1998; 317(7170): 1444–1446.

59. British Medical Association. Housing and health: building for the future. London: British Medical Association, 2003.

60. Watt G. Policies to tackle social exclusion. BMJ 2001; 323(7306): 175–176.

61. Hull S, Boomla K. Primary care for refugees and asylum seekers. BMJ 2006; 332(7533): 62–63.

62. Forrest D, Barrett J. Ethical pitfalls can be hard to avoid. BMJ 2004; 329(7462): 399–400.

63. General Medical Council. Good medical practice. London: General Medical Council, 2004.

64. Hall P. Asylum seekers' health rights. BMA is in denial. BMJ 2007; 335(7621): 629.

65. Sheather J. BMA's response. BMJ 2007; 334: 917.

66. Loewy E. The social nexus of healthcare. Am J Bioeth 2001; 1(2): 37.

QUESTIONS

1. What is the difference between an asylum seeker, a refugee and an internally displaced person (IDP)? Why might the complex sequelae of refugees and asylum seekers be referred to as afflicting "mind, body and spirit"? What is the definition of somatization? What are the implications of this interconnectedness for protection and treatment?

2. Taylor states that "It could be argued that the medical profession is uniquely poised to advocate for the needs of patients, irrespective of issues of citizenship." Why might the medical profession be "uniquely poised" in this regard?

3. Taylor also states that "Some argue that unless care is incentivized, it will succumb to the pressure of competing demands." How can care be incentivized? What are these competing demands, and how could they be addressed?

FURTHER READING

1. Cutts, Mark, *The State of the World's Refugees, 2000: Fifty Years of Humanitarian Action.* Geneva: UNHCR, 2000.

2. Loescher, Gil, Betts, Alexander, & Milner, James, *The United Nations High Commissioner for Refugees (UNHCR): The Politics and Practice of Refugee Protection into the Twenty-First Century.* London: Routledge, 2008.

3. Steiner, Niklaus, Gibney, Mark, & Loescher, Gil, *Problems of Protection: The UNHCR, Refugees, and Human Rights.* New York: Routledge, 2003.

CHAPTER 20

Prevalence and Correlates of Forced Sex Perpetration and Victimization in Botswana and Swaziland

Alexander C. Tsai, Karen Leiter, Michele Heisler, Vincent Iacopino, William Wolfe, Kate Shannon, Nthabiseng Phaladze, Zakhe Hlanze and Sheri Weiser

Male-perpetrated sexual violence against women is recognized as an important human rights concern worldwide.[1] Not only is sexual violence a serious violation of women's human rights, but it is also associated with many adverse health and psychological sequelae,[2,3] including HIV.[4,5] This creates a social context for gender-based power differentials that further limit women's ability to refuse sex or negotiate safe sex practices. Policy and programming discussions about sexual violence prevention should therefore consider the gendered contexts in which sexual violence occurs.[6-10]

The United Nations' Millennium Development Goals explicitly recognize achievement of gender equality as a critical foundation for human development. Gender-based violence is a key manifestation of gender inequality. Thus, identifying its risk factors is critical for devising appropriate preventive strategies. The Sexual Violence Research Initiative and the World Health Organization have also highlighted this as a key area for research.[11-13] Some research in this area has focused on identifying risk factors for sexual violence victimization among women in South Africa,[8,14,15] Uganda,[16] and India.[4,5] A smaller body of work has focused specifically on correlates of sexual violence perpetration among men in South Africa[17-21] and India.[4]

Despite the high priority of research in this area, correlates of gender-based violence have been little studied in Botswana and Swaziland. The prevalence and correlates of sexual violence vary across countries and regions[1,7,22] with different gender-focused policies and legislation, suggesting that effective prevention strategies will be context specific.[23] The context of gender inequality in Botswana and Swaziland is well documented,[24] and these countries also have among the highest HIV prevalence rates in sub-Saharan Africa.[25]

Therefore, our goal in this study was to identify correlates of forced sex victimization among women and forced sex perpetration among men using population-based survey data from Botswana and Swaziland.

METHODS

We conducted a population-based cross-sectional study between November 2004 and May 2005 among adults randomly selected from households in the 5 districts of Botswana with the highest number of HIV-infected individuals (representing a population of 725,000 in the eastern corridor of the country, out of a total population of 1.7 million)[26] and in all 4 regions of Swaziland. We used a stratified 2-stage probability sample design to select the population-based sample of households.

Within each household, one adult member who had a primary residence there and who met the study's inclusion criteria was randomly selected. Up to 2 repeat attempts were made to interview that person if the initial visit was unsuccessful. No replacements were made if participants could not be reached after the repeat attempts. We did not interview more than one member of the household. To be eligible for the study, individuals were required to be 18 to 49 years of age, to have no cognitive disabilities, to be residents of the country where the interview took place, and to be fluent in English, Setswana, or SiSwati. All interviewers were country nationals.

The survey instruments for both countries inquired about multiple domains, including sexual violence, sociodemographic characteristics, health and mental health, and HIV risk behaviors. All surveys and consent forms were translated into Setswana or SiSwati and then back-translated into English to ensure that translations were accurate. All interviews were conducted in private settings, and anonymity was assured. Any study participant who appeared to be in emotional distress after answering sensitive questions was offered the opportunity to speak to one of the study health care providers and was referred to a local health care center for counseling.

The field research team consisted of country nationals who were trained by a team of Physicians for Human Rights research staff along with local field researchers. The supervisory team had extensive expertise in applied research, human rights, gender issues, mental health, and HIV/AIDS. All local field researchers had prior survey experience, and many had expertise in HIV/AIDS work. The training included detailed instruction in the study protocols and research ethics and consisted of classroom teaching and role play followed by field practice in interviewing. Continuous field supervision was provided throughout the study. The survey team received specific training on how to enumerate households (e.g., not counting nonresidential buildings, counting each separate household on the same property separately) and how to ask sensitive questions in an appropriate, nonjudgmental manner. Full details of the survey implementation have been published elsewhere.[24]

Outcome Measures

Among women, we gathered information on 12-month history of forced sex with the question "Were you forced to have sex against your will over the past 12 months?"[11,22] Information on lifetime history of victimization among men and women was obtained with the question "In your lifetime, have you ever been forced to have sex when you did not want to?" Among men, the question "Did you have sex with others when they did not want to over the past 12 months?" was used to gather data on perpetration of forced sex in the preceding year.[19,20] In the Swaziland survey, men were also asked a question about lifetime forced sex perpetration: "In your lifetime, have you ever had sex with someone when they did not want to?" Of note, this survey was implemented as a study of gender equity in general and therefore did not make use of multiple questions to inquire about different aspects of sexual violence.

Prior research has described how the social context in which sex occurs itself shapes women's risk for sexual violence, and sexual violence takes many forms (in addition to the act of forced sex).[8,11] Therefore, in supplementary analyses focusing on women we also examined correlates of lack of control in sexual decision making, which was defined according to a Likert scale-based measure in which women described the extent to which their partners made decisions about when to have sex. Women were categorized as lacking control in sexual decision making if they stated that their partners "usually" or "always" made the decisions about when to have sex.

Key Covariates

Our decisions about which risk factors to investigate were guided by an integrated ecological framework that has been proposed for conceptualizing the etiology of gender- based violence[27] as well as consideration of previously identified risk factors from other developing country settings.[6,8,10,15,17–20] Sociodemographic variables included age, marital status (married, living with partner, other), educational level (high school vs less than high school), monthly household income (more than vs less than 5,000 pula or emalangeni; approximately 800–1,000 U.S. dollars), and area of residence (urban vs rural). On the basis of prior research linking food insufficiency to risky sexual behaviors among women,[28] we included food insufficiency as a potential risk factor. The food insufficiency survey question was adapted from an analysis of data from the Third National Health and Nutrition Examination Survey,[29] in which food insufficiency was defined according to a Likert scale based measure in which participants reported whether they "sometimes" or "often" had not had enough food to eat over the previous 12 months.

We defined problem drinking as consumption of 8 to 14 drinks per week for women and 15 to 21 drinks per week for men, and we defined heavy drinking as consumption of more than 14 drinks per week for women and more than 21 drinks per week for men.[30] We assessed self-reported health status on a Likert scale in which the categories were fair, poor, and other.

We also included 3 variables related to risky sexual behaviors over the preceding 12

months: having had multiple partners (vs 1 or none), having had transactional sex, and having had an intergenerational sexual relationship. The latter 2 variables were defined differently for men and women. Women were asked whether they had exchanged sex for money, food, or other resources and whether they had been involved in a sexual relationship with someone 10 or more years older. Men were asked whether they had paid for or provided resources in exchange for sex and whether they had been involved in a sexual relationship with someone 10 or more years younger. Finally, we also included lifetime history of forced sex victimization. We did not have further data on the sex of the perpetrator.

Statistical Analysis

We used Stata version 11 (StataCorp LP, College Station, Texas) in conducting our statistical analyses. Using univariable logistic regression, we calculated unadjusted odds ratios (ORs) to estimate the degree of association between each of the risk factors and outcomes assessed. We fit separate models by country to identify potential country-level differences, and we also fit pooled models with a binary indicator variable equal to 1 for residence in Botswana. Risk factors significant at $P < .25$ in univariable analyses were identified as candidates for multivariable logistic regression analyses,[31] and the final models retained only variables significant at $P < .05$.

Because of small cell sizes caused by the rarity of the outcome variables, we encountered the problem of separation, that is, covariates perfectly predicting the outcome of interest and therefore yielding infinitely large or infinitely small parameter estimates. To eliminate this small-sample bias, we employed the penalized-likelihood correction proposed by Firth[32–35] when fitting the logistic regression models.

RESULTS

In Botswana, 1433 individuals were randomly selected and approached to take part in the study. Of these individuals, 46 (3.2%) could not be located after 2 repeat visits, 78 (5.4%) refused to take part or did not meet the study criteria, and 41 (2.9%) were unable to complete the survey. We obtained completed surveys from 613 men and 654 women in Botswana (89% response rate). In Swaziland, 876 men and women were randomly selected and approached to take part in the study. Of these individuals, 35 (4.0%) could not be located after 2 repeat visits, 32 (3.7%) refused to take part or did not meet the criteria, and 3 (0.3%) were unable to complete the survey. We obtained completed surveys from 398 men and 407 women in Swaziland (92% response rate).

Among women, 12-month prevalence rates of forced sex victimization were 4.6% in Botswana and 4.7% in Swaziland (Table 20.1). Lifetime prevalence of forced sex victimization was 10.3% in Botswana and 11.4% in Swaziland. Among men, lifetime prevalence rates of forced sex victimization were 3.9% in Botswana and 5.0% in Swaziland. The 12-month prevalence of forced sex perpetration among men was 4.2% in Botswana and 1.8% in Swaziland. In Swaziland, the lifetime prevalence of forced sex perpetration among men was 7.4%. Other characteristics of the sample are provided in Table 20.2.

History of forced sex victimization was strongly correlated with past-year perpetration of forced sex by men in both Botswana (adjusted OR = 13.7; 95% confidence interval [CI] = 4.55, 41.5) and Swaziland (adjusted OR = 5.98; 95% CI = 1.08, 33.1) (Table 20.3). Engaging in transactional sex was also consistently associated with perpetration of forced sex among men in both Botswana (adjusted OR = 2.63; 95% CI = 1.08, 6.40) and Swaziland (adjusted OR = 7.53; 95% CI = 1.25, 45.2).

Other HIV risk behaviors were less consistently associated with perpetration of forced sex. Having multiple sexual partners was a statistically significant correlate of forced sex perpetration by men in Botswana, whereas engaging in transactional sex was statistically significant only in Swaziland. When both country samples were pooled for men, other factors did not emerge as statistically significant; however, the significance levels for factors identified in the country-specific analyses narrowed. The country-level coefficient was of borderline statistical significance (adjusted OR = 2.14; 95% CI = 0.89, 5.15).

Problem or heavy drinking was the risk factor most strongly correlated with past-year victimization among women

Table 20.1 Past-Year and Lifetime Prevalence of Forced Sex Perpetration by Men and Forced Sex Victimization of Men and Women in Botswana and Swaziland, 2004–2005

	Botswana, No. (%; 95% CI)	*Swaziland, No. (%; 95% CI)*
Forced sex perpetration		
Past 12 months	26 (4.3; 2.7, 5.9)	7 (1.8; 0.5, 3.1)
Lifetime	… a	29 (7.4; 4.8, 10.0)
Forced sex victimization		
Past 12 months: women	30 (4.6; 3.0, 6.2)	19 (4.7; 2.6, 6.8)
Lifetime: women	67 (10.3; 7.9, 12.6)	46 (11.4; 8.3, 14.5)
Lifetime: men	24 (3.9; 2.4, 5.5)	20 (5.0; 2.9, 7.2)

Note. CI = confidence interval.

a Question was not asked of male participants in the Botswana survey.

Table 20.2 Characteristics of Male and Female Study Participants: Botswana and Swaziland, 2004–2005

	Men	Women
Botswana[a]		
Age, y, mean (SD)	31.3 (11.3)	31.6 (11.3)
Married, no. (%)	105 (17.2)	136 (20.8)
Living with partner, no. (%)	149 (24.4)	191 (29.3)
Completed high school, no. (%)	335 (55.3)	349 (53.7)
Monthly household income > 5000 pula, no. (%)	114 (18.6)	88 (13.6)
Food insufficiency, no. (%)	113 (18.5)	184 (28.2)
Urban residence, no. (%)	456 (74.4)	478 (73.1)
Problem or heavy drinking, no. (%)	238 (39.3)	163 (25.1)
Fair or poor self-reported health status, no. (%)	191 (31.4)	179 (27.5)
Multiple sexual partners, no. (%)	246 (40.1)	164 (25.1)
Transactional sex, no. (%)	8 (1.3)	45 (6.9)
Intergenerational sexual relationship, no. (%)	55 (9.1)	116 (17.8)
Swaziland[b]		
Age, y, mean (SD)	29.1 (8.6)	29.8 (9.0)
Married, no. (%)	111 (27.9)	156 (38.4)
Living with partner, no. (%)	75 (19.0)	74 (18.5)
Completed high school, no. (%)	189 (47.5)	147 (36.1)
Monthly household income > 5000 emalengeni, no. (%)	66 (16.6)	42 (10.3)
Food insufficiency, no. (%)	113 (28.5)	154 (38.2)
Urban residence, no. (%)	192 (48.2)	221 (54.3)
Problem or heavy drinking, no. (%)	51 (13.0)	14 (3.5)
Fair or poor self-reported health status, no. (%)	126 (31.7)	182 (44.7)
Multiple sexual partners, no. (%)	157 (39.5)	33 (8.1)
Transactional sex, no. (%)	5 (1.3)	5 (1.2)
Intergenerational sexual relationship, no. (%)	49 (12.5)	51 (12.6)

a n = 604; women, n = 649 b n = 393; women, n = 405.

in Botswana (adjusted OR = 2.55; 95% CI = 1.19, 5.49) (Table 20.4). Food insufficiency (adjusted OR = 2.40; 95% CI = 1.03, 5.57) and having multiple sexual partners (adjusted OR = 2.83; 95% CI = 1.17, 6.84) were also associated with past-year victimization. Among women in Swaziland, alcohol use was the only variable identified as a statistically significant risk factor (OR = 14.7; 95% CI = 4.53, 47.6). Pooled analyses among women in both countries confirmed these associations; the country-level coefficient was of borderline statistical significance (adjusted OR = 0.55; 95% CI = 0.25, 1.09), and greater household income was also found to be associated with past-year victimization (adjusted OR = 2.67; 95% CI = 1.20, 5.95).

In supplemental analyses, we identified correlates of lack of control in sexual

Table 20.3 Risk Factors for Forced Sex Perpetration by Men in the Preceding 12 Months: Botswana and Swaziland, 2004–2005

	Botswana (n = 604)		Swaziland (n = 393)		Pooled Analysis (n = 997)	
	Unadjusted OR (95% CI)	Adjusted OR (95% CI)	Unadjusted OR (95% CI)	Adjusted OR (95% CI)	Unadjusted OR (95% CI)	Adjusted OR (95% CI)
Age, y	1.01 (0.97, 1.04)		1.01 (0.94, 1.10)		1.01 (0.98, 1.05)	
Married	0.96 (0.34, 2.71)		1.20 (0.26, 5.43)		0.87 (0.37, 2.08)	
Living with partner	1.19 (0.50, 2.81)		1.92 (0.42, 8.74)		1.35 (0.63, 2.90)	
Completed high school	2.47* (1.00, 6.08)		0.25 (0.04, 1.47)		1.50 (0.73, 3.06)	
Monthly household income > 5000 pula	0.87 (0.31, 2.44)		0.32 (0.02, 5.81)		0.69 (0.25, 1.90)	
Food insufficiency	1.12 (0.43, 2.92)		0.57 (0.10, 3.44)		0.81 (0.34, 1.93)	
Urban residence	1.13 (0.46, 2.78)		16.7 (0.94, 297)		1.87 (0.85, 4.11)	
Problem or heavy drinking	3.49** (1.52, 7.99)		3.17 (0.69, 14.6)		3.89*** (1.93, 7.85)	
Fair or poor self-reported health status	1.27 (0.56, 2.88)		4.85* (1.07, 22.0)		1.73 (0.86, 3.49)	
Multiple sexual partners	10.8*** (3.48, 33.7)	9.41*** (2.91, 30.5)	6.97* (1.17, 41.6)		10.6*** (3.89, 28.7)	8.86*** (3.19, 24.6)
Transactional sex	5.26*** (2.32, 11.9)	2.63* (1.08, 6.40)	10.8* (2.21, 52.5)	7.53* (1.25, 45.2)	7.04*** (3.37, 14.7)	3.13** (1.39, 7.06)
Intergenerational sexual relationship	2.67* (1.00, 7.13)		9.79* (2.34, 41.0)	5.97* (1.36, 26.3)	3.56*** (1.63, 7.75)	
History of forced sex victimization	12.3*** (4.66, 32.3)	13.7*** (4.55, 41.5)	8.96** (1.86, 43.1)	5.98* (1.08, 33.1)	10.1*** (4.44, 23.0)	11.9*** (4.69, 30.0)
Residence in Botswana						2.14 (0.89, 5.15)

Note. OR = odds ratio; CI = confidence interval.
* P < .05;
** P < .01;
*** P < .001.

Table 20.4 Risk Factors for Forced Sex Perpetration by Women in the Preceding 12 Months: Botswana and Swaziland, 2004–2005

	Botswana (n = 604)		Swaziland (n = 393)		Pooled Analysis (n = 997)	
	Unadjusted OR (95% CI)	*Adjusted OR (95% CI)*	*Unadjusted OR (95% CI)*	*Adjusted OR (95% CI)*	*Unadjusted OR (95% CI)*	*Adjusted OR (95% CI)*
Age, y	1.01 (0.98, 1.04)		1.02 (0.97, 1.07)		1.01 (0.99, 1.04)	
Married	0.46 (0.15, 1.43)		1.81 (0.73, 4.45)		0.96 (0.51, 1.82)	
Living with partner	1.68 (0.80, 3.52)		1.27 (0.43, 3.75)		1.49 (0.81, 2.74)	
Completed high school	0.85 (0.41, 1.75)		1.05 (0.42, 2.66)		0.92 (0.52, 1.62)	
Monthly household income > 5000 pula	1.81 (0.73, 4.44)		1.86 (0.56, 6.18)		1.75 (0.84, 3.65)	2.67* (1.20, 5.95)
Food insufficiency	3.09** (1.49, 6.39)	2.81** (1.35, 5.85)	0.70 (0.25, 1.95)		1.77 (0.99, 3.18)	1.95* (1.03, 3.70)
Urban residence	0.53 (0.25, 1.12)		1.49 (0.59, 3.76)		0.76 (0.42, 1.36)	
Problem or heavy drinking	3.64*** (1.75, 7.55)	2.55* (1.19, 5.49)	14.7*** (4.53, 47.6)	14.7*** (4.53, 47.6)	4.06*** (2.26, 7.29)	3.72*** (1.84, 7.50)
Fair or poor self-reported health status	1.38 (0.64, 2.96)		1.12 (0.46, 2.77)		1.25 (0.70, 2.24)	
Multiple sexual partners	4.15*** (1.99, 8.65)	3.01* (1.39, 6.48)	3.51* (1.15, 10.7)		3.55*** (1.98, 6.35)	2.82** (1.45, 5.48)
Transactional sex	4.93*** (2.03, 12.0)		6.66 (0.95, 46.5)		4.75*** (2.13, 10.6)	
Intergenerational sexual relationship	3.94*** (1.88, 8.27)		2.07 (0.69, 6.16)		3.11*** (1.69, 5.70)	
Residence in Botswana						0.55 (0.27, 1.09)

Note. OR = odds ratio; CI = confidence interval.

* P < .05;

** P < .01;

*** P < .001.

decision making. Food insufficiency was a statistically significant risk factor for lack of control in sexual decision making among women in Botswana (adjusted OR = 1.62; 95% CI = 1.07, 2.44) and Swaziland (adjusted OR = 1.67; 95% CI = 1.06, 2.64). Involvement in a sexual relationship with someone 10 or more years older was also consistently associated with elevated odds of lack of control in Botswana (adjusted OR = 2.79; 95% CI = 1.77, 4.41) and Swaziland (adjusted OR = 2.21; 95% CI = 1.19, 4.10). In addition, having multiple sexual partners was a risk factor among women in Botswana (adjusted OR = 2.00; 95% CI = 1.32, 3.04), whereas being married was a risk factor among women in Swaziland (adjusted OR = 1.74; 95% CI = 1.11, 2.74).

DISCUSSION

Using population-based survey data from 2 countries with among the highest HIV prevalence rates in the world, we documented a high lifetime prevalence of forced sex victimization among women in both countries. Sexual victimization was not limited to women. Men who reported a lifetime history of sexual victimization were more likely to report having perpetrated sexual violence. Although we confirmed other previously reported findings such as the association between alcohol use and victimization of women,[28] we found that variables related to women's unequal position in Botswana and Swaziland, including food insufficiency, were also risk factors. Thus, our findings highlight interconnections between sexual violence and social forces that should be addressed in policies and programs targeted at preventing gender-based violence.

More than 10% of women in Botswana and Swaziland had been sexually victimized in their lifetime, and approximately half of these women had been sexually victimized in the preceding year. Data on the national scope of this problem in Botswana have not been reported previously. Only one published study has reported on the scope of the problem in Swaziland. In that investigation, a nationally representative study on the sequelae of sexual violence among girls and young women aged 13 to 24 years, the lifetime prevalence of sexual violence was 33.2% when a broad definition of sexual violence (one that also included coerced sex, attempted unwanted sex, and unwanted touching) was used.[36] When the definition was narrowed to include forced sex only, the lifetime prevalence was 4.9%. This rate was lower than the lifetime prevalence of 11.3% among women in our Swaziland sample; however, this is not unexpected given the higher mean age of the participants in our study.

A second important finding of our study is that nearly 5% of men in Botswana and Swaziland reported having been sexually victimized in their lifetimes, and this was associated with forced sex perpetration even after other potentially influential variables, such as risky alcohol use, had been taken into account. Although the World Health Organization has identified sexual violence against men and boys as "a significant problem," the issue "has largely been neglected in research."[12] An analysis of data from male volunteers in a cluster-randomized HIV prevention trial in South Africa showed that perpetrators of sexual violence were more likely to have experienced childhood physical and sexual abuse.[19] This finding is consistent with prior research on childhood experiences of violence and subsequent perpetration of intimate partner violence during adulthood.[37] Our results thus extend these findings by suggesting an important impact of unaddressed sexual violence among boys and men in Botswana and Swaziland.

A third primary finding of our study is that several factors related to women's inferior and unequal position in Botswana and Swaziland societies were associated with past-year sexual violence victimization. Women who had insufficient food were more likely to have been sexually victimized and were more likely to report that they lacked control in sexual decision making. Given that food insufficiency has also been associated with sex exchange and other HIV transmission risk behaviors among women,[28] our findings emphasize the potential for economic empowerment and hunger alleviation to be integral components of gender-based violence prevention programs worldwide. In Swaziland, food insufficiency was also found to be a risk factor for lack of sexual control, along with marital status. This is consistent with how Swazi women are disadvantaged by customary marriage rites that tie women's social status to their reproductive capabilities and by customary laws that permit polygamy, as well as by property and other civil laws that place them at disadvantaged social status.[24]

Our finding that increased household wealth was associated with greater odds of victimization among women was unexpected and was inconsistent with the results of prior studies. This finding is probably explained by the fact that there was greater reporting of sexual violence in that subpopulation, perhaps because women in wealthier households were more likely to recognize sexual violence as such or felt more comfortable discussing this sensitive topic with field interviewers.

Taken together, our findings suggest multiple targets for primary prevention of gender-based violence. Our study demonstrates that sexual victimization of women in Botswana and Swaziland occurs in a male-dominated economic environment characterized by gender norms that further increase women's susceptibility to sexual violence. Women's lack of control in sexual decision making and compromised ability to negotiate safe sex practices also heighten their susceptibility to HIV.[38] These features strongly argue for addressing sexual violence from human rights and public health perspectives.[10,11]

With regard to human rights, gender-discriminatory norms resulting from gender biases in the customary and civil laws of Botswana and Swaziland are well documented[24] and may be amenable to legal reform. For example, legislative interventions have been shown to induce durable changes in some aspects of gender bias in India.[39] Public health interventions should be considered especially in countries with high HIV prevalence rates. For example, in rural South Africa, a cluster-randomized trial of a microfinance intervention combined with participatory training on HIV prevention, gender norms, domestic violence, and sexuality reduced intimate partner violence[40] as well as risky sexual behaviors.[41] However, our study also highlights the need for targeting sexual victimization of men in addition to women as a strategy to prevent subsequent perpetration of sexual violence.

Limitations

Our findings should be considered in light of the methodological constraints of the study. First, because the risk factors we investigated were all measured concurrently with the outcome, we are by definition limited in our ability to make causal inferences. We are also unable to determine whether these risk factors are predictive of victimization occurring over women's lifetimes. Second, privacy and anonymity were assured by a field research staff that had extensive expertise in applied research, human rights, gender issues, mental health, and HIV/AIDS. However, in light of the high prevalence of sexual violence reported in other sub-Saharan African settings,[1,8,16,22] we believe participants probably underreported their experiences of sexual violence, especially in household settings where women faced fear of reprisal by male partners. This limitation, common to studies in this area of research,[10] suggests that our prevalence estimates are likely underestimates.

Third, small cell sizes weakened our ability to identify statistically significant correlates of forced sex, but this strengthens our confidence in the associations identified. Related to this limitation, we cannot discount the possibility that response bias affected our results. In comparison with data from demographic and health surveys conducted in these countries,[42,43] women 40 to 49 years of age were relatively overrepresented in our Botswana sample, and women younger than 20 years were relatively underrepresented in our Swaziland sample. Survey data were collected only from people who consented to participate in the study, so response rates disaggregated by sex were unavailable. If, for example, women who had recently been victimized were more likely to refuse participation, our prevalence estimates would be downward biased. However, the response rate was very high overall (approximately 90%), suggesting that any potential bias would have limited effects.

A significant risk factor identified in prior work that was not measured in our study was physical violence. We focused specifically on forced sex and did not explicitly address other forms of gender-based violence, including physical violence, sexual exploitation due to economic vulnerability, coerced sex, and unwanted sex due to threats.[8,11] Because the original survey was intended as a general study of gender equity (rather than as a specific study of sexual violence), the survey instrument did not implement some of the research techniques that are standardized in this field for maximizing reporting of sexual violence by women, such as using multiple questions to ask about sexual violence and providing more than one opportunity to report sexual violence. As has been shown previously in Swaziland, broader construals of gender-based violence may yield larger and more accurate prevalence estimates.[36]

The findings related to victimization of men are subject to 2 additional limitations. Our survey instrument did not clarify whether the victimization occurred during childhood or adulthood. Furthermore, prior qualitative work from South Africa has shown that the meaning of men's accounts of forced sex victimization differs considerably depending on whether the perpetrator was a man or woman,[44] and therefore it is questionable whether the 2 sets of experiences should be included in the same category. Future research should confirm our findings with more specific quantitative and qualitative data on the sex of the perpetrator and the timing and context of the encounter.

Conclusions

Sexual violence in Botswana and Swaziland is a major public health and human rights problem. Risk of sexual violence among women is significantly compounded by the high prevalence of HIV in these 2 countries. The impact of past victimization on recent perpetration suggests that gender-transformative work with men and boys[45] may have lasting effects by preventing the long-term psychological sequelae that perpetuate further cycles of violence. However, interventions should not only target the individual psychological dimensions of risk, interpersonal relationships, and behavior. Effectively ending codified gender discrimination in civil, political, and economic rights can also play a role in fundamentally changing gender norms and may be an important lever for gender-based violence prevention in these countries.

REFERENCES

1. Watts C, Zimmerman C. Violence against women: global scope and magnitude. Lancet. 2002; 359(9313):1232–1237.10.1016/S0140-6736(02)08221-1 [PubMed: 11955557]

2. Campbell JC. Health consequences of intimate partner violence. Lancet. 2002; 359(9314):1331–1336.10.1016/S0140-6736(02)08336-8 [PubMed: 11965295]

3. Ellsberg M, Jansen HA, Heise L, Watts CH, Garcia-Moreno C. Intimate partner violence and women's physical and mental health in the WHO multi-country study on women's health and domestic violence: an observational study. Lancet. 2008; 371(9619):1165–1172.10.1016/S0140-6736(08)60522-X [PubMed: 18395577]

4. Decker MR, Seage GR III, Hemenway D, et al. Intimate partner violence functions as both a risk marker and risk factor for women's HIV infection: findings from Indian husband-wife dyads. J Acquir Immune Defic Syndr. 2009; 51(5):593–600.10.1097/QAI.0b013e3181a255d6 [PubMed: 19421070]

5. Silverman JG, Decker MR, Saggurti N, Balaiah D, Raj A. Intimate partner violence and HIV infection among married Indian women. JAMA. 2008; 300(6):703–710.10.1001/jama.300.6.703 [PubMed: 18698068]

6. Jewkes R, Levin J, Penn-Kekana L. Risk factors for domestic violence: findings from a South African cross-sectional study. Soc Sci Med. 2002; 55(9):1603–1617.10.1016/ S0277-9536(01)00294-5 [PubMed: 12297246]

7. Jewkes R. Intimate partner violence: causes and prevention. Lancet. 2002; 359(9315):1423–1429.10.1016/S0140-6736(02)08357-5 [PubMed: 11978358]

8. Jewkes R, Abrahams N. The epidemiology of rape and sexual coercion in South Africa: an overview. Soc Sci Med. 2002; 55(7):1231–1244.10.1016/ S0277-9536(01)00242-8 [PubMed: 12365533]

9. Zierler S, Krieger N. Reframing women's risk: social inequalities and HIV infection. Annu Rev Public Health. 1997; 18:401–436.10.1146/annurev.publhealth.18.1.401 [PubMed: 9143725]

10. Heise LL, Raikes A, Watts CH, Zwi AB. Violence against women: a neglected public health issue in less developed countries. Soc Sci Med. 1994; 39(9):1165–1179.10.1016/0277-9536(94)90349-2 [PubMed: 7801154]

11. Garcia-Moreno, C.; Jansen, HA.; Ellsberg, M.; Watts, C. WHO Multi-Country Study on Women's Health and Domestic Violence Against Women: Initial Results on Prevalence, Health Outcomes, and Women's Response. Geneva, Switzerland: World Health Organization; 2005.

12. Krug, E.; Dahlberg, LL.; Mercy, JA.; Zwi, A.; Lozano, R. World Report on Violence and Health. Geneva, Switzerland: World Health Organization; 2002.

13. Violence Against Women and HIV/AIDS: Setting the Research Agenda. Geneva, Switzerland: World Health Organization; 2000.

14. Jewkes R, Penn-Kekana L, Levin J, Ratsaka M, Schrieber M. Prevalence of emotional, physical and sexual abuse of women in three South African provinces. S Afr Med J. 2001; 91(5):421–428. [PubMed: 11455808]

15. Jewkes R, Levin J, Mbananga N, Bradshaw D. Rape of girls in South Africa. Lancet. 2002; 359(9303): 319–320.10.1016/S0140-6736(02)07530-X [PubMed: 11830201]

16. Koenig MA, Lutalo T, Zhao F, et al. Coercive sex in rural Uganda: prevalence and associated risk factors. Soc Sci Med. 2004; 58(4):787–798.10.1016/S0277-9536(03)00244-2 [PubMed: 14672593]

17. Gupta J, Silverman JG, Hemenway D, Acevedo-Garcia D, Stein DJ, Williams DR. Physical violence against intimate partners and related exposures to violence among South African men. CMAJ. 2008; 179(6):535–541. [PubMed: 18779527]

18. Dunkle KL, Jewkes RK, Nduna M, et al. Perpetration of partner violence and HIV risk behaviour among young men in the rural Eastern Cape, South Africa. AIDS. 2006; 20(16):2107–2114.10.1097/01.aids.0000247582.00826.52 [PubMed: 17053357]

19. Jewkes R, Dunkle K, Koss MP, et al. Rape perpetration by young, rural South African men: prevalence, patterns and risk factors. Soc Sci Med. 2006; 63(11):2949–2961.10.1016/j.socscimed.2006.07.027 [PubMed: 16962222]

20. Abrahams N, Jewkes R, Hoffman M, Laubsher R. Sexual violence against intimate partners in Cape Town: prevalence and risk factors reported by men. Bull World Health Organ. 2004; 82(5): 330–337. [PubMed: 15298223]

21. Jewkes, R.; Sikweyiya, Y.; Morrell, R.; Dunkle, K. Understanding Men's Health and Use of Violence: Interface of Rape and HIV in South Africa. Pretoria, South Africa: Medical Research Council of South Africa; 2009.

22. Garcia-Moreno C, Jansen HA, Ellsberg M, Heise L, Watts CH. Prevalence of intimate partner violence: findings from the WHO multi-country study on women's health and domestic violence. Lancet. 2006; 368(9543):1260–1269.10.1016/S0140-6736(06)69523-8 [PubMed: 17027732]

23. Garcia-Moreno C. Dilemmas and opportunities

for an appropriate health-service response to violence against women. Lancet. 2002; 359(9316):1509–1514.10.1016/S0140-6736(02)08417-9 [PubMed: 11988263]

24. Epidemic of Inequality: Women's Rights and HIV/AIDS in Botswana and Swaziland. Cambridge, MA: Physicians for Human Rights; 2007.

25. Gouws E, Stanecki KA, Lyerla R, Ghys PD. The epidemiology of HIV infection among young people aged 15–24 years in southern Africa. AIDS. 2008; 22(suppl 4):S5, S16.10.1097/01.aids.0000341773.86500.9d [PubMed: 19033755]

26. Botswana 2003 Second Generation HIV/AIDS Surveillance. Gaborone, Botswana: National AIDS Coordinating Agency; 2003.

27. Heise LL. Violence against women: an integrated, ecological framework. Violence Against Women. 1998; 4(3):262–290.10.1177/1077801298004003002 [PubMed: 12296014]

28. Weiser SD, Leiter K, Bangsberg DR, et al. Food insufficiency is associated with high-risk sexual behavior among women in Botswana and Swaziland. PLoS Med. 2007; 4(10):1589–1597.10.1371/ journal.pmed.0040260 [PubMed: 17958460]

29. Alaimo K, Olson CM, Frongillo EA. Family food insufficiency, but not low family income, is positively associated with dysthymia and suicide symptoms in adolescents. J Nutr. 2002; 132(4):719–725. [PubMed: 11925467]

30. The Physician's Guide to Helping Patients With Alcohol Problems. Bethesda, MD: National Institute on Alcohol Abuse and Alcoholism; 1995.

31. Hosmer, D.; Lemeshow, S. Applied Logistic Regression. New York, NY: John Wiley & Sons Inc; 2000.

32. Zorn C. A solution to separation in binary response models. Polit Anal. 2005; 13(2):157–170.10.1093/pan/mpi009

33. Heinze G, Ploner M. Fixing the nonconvergence bug in logistic regression with SPLUS and SAS. Comput Methods Programs Biomed. 2003; 71(2):181–187.10.1016/S0169-2607(02)00088-3 [PubMed: 12758140]

34. Heinze G, Schemper M. A solution to the problem of separation in logistic regression. Stat Med. 2002; 21(16):2409–2419.10.1002/sim.1047 [PubMed: 12210625]

35. Firth D. Bias reduction of maximum likelihood estimates. Biometrika. 1993;80(1):27–38.10.1093/biomet/80.1.27

36. Reza A, Breiding MJ, Gulaid J, et al. Sexual violence and its health consequences for female children in Swaziland: a cluster survey study. Lancet. 2009; 373(9679):1966–1972.10.1016/ S0140-6736(09)60247-6 [PubMed: 19428100]

37. Gil-Gonzalez D, Vives-Cases C, Ruiz MT, Carrasco-Portino M, Alvarez-Dardet C. Childhood experiences of violence in perpetrators as a risk factor of intimate partner violence: a systematic review. J Public Health (Oxf). 2008; 30(1):14–22.10.1093/pubmed/fdm071 [PubMed: 17986717]

38. Dunkle KL, Jewkes RK, Brown HC, Gray GE, McIntryre JA, Harlow SD. Gender-based violence, relationship power, and risk of HIV infection in women attending antenatal clinics in South Africa. Lancet. 2004; 363(9419):1415–1421.10.1016/S0140-6736(04)16098-4 [PubMed: 15121402]

39. Beaman L, Chattopadhyay R, Duflo E, Pande R, Topalova P. Powerful women: does exposure reduce bias? Q J Econ. 2009; 124(4):1497–1540.10.1162/qjec.2009.124.4.1497

40. Pronyk PM, Hargreaves JR, Kim JC, et al. Effect of a structural intervention for the prevention of intimate-partner violence and HIV in rural South Africa: a cluster randomised trial. Lancet. 2006; 368(9551):1973–1983.10.1016/S0140-6736(06)69744-4 [PubMed: 17141704]

41. Pronyk PM, Kim JC, Abramsky T, et al. A combined microfinance and training intervention can reduce HIV risk behaviour in young female participants. AIDS. 2008; 22(13):1659–1665.10.1097/QAD.0b013e328307a040 [PubMed: 18670227]

42. Botswana Family Health Survey II: 1988. Gaborone, Botswana: Central Statistics Office and Institute for Resource Development/Macro Systems Inc; 1989.

43. Swaziland Demographic and Health Survey 2006–07. Mbabane, Swaziland: Central Statistical Office and Macro International Inc; 2008.

44. Sikweyiya Y, Jewkes R. Force and temptation: contrasting South African men's accounts of coercion into sex by men and women. Cult Health Sex. 2009; 11(5):529–541.10.1080/13691050902912783 [PubMed: 19499390]

45. Dunkle KL, Jewkes R. Effective HIV prevention requires gender-transformative work with men. Sex Transm Infect. 2007; 83(3):173–174.10.1136/sti.2007.024950 [PubMed: 17569718]

QUESTIONS

1. Do you believe that this study overestimates or underestimates the extent of sexual violence? Why? Consider that approximately 90% of people contacted participated in the survey. Who do you believe participated and why? Do you believe that the survey can be assumed to be equally reliable for all who participated? Review the results of this study. Are any of these findings surprising to you? For instance, was having multiple sexual partners found to be a risk factor? What were the major risk factors found in this study? Consider the effects of chance, bias and confounding factors that may have influenced these results.

2. The authors state that the World Health Organization (WHO) has identified "the issue of sexual violence against men and boys as a 'significant problem' that has been largely neglected." Why do you think this topic has been neglected?

3. In the conclusion, the authors state that the "risk of sexual violence among women is significantly compounded by the high prevalence of HIV in these two countries." Do you believe that sexual violence contributed to high rates of HIV and vice versa? Why or why not?

FURTHER READING

1. Kara, Siddharth, *Sex Trafficking: Inside the Business of Modern Slavery.* New York: Columbia University Press, 2009.
2. Kempadoo, Kamala, Sanghera, Jyoti, & Pattanaik, Bandana, *Trafficking and Prostitution Reconsidered: New Perspectives on Migration, Sex Work, and Human Rights.* Boulder, CO: Paradigm Publishers, 2005.
3. Pinker, Steven, *The Better Angels of Our Nature: Why Violence Has Declined.* New York: Viking, 2011.

POINT OF VIEW

Indigenous Health Is a Matter of Human Rights

Tom Calma

The lethargy with which we have faced the apparently intractable crisis of Indigenous health is not forever. We know that in a relatively short time frame the fortunes of Maoris and Native Americans have been improved. In my *2005 Social Justice Report* I argued that Indigenous health inequality was an urgent human rights issue and I called on the Australian Government to commit to closing the 17-year life expectancy gap within a generation—that is, by 2030.

Indigenous health inequality is the result of a failure to realise the right to health of Indigenous Australians. We have not ensured Indigenous Australians have the same opportunities to be as healthy as other Australians, or taken effective action to remedy long-standing and substantial health inequalities. Indigenous Australians are dying between 10 and 17 years before other Australians. Chronic disease, notably heart disease, kills Indigenous Australians at between two and three times the rate of death in the non-Indigenous population. Deaths from diabetes are more than 10 times higher and smoking related diseases account for 20% of all Indigenous Australian deaths.

To date governments have tackled the Indigenous health problem by pouring in more funding or services. But we know that programs are more successful if people are actively involved in their own development, rather than being passive recipients. That's why a human rights-based approach to Indigenous health holds the promise of real success where other campaigns have failed.

Addressing health as a human rights issue holds governments accountable for health by treating outcomes as a matter of legal obligation. It also guards against threats to health such as discrimination and inequality, and ensures that the determinants of health, such as education, adequate housing and nutrition, are dealt with effectively.

The human rights-based approach to health is one of the most cutting edge developments I have seen in the international sphere. The right to health has been acknowledged for more than 60 years, dating back to the Constitution of the World Health Organization, the Universal Declaration of Human Rights and the International Covenant on Economic, Social and Cultural Rights. But health programming has only now begun to catch up, and to talk seriously about what a rights-based approach to health means.

When we launched the Close the Gap Campaign for Indigenous Health Equality in Australia in April 2007, I said governments cannot guarantee that their citizens will be healthy; that involves individual choice and freedom. But they can guarantee that every opportunity has been provided to facilitate this outcome. The campaign was built on evidence that shows that significant improvements in the health status can be achieved within short timeframes. For example, the life expectancy of Native Americans increased by about nine years between the 1940s and the 1950s, and in New Zealand, the life expectancy of Maori increased by about 12 years over the two decades from the 1940s to the 1960s, when primary health care services were provided. In Australia, death rates among Aboriginal people from pneumonia have dropped by 40 per cent since 1996, following the roll-out of pneumococcal vaccinations. And a program known as the "Strong Babies, Strong Culture" maternal health program has shown that significant reductions in the number of low birth weight babies can occur within a matter of years.

The challenge ahead for us remains to hold governments to their commitments to a comprehensive national planning process and to also embrace a true partnership with Indigenous people. It is absolutely vital that the people whom governments are hoping to help in any given policy context are active players in the design and delivery of the policies and programs that result.

The plan should include a co-ordinating body to oversee and guide the work of the many Australian, State and Territory government agencies responsible for delivering health and allied services for the Aboriginal and Torres Strait Islander population, and a monitoring body, as accountability is essential to the human rights approach. The plan, too, should address all the factors that contribute to Indigenous health inequality. This is a fundamental human rights obligation of governments, and particularly when faced with extreme inequality along racial lines. In that regard, the campaign can be viewed, in human rights terms, as a special measure to address inequality.

This is not just a matter of rights for rights' sake. Human rights are practical and grounded in common sense from a policy perspective. By partnering with Indigenous people, introducing a national plan and setting ambitious but realistic targets we will be able, I believe, to see a day when the gap between indigenous and non-Indigenous health in Australian, and around the world, will be closed for good.

POSTSCRIPT

In November 2011, the Minister for Health and the Minister for Indigenous Health announced the development of a new health plan for Aboriginal and Torres Strait Islander Australians. The *National Aboriginal and Torres Strait Islander Health Plan* is being established by the Australian Government working in partnership with Aboriginal and Torres Strait Islander peoples and organisations, and with the participation of state and territory governments. The National Aboriginal and Torres Strait Islander Health Equality Council will provide strategic policy advice on the plan. An advisory group co-chaired by the Department of Health and Ageing and the National Congress of Australia's First Peoples will inform the development and content of the plan.

Tom Calma is an Aboriginal elder from the Kungarakan tribal group and a member of the Iwaidja tribal group, National Coordinator, Tackling Indigenous Smoking, and the former Australian Aboriginal and Torres Strait Islander Social Justice Commissioner.

CHAPTER 21

Solitary Confinement and Mental Illness in U.S. Prisons: A Challenge for Medical Ethics

Jeffrey L. Metzner and Jamie Fellner

Physicians who work in U.S. prison facilities face ethically difficult challenges arising from substandard working conditions, dual loyalties to patients and employers, and the tension between reasonable medical practices and the prison rules and culture. In recent years, physicians have increasingly confronted a new challenge: the prolonged solitary confinement of prisoners with serious mental illness, a corrections practice that has become prevalent despite the psychological harm it can cause. There has been scant professional or academic attention to the unique ethics-related quandary of physicians and other healthcare professionals when prisons isolate inmates with mental illness. We hope to begin to fill this gap.

Solitary confinement is recognized as difficult to withstand; indeed, psychological stressors such as isolation can be as clinically distressing as physical torture.[1,2] Nevertheless, U.S. prison officials have increasingly embraced a variant of solitary confinement to punish and control difficult or dangerous prisoners. Whether in the so-called supermax prisons that have proliferated over the past two decades or in segregation (i.e., locked-down housing) units within regular prisons, tens of thousands of prisoners spend years locked up 23 to 24 hours a day in small cells that frequently have solid steel doors. They live with extensive surveillance and security controls, the absence of ordinary social interaction, abnormal environmental stimuli, often only three to five hours a week of recreation alone in caged enclosures, and little, if any, educational, vocational, or other purposeful activities (i.e., programs). They are handcuffed and frequently shackled every time they leave their cells.[3-5] The terms segregation, solitary confinement, and isolation will be used interchangeably to describe these conditions of confinement.

Isolation can be psychologically harmful to any prisoner, with the nature and severity of the impact depending on the individual, the duration, and particular conditions (e.g., access to natural light, books, or radio). Psychological effects can include anxiety, depression, anger, cognitive disturbances, perceptual distortions, obsessive thoughts, paranoia, and psychosis.[6]

The adverse effects of solitary confinement are especially significant for persons with serious mental illness, commonly defined as a major mental disorder (e.g., schizophrenia, bipolar disorder, major depressive disorder) that is usually characterized by psychotic symptoms and/or significant functional impairments. The stress, lack of meaningful social contact, and unstructured days can exacerbate symptoms of illness or provoke recurrence.[7] Suicides occur disproportionately more often in segregation units than elsewhere in prison.[8-10] All too frequently, mentally ill prisoners decompensate in isolation, requiring crisis care or psychiatric hospitalization. Many simply will not get better as long as they are isolated.

Mental health professionals are often unable to mitigate fully the harm associated with isolation. Mental health services in segregation units are typically limited to psychotropic medication, a health care clinician stopping at the cell front to ask how the prisoner is doing (i.e., mental health rounds), and occasional meetings in private with a clinician.[7] Individual therapy; group therapy; structured educational, recreational, or life-skill-enhancing activities; and other therapeutic interventions are usually not available because of insufficient resources and rules requiring prisoners to remain in their cells.[11]

The use of segregation to confine the mentally ill has grown as the number and proportion of prisoners with mental illness have grown. Although designed and operated as places of punishment, prisons have nonetheless become *de facto* psychiatric facilities despite often lacking the needed mental health services.[7] Studies and clinical experience consistently indicate that 8 to 19 percent of prisoners have psychiatric disorders that result in significant functional disabilities, and another 15 to 20 percent require some form of psychiatric intervention during their incarceration.[12] Sixty percent of state correctional systems responding to a survey on inmate mental health reported that 15 percent or more of their inmate population had a diagnosed mental illness.[13]

Despite significant improvements in correctional mental health services, often related to litigation and development of standards and guidelines by the National Commission on Correctional Health Care (NCCHC), the American Psychiatric Association (APA), and other professional organizations, in many prisons the services remain woefully inadequate. Relative to the number of prisoners needing help, there is an insufficient number of qualified staff, too few specialized facilities, and few programs.[7] Mindful of budget constraints and scant public support for investments in the treatment (as opposed to punishment) of prisoners, elected officials have been reluctant to provide the funds and leadership needed to ensure that prisons have sufficient mental health resources. Twenty-two of 40 state correctional systems reported in a survey that they did not have an adequate mental health staff.[13]

Persons with mental illness are often impaired in their ability to handle the stresses of incarceration and to conform to a highly regimented routine. They may exhibit bizarre, annoying, or dangerous behavior and have higher rates of disciplinary infractions than other prisoners. Prison officials generally respond to them as they do to other prisoners who break the rules. When lesser sanctions do not curb the behavior, they isolate the prisoners in the segregation units, despite the likely negative mental health impact. Once in segregation, continued misconduct, often connected to mental illness, can keep the inmates there indefinitely.[7,14]

In class action cases challenging the segregation of inmates with serious mental illness as unconstitutionally cruel because of the psychological harm it can inflict, U.S. federal courts have either issued rulings or accepted settlements that prohibit or sharply curtail the practice. According to one federal judge, putting mentally ill prisoners in isolated confinement "is the mental equivalent of putting an asthmatic in a place with little air...."[15] Unfortunately, except in the small number of prisons governed by the outcome of such litigation, mentally ill prisoners continue to be sent to segregation; indeed, they are often disproportionately represented in segregation units.[16,17]

International treaty bodies and human rights experts, including the Human Rights Committee,[18] the Committee against Torture,[19,20] and the U.N. Special Rapporteur on Torture,[21] have concluded that solitary confinement may amount to cruel, inhuman, or degrading treatment in violation of the International Covenant on Civil and Political Rights[22] and the Convention against Torture and other Cruel, Inhuman, and Degrading Treatment or Punishment.[23] They have specifically criticized supermax confinement in the United States because of the mental suffering it inflicts.[19,20] Whatever one's views on supermax confinement in general, human rights experts agree that its use for inmates with serious mental illness violates their human rights.

Principles of ethics regarding beneficence, nonmaleficence, and respect for the rights and dignity of all patients have led international and national professional organizations to affirm that physicians are ethically obligated to refrain from countenancing, condoning, participating in, or facilitating torture or other forms of cruel, inhuman, or degrading treatment.[24–27] Involvement of healthcare practitioners in abusive interrogations recently prompted the American Medical Association[28] and the APA[29] to oppose the participation of physicians in interrogations. Two years ago, the NCCHC issued a position statement that correctional health care professionals "should not condone or participate in cruel, inhumane or degrading treatment of inmates."[30] To date, however, the medical organizations have not formally acknowledged that prolonged isolation of the mentally ill constitutes cruel or inhuman treatment in violation of human rights, nor have they addressed health professionals' ethics-related responsibilities when faced with such cases.

Correctional health care professionals struggle with constrained resources and large caseloads that limit the services they can provide their patients. It is ethical for them to do the best they can under the circumstances rather than resigning, which would result in even fewer services for their patients. But what are practitioners' ethics-related responsibilities when prison officials impose conditions of confinement that exacerbate the symptoms of a prisoner's mental illness?

The ethics-based calculus physicians face when prisoners are isolated for disciplinary or security reasons is different than that created by the struggle with limited resources. Segregation of mentally ill prisoners (or any other prisoner) is not an unintended consequence of tight budgets, for example. It reflects a penal philosophy and the conscious decision by prison officials about whom to isolate, for how long, and under what conditions. If health professionals simply do their rounds but say nothing, are they implicitly legitimizing the segregation of mentally ill prisoners and thereby contributing to the continuation of the harm? What must they do to avoid being complicit in conditions of confinement that may well constitute a human rights violation?

We believe it is ethical for physicians to treat prisoners who have been abused, but they must also take measures to end the abuse. In addition to providing whatever services they can to segregated patients, they should advocate within the prison system for changed segregation policies and, if that fails, they should undertake public advocacy.[31–33]

Publically exposing and urging change in harmful prison practices is difficult and, needless to say, can threaten job security, but individual practitioners should not have to wrestle alone with a prison practice that violates human rights norms. Their professional organizations should help them. Through the organizations, health professionals collectively can support colleagues who work in prisons in the quest to ensure ethically defensible correctional policies. The APA[34] and the NCCHC[35] have provided basic frameworks for increased mental health monitoring and treatment of segregated inmates. They must do more, however.

Professional healthcare organizations should acknowledge that prolonged segregation of inmates with serious mental illness violates basic tenets of mental health treatment. The mental health standards of the NCCHC include the "optional recommendation" that mentally ill prisoners be excluded from extreme isolation,[35] noting in an appendix that clinicians "generally agree that placement of inmates with serious mental illnesses in settings with 'extreme isolation' is contraindicated because many of these inmates' psychiatric conditions will clinically deteriorate or not improve."[36,37] In light of that general consensus, shouldn't the NCCHC make the exclusion mandatory, instead of optional? The APA and AMA should also formally adopt a similar position.

However, adopting a similar position is easier said than done. Very few physicians in the APA and AMA have experience or knowledge regarding correctional mental health care, let alone correctional environments in general. They are not familiar with the differences between a general population housing unit and a disciplinary segregation housing unit. Administrative segregation, supermax, rules infractions, mental health rounds, and "kites" are terms most noncorrectional physicians do not understand. In short, we recognize that a serious educational effort must be mounted so that noncorrectional mental health practitioners have a better understanding of the world in which their correctional colleagues work and the unique challenges they face, including the isolation of seriously ill patients for months, even years, that would never be condoned in a noncorrectional mental health setting.

No doubt some correctional mental health clinicians will not agree with us. They may believe the isolation of volatile mentally ill prisoners is necessary for security reasons. They may believe they are guests in the house of corrections who have no business addressing custody policies, or they may have become so accustomed to the extended use of isolation that they have lost sight of its potential to cause psychological harm.

Experience demonstrates that prisons can operate safely and securely without putting inmates with mental illness in typical conditions of segregation. Because of litigation, in some prisons, mentally ill prisoners who would otherwise be locked in their cell for 23 to 24 hours a day are given more time outside their cells, including time in group therapy and other therapeutic interventions.[11] The improved clinical responses of prisoners with mental illness have been achieved without sacrificing needed controls or relinquishing the goal of holding those accountable, whether mentally ill or not, who willfully violate prison rules.

The professional organizations should acknowledge that it is not ethically defensible for health care professionals to acquiesce silently to conditions of confinement that inflict mental harm and violate human rights. They should affirm that practitioners are ethically obligated, not only to treat segregated inmates with mental illness, but also to strive to change harmful segregation policies and practices.[31-33] Finally, the organizations should not be content with clarifying the ethics-related responsibilities of individual practitioners in these circumstances. They should actively support practitioners who work for changed segregation policies, and they should use their institutional authority to press for a nationwide rethinking of the use of isolation. The medical professions' commitment to ethics and human rights would be well served by such steps.

REFERENCES

1. Reyes H: The worst scars are in the mind: psychological torture. Int Rev Red Cross 89:591–617, 2007
2. Basoglu M, Livanou M, Crnobaric C: Torture vs. other cruel, inhuman and degrading treatment: is the distinction real or apparent? Arch Gen Psychiatry 64:277–85, 2007
3. Riveland C: Supermax prisons: overview and general considerations. Washington, DC: U.S. Department of Justice, National Institute of Corrections, January 1999
4. Fellner J, Mariner J: Cold storage: supermaximum security confinement in Indiana. Human Rights Watch, October 1997
5. Commission on Safety and Abuse in America's Prisons: Confronting confinement: a report of the Commission on Safety and Abuse in America's Prisons. Washington, DC: Vera Institute of Justice, June 2006, pp 52–61.
6. Smith PS: The effects of solitary confinement on prison inmates: a brief history and review of the literature. Crim Just 34:441–568, 2006
7. Abramsky S, Fellner J: Ill-equipped: US prisons and offenders with mental illness. Human Rights Watch, 2003, pp 145–68
8. Patterson RF, Hughes K: Review of completed suicides in the California Department of Corrections and Rehabilitation, 1999 to 2004. Psychiatr Serv 59:677–81, 2008
9. White T, Schimmel D, Frickey R: A comprehensive analysis of suicide in federal prisons: a fifteen-year review. J Correct Health Care 9:321–43, 2002
10. Hayes LM: Prison guide: an overview and guide to prevention. Washington, DC: U.S. Department of Justice, National Institute of Corrections, 1995.
11. Metzner JL, Dvoskin JA: An overview of correctional psychiatry. Psychiatr Clin North Am 29:761–72, 2006
12. Metzner JL: Class action litigation in correctional psychiatry. J Am Acad Psychiatry Law 30:19–29, 2002
13. Hill C: Inmate mental health care. Correct Compend 29:15–31, 2004
14. Fellner J: A corrections quandary: mental illness and prison rules. Harv CR-CL L Rev 41:391–412, 2006
15. Madrid v. Gomez, 889 F. Supp. 1146, 1265 (N.D. Cal. 1995)
16. Lovell D: Patterns of disturbed behavior in a supermax prison. Crim Just Behav 35:985–1004, 2008
17. O'Keefe M, Schnell MJ: Offenders with mental illness in the correctional system. J Offend Rehabil 45:81–104, 2007
18. United Nations Human Rights Committee: CCPR General comment No. 20: replaces general comment 7 concerning prohibition of torture, or other cruel, inhuman or degrading treatment or punishment. New York: UNHRC, 1992
19. United Nations Human Rights Committee: Consideration of reports submitted by States parties under Article 40 of the Covenant, concluding observations of the Human Rights Committee, United States of America. New York: UNHRC, UN Doc. CCPR/C/USA/CO/3, 2006
20. United Nations Committee Against Torture: Consideration of reports submitted by States parties under Article 19 of the Convention, Conclusions and Recommendations of the Committee Against Torture, United States of America. New York: UN Committee Against Torture, UN Doc. CAT/C/USA/CO/2, 2006
21. Interim Report of the Special Rapporteur on Torture and Other Cruel, Inhuman or Degrading Treatment or Punishment. UN General Assembly. New York: United Nations, UN Doc. A/63/175:18–21, 2008
22. International Covenant on Civil and Political Rights.
23. Convention Against Torture and Other Cruel, Inhuman or Degrading Treatment or Punishment.
24. World Medical Association: Guidelines for medical doctors concerning torture and other cruel, inhuman or degrading treatment or punishment in relation to detention and imprisonment. Adopted by the 29th WMA Assembly, Tokyo, Japan, October 1975
25. American Medical Association: Code of Medical Ethics. Opinion 2.067, Torture, 1999
26. The World Psychiatric Association: Madrid Declaration on Ethical Standards for Psychiatric Practice. Approved by the WPA General Assembly, 1996
27. American Medical Association: H-65.997, Human Rights. Health and ethics policies of the AMA House of Delegates. Adopted December 1978
28. American Medical Association: Code of Medical Ethics. Opinion 2.068, Physician participation in interrogation. Issued November 2006
29. American Psychiatric Association: Position state

ment: Psychiatric participation in interrogation of detainees. Adopted May 2006

30. National Commission on Correctional Health Care: Position statement: correctional health care professionals' Response to Inmate Abuse. Adopted October 14, 2007

31. Dual loyalty and human rights in health professional practice: proposed guidelines and institutional mechanisms. Physicians for Human Rights and School of Public Health and Primary Health Care, University of Cape Town, 2003.

32. Nielsen NH, Heyman JM: Letter from the American Medical Association President and Chair of the Board of Trustees (respectively) to the Honorable Barak Obama, April 17, 2009.

33. World Medical Association: Declaration concerning support for medical doctors refusing to participate in, or to condone, the use of torture or other forms of cruel, inhuman or degrading treatment. Adopted by the 49th WMA Assembly. Hamburg, Germany, November 1997.

34. National Commission on Correctional Health Care: Standards for mental health services in correctional facilities. Standard MHE-07, 2008

35. American Psychiatric Association: Psychiatric services in jails and prisons: a task force report of the American Psychiatric Association (ed 2). Washington, DC: American Psychiatric Association, 2000, pp 4–5

36. Metzner JL: Mental health considerations for segregated inmates. Appendix E to Standards for Mental Health Services in Correctional Facilities. Chicago, IL: National Commission on Correctional Health Care, 2008, pp 129–31

37. Work Group on Schizophrenia: American Psychiatric Association practice guidelines: practice guideline for the treatment of patients with schizophrenia. Am J Psychiatry 154(April Suppl.):1–63, 1997

QUESTIONS

1. The authors state that "by simply doing rounds, health care professionals are implicitly legitimizing the segregation of the mentally ill." Comment on this statement. Does the medical profession's commitment to "do no harm" necessitate advocacy? Why is there limited precedence for such advocacy in prison settings? Consider other historical instances in which physicians have "implicitly legitimized" human rights violations.

2. What role do the authors recommend NGOs take in addressing solitary confinement in prisons? Do you agree? Do prison physicians have special obligations for the welfare of their patient/prisoners? Why or why not?

3. The authors state, "We conclude by urging professional organizations to adopt formal positions against the prolonged isolation of prisoners with serious mental illness." Do you believe we should go further and abolish solitary confinement?

FURTHER READING

1. Dudley, Michael, Silove, Derrick, & Gale, Fran, *Mental Health and Human Rights: Vision, Praxis, and Courage.* Oxford: Oxford University Press, 2012.
2. Stuntz, William J., *The Collapse of American Criminal Justice.* Cambridge: Harvard University Press, 2011.
3. Drucker, Ernest, *A Plague of Prisons: The Epidemiology of Mass Incarceration in America.* New York: New Press, 2011.

POINT OF VIEW

Dual Loyalty in Clinical and Public Health Settings—the Imperative to Uphold Human Rights

Leslie London, Laurel Baldwin-Ragaven and Leonard Rubenstein

Dual loyalty describes a situation in which a health professional allows third party pressures to induce complicity in human rights violations of patients. Such conflicts are commonplace in contexts of closed institutions where secrecy and invisibility tend to foster subordination of clinical independence to the interests of a state security authority. For example, health professionals assisted in the interrogation of prisoner-detainees in US bases in Iraq and Guantánamo Bay by disclosing confidential medical information and advising on interrogation techniques.

Characteristic of divided loyalty is the use of professional skills to advance third party interests, where third party interests are thought to fulfill a social objective. Resolution of these conflicts is poorly addressed in health professional ethical codes and conflicts may be masked by lip service to the Hippocratic notion that, "The health of my patient shall be my first consideration"; since, in reality, third parties frequently do have considerable stake in the outcomes of health professional practice. Such situations are exacerbated by employment relationships, professional isolation, reimbursement mechanisms, class position, stigma and institutional discrimination against vulnerable groups.

In response, an international working group developed guidelines in 2002 that drew on both existing international ethical codes and human rights standards in a booklet entitled "Dual Loyalty and Human Rights." Central to the guidelines approach is the conclusion that health personnel should not become instruments by which third parties commit human rights violations. Procedurally, the clinician does not attempt to balance these competing interests through an ethics paradigm chosen by the individual, but strives to follow global human rights standards, and, ideally, does so in an environment with institutional mechanisms to protect clinical independence structurally.

It is difficult to extend this framework to public health professionals. First, many public health professionals provide services to vulnerable communities or populations, rather than individuals, and human rights obligations to populations are less fully articulated. Second, many public health professionals work in a context where professional accountability does not exist in the same manner as where direct patient care is involved.

Nonetheless, because public health policy decisions, often couched in the language of equity, efficiency and effectiveness, have widespread ramifications for the rights of communities, there should be human rights standards and professional accountability for public health actions. Health professionals are often asked to interpret the interests of the state (or a third party) as being more morally compelling than that of a single vulnerable individual (clinical conflict) or a vulnerable population (public health conflict). Aside from ethical considerations, health professionals typically do not possess the information or skills to make such an interpretation. For example, how is a health professional to judge a claim that a detainee is a 'terrorist' who has planned mass destruction, and who security officials suggest should be subjected to harsh and inhuman interrogation to foil the plan.

Where limitations of individual rights are proposed to benefit the public good, often framed by utilitarian arguments, in the clinical context any decision to depart from fidelity to the patient should be within a recognized framework of exceptions, such as suicide prevention. Translated into the public health context, this means: (a) the application of well established tools for measuring the justification for such limitations; and (b) working in the context of a recognized framework for evaluating policies that are transparent and trustworthy.

The public health practitioner needs to understand a rights-based approach to balancing the public good against individual rights in the rare cases where these conflict. Public health practice recognises that health is both an individual right and a government instrumental to human development, and thee may be circumstances where limits may justifiably be placed on individual rights in order to advance the public good, and where the public good is itself the realization of public health as a right (such as universally fluoridating water, or adding folic acid to flour to prevent caries or neural tube defects, respectively). But such limitations must be consonant with human rights principles and must recognize the indivisibility of civil and political rights with socio-economic entitlements, even in the context of priority setting among competing public health needs. Public

health professionals need skills and support to make such assessments. They will usually, for example, require use of the least intrusive intervention to meet the public health goal.

When confronted with requirements to develop or implement public health policies that infringe human rights, the public health official is required to resist them just as a clinician faced with a demand to participate in torture should; and professional peers and organisations should offer support to maintaining a human rights stance.

Public officials and leaders who are also themselves health professionals must be accountable. If ordinary citizens are expected to act in accordance with a rights-based social contract and officials, as agents of the state, must also respect, protect and fulfill human rights, then particular and additional responsibilities for health professionals in relation to human rights exist both in clinical and public health roles. Such commitment is consistent with the ideals of a public health tradition with deep historical roots in social processes that recognize the social determinants of health, and the role that health plays not only as an end in itself but as essential to human development.

Leslie London is Head, Health and Human Rights Division, and Professor and Director, School of Public Health and Family Medicine, and Associate Director, Occupational and Environmental Health Unit, University of Cape Town, Cape Town, South Africa.
Laurel Baldwin-Ragaven MD, is Professor of Family Medicine, University of Witwatersrand, Johannesburg, South Africa.
Leonard Rubenstein JD, is Senior Scholar at the Center for Public Health and Human Rights, Johns Hopkins Bloomberg School of Public Health, Baltimore, Maryland.

CHAPTER 22

American Vertigo: "Dual Use," Prison Physicians, Research and Guantánamo

George J. Annas

The concept of "divided loyalties" is an inherently perverse one, suggesting that loyalty is negotiable and never trustworthy. This is how many Americans felt about the Japanese-Americans in World War II, and is why Japanese were confined in concentration camps, even though there was no evidence that they were disloyal to the United States.[1] The terms "divided loyalty" and "dual loyalty" were used as a rationalization for taking action against them. Something similar is going on when this term is deployed to describe physicians in the United States military: that they have divided or dual loyalties because they face inherent conflicts between their obligations as physicians and their obligations as military officers. My own view is that this is simply false; the entire rationale for having a military medical service is to provide the best medical care possible to the U.S. military—and that such care can only be provided if soldiers trust military physicians to follow medical ethics without exception.[2]

Military commanders in charge of prisons do, however, attempt to use military physicians for nonmedical, security purposes. In this regard, it is more analytically useful to think about this as a case of "dual use," in the same sense that medically beneficial products and processes can also be used as weapons to harm people. Physicians, both military and civilian, can also make "dual use" of people when practicing medicine: treating them for their medical condition, and thus as a patient, but also using them as research subjects to test a hypothesis. It is also possible that military physicians could find themselves confronted by both types of dual use; for example, ordered to experiment on their patient-prisoners by their superiors. Thus, it makes sense when reviewing attempts to make dual use of military physicians in prisons that we simultaneously look at the dual use of prisoners—as patients and research subjects—that some physicians propose themselves.[3]

The primary places where dual use of military physicians has occurred is in the post 9/11 prisons at Bagram Air Force Base, Abu Ghraib, and Guantánamo.[4] The first two have been renamed in an unrealistic attempt to rehabilitate them.[5] Guantánamo, however, seems likely to stay open and functioning with its original name indefinitely.[6] The role of military physicians there is doubly complicated by the fact, recognized by the U.S. Department of Defense, that the continued force feeding of competent hunger strikers at Guantánamo is a direct violation of medical ethics as articulated by the World Medical Association (WMA) and the American Medical Association.[7] This situation (officially requiring military physicians to ignore medical ethics precepts) is unique in American military history, and one that I have written about before.[8] In this chapter, I will say more about hunger strikes at Guantánamo, but I will also examine another duality, refuting the claim that military prison at Guantánamo, and the dual use of physicians there, is so unique that it should be seen as an aberration in the American justice system, rather than as a mirror image of the worst aspects of U.S. mainland prisons. The way wardens, physicians, expert commentators, and the courts have justified nonmedical and coercive acts by physicians is bizarre enough to cause vertigo, and this helps explain my title for this chapter. And because the anti-prisoner actions seem to me to be entirely consistent with America's view of the dangerousness of its large prison population, "American vertigo" seems appropriate as well.

American Vertigo is also the title French philosopher and journalist, Bernard-Henri Levy, gave to his observations of America that he made after retracing the footsteps of Tocqueville.[9] Like a leading U.S. expert group that championed doing more medical research on prisoners—the Institute of Medicine's (IOM) Committee on Prisoner Research (Committee)[10]—Levy began his journey in 2005. This was four years after 9/11 and the commencement of our "global war on terror," and three years after Guantánamo was opened. The centerpiece of this war has been to capture would-be terrorists and interrogate them in our greatly expanded global prison system, especially, as previously noted, in Afghanistan, where the most infamous was Bagram Air Force Base; in Iraq, which featured Abu Ghraib; and in Cuba, which features Guantánamo. At all of these prisons, the Central Intelligence Agency and the American military have inflicted tortuous acts and cruel and degrading treatment on prisoners.[11] At home, the U.S. prison population continues to grow, and the United States has set a new world-record in terms of the percentage of the civilian population in prison.[12]

In March 2011, President Barack Obama, reversing his promise and position that he would close the prison in Guantánamo Bay, decided instead to reinitiate military trials there and keep the prison open indefinitely.[13] The reason the President originally pledged to close Guantánamo was his belief that it was a uniquely horrible prison, "quite simply a mess, a misguided experiment."[14] He is not the only one to refer to Guantánamo as an experimental prison. A Senate investigation found that commanders at the prison often referred to it as "America's Battle Lab" where untested methods of interrogation, which were to some degree experimental, were tried out.[15] I have also previously suggested that the use of "restraint chairs" by the medical staff at the prison to break the 2005–06 mass hunger strike there could also be seen as "experimental," since they had never before been used for this purpose.[16] In this chapter, I will use this "experimental" designation to explore the question of whether the President was right initially to see Guantánamo as an aberration of American justice and the American prison system, or whether Guantánamo is more properly seen as a logical extension of the American prison system, as Levy maintained, and as President Obama now seems to accept as well. I will approach this question by examining in some depth an IOM report on human experimentation in American prisons issued during the Bush administration, with a view to determine how Guantánamo "fits" into the landscape of American prisons, American justice, and American research.

THE IOM PRISON RESEARCH COMMITTEE

The IOM Committee described its charge: "to examine whether the conclusions reached by the national commission

[National Commission for the Protection of Subjects of Biomedical and Behavioral Research] in 1976 remain appropriate today."[17] There was no identification of any major problems with prison research in the United States that would have provided a framework for the committee's work.[18] Instead, the structure was to consider changes in prisons and medical research that might lead to a reconsideration of existing rules, and to suggest an approach that would permit more research on prisoners. To oversimplify somewhat, the committee's report follows a syllogism:

1. Research is beneficial.
2. Prisoners should have access to that which is beneficial.
3. Therefore prisoners should have (more) access to research.

A parallel syllogism seems to have been applied at Guantánamo in response to the hunger strikes:

1. Hunger striking risks the prisoner's life.
2. Physicians should prevent prisoners from risking their lives.
3. Therefore, physicians should prevent prison hunger strikes.

Both syllogisms have problems. The primary one with the first syllogism is that it conflates research with treatment (usually woefully inadequate in prisons), thereby making a dual use seem like a single use. The same is true of the second syllogism, where force-feeding hunger strikers is equated with medical treatment. But there are others: prisoners are not granted all the benefits of free living people, and prisoners are uniquely situated in ways that compromise their autonomy and make voluntary consent especially problematic.

But even this syllogism structure is grossly oversimplified, as the IOM report itself provides support for almost every position one might have to either promote or restrict research on prisoners. Most often, the goal is stated as expanding research on prisoners, but at other times the stated goal is to protect prisoners from exploitation.[19] Sometimes informed consent is seen as too important in current regulations and replaceable, other times it is seen as central and nonnegotiable.[20] Sometimes prisons are seen as the new mental health institutions; other times the as yet unadopted regulations on research on the mentally disabled are viewed as irrelevant in the prison setting.[21] Children are excluded from the analysis, but the children's research regulations are sometimes viewed as a model for changing the prisoner regulations.[22] No specific language is ever suggested as to how the current prisoner regulations might be modified.

How did the Committee adopt such a confused and internally inconsistent report? My own view is that by abstracting the issue of research on prisoners from the questions of how they became prisoners, why we have more prisoners per capita than any country in the world, why African Americans and Hispanics are so overrepresented in prisons, and what the impact of the global war on terror is on our view of prisoners and their rights, the entire exercise became so disconnected from the real world that it could produce no useful public policy recommendations. As will be addressed later, similar observations apply to breaking the hunger strikes at Guantánamo.

The definition of prisoner is the central issue in any discussion of research on prisoners. The Committee knows this, but nonetheless insists on expanding the definition of "prisoner" from the current one that includes those "involuntarily confined or detained in a penal institution" to include an additional five million non-prisoners (unconfined people on probation and parole).[23] This begs the question of why we should have separate rules for prisoners at all (if not because their involuntary confinement makes voluntary consent extremely unlikely), and why we should not just include all potential research subjects under the term "prisoner"? This is the central conceptual problem with the IOM's report.

Two more concrete operational problems undermine the report's credibility. The first is that while expanding the definition of prisoner radically, the report simultaneously contracts it by excluding from consideration not only children and involuntarily confined mental patients, but also prisoners held under the U.S.A. Patriot Act.[24] The report did not specifically exclude Guantánamo and Abu Ghraib, but nonetheless fails to even mention these two American prisons.[25] The second concrete problem with the report is its internal incoherence. There are, for example, only two chapters devoted to "ethics," and these often read as if they were written by two separate committees (or study directors) that had fundamental disagreements. The report really does induce vertigo. Each of the two major operational flaws merits discussion.

AMERICAN PRISONS AT HOME AND ABROAD

Writing a report about research on prisoners without acknowledging the increasing role of prisons and mistreatment of prisoners can only paint a partial picture. By far the most famous prison in the world is Guantánamo Bay, and the most infamous prison in the world is Abu Ghraib. This was also true when the Committee was working on their report.

How is it possible that an IOM committee on the ethics of prison research could proceed as if these prisons did not exist? It was, of course, Bush Administration doc-trine that "we do not torture," that Abu Ghraib was the result of a few bad apples on the night shift, and that Guantánamo only holds the "worst of the worst" and is necessary to prevent another 9/11.[26] But IOM study committees should proceed from science and data, not from the political ideology of the administration in power. Nonetheless, these prisons were so central to the Bush Administration's view of what is and is not acceptable to do to prisoners (both under domestic and international law) that it would be unthinkable to prepare a report on U.S. research on prisoners without at least mentioning, if not analyzing, them.[27]

The Committee's chairman, Professor Lawrence Gostin, seems to agree with this assessment. In a summary of the report for the readers of the *Journal of the American Medical Association*, written in the wake of criticisms of the report, he wrote that "[t]he IOM report recounted the painful history of medical mistreatment in the Tuskegee syphilis trials and Holmesberg prison, as well as prisoner abuse at Guantánamo Bay and Abu Ghraib."[28] I do not believe that Professor Gostin meant to intentionally misrepresent his Committee's report to an audience of physicians unlikely to ever read the report itself. Rather, I think he was simply reflecting his view that the report would have no legitimacy if it did not include reflection on these prisons; therefore, it must have included them, even though it did not. But there is a logical and reasonable rationale for either not treating Guantánamo at all or treating it as an afterthought: the IOM Committee members really did see Guantánamo as nothing special or different than other U.S. prisons, and thus did not see it as necessary to make any specific comments on it.

Gostin also mentions Nuremberg, Holmesberg prison, and Tuskegee. The latter, of course, did not involve research on prisoners, but on free-living African

Americans. It is nonetheless relevant because of its racism, which is mirrored in the American prison population, which is disproportionately comprised of African American males found guilty of drug-related crimes.[29] Racial disparities in medicine are now widely condemned, but grossly disproportionate racial distributions in prisons seem well accepted. The IOM report reflects this view. The Committee recognizes the incredibly disproportionate numbers of African Americans and Hispanics in our prisons, but the report never addresses the issue or makes any suggestions of why it might matter, even concerning virtually all-African American prisons like Holmesberg.[30]

THE NUREMBERG CODE AND INTERNATIONAL LAW

Using Tuskegee as a cipher to represent racial injustice without actually dealing with the problem of race may have made it seem reasonable to use Nuremberg as a cipher as well and to ignore its meaning. The Committee writes simply that "[t]he commission's [National Commission] deliberations took place against a background that included the Nazi experiments with concentration camp prisoners followed by the adoption of a stringent standard of voluntary consent in the Nuremberg Code."[31] There is no discussion of what research was actually conducted by Nazi physicians in the concentration camps, of the prosecution of these physicians by American prosecutors to a court composed of American judges, or of the rationale for the Nuremberg Code and its direct application to the American military, American prisoners, and American researchers. Instead, the Committee seems to view the Nuremberg Doctors' Trial and its resultant Nuremberg Code as an historical anomaly rather than as the foundational ethical and legal text for the worldwide regulation of all experimentation on humans.[32]

Because the Bush Administration was trying to marginalize related international treaties, including the Geneva Conventions and the Convention against Torture, it may have seemed reasonable to the IOM Committee to simply adopt the Bush administration's dismissal of international humanitarian and human rights laws. Gostin suggests this explanation in writing about his own change of philosophy regarding human rights and civil liberties. In accepting an invitation to rewrite public health laws to give public health officials more power over Americans after 9/11, Gostin writes: "I had no desire to work for the Bush Administration, but when I was informed that if I did not accept, the White House planned to draft the law internally, I reluctantly accepted, after seeking whatever assurances I could of non-interference."[33]

My point here is not whether the Chairman is right or wrong, or even whether he (or the Committee) is credible as a spokesperson for the imprisoned poor. Rather, it is that the report is consistent with Gostin's stated philosophy: accept, even advocate, infringing on individual rights (for example, voluntary consent) as long as your intentions (for instance, to improve health status through beneficial research) are good. Dual use of prisoners under this rationale is not only permissible, it is desirable. This seems to be precisely the ethic that is at work in Guantánamo that permits physicians to rationalize force-feeding competent hunger strikers in restraint chairs: dual use of military physicians is justified, even required, to prevent prisoners from "harming themselves."

GUANTÁNAMO HUNGER STRIKES AND EXPERIMENTATION

Even if the IOM Committee wanted to avoid any criticism of the Bush Administration's anti-human rights prison policies, it should have at least examined the military's suppression of a mass hunger strike at Guantánamo in early 2005. The U.S. military adopted a novel strategy of using a "restraint chair" to break a mass hunger strike by placing hunger strikers in eight point restraints and then forcing a nasogastric tube up their nose and down their esophagus.[34] This basic technique had been labeled torture by the President's Bioethics Council—albeit when done to prisoners in the Soviet Union using a straightjacket instead of a restraint chair.[35] But even if not considered torture, it seems correct to me to label it as a form of human experimentation since this "medical device" (the restraint chair) had never been used for the purpose of breaking a mass hunger strike before, and the U.S. military was "studying" it to see if it was safe and effective.[36]

The argument that the procedures followed, whether research or discipline, at Guantánamo are irrelevant to what goes on in U.S. mainland prisons is not persuasive. Levy, who visited six American prisons in the footsteps of Tocqueville, again helps give us perspective. Reflecting on his visit to Guantánamo near the end of his U.S. journey, he writes:

> You can argue about whether or not Guantanamo should be closed. . . . What you cannot possibly say is that *Guantanamo* is a UFO, fallen from some unknown, obscure disaster. What you are bound to recognize is that it *is a miniature, a condensation, of the entire American prison system.*[37]

Levy seems correct. One could go even further and argue that the "supermax" prisons in the United States violate basic international human rights. This argument is currently being made to the European Court of Human Rights—but, of course, international human rights apply in U.S. prisons only insofar as they are consistent with the U.S. Constitution and the Eighth Amendment.[38] Nonetheless, it should be of great interest that almost simultaneously with the large Guantánamo 2005 hun-

ger strike, there was a coordinated hunger strike at the federal supermax prison in Florence, Colorado by the convicted al-Qaeda terrorists being held there.[39] Because almost no information ever gets out of supermax prisons, we know virtually nothing about this hunger strike, except that unlike Guantánamo, it was "successful" in that the convicted terrorists were transferred from high security detention.[40]

The newest Justice on the U.S. Supreme Court, Justice Sonia Sotomayor, can be viewed as the Justice most concerned with prisoners' rights. In 2010, there were only seven occasions in which any Justice wrote a dissent to the Court's refusal to hear a case and she wrote three of them—more than any other Justice—and all were about the rights of criminal defendants or prisoners.[41] The most important one involved a Louisiana prisoner, Anthony C. Pitre, an AIDS patient, who stopped taking his antiretroviral medication to protest his transfer to another prison.[42] In response, prison officials assigned him to perform hard labor in one-hundred degree heat—labor that caused him to collapse and require emergency treatment.[43] The prison physician, nevertheless, approved the hard labor punishment as a reasonable way to get him to change his mind and go back to taking his medications.[44] A lower court also approved of the punishment, saying that the prisoner could stop it at any time by taking his medications voluntarily.[45] In Sotomayor's view, the Court should have at least heard his appeal because, as she saw it,

> Pitre's decision to refuse medication may have been foolish and caused a significant part of his pain. But that decision does not give prison official license to exacerbate Pitre's condition further as a means of punishing or coercing him—just as a prisoner's disruptive conduct does not permit prison officials to punish the prisoner by handcuffing him to a hitching post.[46]

Of course, a completely analogous punishment is ongoing at Guantánamo, where prisoners are force-fed in restraint chairs as punishment for refusing to eat, and the rationale can also be that they can stop this punishment at any time by their own action of starting to eat again. It is also of note that military officials at Guantánamo and in the Pentagon have also rationalized their force-feeding behavior by saying that the Standard Operating Procedure in hunger strikes is based on the U.S. Bureau of Prisons hunger strike regulations.[47] While I have in the past argued that this was not accurate—given that in the U.S. prison all decisions about force-feeding are to be made solely by the prison physician on the basis of the prisoner's health needs, and the prisoner has been tried, convicted of a crime, and sentenced, and continues to have access to an attorney—these are all differences without a distinction if the prison physician is willing to force-feed a competent prisoner.[48] Unfortunately, as the case of William Coleman in Connecticut illustrates, this can be the case.[49] It should nonetheless be underlined that although the method of breaking hunger strikes by using restraint chairs has also been adopted in the U.S. prison system, there is no prison hunger strike on record anywhere in the world of the length (sometimes years) that some Guantánamo prisons have refused to eat.

In addition, while not available to the IOM Committee, the treatment of an American soldier in a U.S. mainland military prison confirms the similarities with Guantánamo. As is now well-known, the first set of classified Standard Operating Procedures at Guantánamo, including instructions on how to halt a hunger strike, were posted on the Internet by WikiLeaks in 2007.[50] WikiLeaks later became seen as a much more direct threat to American security when it posted a large batch of internal U.S. government documents in 2010.[51] These documents were thought to have been provided to WikiLeaks by an active duty U.S. soldier, Private First Class (Pfc) Bradley E. Manning.[52] Manning was arrested in May 2010 and has since been held in solitary confinement in a Marine Corps jail cell.[53] He is said to be stripped naked every night, forced to stand at attention naked, and sleeps in a "suicide-proof" smock under constant suicide-watch.[54] The military psychiatrist asked to determine whether or not Manning was suicidal or likely to hurt himself, originally determined that he was.[55] But in January 2011, the psychiatrist withdrew his suicide-watch recommendation, saying Manning was actually a "low risk" prisoner.[56] In this case, the military physician seems to have successfully resisted being used for security purposes. The case of Pfc. Manning is ongoing, and even President Obama had to comment on it after the State Department's top spokesperson, Philip J. Crowley, called Manning's treatment "ridiculous, counterproductive and stupid."[57] Obama's unsatisfactory response could have been provided by President George W. Bush. Obama said he asked the Pentagon whether the procedures being used to confine Manning "are appropriate and are meeting our basic standards [and] [t]hey assure me that they are."[58] Put another way, Guantánamo standards are consistent with U.S. "basic standards." And, of course, to the extent that President Obama adopts the approaches to the "war on terror" first implemented by President George W. Bush, these approaches become official U.S. policy rather than a one-president aberration.

INTERNAL INCONSISTENCIES

Just as Americans and Supreme Court Justices (but not Presidents) are often of two minds in comparing Guantánamo to the U.S. prison system in general, the IOM was of two minds in applying the core doctrine of informed consent to research on American prisoners (it obviously has had no application to the hunger strike response at Guantánamo, but is, of course, critical to the WMA's hunger strike ethics policy). A central example is the IOM Committee's view of the Nuremberg Code and the Code's insistence on informed consent. The American judges at Nuremberg did make informed consent of prisoner research subjects their number one item in the Nuremberg Code, but that was not the end of it.[59] The judges, looking forward, also insisted that although informed consent is necessary, it is never sufficient—there are nine additional requirements for legal and ethical research in the ten-point Nuremberg Code.[60]

The Nuremberg Code insists that consent be "voluntary, competent, informed and understanding."[61] In the prison context, of course, the primary issue is voluntariness, as the Committee recognized.[62] Nonetheless, instead of thinking hard about how consent might be judged to be voluntary in the prison context, the Committee spends almost an entire chapter in the report denigrating consent as a meaningful or useful protection against the exploitation of human subjects.[63] Paradoxically, in the next and final chapter of the report, "Systems of Oversight, Safeguards, and Protections," the Committee sets forth a ringing endorsement of the consent requirement of the Nuremberg Code:

> Recommendation 6.1. *Ensure voluntary informed consent. Human research participant protection programs should ensure voluntary informed consent is obtained from subjects in all research involving prisoners.*[64]

This recommendation, which is also consistent with the WMA's 2006 position on care for hunger striking prisoners, is directly on target. The Committee merits commendation for its insights on informed consent, which are worth quoting at some length:

> *Informed consent is vital to autonomous decision making and respect for persons* and is considered a bedrock of ethical research—whether it involves prisoners or non-prisoners. Informed consent is an interactive and ongoing process. . . . The written consent form—one part of the process—is the mechanism for documenting that communication with the participants regarding relevant considerations to enrollment in a protocol has taken place. *The informed consent process must help the prisoner to exercise autonomous decision making.* The process poses special challenges in the correctional setting, where autonomy may be inconsistent with institutional order and judicially imposed limitations on liberty. . . . There is no question that, within correctional settings, it is more difficult to provide integrity to the process of informed consent, but this does not remove the obligation. *If it is determined that voluntary informed consent is not obtainable, then a research protocol should not go forward.*[65]

The centrality of prisoner autonomy to the doctor-patient relationship is, of course, also the foundational rationale for the WMA's insistence that prison physicians not force-feed competent hunger strikers. Only the informed consent of a competent prisoner can justify a physician to provide treatment (or engage in research), including "physician-assisted" feeding.

JUSTICE AND PRISON RESEARCH REGULATIONS

There are other examples of inconsistencies in the IOM report that induce vertigo. The report begins by underlining in its preface that "The charge of our Committee . . . was to explore whether the conclusions reached in 1976 by the National Commission . . . remain appropriate today."[66] Nonetheless, in the one-hundred and seventy-four pages that follow, virtually no attempt is made to address this charge. The 1976 report, for example, is never analyzed.

My colleagues Leonard Glantz and Barbara Katz and I wrote the informed consent background paper for the National Commission's prisoners report, which covered—in much more detail than the IOM report—the issues of voluntariness, including the meaning of coercion and undue influence in the prison setting, as well as detailed discussions contrasting behavioral research from biomedical research.[67] The point is not that the Committee did not read our background paper; the Committee does not seem to have read any of the fifteen background papers or the four staff papers and reports that were prepared for the National Commission on the subject of research involving prisoners.[68]

One can conclude, as the National Commission did, that it is possible to do ethical research in prisons, without concluding either that emphasis on consent is "myopic" (both the IOM and National Commission discussions with prisoners actually support the opposite conclusion), or that we should approve of research simply because prisoners want it. Neither conclusion follows. Prisoners support informed consent as much as ethicists do; and what prisoners want most, including, and perhaps especially those at Guantánamo who have no release date, is not to be research subjects, or to be on a hunger strike, but to be out of prison.

This suggests another vertigo-inducing problem in the IOM report (and at Guantánamo): the conclusion that we should focus more on "justice"(the procedural task of weighing risks versus benefits) than "consent" (the substantive rule of prisoner self-determination) in prison research. Committee member Jonathan Moreno wrote about this issue in a book cited by the Committee for this proposition.[69] But the Committee's incoherent emphasis on procedural "cost/benefit justice"[70] in this context cannot be attributed to him. As Moreno concludes:

Generalized discussions about justice are sorely limited concerning specific groups. . . . The respective situations of prisoners, institutionalized persons, military personnel, and students are quite different and require analyses tailored to each of them. Underlying all these cases are complex issues of social status and power as well as medical ethics.[71]

Moreno seems correct here, and these justice considerations are central to the Committee's conclusion that some studies would simply not be allowable under the Committee's "risk-benefit analysis." Specifically, in the Committee's words:

The potential benefit of an experimental intervention must be established before engaging in a risk-benefit analysis. As such, phase l and phase 2 studies, as defined by the FDA to determine safety and toxicity levels, would not be allowable . . . only phase 3 studies would be allowed [in prisons].[72]

This seems clear enough. Thus, it is at least surprising that in the very next chapter the most controversial example of a study that the Committee believes should be able to be done under its new ethical framework is "[a] phase I study of a medication [that] may reduce repetitive sexual assaults."[73] The Committee at least realizes that this study would not be justifiable under its risk-benefit framework, and so suggests it as an exception that is "necessary as there are no alternative candidate research populations to draw from."[74] But repetitive sexual assault is hardly a unique problem of prisoners, and the prison sample is skewed, representing as it does only those who got caught by the criminal justice system. In Moreno's terms, such subjects seem to be mostly targeted because they are "captive and convenient" rather than the most scientifically relevant. This again is consistent with the Guantánamo prisoners where actions taken against them are justified primarily because they are "captive," and the only effective way they have to protest their confinement is by going on a hunger strike. The "justice" justification for force-feeding them is the military's weighing of risks and benefits to their health of not eating; the justice of their confinement is never addressed.

CONCLUSION

A contemporary report on the ethics of prisoner research, including "research" on breaking prison hunger strikes, has yet to be written. The IOM report will survive mostly as a relic of the Bush Administration because it identified no real problem to address, both expanded and contracted the definition of prisoners, ignored the context of the global war on terror and international law, and failed to develop either a consistent ethical framework or a draft of recommended changes in statutory or regulatory law. Nonetheless, it can help us understand what is happening at Guantánamo, and why it is accurate to see Guantánamo as a mirror of official U.S. prison policy and practice, not an exception or aberration. Dual use of physicians in prisons has a formidable pedigree in the United States, and the only "solution" to it is for prison physicians to refuse to comply with any order or request from prison officials, including military commanders in charge of military prisons, that is inconsistent with medical ethics. Such orders should also be explicitly labeled "unlawful" orders by the U.S. Department of Defense. Military physicians should no more be expected to violate medical ethics than military lawyers should be expected to violate the U.S. Constitution, or than military chaplains should be expected to violate the tenets of their religions. Military physicians should not, however, be expected to do this alone; medical professional organizations, state licensing boards, and the public all have a stake in the medical profession and all should actively support physicians who take medical ethics seriously. This is one reason (patient health is another) why military and prison physicians should be able to call in independent civilian medical consultants as they see fit.

The IOM Committee was right to quote an observation usually attributed to Dostoyevsky, although it is impossible to identify where the author actually wrote these words: "The degree of civilization in a society can be judged by entering its prisons." In the case of the United States, those prisons have names, including Abu Ghraib and Guantánamo. And our civilization deserves to be judged by our fidelity to international human rights law and medical ethics practice as reflected in those prisons. We cannot credibly reform Guantánamo alone; we must reform our entire prison system, especially our system of prison healthcare, of which Guantánamo is just a reflection. In commenting about his visit to Alcatraz, Levy could have been making an observation about Guantánamo and the Marine Corp brig holding Private Bradley Manning: "No escapees from Alcatraz. Just the damned of Alcatraz. And perhaps, beyond Alcatraz, a whole segment of the American penal system [modeled on the leper colony]."[75]

REFERENCES

1. Ilan Zvi Baron, *The Problem of Dual Loyalty*, 41 Canadian J Political Sci 1025, 1033 (2009).
2. George J. Annas, *Military Medical Ethics: Physician First, Last, Always*, 359 New England J. Med. 1089–90 (2008).
3. *Cf.* George J. Annas, *Worst Case Bioethics*, 68–69 (Oxford, 2010).
4. *See, e.g.*, Workshop Summary, *Institute of Medicine, Military Medical Ethics: Issues Regarding Dual Loyalties*, ix (Sep. 8, 2008)
5. *See, e.g.*, Michael Phillips, *U.S. Seeks Friends in Afghan Detainees*, Wall St. J., Mar. 5–6, 2011, A11.
6. Scott Shane & Mark Landler, *Obama, in Reversal, Clears Way for Guantanamo Trials to Resume*, N.Y. Times, March 8, 2011, A19; Hendrik Hertzberg, *Prisoners*, New Yorker, Apr. 18, 2011, 45–46.

7. Annas, *Worst Case Bioethics, supra* note 3 at 64. *See also, Media Roundtable with Assistant Secretary Winkenwerder,* Department Of Defense (June 7, 2006), http://www.defense.gov/transcripts/transcript.aspx?transcriptid=33.

8. Annas, *Worst Case Bioethics, Supra* Note 3, At 59–74.

9. Bernard-Henri Levy, American Vertigo: Traveling America In The Footsteps Of Tocqueville (Charlotte Mandell, trans., 2006).

10. The Committee's formal name is longer, "Committee on Ethical Considerations for Revisions to DHHS Regulations for Protection of Prisoners Involved in Research." *Project Information,* Institute Of Medicine

11. Annas, *Worst Case Bioethics supra* note 3, 41–57 and sources cited therein.

12. *See, e.g.,* Adam Liptak, *US Prison Population Nears 1.6 Million,* N.Y. Times, Feb. 29, 2008.

13. Exec. Order 13,567, 76 Fed. Reg. 13,277 (Mar. 7, 2011)

14. Annas, *supra* note 3, at 69; *see also* Physicians For Human Rights, Experiments In Torture: Evidence Of Human Subject Research And Experimentation In The "Enhanced" Interrogation Program 3 (2010).

15. Annas, *supra* note 3, at 69.

16. *Id.* at 60.

17. Comm. on Ethical Considerations for Revs. to Dhhs Regs. For Protection of Prisoners Involved In Res., Inst. of Med. of The Nat'l Acads., Ethical Considerations For Research Involving Prisoners (Nat'l Acads. Press, 2007).

18. Although the IOM Committee itself found prison research acceptable, critics disagreed. See, e.g., Osagie Obasogie, Prisoners as Human Subjects: A Closer Look at the Institute of Medicine's Recommendations to Loosen Current Restrictions on Using Prisoners in Scientific Research, 82 Stan. J. C.R. & C.L. 41 (2010).

19. *See* IOM Committee, *supra* note 17, at 4, 115.

20. *See id.* at 4, 147.

21. *See id.* at 44, 57.

22. *See id.* at 3 n.1, 79.

23. *See id.* at 102–03.

24. *Id.* at 26 n.1.

25. The committee itself seems to have been conflicted on this topic.

26. Richard Benedetto, *Bush Defends Interrogation Practices: "We Do Not Torture",* USA Today, Nov. 7, 2005.

27. *See, e.g.,* Elie Wiesel, *Without Conscience,* 352 New Engl J. Med. 1511, 1511–13 (2005).

28. Lawrence O. Gostin, *Biomedical Research Involving Prisoners: Ethical Values and Regulation,* 297 JAMA 737, 739 (2007).

29. *See* Annas, *supra* note 3.

30. A. M. Hornblum, *Acres Of Skin: Human Experiments At Holmesburg Prison* (Routledge, 1998).

31. Ethical Considerations, *supra* note 17, at 114.

32. International Covenant on Civil and Political Rights, which, among other provisions, states clearly, in article 7 that "[n]o one shall be subjected to torture or to cruel, inhuman or degrading treatment or punishment. *In particular, no one shall be subjected without his free consent to medical or scientific experimentation."* (emphasis added).

33. Lawrence O. Gostin, *From a Civil Libertarian to a Sanitarian,* 34 J. Law & Society 594, 614–615 (2007).

34. *See* Letter from The Center for Constitutional Rights (CCR) to Mr. Manfred Nowak, United Nations Special Rapporteur, Mr. Anand Grover, United Nations Special Rapporteur, and Martin Scheinin, United Nations Special Rapporteur (Apr. 2, 2009).

35. *See* George J. Annas, *The Legacy of the Nuremberg Doctors' Trial to American Bioethics and Human Rights,* 19 Minn. J.L. Sci. & Tech. 19 (2009).

36. Annas, *supra* note 3. *See also* Vincent Iacopino, Scott Allen & Allen Keller, *Bad Science Used to Support Torture and Human Experimentation,* 331 Science 34 (2011).

37. Levy, *supra* note 9, at 227 (emphasis added).

38. Jean Casella and James Ridgeway, *U.S. Supermax Prisons are Challenged in the European Court of Human Rights—and Lose the First Round,* Solitarywatch, July 8, 2010. *See also* Atul Gawande, *Hellhole: The United States hold tens of thousands of inmates in long-term solitary confinement. Is this torture?,* New Yorker, Mar. 30, 2009.

39. Joby Warrick and Peter Finn, *'06 Memo cites Food Strike by Detainees,* Wash. Post, Aug. 28, 2009, at A03.

40. Memorandum from U.S. Dep't of Justice, Office of Legal Counsel, for John A. Rizzo, Acting General Counsel, Central Intelligence Agency Re: Application of the Detainee Treatment Act to Conditions of Confinement at Central Intelligence Agency Detention Facilities, 13 n.11 (Aug. 31, 2006).

41. Adam Liptak, *Sotomayor Guides Court's Liberal Wing,* N.Y. Times, Dec. 28, 2010, at A10.

42. Pitre, 131 S. Ct. at 8.

43. *Id.*

44. *Id.* at 9.

45. *Id.* at 8.

46. *Id.* at 9.

47. 28 C.F.R. § 549.60 (1994).

48. *See* Annas, *supra* note 8, 60–70.

49. Lantz v. Coleman, 978 A.2d 164 (Conn. 2008).
50. *U.S. Says Wikileaks Could "Threaten National Security"*, BBC (July 26, 2010), *See generally*, David Leigh & Luke Harding, Wikileaks: Inside Julian Assange's War On Secrecy 20–31 (Guardian Books 2011).
51. Glenn Greenwald, *The Inhumane Conditions of Bradley Manning's Detention*, Salon.Com (Dec. 15, 2010).
52. Scott Shane, *Obama Defends Detention Conditions for Soldier Accused in WikiLeaks Case*, N.Y. Times, Mar. 11, 2011.
53. *Id.*
54. *Id.*
55. *Id.*
56. *Id.*
57. *Id.*; After making this statement, the spokesman resigned two days later. Jeffrey Young, *State Department's Philip J. Crowley Resigns, Citing WikiLeaks Comments*, Bloomberg (Mar. 14, 2011).
58. Shane, *supra* note 53.
59. National Institute of Health, *Regulations and Ethical Guidelines, Nuremberg Code*, http://ohsr.od.nih.gov/guidelines/nuremberg.html.
60. *Id.*
61. *Id.*
62. *Id.*
63. Ethical Considerations, *supra* note 17. *Id.* at 117–122.
64. *Id.* at 147 (emphasis added).
65. *Id.* at 147–48 (emphasis added).
66. *See* Ethical Considerations, *supra* note 17, at ix.
67. *See generally* G.J. Annas, L.H. Glantz & B.F. Katz, *The Law of Informed Consent in Human Experimentation: Prisoners, in Research Involving Prisoners: Appendix to Report and Recommendations* 7-1–7-60 (1976), *in* Informed Consent to Human Experimentation: The Subject's Dilemma 1–55 (Ballinger, 1977).
68. *See generally* Ethical Considerations, *supra* note 17.
69. J.D. Moreno, *Convenient and Captive Populations in* J.P. Kahn, A.C. Mastroianni, J. Sugarman, Beyond Consent: Seeking Justice In Research 111–130 (New York: Oxford U. Press, 1998).
70. *See* Ethical Considerations, *supra* note 17, at 65–66.
71. Ethical Considerations, *supra* note 17, at 126.
72. *Id.* at 127.
73. *Id.* at 167. The only specific comment on the National Commission's own report occurs at pages 121 and 122 of the IOM report.
74. Ethical Considerations, *supra* note 17, at 167.
75. Levy, *supra* note 9, at 167.

QUESTIONS

1. In describing the position of physicians working for the state, it is often said that they are in a position of having "conflicting loyalties," as in they must be loyal to their employer and to their patients. The author argues that we should replace this term with dual use," as in the state wants to take advantage of the "do no harm" beneficent view most of the public has of physicians to "use" them for the state's agenda in ways that are harmful to their patients (torture being the most extreme). Which description do you think is more accurate, and why does it matter? Would it be more helpful in sorting out the physician's ethical and human rights obligations to simply say the physician has a "conflict of interest?"

2. The author suggests that the prison physician is in an analogous position to that of a medical researcher in that physicians in both of these roles may devalue the interests of their patients in ways that could harm the patients. In research it has been suggested that patients should have their own personal physician who has no interest in the research to advise them. Similarly, should prisoners have access to independent physicians to counsel them or give them a second opinion?

3. Informed consent is said to be the most important legal and bioethical doctrine in the doctor–patient relationship. Can the doctrine of informed consent also be described as a basic human right? Explain.

FURTHER READING

1. Institute of Medicine, *Military Medical Ethics: Issues Regarding Dual Loyalties.* Washington DC: IOM, 2009.
2. Miles, Steven, *Oath Betrayed: Torture, Medical Complicity, and the War on Terror.* New York: Random House, 2006.
3. Goodman, Ryan & Roseman, Mindy Jane, *Interrogations, Forced Feedings, and the Role of Health Professionals.* Cambridge: Human Rights Program, Harvard Law School, 2009.
4. British Medical Association, *Medicine Betrayed: The Participation of Doctors in Human Rights Abuses: Report of a Working Party.* London: Zed in association with the BMA, 1992.

PART IV

*A*ddressing System Failures

Introduction

The term "system failures" refers to situations where the rights, needs and capacities of populations are well known but national and international efforts to address them are insufficient, inadequate or ineffective. The emphasis is on the structural and systemic failures of states and the international community to meet their obligations. Inaction may be the result of denial, unwillingness, neglect or incapacity. Prominently featured in this part is the inaction of states in delivering on their obligations to *protect* human rights impacting on health and well-being when the abuses are perpetrated by non-State actors, including groups motivated by cultural or religious agendas and transnational corporations. This part features works that help to highlight issues of concern for key populations across a range of topics and experience, not work devoted to specific populations.

Addressing system failures necessitates ardent governmental support for implementation of existing treaties, and an ability to move forward in protecting the rights and health of populations not initially considered such as sexual minorities, the mentally disabled, and drug users. However, as history has shown, putting total responsibility on governments is an incomplete solution. The question remains: why, even with new language, advocacy structures and infrastructure in place, do systems persist in allowing people to suffer marginalization and victimization, and what additional body of evidence is needed to persuade state and non-state actors to redress such situations and, critically, what can we do about it?

In the first chapter, Cook proposes a framework for considering issues of gender, health and human rights. She provides historical context to the approaches taken to address the needs and rights of women and girls by the international community. Questions of gender, health and human rights are furthered by Miller's Point of View that follows.

O'Flaherty and Fisher bring this question into the new millennium, addressing the creation of international norms to promote and protect human rights in relation to sexual minorities and gender identity. While there have been many positive developments, reproductive and sexual rights remain a battleground in the development of international standards to fully support the rights and health of all populations.

In his Point of View, Beyrer extends the discussion of sexuality and human rights to men who have sex with men. The next two chapters both address system failures in this important area. Davies highlights the implications of different approaches to understanding the human rights protections that exist in the reproductive health arena while Cottingham and colleagues point to specific gaps in protection and suggest ways forward. This is followed by Annas' chapter "Global Baby," which explores a relatively new dimension of health-related human rights, and the lack of coherent international policy to adequately address the fast growing area of assisted reproduction, and the need for new protections of women acting as egg donors and "surrogate mothers," as well as the resulting children. Touré's Point of View identifies the critical role men must play in the advocacy to gain gender equality and reproductive rights of women.

Using maternal deaths to highlight the system failures inadequately addressed by the Millennium Development Goals (MDGs), Pinho not only provides specific examples but suggests issues which ought to be addressed through a rights-based approach in global development frameworks going forward. Garcia-Moreno and Stöckl's chapter addresses violence against women and its impact on gender equality. While they note that violence can take place in multiple settings and be perpetrated by a wide array of parties, the chapter focuses on intimate partner violence and sexual violence.

The final chapter raises questions about the ability of systems to support an increasing array of issues and populations that have historically been marginalized by health care institutions, and governments more generally. Burns proposes using a human rights approach to address discrimination related to mental disability. The Point of View by Solón focuses on the right to water and sanitation, noting the devastating public health problems which arise from a lack of clean drinking water and safe sewage. Associated with the need for clean water is the need for adequate nutrition. Schuftan's powerful chapter notes that over a billion people live in hunger at a time of record global harvests and profits for the world's major agribusiness corporations. He notes that the global food crisis is not caused by actual food shortages but by a crisis of food price inflation and market forces. The last chapter in this part by Dresler and colleagues proposes a rights-based approach to the issue of tobacco control.

TOPICS FOR DISCUSSION

1. What are the root causes of system failures in relation to health and human rights?
2. Readers are encouraged to consider the shared characteristics of the various populations presented here, as well as the implications of these similarities for addressing systemic issues. For example, can experience in advocacy around the rights of the child be used to strengthen advocacy for the aged and/or for the mentally ill?
3. Should a rights-based approach be implemented for the protection of all vulnerable populations in the same manner? What could be the potential pitfalls of Special Protection measures? What are the implications of exceptionalism? Could this enhance isolation, differentiation, disempowerment, or could this create grounds for inequity for some populations?
4. The readings address a number of system failures, but implicitly also point to advances and successes in recent years. What do you consider to be the most exciting developments in improving rights and health at a systems level in the last decade?

CHAPTER 23

Gender, Health and Human Rights

Rebecca J. Cook

Motherhood can take a woman to the heights of ecstasy and the depths of despair; it can offer her protection and reverence. But it can also deny a woman consideration as anything more than a vehicle for human reproduction. Women's reproductive function fits within a social framework of gender that affects women's capacities and health. While traditional cultures established laws to protect women's reproductive functions, these laws have confined women to the extent that they have been denied almost all additional and alternative opportunities to flourish as individuals and to achieve complete health in their communities and wider societies. Emphasizing that health is more than a matter of an individual's medical condition, the World Health Organization (WHO) asserts that "health is a state of complete physical, mental and social well-being and not merely the absence of disease or infirmity."[1]

It has been only recently recognized that states must address the protection and advancement of women's health interests through gender planning, to achieve not simply the abstract value of justice, but to conform to legally binding international human rights obligations as well. Gender planning concerns both practical and strategic needs of women in developing and industrialized countries.[2] Their prac-tical needs are addressed through programs like the Safe Motherhood Initiative, co-sponsored by several UN agencies and international nongovernmental organizations.[3] This program focuses on reducing the rates of maternal mortality, unwanted pregnancy, and sexually transmitted diseases, including HIV infection. Comparable programs address women's health and nutritional needs throughout the life cycle.[4]

Women's strategic needs transcend such practical needs however, because they address the value of women to society—a value extending beyond motherhood and service in the home. Focusing on strategic needs promotes women's roles in such areas as the economic, political, spiritual, professional and cultural life of communities. Most importantly, it opens the way to women's achievement of complete health as defined by WHO.

There is a paradox in addressing women's practical and strategic needs: those concerned with practical needs may develop concepts whose effects, and perhaps whose purpose, confine women to maternal, domestic and subordinate social roles. This denies women's legitimate strategic needs and prevents them from flourishing to their full capacity within the family, community and society.

This chapter addresses how the gender role in society occupied primarily by women has constrained women's growth to the detriment of their complete health. It also outlines how international human rights law obliges states to liberate women from this constraint to permit women's pursuit of health and achievement in areas of their own choice.

SEX AND GENDER

Medicine has historically used male physiology as the model for medical care, based on research studies involving exclusively men.[5] Accordingly, women have been considered only to the extent that they are different from men, focusing medical attention on reproductive characteristics.

Further, medicine progressed from being an art of human interaction to a science dominated by biological revelations achieved in laboratories. More and more, it is driven by the institutional demands of hospital-based medicine, where results of laboratory science and, more recently, medical engineering and technology, can be applied. In moving the locus of their functions from the community to the laboratory and hospital, doctors have become isolated from those social realities that condition the lives and health status of their patients.

In many regions of the world, health agencies are increasingly recognizing how functions performed by community members can protect and enhance people's health, and how important it is to reassess how an individual woman's self-esteem and health status are affected by the value placed on women by her community.[6] Health professionals themselves are becoming more sensitive to the health impact of patients' social experiences. For example, the 1994 World Report on Women's Health, issued by the International Federation of Gynecology and Obstetrics, concluded that future improvements in women's health require not only improved science and health care, but also social justice for women and removal of socially and culturally conditioned barriers to women's equal opportunity.[7]

The experiences of women in their families and communities are different from those of men. The difference transcends reproductive functions, although the reproductive role of women in the creation and maintenance of families has commonly been used to justify women's subordination and denial of equal opportunity. The dominant view that women are distinguishable from men only as regards their biological constitution and reproductive role hides the profound psychological and social differences based on gender that societies have created, and that compromise women's complete health.[8]

The terms *sex* and *gender* are frequently used interchangeably. The latter is often preferred over the crude and salacious connotations of the former; but strictly speaking, the terms are different. *Sex* is a matter of biological differentiation, whereas *gender* is a social construct by which various activities and characteristics are associated with one or the other sex. For instance, leadership through success in battle is male gendered, whereas caring for the dependent young, sick, and elderly is female gendered. Popular imagery of leadership in, for example, politics, commerce, industry, the military, and religion is male gendered, whereas nursing and domestic service are female gendered. It is obvious that women can be political and industrial leaders, and that men can be care-givers, but it has been considered exceptional for people to assume a gender role at variance with their sex. Activities and characteristics are preconceived via gender stereotypes, which determine the parameters of the normal. "Masculine" behavior in women, and "feminine" behavior in men have long been considered deviant. That which is normal or self-evident escapes special attention, because it is taken as the norm from which only departures are of interest. Behavior that is in accordance with conventional expectations and presuppositions of gender roles is generally unremarkable.

WOMEN'S SUBORDINATION AND EXCLUSION

In societies around the world, female-gendered status is inferior and subordinate to male-gendered status. The male protects the female through the attributes of gallantry and chivalry, he is bold in courtship, aggressive in initiative, and forthcoming among peers. The female is passive, renders service in modest fulfillment of duty, and offers comfort in responsive obedience. Societies have modelled their role expectations on these assumptions of the natural order of humankind. Historic social structures, including the organization and conduct of warfare, the hierarchical ordering of influential religious institutions, the attribution of political power, the authority of the judiciary, and the influences that shape the content of the law, reflect this gender difference of male dominance and female subordination.

Because women naturally tend to behave in female-gendered ways, they have been vulnerable to confinement to female status by social, political, religious and other institutions, populated exclusively by men, that act in male-gendered ways. Women have accordingly been subordinated to assume only inferior, servile social roles, and have traditionally been excluded from centers of male-gendered power by legal and other instruments. These include legislatures, military institutions, religious orders, universities, and the learned professions, including medicine. This is still the age of "first women,"

such as the first woman medical school dean, the first woman Supreme Court justice, and the first woman head of a medical association.

The historic subordination, silencing, and imposed inferiority of women (beginning at birth as an expendable and often unwanted girl child) has been invisible because it has been considered not simply a natural feature of society, but the very condition by which society can exist. Traditional forces emphasizing that women's "natural place" is in the home and that their natural functions in the rearing of children must always be protected, cannot envisage that women can aspire to and achieve the same advances in areas of male-gendered activities as men; nor do they acknowledge that it is oppressive of women's human rights to confine them to servile functions traditionally considered natural to their sex.

It is becoming increasingly recognized that an individual's health status is determined not only by chance genetic inheritance and the geographical availability of nutritional resources, but also by socioeconomic factors.[9] Relatively affluent people, and those content with their lives, enjoy better health status than impoverished, frustrated, and oppressed people who suffer disrespect in their communities and poor self-image. The determinants of earned income, including education, literacy, employment opportunities, and, for instance, financial credit for launching income initiatives, all show how women have been disadvantaged by their inferior gender role. Even within affluent families, women have often suffered frustrations-through male preference in inheritance, education preceding marriage, and training to occupy positions of influence and power within their communities. Women have been denied a commitment of family resources for these opportunities, in the belief that upon marriage, they will attenuate association with their own families (reflected, for example, in their shedding family names) and will assume a role of service within their husbands' families.

Complex social dynamics have produced a modern reality, common to communities across the full spectrum of economic and industrial development, of women being primary or sole economic supports of their families, and also being unmarried, widowed, or abandoned mothers of their children. Women's unequal opportunities to participate in the resources and well-being of their communities, and to contribute to political, economic, spiritual, and related leadership has a serious impact. It deprives those families that financially depend on women of equal opportunities for well-being; and it robs women themselves of the economic, psychological, and social determinants of health. Women's vulnerability to sexual subordination through the greater physical, military, and social force of men produces harmful health consequences in women extending beyond pain, indignity, unwanted pregnancy, and venereal infection.

HOW HEALTH PROFESSIONS HAVE CONSTRUCTED WOMEN

Members of the health professions have done much to mitigate the health consequences of women's gendered disadvantage. They have cared for the distressed and violated, relieved physical pain, and eased women through unwanted and, at times, violently imposed pregnancy. As participants in traditional communities, however, undertaking the male-gendered functions of decision-making and leadership, doctors have tended to share prevailing perceptions of women's natural role, and exhibit blindness toward women's gender-specific health risks. Indeed, in the past, doctors have considered women constitutionally unsuited to political, commer-

cial, and professional life, prone to swoon under stress and to require nine months of bed rest while pregnant.

When society blamed women for resorting to prostitution as a means of economic maintenance, while denying them alternative opportunities to support themselves and their families, doctors, among others, promoted the image of women as vectors of disease. Accordingly, when, for instance, victorious soldiers returned to the United States from 1918 to 1920, 18,000 women-alleged to be prostitutes were detained in a medically supported governmental initiative, for fear that they would spread venereal infection.[10] Women's image as vectors of disease to sexual partners and to children they conceive has been recycled in the modern pandemic of AIDS.[11]

In many parts of the world, medicine retains marks of its gendered practice, for instance in placing women under the patriarchal control of men and others who exercise male-gendered authority. For example, in some countries, a woman's request for health care is accepted only with the express authorization of her husband.[12] Women's requests for control over their reproduction have so threatened male dominance of women's fertility that birth control and voluntary sterilization were condemned until recently, as Crimes Against Morality.[13] Voluntary abortion remains a major point of contention almost universally within institutions of traditional power, which are male-gendered. Whether it is discriminatory and socially unconscionable to criminalize a medical procedure that only women need is a question that usually goes not simply unanswered, but unasked.

MEDICINE SERVING THE STATUS QUO

By focusing its attention on the distress of individual women in clinical settings, medicine in general and psychiatry in particular have inadvertently served as agents of the continued subordination and oppression of women.[14] Women have suffered feelings of ill health and emotional dissonance with family and community, as a reaction to denial of equal opportunities to seek their own achievements and their confinement to seeking satisfaction in the care of children, the sick and the dependent. Health professionals have conscientiously looked for physiological and psychiatric causes of maladjustment in patients' lives, and for other medical reasons for unhappiness and discontent.[15] Illness alone was used to explain women's unhappiness in the midst of affluence and caring family members, a situation that by conventional standards should produce contentedness.

One effect of modern feminist sensitivity has been to expose feelings of frustration and anger as not being unnatural reactions to natural conditions, but as natural healthy reactions to social injustice. By diagnosing women's discontent and "disorders" as medical problems, physicians have reinforced and perpetuated the injustice of the prevailing social order, which prejudices women's health, rather than acting as instruments of remedy.

Medicine has a history of paternalism. Patients have been infantilized and denied social status, for example, by being called by their first names and presumed incapable of exercising informed choice among treatment options. A legal recognition of only recent evolution is that treatment choices are not to be medically dictated, but are to be medically-informed personal choices made by patients as an act of self-determination. Physicians are increasingly required by law to afford patients respect as equals—capable of and responsible for making critical life decisions—by providing them the medical information they need to fully exercise choice.

However, while meeting this objective standard of medical disclosure, doctors must recognize how women's experiences in female-gendered roles have affected their medical histories and health prospects. The critical transition is from doctors treating women as inferior to men, physiologically different only in reproductive functions, to recognizing women as equal to men, only different because of the gendered experiences that affect their health.

As the health care system moves from a biomedical model of practice to a health promotion model, health professionals must meet the challenge and opportunity of reshaping their understanding of how women's experiences affect health. Restoration of health in reaction to illness and dysfunction can no longer concentrate only on the sciences, including physiology, biology, chemistry, and pharmacology. At the clinical level, these disciplines are essentially impersonal and neutral to the social, political, and environmental conditions that influence health. When health professionals concentrate on promoting health rather than just treating disease and dysfunction, they are compelled to consider the social, economic, and, for instance, environmental determinants of health. They must confront among other influences, gender-based discrimination which denies women opportunities for achieving physical and mental health.[16]

Clinically trained health professionals enhance their diagnostic and therapeutic capacities via recognition of the links between women's health status and the social environments they inhabit. Their knowledge about gender-based vulnerabilities to, for example, domestic violence and unwanted pregnancy, and their awareness of gender-based social constraints on career ambitions, will educate health professionals about the many factors beyond clinical services which contribute to women's health. As health professionals come to realize the extent to which health is compromised as a result of gender discrimination, they may turn to human rights principles and instruments in order to find ways in which discrimination may be remedied or even prevented.

THE DEVELOPMENT OF HUMAN RIGHTS

The function of modern human rights is to redress the imbalance between society's privileged and unempowered members.[17] Countries may now be held to international account for internal policies, practices, and failures of public intervention, by which an individual's human dignity is violated. It usually falls to the weak and vulnerable of a society, and to those who advocate on their behalf, to invoke inherent human rights for the protection and promotion of their interests. Similarly, those who enjoy the privilege of power and protection resist challenges to their conventional authority. While at times sympathetic to rights rhetoric that may advance their own claims to entitlement, the privileged often resist service to rights that requires them to yield or share their privilege, observe duties related to rights, or support action that would reduce their privilege to no more than the rights that are shared by all others.

The United Nations was founded in 1945 on principles of respect for individual human rights, and paid tribute to its inspiration in its 1948 Universal Declaration of Human Rights. Post-war reconstruction and the Cold War preoccupied much of the early UN work to advance human rights. Rights of sexual equality were submerged in efforts against colonialism, of relieving the plight of refugees, and of resisting Apartheid. General international human rights conventions that gave legal substance to the Universal Declaration, namely the International Covenant on Civil and Political Rights and the International Covenant on Economic, Social and Cultural Rights,

condemned sexual discrimination in only nominal terms. The several related regional human rights conventions were no more vigorously applied in this area.

It was not until 1966 that the UN adopted the International Convention on the Elimination of Racial Discrimination. The move to advance women's equality was more prolonged, because violations of women's rights were not as visible to male authorities as those suffered on racial grounds. However, one of the most dynamic perceptions of the late 20th century has been growing recognition of the unjust exclusion, oppression, and subordination of women through gender stereotyping practiced by such reputable institutions as, for instance, democratic governments, organized religions, and higher education, as well as such professions as medicine and law.

In 1979, the UN adopted the Convention on the Elimination of All Forms of Discrimination against Women (the Women's Convention), and ratifications brought the Convention into legal effect with unusual speed. The Convention is currently ratified by at least 140 countries, although it remains subject to such extensive exceptions of applicability by some ratifying states that it is legitimate to ask whether, by tests of international treaty law, these states are truly parties.[18] Nevertheless, the Women's Convention reinforces previous general and regional human rights conventions, and provides language to express those specific and binding entitlements to respect for individual dignity that constitute the human rights of women.

The points at which women's social inequality and negative stereotyping can be demonstrated are recognized more and more. Modern analysis has shown systemic denial and suppression of information concerning women's victimization by violence and rape in their homes.[19] In fact, rape has been re-characterized by feminist scholarship not as a sexual act perpetrated by force, but as a violent act perpetrated through sex.[20] Certain countries, including Canada, now grant refugee status to women fleeing their countries due to a well-founded fear that they or their daughters would be circumcised. [21]Sexual abuse in military conflict has been exposed as an act of dominance against women that amounts to torture. Additionally, it is often intended as a means of aggression towards men, who consider the chastity and sexual availability of women in their communities to be their exclusive possession. Recently, the Inter-American Commission on Human Rights, in a report on the situation of human rights under the administration of Raoul Cedras, determined that the rape and abuse of Haitian women constituted violations of their rights to be free from torture and inhuman and degrading treatment, and their right to liberty and security of the person.[22]

HUMAN RIGHTS RELATING TO WOMEN'S HEALTH

The International Covenant on Economic, Social and Cultural Rights explicitly names the right to the highest attainable standard of health, and to enjoyment of the benefits of scientific progress. But because the determinants of health, including socioeconomic status and the capacity to realize reasonable life ambitions, are multifaceted, most, if not all, named human rights contribute in differing degrees to the protection and promotion of health.[23] In its Preamble, the Women's Convention observes that the need for this separate legal instrument to reinforce the sexual nondiscrimination provisions of previous international conventions arises from the concern that "despite these various instruments, extensive discrimination against women continues to exist." It goes on to state that, "in situations of poverty, women have the least access to food, health, education, training

and opportunities for employment and other needs." By Article 12(1) of the Women's Convention, States parties agree that they will "take all appropriate measures to eliminate discrimination against women in the field of health care in order to ensure, on a basis of equality of men and women, access to health care services, including those related to family planning."

Promotion of women's health depends upon the interaction of most, if not all, human rights. Rights relevant to health include those to protect women's employment and grant equal pay for work of equal value; to education; to information; and to political participation, influence, and democratic power within legislatures. These last rights permit women's rights to be respected in the general conduct of states.

In international and regional human rights conventions, the common prohibition of discrimination on grounds of sex has not been applied to condemn discrimination on grounds of gender. Elimination of sexual discrimination alone would bring women's status closer to that of men, and afford women the means that men enjoy to protect and advance their health. However, the wider health disadvantage that women suffer on grounds of gender must be tackled. Further, it must be based not only on the biological difference between the sexes, but on socially-structured gender differences that compromise women's achievement of "the highest attainable standard of health." By Article 5(1) of the Women's Convention, States parties agree to deconstruct gender discrimination by taking appropriate measures to modify the social and cultural patterns of conduct of men and women. This is agreed upon with a view toward eliminating prejudices, and customary and all other practices based on the inferiority or superiority of either sex, or on stereotyped roles for men and women.

Women's poor physical and psychological health may represent a metaphor for the poor health of women's rights in the body politic and in influential community institutions, whether political, economic, religious, or health care. Application of human rights law may provide a remedy that results in improvements in women's health status. While this legal application faces formidable challenges, these challenges are increasingly being addressed by developments in legal doctrine.

LEGAL APPROACHES TO APPLY HUMAN RIGHTS TO HEALTH

Human rights law makes an important distinction between *negative* and *positive* rights. Of the two, negative rights are more easily applied, as they require states to do nothing but permit individuals to pursue their own preferences. In fact, states have not trusted women to make decisions affecting their own lives—rather, they have encumbered those women pursuing reproductive and other health interests with burdens, conditions, and at times, ferocious penalties.

Male-gendered institutions of government, religion, and the health professions have justified intervention in women's reproductive self-determination by invoking their own principles of public order, morality, and public health. Laws have been developed in many countries that punish women, and those who assist them, for resorting to contraception or abortion, and women's access to health examinations and services have been made dependent upon authorization by husbands and fathers. Women's negative human rights require that states remove all such barriers to women's pursuit of their health interests, except for those governing safety and efficacy of health services in general.

Positive rights require more of states—

even amounting in some cases to social reconstruction. For example, the Colombian Ministry of Health's interpretation of the Women's Convention led it to introduce a gender perspective into national health policies. These policies consider "the social discrimination of women as an element which contributes to the ill-health of women."[24] One Ministerial resolution orders health institutions to respect women's decisions on all issues that affect their health, lives, and sexuality, and rights "to information and orientation to allow the exercise of free, gratifying, responsible sexuality which cannot be tied to maternity."[25]

Human rights regarding health require that the state provide health care that individuals are not able to obtain or provide on their own. This includes clinic and hospital-based services dependent on specialized skills of health care professionals, surgical interventions, and medical technologies. It also includes less sophisticated means, such as the supply of routine antibiotics and contraceptives that require little more than minimum counselling, nursing, and pharmaceutical services.

Positive rights may be difficult to observe in states with strained resources. However, it is a notorious fact that states invoking poverty to justify nonobservance of duties to defend women's health often provide disproportionately large military budgets. This is consistent with male-gendered perceptions of a population's needs.

Epidemiological data can be used to show how human rights can be made relevant to women's health. For example, international law has not yet developed the right to life beyond the duty to apply due process of law in cases of capital punishment. The right to life has not been invoked on behalf of the estimated 500,000 women annually who die of pregnancy-related causes because of lack of appropriate care.[26] Supplying appropriate care for women may be characterized as a duty of positive human rights to which states must allocate resources. An estimated 200,000 of these deaths are due to unsafe abortion alone.[27] Health indications for abortion include pregnancies that come too early, too late, too frequently, and too closely spaced. Permitting women access to qualified health personnel willing to perform the procedure is a negative human right that states are increasingly recognizing. The challenge remains of requiring states to satisfy the positive duty of providing qualified services when women have no access to them on their own.

Feminist legal analysis exposes further areas of human rights observance to which states can be held. A distinction is commonly drawn between public and private law. Typically, the state engages its machinery for public law concerns such as governmental administration and maintenance of public order, but excludes itself from such private law matters as family relationships and functioning. Feminists identify domestic violence, discrimination against female children, women's exclusion from family inheritance, and demands for husbands' authorization of wives' medical care, as oppression and subordination. They point out that these impair women's health, but are not observed and remedied by the state.[28] In many countries, laws excluded husbands from liability for rape of their wives until recently, while these laws are still maintained in others. Feminist theories show how such male-gendered laws are structured and enforced at a cost to women's health. Similarly, laws permitting younger marriage of girls than boys promote the stereotyping of women in childbearing and service roles, and exclude them from the education and training that boys receive to fulfill their masculine destiny as family and social leaders.

CONCLUSION

Recognition of gender stereotyping exposes the underlying social conditions that compromise women's health. International human rights law requires state action to remove stereotyping that negatively affects women's status and health. Further, it justifies individual and nongovernmental organization initiatives to both assist states in conforming to the law, and to hold states accountable for their failures.

Achieving respect for each person's right to the highest attainable standard of health is in itself an important goal of international law, but that right is interdependent with many other human rights. Good health is the precondition to individuals' exercise of rights to equal participation in communal and social life. At the same time, an individual's capacity for participation in activities of their choice enhances their health status.

REFERENCES

1. Constitution of the World Health Organization, signed July 22, 1946 and entered into force on April 7, 1948, in Basic Documents, 39th ed. (Geneva: World Health Organization, 1993).
2. C.O.N. Moser, "Gender planning in the Third World: Meeting practical and strategic needs," World Dev. 17(1989): 1799–1825.
3. See generally, T. Turman, C. AbouZahr, and M. Koblinsky, eds., "Reproductive Health: The MotherCare Experience," International Journal of Gynecology & Obstetrics Vol. 48, Supp (1995).
4. See generally, World Bank, A New Agenda for Women's Health and Nutrition (Washington DC: World Bank, 1994).
5. A.C. Mastroianni, R. Faden, and D. Federman, Women and Health Research, Vols. 1 and 2 (Washington, D.C.: National Academy Press, 1994).
6. R. de los Rios, "Gender, Health, and Development: An Approach in the Making," in Gender, Women, and Health in the Americas (Washington, D.C.: Pan American Health Organization, 1993): 3–17.
7. M.F. Fathalla, "Women's Health: An Overview," International Journal of Gynecological Obstetrics Vol. 46 (1994): 105–118.
8. C. Gilligan, In A Different Voice: Psychological Theory and Women's Development (Cambridge, Mass.: Harvard University Press, 1982).

9. J.S. Stein, Empowerment and Women's Health: A New Framework (London: Zed Press, forthcoming 1996).

10. A.M. Brandt, No Magic Bullet: A Social History of Venereal Disease (New York: Oxford University Press, 1985).

11. G. Seidel, "The Competing Discourses of HIV/AIDS in Sub-Saharan Africa: Discourses of Rights and Empowerment v Discourses of Control and Exclusion," Soc. Sci. Med. 36 (1993): 175–194.

12. R.J. Cook and D. Maine, "Spousal Veto over Family Planning Services," American Journal of Public Health 77 (1987): 339–344.

13. On Canada, see B.M. Dickens, Medico-Legal Aspects of Family Law (Toronto: Butterworths, 1979): 28.

14. V. Franks and E.D. Rothblum, eds., The Stereotyping of Women: Its Effects on Mental Health (New York: Springer Publishing Co., 1983).

15. E.D. Rothblum, "Sex-Role Stereotypes and Depression in Women," in V. Franks and E.D. Rothblum, ibid.: 83–111.

16. N. Lewis, S. Huyer, B. Hettel, L. Marsden, Safe Womanhood: A Discussion Paper (Toronto: Gender, Science and Development Program, The International Federation of Institutes for Advanced Study, 1994).

17. R. Dworkin, Taking Rights Seriously, (Cambridge, Mass.: Harvard University Press, 1977).

18. R.J. Cook, "Reservations to the Convention on the Elimination of All Forms of Discrimination against Women," Virginia Journal of International Law 30 (1990): 645–716.

19. Human Rights Watch, Criminal Injustice: Violence Against Women in Brazil (New York: Human Rights Watch, 1991).

20. S. Brownmiller, Against Our Will: Men, Women and Rape (New York: Simon and Schuster, 1975).

21. C. Farnsworth, "Canada Gives a Somali Refuge from Genital Rite," The New York Times, July 21, 1994.

22. OEA/Ser.L/V/II.88, February 9, 1995: 12–13, 39–47, 93–97.

23. R.J. Cook, Women's Health and Human Rights (Geneva: World Health Organization, 1994).

24. M.I. Plata, "Reproductive Rights as Human Rights: the Colombian Case," in Human Rights of Women: National and International Perspectives, ed. R.J. Cook (Philadelphia: University of Pennsylvania Press, 1994): 515–531.

25. Ibid.

26. C. AbouZahr and E. Royston, Maternal Mortality: A Global Factbook (Geneva: World Health Organization, 1991) p. 1.

27. World Health Organization, Coverage of Maternity Care: A Tabulation of Available Information, Third edition (Geneva: World Health Organization, WHO/FHE/MSM/93.7, 1993) p. 12.

28. S. Goonesekere, Women's Rights and Children's Rights: The United Nations Conventions as Compatible and Complementary International Treaties (Florence: UNICEF, 1992).

QUESTIONS

1. Cook argues that "Laws obstruct women's access to reproductive health services." However, Cook also advocates for greater governmental involvement in ensuring women's rights and reproductive health. Do you think it is possible to reconcile this seeming contradiction?

2. Cook notes that in some countries the legal age of marriage is lower for women than for men and that in some countries health clinics require the consent of a husband for a wife to access health care. Consider examples of countries where this is practiced. What are the implications for health and human rights? How would you effectively work for change?

3. This work was published in 1993. Using additional resources as necessary, comment on what you think has changed in guaranteeing womens' human rights since this article was written. If you were to provide an update to this article, what new issues would you raise?

FURTHER READING

1. Baptiste, Donna, Kapungu, Chisina, Khare, Manorama H., Lewis, Yvonne, & Barlow-Mosha, Linda, Integrating Women's Human Rights into Global Health Research: An Action Framework. *Journal of Women's Health*, 2010; 19: 2091–99 http://online.liebertpub.com/doi/abs/10.1089/jwh.2010.2119
2. Pollack Petchesky, Rosalind, *Global Prescriptions Gendering Health and Human Rights.* London: Zed Books, 2003.
3. Bunch, C., Beijing, Backlash, and the Future of Women's Human Rights. *Health and Human Rights*, 1995; 1: 449–453.
4. *Roe v. Wade*, 410 U.S. 113 (1973).

POINT OF VIEW

Sexuality, Health and Human Rights: Nothing Sacred, Nothing Assumed

Alice Miller

A "health and human rights" approach to sexuality can be useful to the project of realizing sexual rights, but its application requires careful analysis. The last decade of global sexual rights work has been productive, but also contentious and fractured, with some aspects gaining more traction than others. Given the significant but checkered status of sexual rights, particularly in the context of health-based claims, I seek here to raise cautions around some of the assumptions and foci—shorthanded as GBV, LGBT, SOGI, SRH—on which advocates and policy makers have relied in advancing different versions of sexual rights. The ideas and approach presented here draw heavily on insights gained in interactions with other scholars and advocates who are raising these concerns globally.

With a critical but ultimately optimistic perspective, I suggest that neither "sexuality" nor "health" should be employed without close examination of the ways in which each concept functions and connects to others. Overall, the process of theorizing and practicing an integrated approach to sexuality by linking the worlds of health and human rights should prioritize understandings that support broader social justice claims, and engage with power differentials between and within nations, especially attending to hierarchies of race, ethnicity, religion, disability, sex, gender and age. This would place sexual rights work squarely in the domain of political analysis, which along with epidemiology and other traditional tools of public health, can support inclusive global advocacy and programming in sexuality and rights.

One of the most comprehensive frameworks for sexual rights is found in the International Planned Parenthood Federation's "Sexual Rights: A Declaration" (found at: www.ippf.org/en/Resources/Statements/Sexual+rights+an+IPPF+declaration.htm). This framework, which I played a role in developing, stresses that sexual rights must engage with the full range of existing human rights. It frames sexual rights to include the diversity of people and practices, with a focus on the rights necessary for all persons to determine their own sexualities, not only their conduct but also the meaning of sexuality to them and to their communities. It also stresses rights to participate in debates over the policies, material and political conditions, and state and non-state practices that govern sexuality.

UNDERSTANDING HUMAN SEXUALITY (HETEROSEXUALITY AS WELL AS HOMOSEXUALITY) AS A PRODUCT OF HISTORY, CULTURE, IDEAS, POLITICS AND THE MARKET, AND NOT JUST PHYSIOLOGY, HORMONES AND HEALTH

Contemporary work on sexuality stresses its socially constructed nature—that beliefs, practices and identities around sexuality (including terminology such as "gay" and "straight") are a product of history and place. It is not so much that bodies and sexual acts have changed so radically over time, but that the priority and meaning attached to those practices have changed. Sexual practices did not always produce the social identities we give them today. As many scholars have noted, the categories of both heterosexuality and homosexuality were invented in the 19th century, as newly-minted European and American "sexuality experts" sought to distinguish respectable from disreputable citizens in their rapidly changing nations. Women liking sex with men too much were deemed perverse heterosexuals, for example. Moreover, in other cultures, men having sex with men were not deemed to have a "homosexual orientation," let alone called "gay" because their societies didn't organize people and sexual practices that way. Historical and culturally grounded understandings of sexuality do not assume people are "hiding" their true natures. Rather, they seek to develop analyses which pay careful attention to how meaning is constructed around sexuality in each place and time, giving biology and the body *a* role in sexuality but *not the exclusive* role, and not claiming any transnational truth.

Contemporary human rights' underlying theory promotes *decision-making* and *conscience* as key elements of human dignity. Thus, it is consistent with a social construction/historically grounded approach to sexuality. This version of rights does not lose power by not requiring sexual preferences be inborn; moreover while it includes protections for diverse sexual orientations, rights protections are not limited to any identity—they include rights of child "brides," persons in sex work, anyone facing sexual violence or coercion, people in detention or facing penal sanctions for real or imagined sexual practices, persons seeking to link or delink their sexual practices from reproduction, men having sex with men (and women) etc. The limits to sexual rights are set by the same rules as the carefully-scrutinized limits to all rights: evidence of actual harm to others.

HEALTH AND HUMAN RIGHTS AS (PARTIAL) INCUBATORS OF SEXUAL RIGHTS?

It is no accident that some of the earliest interpretations of international human rights law giving protection for some sexual rights occurred in the context of health. Progressive health-based responses to HIV/AIDS, and recognition of the existence of (sexual) violence against women, made health a relatively accessible site for sexual rights. By acknowledging the diversity of sexual practices, and engaging with the complex flow of power differentials that shape sexual encounters, including in marriage, health-focused analyses provided critical support for new sexual rights claims.

One of the first breakthroughs in international standards on sexuality, in this case, on homosexual behaviour, was issued in 1994 by the Human Rights Committee, the United Nations expert body which reviews implementation of the International Covenant on Civil and Political Rights. This opinion stated that the "criminalization of homosexual practices cannot be considered a reasonable means nor proportionate measure to achieve the aim of preventing the spread of HIV/AIDS," and found punitive laws in Australia violated rights to privacy and non-discrimination. In 2000, the Committee that monitors the Covenant on Economic, Social and Cultural Rights issued an authoritative statement on health, including a first-ever reference to sexual orientation in this kind of general interpretation. Since then, many treaty bodies have taken on protection of "sexual orientation"

—including the Committee that monitors the Convention on the Rights of the Child and most recently, in 2011, the Committee responsible for oversight of the Convention on the Elimination of All Forms of Discrimination against Women (CEDAW). CEDAW's adoption of a statement on non-discrimination on sexual orientation and gender identity ended a rather deafening silence in the treaty bodies on diversity in sexual and gender orientations for persons deemed female.

In regard to heterosexual behaviour and sexual rights, health has been a useful, but arguably less fully productive, site, especially for the category of "woman." (The persistent presumption that the category of 'woman' is biologically unified and heterosexual must be noted.) By 1993, sexual violence had been flagged in the U.N. as a violation of health, autonomy and bodily integrity rights (for women). By 1995, the Beijing Platform for Action, a global political consensus document stated in its *health* chapter that "the human rights of women include their right to have control over and decide freely and responsibly on matters related to their sexuality, including sexual and reproductive health, free of coercion, discrimination and violence." Yet nearly 20 years later, there is remarkably little human rights law that moves beyond a violence/protection and a "safe to reproduce" health focus. Indeed, standards generally stop short of supporting a woman's right to have or not have sex as an aspect of her personhood. Nor are there yet unequivocal standards supporting the termination of pregnancy as a free-standing right of women: a confrontative report by the independent UN expert on health claiming abortion rights as health rights stands alone. Thus, the articulation of a rights-based choice to link, or separate, sexuality and reproduction on an equal basis for all persons, regardless of gender and sex, remains a major challenge.

HEALTH AND HUMAN RIGHTS: A NECESSARY, NOT SUFFICIENT AND SOMETIMES CONSTRAINING SITE FOR SEXUAL RIGHTS

While health, especially with respect to HIV, has driven the attention of the human rights community to diversity of sexual practices and orientations, health is neither the sole nor always most appropriate domain of protection. Addressing only health rights or access to health services as sexual rights can hide the ways that autonomy and conscience in regard to sexuality goes beyond health services and health information. Control of sexuality is deeply political: national and international debates over sexual mores and practices should be recognized as processes through which sexual behaviours are given meaning, and governed.

Although health has been an undeniably productive site for promoting sexual rights, especially for previously stigmatized practices or invisible persons such as men who have sex with men, or persons in sex work etc, interventions using "health" cannot be presumed as always benign. Both governmental deployment of medicine and public health, and the medical professions' own gate-keeping, have documented histories of oppression for same sex behaviours and persons deemed as lesbian, gay, bisexual or trans persons. This history intertwines with the history of states' and medical establishments' control of women's sexuality through surveillance and reproductive controls. Although it may appear politically tempting to advance sexual rights through health approaches alone, sidestepping condemnations based on religion, culture, or morality, medicalizing sexuality to hide the politics of sexuality can backfire, entrenching already powerful perspectives.

CONCLUSION

A health and human rights approach to sexuality can, if used with care, support strategies for coalition building among groups claiming disconnected corners of sexual rights work. We can present the relevance of sexual rights for all, fighting its assignment it to any one sub-group of people, and countering arguments that sexual rights are rights of "privilege" or special, needing to wait until other rights are realized. If done with self-reflection and generosity of outlook, it can contribute to reviving calls for sexual justice as social justice, helping to ensure that sexual rights function effectively for the most diverse range of people. An integrated approach can be used to transform the practice of rights-based accountability to make states truly responsive to sexuality and gender in their efforts to "ensure the conditions in which all persons can be healthy," equal, committed and free.

Alice Miller is Associate Research Scientist in Law and Robina Foundation Human Rights Fellow, Yale Law School, Clinical Professor of Epidemiology, Yale School of Public Health, and Lecturer in Faculty of Arts and Sciences, Yale University, New Haven, CT, USA.

CHAPTER 24

Sexual Orientation, Gender Identity and International Human Rights Law: Contextualising the Yogyakarta Principles

Michael O'Flaherty and John Fisher

INTRODUCTION

Worldwide, people are subject to persistent human rights violations because of their actual or perceived sexual orientation and gender identity. These human rights violations take many forms, from denials of the rights to life, freedom from torture, and security of the person, to discrimination in accessing economic, social and cultural rights such as health, housing, education and the right to work, from non-recognition of personal and family relationships to pervasive interferences with personal dignity, suppression of diverse sexual identities, attempts to impose heterosexual norms, and pressure to remain silent and invisible.

At least seven countries maintain the death penalty for consensual same-sex practices,[1] and numerous reports have documented persons killed or sentenced to death because of their sexual orientation or gender identity,[2] including a gay man sprayed with gasoline and set on fire in Belgium, the murder of a transgender human rights defender in Argentina, a nail bomb explosion in a gay bar in the United Kingdom, killing three people and injuring dozens of others, the murder of a gay rights activist by multiple knife wounds in Jamaica, prompting a crowd to gather outside his home, laughing and calling out 'let's get them one at a time', and the recent execution-style murder of two lesbian human rights defenders in South Africa. Often killings based on sexual orientation or gender identity are perpetrated 'by agents of the State, and their murders go unpunished. Indeed no prosecution is ever brought'.[3]

In a recent report,[4] Amnesty International documents serious patterns of police misconduct directed against individuals in the United States because of their sexual orientation or gender identity, including profiling of such individuals as criminal, selective enforcement of laws, sexual, physical and verbal abuse, failure to respond or inadequate responses by the police to hate crimes and violence, as well as to situations of domestic violence that involve same-sex partners, inappropriate searches and mistreatment in detention and a lack of accountability for perpetrators.

Those who transgress gender norms are particularly likely to be targeted for violence. The organisation 'Transgender Day of Remembrance' estimates that one transgender person is killed every month in the US.[5] In Nepal, métis (people born as men who identify as women) have been beaten by police with batons, gun butts and sticks, burnt with cigarettes and forced to perform oral sex.[6]

Transgender people are 'often subjected to violence . . . in order to "punish" them for transgressing gender barriers or for challenging predominant conceptions of gender roles',[7] and transgender youth have been described as 'among the most vulnerable and marginalized young people in society'.[8] As one Canadian report underlines:

> The notion that there are two and only two genders is one of the most basic ideas in our binary Western way of thinking. Transgender people challenge our very understanding of the world. And we make them pay the cost of our confusion by their suffering.[9]

Violations directed against lesbians because of their sex are often inseparable from violations directed against them because of their sexual orientation.[10] Community restrictions on women's sexuality result in a range of human rights violations, such as the multiple rape of a lesbian in Zimbabwe, arranged by her own family in an attempt to 'cure' her of her homosexuality.[11] The Institute for Democracy in South Africa has reported that lesbians face violence twice as frequently as heterosexual women, and are at increased risk of being raped precisely because of their sexual orientation, often by someone they know.[12] According to the Institute, the reason most frequently cited for rape of lesbians was that the man needed to 'show her' she was a woman.[13]

The linkages between violence based on sex, sexual orientation, gender identity and gender expression are illustrated by a recent case in which a teenager in Dublin attacked a woman he mistook for a gay man because of her hairstyle. Approaching the woman and her male companion with the inquiry 'are you two gay guys?' he proceeded to strike the couple, knocking them to the ground, before kicking the woman in the back and stomach, and jumping on the man's back.[14]

More than 80 countries still maintain laws that make same-sex consensual relations between adults a criminal offence.[15] Recently, such laws were used in Morocco to convict six men, after allegations that a private party they had attended was a 'gay marriage',[16] and in Cameroon 11 men were arrested in a bar believed to have a gay clientele in May 2005, and sent to prison where they spent more than a year, and a further six men were arrested on 19 July 2007, after a young man who had been arrested on theft charges was coerced by police into naming associates who were presumed to be homosexual.[17] In other countries, laws against 'public scandals', 'immorality' or 'indecent behaviour' are used to penalise people for looking, dressing or behaving differently from enforced social norms.[18] Even where criminal sanctions against homosexuality or 'immorality' are not actively enforced, such laws can be used to arbitrarily harass or detain persons of diverse sexual orientations and gender identities, to impede the activities of safer sex advocates or counsellors, or as a pretext for discrimination in employment or accommodation.[19]

Those seeking to peaceably affirm diverse sexual orientations or gender identities have also experienced violence and discrimination. Participants in an Equality March in Poland, for example, faced harassment and intimidation by police as well as by extremist nationalists who shouted comments such as 'Let's get the fags', and 'We'll do to you what Hitler did with Jews',[20] and attempted suppression of Pride events has been documented in at least 10 instances in Eastern Europe.[21] State interference with such exercise of the freedoms of expression, assembly and association have included banning of Pride marches, conferences and events, condemnatory anti-homosexual comments by political representatives, police failure to protect participants from violence or complicity in such violence, and discriminatory or arbitrary arrests of peaceful participants.[22]

Discrimination in accessing economic, social and cultural rights has been widely documented. People have been denied employment, employment-related benefits or faced dismissal because of their sexual orientation or gender identity.[23] In the context of the right to adequate housing, lesbian and transgender women have been found to be at increased risk of homelessness, discrimination based on sexual orientation or gender identity in renting accommodations has been experienced both by individuals and same-sex couples, and persons have been forced from their homes and communities when their sexual orientation or gender identity has become known.[24] Transgender persons may face particular obstacles in seeking to access gender-appropriate services within homeless shelters.[25] Materials referencing issues of sexual orientation and gender identity have been banned from school curricula, student groups addressing sexual orientation and gender identity issues have been prohibited, students have faced high levels of bullying and harassment because of their actual or perceived sexual orientation or gender identity, and in some cases young persons who express same-sex affection have been expelled.[26] In some countries, laws have prohibited the 'promotion of homosexuality' in schools.[27]

Multiple health-related human rights violations based on sexual orientation and gender identity have also been documented. Lesbian, gay, bisexual and transgender persons have been forcibly confined in medical institutions, and subject to 'aversion therapy', including electroshock treatment.[28] Criminal sanctions against homosexuality have had the effect of suppressing HIV/AIDS education and prevention programs designed for men who have sex with men or persons of diverse sexual orientations or gender identities.[29] Trans-

gender people report having been referred to by health professionals as 'thing', 'it', or 'not a real man/woman'.[30] Intersex people have been subjected to involuntary surgeries in an attempt to 'correct' their genitals.[31]

In the health-sector and elsewhere, same-sex relationships are frequently unrecognised and devalued, with same-sex partners denied a broad range of entitlements available to heterosexuals, such as the right to make medical decisions for an incapacitated partner, to visit a partner or partner's child in hospital, to inherit property or be involved in funeral arrangements when a partner dies, to have equal pension benefits, file joint tax returns, obtain fair property settlement if a relationship ends, or be recognised as a partner for immigration purposes.[32]

Those who seek to advocate for an end to such violations or affirm the human rights of persons of diverse sexual orientations or gender identities are particularly at risk:[33]

> Defenders [of the rights of lesbian, gay, bisexual, transgender and intersex persons (LGBTI)] have been threatened, had their houses and offices raided, they have been attacked, tortured, sexually abused, tormented by regular death threats and even killed. . . . In numerous cases from all regions, police or government officials are the alleged perpetrators of violence and threats against defenders of LGBTI rights. In several of these cases, the authorities have prohibited demonstrations, conferences and meetings, denied registration of organisations working for LGBTI rights and police officers have, allegedly, beaten up or even sexually abused these defenders of LGBTI rights.

Although less tangible, perhaps even more systemic and far-reaching in consequence is the net result of such endemic human rights violations: the constant fear in which many persons of diverse sexual orientations and gender identities have to live.[34] As one man arrested and subsequently tortured following a police raid of a gay discotheque in Egypt noted: 'I used to think being gay was just part of my life and now I know it means dark cells and beatings.'[35]

Faced with obstacles to familial and social acceptance that may seem overwhelming, many lesbians, gays, bisexuals, transgender and intersex people remain invisible and isolated. The high rates of documented suicide by such people are consequently unsurprising.[36]

REVIEW OF LAW AND JURISPRUDENCE

There is a growing jurisprudence and other law-related practice that identifies a significant application of human rights law with regard to people of diverse sexual orientations and gender identities. This phenomenon can be observed at the international level, principally in the form of practice related to the United Nations-sponsored human rights treaties, as well as under the European Convention on Human Rights. The development of this sexual orientation and gender identity-related human rights legal doctrine can be categorised as follows: (a) non-discrimination, (b) protection of privacy rights, and (c) the ensuring of other general human rights protection to all, regardless of sexual orientation of gender identity. In addition, it is useful to examine (d) some general trends in human rights law that have important implications for the enjoyment of human rights by people of diverse sexual orientations and gender identities.

Non-Discrimination

The practice of the bodies that monitor implementation of the United Nations-sponsored human rights treaties relates to sexual orientation-related discrimination rather than to discrimination on the basis of gender identity.

The Committee on Economic, Social and Cultural Rights (CESCR) has dealt with the matter in its General Comments, the interpretative texts it issues to explicate the full meaning of the provisions of the Covenant on Economic, Social and Cultural Rights. In General Comments Nos 18 of 2005 (on the right to work),[37] 15 of 2002 (on the right to water)[38] and 14 of 2000 (on the right to the highest attainable standard of health),[39] it has indicated that the Covenant proscribes any discrimination on the basis of, inter-alia, sex and sexual orientation 'that has the intention or effect of nullifying or impairing the equal enjoyment or exercise of [the right at issue]'. The CESCR has consistently based this prohibition on the terms of the Covenant's anti-discrimination provision, Article 2.2, which lists invidious categories of discrimination as including 'sex' and 'other status'. Presumably, since the CESCR distinguishes 'sex' and 'sexual orientation' in its General Comments, it locates sexual orientation within the rubric of 'other status'. The CESCR, in the General Comments, also invokes the article addressing equal rights of men and women, Article 3, as a basis for its prohibition of sexual orientation-related discrimination. This linkage of the categories of sex and sexual orientation-related discrimination is discussed subsequently in the context of the practice of the Human Rights Committee (HRC).

The Committee on the Rights of the Child (CRC) has also dealt with the issue in a General Comment. In its General Comment No. 4 of 2003,[40] it stated that, 'State parties have the obligation to ensure that all human beings below 18 enjoy all the rights set forth in the Convention [on the Rights of the Child] without discrimination (Article 2), including with regard to "race, colour, sex, language, religion, political or other opinion, national, ethnic or social origin, property, disability, birth or other status". These grounds also cover [inter alia] sexual orientation'. The CRC thus appears to adopt the same approach as the CESCR in locating sexual orientation within the category of 'other status'.

Both the CESCR and the CRC very occasionally raise issues of sexual orientation-related discrimination in the Concluding Observations they adopt on the periodic reports submitted to them by States parties on their record of implementation of the treaties (CESCR: regarding eight of the 70 States considered between 2000 and 2006, CRC: regarding five of the 186 States considered in the same period). These Concluding Observations have a non-binding and flexible nature. As such, they are not always a useful indicator of what a Committee may consider to be a matter of obligation under the Covenant. Nevertheless, where the Committee expresses concern or makes a specific recommendation for correction of a practice, we can discern that serious issues under the treaty are at issue.[41] It is in this context that we may observe the CESCR's regret, in 2005, that Hong Kong's anti-discrimination legislation failed to cover sexual orientation-related discrimination[42] and its concern, in 2000, that Kyrgyzstan classified lesbianism as a sexual offence in its penal code.[43]

The Committee on the Elimination of Discrimination against Women (CEDAW), notwithstanding that it has not addressed the matter in a General Comment or otherwise specified the applicable provisions of the Convention on the Elimination of All Forms of Discrimination Against Women, on a number of occasions has criticised States for discrimination on the basis of sexual orientation. For example, it also addressed the situation in Kyrgyzstan and recommended that, 'lesbianism be reconceptualised as a sexual orientation and that penalties for its practice be abolished'.[44] The Committee on the Elimination of Racial

Discrimination (CERD) appears never to have engaged with issues of discrimination against persons who belong to both racial and sexual minority groups. This gap is startling when one considers the authoritative evidence of such persons facing forms of 'double discrimination', as reported, for instance, by the UN Human Rights Council's Special Rapporteur on contemporary forms of racism, racial discrimination, xenophobia and related intolerance.[45]

Issues of sexual orientation have received the most extensive attention in the work of the monitoring body under the International Covenant on Civil and Political Rights, the HRC. In the individual communication, Toonen v Australia, in 1994, it considered that, 'the reference to "sex" in articles 2, paragraph 1, and 26 is to be taken as including sexual orientation'.[46] The HRC thus decided that sexual orientation-related discrimination is a suspect category in terms of the enjoyment of Covenant rights (Article 2) and, more generally, for equality before and equal protection of the law (Article 26). The HRC has persistently observed, however, that discrimination on the basis of sexual orientation, as is the case for all the other discrimination categories listed in Articles 2 and 26, is not inherently invidious, since 'not every distinction amounts to prohibited discrimination under the Covenant, as long as it is based on reasonable and objective criteria'.[47]

The HRC, in individual communications subsequent to Toonen, while reaffirming the scope of the Article 2.1 and 26 provisions to embrace sexual-orientation-related discrimination, has avoided specifying that this is by means of a reading of the term 'sex', albeit an individual concurring opinion of two HRC members in the case of Joslin v New Zealand, in 2002, categorically states that, 'it is the established view of the Committee that the prohibition against discrimination on grounds of "sex" in article 26 comprises also discrimination based on sexual orientation'.[48] The apparent reliance on the 'sex' category has been criticised by the European Court of Justice,[49] on the basis that matters of sexual orientation are substantively different from binary men/ women issues which the category of 'sex' is often perceived to address. However, in support of the HRC's approach it may be recalled[50] that much discrimination based on sexual orientation or gender identity is directed against those who violate social or cultural conceptions of gender. Also, taking account of how sexual discrimination has an elevated status in the Covenant, being addressed also in Article 3, the reliance on the 'sex' category appears to elevate the suspect nature of sexual orientation-related discrimination to a higher level than that of the other listed categories. Perhaps it is with considerations such as these in mind that Jack Donnelly described the HRC's approach as 'radical and provocative'.[51] The approach adopted by the HRC has the additional merit of avoiding an invocation of the category of 'other status' in the absence of clearly established criteria for when a non-specified form of discrimination can be so designated.

A small number of cases have illustrated the HRC's application of its nondiscrimination doctrine. In Young v Australia[52] and X v Colombia[53] the HRC impugned a distinction made in law between same-sex partners who were excluded from pension benefits, and unmarried heterosexual partners who were granted such benefits. In Joslin the denial of the right to marry to same-sex couples was considered not to constitute a violation of Article 26. However, an individual concurring opinion of two members observed that the authors had not sought to identify any difference in treatment arising from their inability to marry and, 'the Committee's jurisprudence supports the position that such differentiation may very well, depending on the cir-

cumstances of a concrete case, amount to prohibited discrimination'.[54]

The breadth of the application of the HRC approach is best seen in its practice under the report review procedure. HRC frequently raises the issue of discrimination on the basis of sexual orientation: during the period 2000–06, it did so regarding 13 of the 84 countries under review. It criticised the criminalisation of homosexual sexual relations (multiple countries),[55] a failure to prohibit employment-related discrimination,[56] failure to include the category of sexual orientation in broad anti-discrimination legal regimes (multiple countries),[57] a lack of education programs to combat discriminatory attitudes[58] and unequal ages of consent for sexual activity.[59]

At the regional level, the European Court of Human Rights (ECtHR) has been invited to consider issues of discrimination with regard to both sexual orientation and gender identity. The ECtHR, while reiterating that the nondiscrimination provision of the European Convention on Human Rights (ECHR), Article 14, unlike Article 26 of the International Covenant on Civil and Political Rights, does not erect an autonomous anti-discrimination provision, but rather one that can only be applied in conjunction with a substantive provision of the ECHR (albeit it embraces those additional rights, falling within the general scope of any ECHR article, for which a State has voluntarily decided to provide),[60] has consistently stated that differences based on sex and sexual orientation must 'have particularly serious reasons by way of justification'.[61] And the ECtHR, and the former European Human Rights Commission, have not been concerned to identify whether the identification of such forms of suspect discrimination derives from the categories of 'sex', 'other status' or otherwise.[62]

In Salgueiro da Silva Mouta v Portugal the ECtHR held that a judge's denial of child custody to a homosexual father on the grounds of his sexual orientation created a discriminatory enjoyment of privacy.[63] In Karner v Austria the ECtHR was of the view that the failure of Austria to permit a homosexual man to continue occupying his deceased partner's flat was discriminatory, since this right, enjoyed by other family members under Austrian law, did not apply to same-sex partners. Although the government claimed that excluding homosexuals aimed to protect 'the family in the traditional sense', the ECtHR held Austria had not demonstrated how the exclusion was necessary to that aim.[64] In L. and V. v Austria[65] and S.L. v Austria[66] the ECtHR considered that Austria's differing age of consent for heterosexual and homosexual relations was discriminatory; it 'embodied a predisposed bias on the part of a heterosexual majority against a homosexual minority', which could not 'amount to sufficient justification for the differential treatment any more than similar negative attitudes towards those of a different race, origin or colour'.[67]

One instance in which a discrimination-based claim failed was that in Fretté v France. In this case a homosexual man argued that a refusal to allow him to adopt a child for reasons of his sexual orientation constituted a violation of the ECHR.[68] In finding against him, the ECtHR referred to the fast evolving and very diverse practice across Europe as well as the conflicting views of experts as to what would be in the best interests of the child. The judgment is problematic. The reasoning is inconsistent and posits false dilemmas such as a supposed tension between the rights of the man and the child. There is no such tension. The tension is between the rights of homosexual and heterosexual prospective adoptive parents, with the rights of the child, especially its best interests, always being paramount. Issues such as these were handled in a more consistent and comprehensible manner in the very recent

decision in E.B. v France. The ECtHR, while assiduously maintaining the paramount principle of the best interests of the child, held that 'in rejecting the applicant's application for authorisation to adopt, the domestic authorities made a distinction based on considerations regarding her sexual orientation, a distinction which is not acceptable under the Convention'.[69]

It is unclear how far a non-discrimination approach can go in terms of the regulation of practices of non-state actors, not least since the existing jurisprudence and practice only addresses instances of discrimination that fall clearly within well established jurisprudential limits. Taking account of the extensive literature on the subject of the reach of anti-discrimination law into the private sphere, the applicable principles are well-articulated by Jack Donnelly: '[T]he internationally recognized human right to non-discrimination prohibits invidious public (or publicly supported or tolerated) discrimination that deprives target groups of the legitimate enjoyment of other rights.... Only when ... social contacts systematically influence access to economic or political opportunities do they become a matter of legitimate state regulation.'[70]

Protection of Privacy Rights

The first successful international human rights cases on issues of sexual orientation were taken under the ECHR and concerned the privacy of same-sex sexual relations. In Dudgeon v United Kingdom[71] and Norris v Ireland,[72] the criminalisation of such practices was deemed a violation of the privacy protection in Article 8 of the ECHR. In Modinos v Cyprus the ECtHR again held that such a law violated the right to privacy, and maintained that even a 'consistent policy' of not bringing prosecutions under the law was no substitute for full repeal.[73] Privacy arguments were also successfully invoked in cases concerning a ban on recruitment to the military of homosexuals: Smith and Grady v United Kingdom[74] and Lustig-Prean and Beckett v United Kingdom.[75] The ECtHR has also recognised privacy protection under the ECHR for transsexual persons. In Goodwin v United Kingdom[76] and I. v United Kingdom[77] it considered the cases of two transsexual women who claimed that the United Kingdom's refusal to change their legal identities and papers to match their post-operative genders constituted discrimination. Reversing a number of its previous decisions, the ECtHR held that their right to respect for their private lives, and also their right to marry, had been violated (Articles 8 and 12 of the ECHR). In Van Kuck v Germany[78] the ECtHR considered the case of a transsexual woman whose health-insurance company had denied her reimbursement for costs associated with sex-reassignment surgery and who had unsuccessfully sought redress in the domestic courts. It found violations of the right to a fair hearing (Article 6(1) of the ECHR) and of the right to private life, holding that the German civil courts had failed to respect 'the applicant's freedom to define herself as a female person, one of the most basic essentials of self-determination'. In a powerful statement of the entitlement to an autonomous gender identity the ECtHR spoke of 'the very essence of the ECHR being respect for human dignity and human freedom, protection is given to the right of transsexuals to personal development and to physical and moral security'.[79] In L. v Lithuania, the ECtHR considered that the State was required to legislate for the provision of full gender-reassignment surgery whereby a person in the 'limbo' of partial reassignment could complete the process and be registered with the new gender identity.[80]

The HRC, in Toonen, adopted the Dudgeon/Norris approach in finding a violation by Australia of Article 17 of the Covenant.

It considered that a criminal prohibition on same-sex sexual activity, even if unenforced, constituted an unreasonable interference with Mr Toonen's privacy.[81] The HRC has not had the occasion since, in its consideration of individual cases, to address other applications of the right to privacy in the context of sexual orientation or gender identity. One possible opportunity, in Joslin, was missed since Ms Joslin was unsuccessful in arguing the primordial claim that Article 23 of the Covenant on marriage extended protection to same-sex relationships on the same basis as heterosexual relationships.[82] Nor has the HRC taken the opportunity to itself explore the range of applications of a privacy approach in the context of its review of periodic reports. Here it has addressed privacy rights exclusively in the context of the criminalisation of same-sex sexual activity (as is the case, also, in CESCR, CEDAW and CRC). Taking account of the relatively vigorous and wide-ranging engagement with privacy issues in the European context, this dearth of practice is notable. It may reflect unease with the issues on the part of the treaty bodies or a failure of civil society groups to bring situations of concern to their attention.

The Ensuring of Other General Human Rights Protection to All, Regardless of Sexual Orientation or Gender Identity

In 2006, during the HRC's consideration of a periodic report, a representative of the State party, while replying to a question of a committee member on police violence against transsexuals,[83] observed that there was no mention of such people in the Covenant. The inference seemed to be that these people had a lesser entitlement to protection. Any such view is, of course, untenable. The HRC and the other treaty bodies, in the review of periodic reports, on a number of occasions, have insisted on the entitlement of people of diverse sexual orientations and gender identities to benefit from the protection of human rights of general application. The HRC has addressed various aspects: 'violent crime perpetrated against persons of minority sexual orientation, including by law enforcement officials [and] the failure to address such crime in the legislation on hate crime';[84] '[t]he State party should provide appropriate training to law enforcement and judicial officials in order to sensitive them to the rights of sexual minorities';[85] '[t]he Committee expresses concern at the incidents of people being attacked, or even killed, on account of their sexual orientation (art.9), at the small number of investigations mounted into such illegal acts'.[86] The CRC has expressed concern that homosexual and transsexual young people 'do not have access to the appropriate information, support and necessary protection to enable them to live their sexual orientation'.[87] The practice of the Committee Against Torture (CAT) is also notable. On a number of occasions it has expressed concern about the torture of homosexuals (for instance, Argentina[88] and Egypt[89]), and, in 2002, regarding, 'complaints of threats and attacks against sexual minorities and transgender activists' in Venezuela.[90]

The proceedings of the Special Procedures of the former UN Human Rights Commission and the current Human Rights Council constitute a valuable repository of examples of the application for people of diverse sexual orientations and gender identities, of general human rights protections, as well as of the principle of non-discrimination. The Working Group on Arbitrary Detention has frequently invoked Toonen as a basis for its finding of arbitrary detention of homosexuals. The Special Representative of the Secretary-General on the situation of human rights defenders has been assiduous in condemning the intimidation of and attacks on lesbian, gay, bisexual, transgender and intersex activists.[91] She has drawn attention to such human rights violations as arbitrary detention, torture, summary execution, arbitrary and unreasonable impediments to freedom of expression, movement, association and participation in political and public life.

The Special Representative has referred to the phenomenon of multiple victimisation, where already vulnerable people face heightened risk when promoting the rights of people of diverse sexual orientations and gender identities. In 2002, she reported about women human rights defenders as follows: 'women human rights defenders are paying a heavy toll for their work in protecting and promoting the human rights of others. . . . For women human rights defenders standing up for human rights and the victims of human rights abuses—be they migrants, refugees, asylum-seekers or political activists, or simply people unwillingly relegated to the margins of society, such as ex-offenders and member of sexual minorities—can result in intimidation, harassment, unfair dismissal, death threats, torture and ill-treatment, and even death'.[92] A similar point was made by the Independent Expert on minority issues, who referred to the 'multiple forms of exclusion' of members of minority communities, 'based on aspects of their identities and personal realities such as sexual orientation or gender expression that challenge social or cultural norms'.[93] The Special Rapporteur on contemporary forms of racism, racial discrimination, xenophobia and related intolerance, has drawn attention to problems within racial minority groups: '[b]lack homosexuals suffer from double discrimination, because of their colour and sexual orientation'.[94]

Among the other Special Procedures that have engaged with the issues are those on extrajudicial, summary or arbitrary executions; torture and other cruel, inhuman or degrading treatment or punishment; freedom of religion; promotion and protection of the right to freedom of opinion and expression; violence against women; and sale of children, child prostitution and child pornography.

Those Special Procedures that address issues of economic, social and cultural rights have frequently drawn attention to the extent to which violations of these rights are at issue for people of diverse sexual orientations and gender identities. The Special Rapporteur on the right of everyone to the enjoyment of the highest attainable standard of physical and mental health has drawn wide-ranging consequences from his analysis of the state of international human rights law. For instance, in 2004, he observed that 'fundamental human rights principles, as well as existing human rights norms, lead ineluctably to the recognition of sexual rights as human rights. Sexual rights include the right of all persons to express their sexual orientation, with due regard for the well-being and rights of others, without fear of persecution, denial of liberty or social interference'.[95]

The regional level has also presented instances of attention by human rights mechanisms and procedures to sexual orientation and gender identity-related issues of the general application of human rights. For instance, country reports and follow-up reports of the Inter-American Commission on Human Rights have drawn attention to such violations as 'social-cleansing' (killing) of homosexuals and the treatment of lesbian prisoners.[96] The current Council of Europe Commissioner for Human Rights, Thomas Hammarberg, repeatedly addresses country-level sexual orientation-related concerns. His detailed and expansive treatment of such issues in a 2007 'memorandum' to the Polish government is noteworthy.[97]

The question arises of when a generally stated human right is actually limited in terms of who may benefit. For our purposes, the issue concerns when a right exclusively addresses the situation and choices of what we might term sexual majorities. The matter has been considered with regard to the right to marry. The HRC, in Joslin, stated that the 'use of the term "men and women" rather than the general terms used elsewhere in Part III of the Covenant, has been consistently and uniformly understood as indicating that the treaty obligation of States parties stemming from article 23, paragraph 2 of the Covenant is to recognize as marriage only the union between a man and a woman wishing to marry each other'.[98] It is less clear whether the Covenant recognises the rights of same-sex unmarried families. Article 23, paragraph 1 states the fundamental importance of the family and its entitlement to protection by the State, without reference to the form of family under consideration. Only in Article 23 paragraph 2 do we find reference to the right of men and women to marry and found families. It does not follow, however, that Article 23 paragraph 2 restricts the meaning of the word 'family' in Article 23 paragraph 1, and in this regard it may be observed that in its General Comment No. 19, the HRC has acknowledged the existence of various forms of family.[99] The HRC has been willing to impugn State practices that impede same sex couples from benefiting from family-related benefits, such as transfer of pension entitlements (Young and X, referred to before). These cases, however, only addressed Article 26-based issues and, in X, in a dissenting opinion of two members, it was observed that 'a couple of the same sex does not constitute a family within the meaning of the Covenant and cannot claim benefits that are based on a conception of the family as comprising individuals of different sexes'.[100]

The ECtHR, in a number of cases, had held that marriage, for purposes of the ECHR is the union of two persons of the 'opposite biological sex'[101] but, in Goodwin, it indicated that the determination of sex cannot be undertaken with solely biological criteria, so that an individual who has had a sex change operation has a right to marry someone of the now opposite sex.[102] While not specifically addressing the issue of any distinction between families and marriages, the ECtHR has frequently indicated that homosexual stable relationships are not equivalent in rights to heterosexual relationships.[103] However, in the Salguiero da Silva Mouta case, the ECtHR found a violation of the right to family life of a man in a homosexual relationship, albeit the family unit under consideration was that of the man and his daughter rather than that of him and his partner.[104] And, in Goodwin, the ECtHR was willing to interpret the term in Article 8 of the ECHR, 'the right of a man and a woman to marry' in a flexible manner taking account of changes in society.[105] It is beyond the scope of the present chapter to explore this issue further, other than to take account of the various other sources which lean towards flexible understanding of the term 'family',[106] as well as the increasing recognition by States of diversity of family forms, as reflected in the Declaration on the International Year of the Family.[107]

Some General Trends in Human Rights Law That Have Important Implications for the Enjoyment of Human Rights by People of Diverse Sexual Orientations and Gender Identities

An examination of the human rights of people of diverse sexual orientations and gender identities would be incomplete without a brief reference to the evolving understanding of the duties that fall to States and the entitlements of the rights holder. Reference has already been made to those wide-ranging aspects of the human rights obligations that have been charted by the UN Special Procedures. Of more immediate normative significance are those recent General Comments of the United Nations human rights treaty bodies[108] that have emphasised that States are obliged to undertake effective programs of education and public awareness about human rights and must otherwise seek to enable people to fully enjoy their entitlements. They must be assiduous in protecting rights, establishing appropriate monitoring and promotional institutions, as well as investigating and disciplining violations. Victims of human rights violations are entitled to redress and reparation and those who defend and promote human rights must be protected.

More generally, the programmatic implications of the duty that falls on States are being clarified within the context of the theory and practice of the human rights-based approaches to development (RBAD). The principal elements of the rights-based approach have been indicated in a statement of a common position of all of the UN agencies engaged in the work of human development, the Statement of Common Understanding, adopted at Stamford, Connecticut, USA (the Stamford Statement) in May 2003.[109] The Stamford Statement asserts that all programs of development co-operation, policies and technical assistance should further the realisation of human rights as laid down in the Universal Declaration of Human Rights (UDHR) and other international human rights instruments and that development co-operation contributes to the development of the capacity of 'duty-bearers'[110] to meet their obligations and/or of 'rights-holders' to claim their rights. The Statement identifies a number of elements which it considers as 'necessary, specific and unique to a RBAD:

1. Assessment and analysis in order to identify the human rights claims of

rights-holders and the corresponding human rights obligations of duty-bearers[111] as well as the immediate, underlying, and structural causes of the non-realisation of rights.

2. Programs assess the capacity of rights-holders to claim their rights and of duty-bearers to fulfil their obligations. They then develop strategies to build these capacities.
3. Programs monitor and evaluate both outcomes and processes guided by human rights standards and principles.
4. Programming is informed by the recommendations of international human rights bodies and mechanisms'.

Of most direct interest for the present discussion are the principles derived from human rights law which are identified as integral to a RBAD. These are described in the Stamford Statement to be: universality and inalienability; inter-dependedness and interrelatedness; non-discrimination and equality; participation and inclusion; and accountability and the rule of law.

This elaboration in General Comments as well as in RBAD theory of the nature of human rights entitlements and duties has obvious implications for the human rights of people of diverse sexual orientations and gender identities. They can, as a matter of right, demand that the promotion and protection of their rights be undertaken in a vigorous, consistent and comprehensive manner. They are entitled to have their welfare and well-being placed at the heart of the state's policy making and public programming. Moreover, they have the right to be participants in the elaboration and implementation of such policies and programs. Indeed, one can, without hyperbole, refer as a matter of law to the human right of all persons, regardless of and in full respect for their sexual orientations and gender identities, to live honoured and dignified lives within society.

IMPACT OF THE LAW AND JURISPRUDENCE FOR THE PROTECTION OF THE HUMAN RIGHTS OF PEOPLE OF DIVERSE SEXUAL ORIENTATIONS AND GENDER IDENTITIES

Notwithstanding the extent to which applicable legal standards have been clarified and articulated, the response of States and intergovernmental organisations to human rights violations based on sexual orientation or gender identity has been equivocal and inconsistent. The Special Representative of the Secretary General on human rights defenders has expressed concern at the 'almost complete lack of seriousness' with which human rights violations based on sexual orientation or gender identity are treated by the concerned authorities.[112] The High Commissioner for Human Rights has noted the 'shameful silence' surrounding such violations and the fact that 'violence against LGBT persons is frequently unreported, undocumented and goes ultimately unpunished'.[113] A number of States do not acknowledge that human rights violations based on sexual orientation or gender identity constitute legitimate areas of human rights concern. For example, a letter distributed to all State Missions in Geneva by Pakistan on behalf of the Organization of the Islamic Conference asserted that 'sexual orientation is not a human rights issue'.[114] When criticised by the Special Rapporteur on extrajudicial executions for maintaining the death penalty for homosexuality,[115] Nigeria responded that 'the death penalty by stoning under Shari'a law for unnatural sexual acts . . . should not be equated with extrajudicial killings, and indeed should not have featured in the report'.[116] Similarly, the United Republic of Tanzania opposed granting UN accreditation to nongovernmental organisations (NGOs) working to address human rights violations based on sexual orientation, on the grounds that such matters were 'not relevant to our work'.[117]

NGOs working on issues of sexual orientation and gender identity have faced challenges to their participation in UN activities. At the UN General Assembly Special Session on HIV/AIDS in June 2001, a representative of the International Gay and Lesbian Human Rights Commission had been chosen, along with other representatives from governments, NGOs and UN agencies, to participate in an official roundtable discussion on HIV/AIDS and human rights. Following objections from a number of States, she was excluded and only allowed to take the floor after debate and vote in the General Assembly.[118] The same year, the International Lesbian and Gay Association, along with hundreds of other NGOs, sought accreditation to the United Nations World Conference against Racism, Racial Discrimination, Xenophobia and Related Intolerance. Following an objection by Malaysia on behalf of the Organization of the Islamic Conference, its accreditation was put to a vote, resulting in a 43–43 tie and the denial of accreditation.[119] The NGO Committee of the UN Economic and Social Council (ECOSOC) has persistently denied UN consultative status to NGOs working on issues of sexual orientation and gender identity, a decision seemingly inconsistent with an ECOSOC resolution requiring that the 'full diversity of nongovernmental organisations' be taken into account when determining matters of accreditation.[120] Such status governs whether NGOs can participate in UN activities, including by accessing UN premises, attending international meetings, submitting written statements, making oral interventions and hosting parallel panel discussions. The plenary ECOSOC has reviewed and overturned these rejections,[121] although in subsequent meetings the NGO Committee has continued to defer or deny applications submitted by NGOs working on these issues, with the result that NGOs seeking to address matters of sexual orientation or gender identity must continue to fight for the recognition routinely granted to NGOs working on other issues.

States that have sought to promote the human rights of people of diverse sexual orientations and gender identities in international fora have also faced difficulties. When Brazil presented a resolution at the former UN Commission on Human Rights in 2003 condemning human rights violations based on sexual orientation, States opposed to consideration of the resolution brought a 'no action' motion in an attempt to prevent the Commission from considering the issue. When the motion was narrowly defeated, these States threatened to bring hundreds of amendments to the text, resulting in a decision by the Commission to defer the resolution until its 2004 session.[122] At the 2004 session, Brazil was pressured to further defer consideration of the resolution, indicating in a press release that it had 'not yet been able to arrive at a necessary consensus'.[123] A statement of the Chair was adopted, carrying the resolution over until 2005. In 2005, Brazil did not proceed with the resolution, which therefore lapsed on the Commission agenda.

Although ultimately not pursued, the Brazilian resolution on sexual orientation and human rights did raise States' awareness of the issues, and mobilised NGOs from all regions to engage in UN processes.[124] When it became apparent that the resolution would not be discussed in 2005, New Zealand delivered a joint statement on sexual orientation and human rights on behalf of a cross-regional grouping of 32 States,[125] asserting that States 'cannot ignore' the evidence of human rights violations based on sexual orientation, and calling for the Commission to respond. By the December 2006 session of the Human Rights Council, support for a similar joint statement delivered by Norway had grown to 54 States, from four of the five UN regions.[126] This statement acknowledged that the Council had received extensive evidence of human rights violations based on sexual orientation and gender identity, commended the work of NGOs, Special Procedures and treaty bodies in this area, called upon all Special Procedures and treaty bodies to integrate consideration of human rights violations based on sexual orientation and gender identity within their relevant mandates, and urged the President of the Council to allocate time for a discussion of these issues at an appropriate future session. The Norwegian joint statement also represented the first time that 'gender identity' had been included in a UN statement.

Some recognition of these concerns had already been articulated in UN resolutions, although this has thus far been limited to resolutions addressing matters of extrajudicial executions and the death penalty, rather than the full range of human rights violations identified by the Special Procedures. The former Commission on Human Rights adopted a resolution on extrajudicial executions in each of 2000, 2002, 2003, 2004 and 2005, expressly affirming the obligation of States to 'protect the inherent right to life of all persons under their jurisdiction' and calling upon States to investigate promptly and thoroughly 'all cases of killings including those ... committed for any discriminatory reason, including sexual orientation'.[127] 'Gender identity' was also included in a draft of this resolution in 2005, and received widespread support, representing the first time that language to explicitly protect the rights of transgender people has been presented in a UN forum, although the reference was removed from the text by sponsoring States before the resolution came to a vote in order to ensure adoption of the resolution. The resolution on the death penalty, adopted each year by the former Commission, recalled that the death penalty may not be imposed for any but the 'most serious crimes', and called

upon States 'to ensure that the notion of "most serious crimes" does not go beyond intentional crimes with lethal or extremely grave consequences and that the death penalty is not imposed for non-violent acts such as ... sexual relations between consenting adults'.[128]

Although, as already noted, a number of Special Procedures have consistently addressed relevant sexual orientation and gender identity issues falling within their mandate,[129] practice, overall, is inconsistent. During the Interactive Dialogue at the September 2006 session of the Human Rights Council, for example, the Special Rapporteur on the promotion and protection of the right to freedom of opinion and expression indicated that the question of sexual orientation 'was not debated' when his mandate was created, and he appeared to believe he required more explicit authorisation before addressing human rights violations on this ground.[130] Similarly, although a number of the treaty bodies regularly address issues of sexual orientation and gender identity, and engage States in discussion of these issues during consideration of country reports, there is a great deal of room for them to integrate these issues more systematically within consideration of State reports, Concluding Observations and General Comments.

THE YOGYAKARTA PROCESS

The High Commissioner for Human Rights, Louise Arbour, has expressed concern about the inconsistency of approach in law and practice. In an address to a lesbian, gay, bisexual and transgender forum, she suggested that although the principles of universality and non-discrimination apply to the grounds of sexual orientation and gender identity, there is a need for a more comprehensive articulation of these rights in international law, '[i]t is precisely in this meeting between the normative work of States and the interpretive functions of international expert bodies that a common ground can begin to emerge'.[131] Furthermore, commentators have suggested that international practice could also benefit from the application of more consistent terminology to address issues of sexual orientation and gender identity.[132] While some Special Procedures, treaty bodies and States have preferred speaking of 'sexual orientation' or 'gender identity', others speak of 'lesbians', 'gays', 'transgender' or 'transsexual' people, and still others speak of 'sexual preference' or use the language of 'sexual minorities'. In addition, issues of gender identity have been little understood, with some mechanisms and States referencing transsexuality as a 'sexual orientation', and others frankly acknowledging that they do not understand the term.[133]

It is in this context of such diverse approaches, inconsistency, gaps and opportunities that the Yogyakarta Principles on the application of international human rights law in relation to sexual orientation and gender identity (the Yogyakarta Principles)[134] were conceived. The proposal to develop the Yogyakarta Principles originated, in 2005, with a coalition of human rights NGOs that was subsequently facilitated by the International Service for Human Rights and the International Commission of Jurists. It was proposed that the Principles have a tri-partite function.[135] In the first place they should constitute a 'mapping' of the experiences of human rights violations experienced by people of diverse sexual orientations and gender identities. This exercise should be as inclusive and wide ranging as possible, taking account of the distinct ways in which human rights violations may be experienced in different regions of the world. Second, the application of international human rights law to such experiences should be articulated in as clear and

precise a manner as possible. Finally, the Principles should spell out in some detail the nature of the obligation on States for effective implementation of each of the human rights obligations.

Twenty-nine experts were invited to undertake the drafting of the Principles. They came from 25 countries representative of all geographic regions. They included one former UN High Commissioner for Human Rights (Mary Robinson, also a former head of state), 13 current or former UN human rights special mechanism office holders or treaty body members, two serving judges of domestic courts and a number of academics and activists. Seventeen of the experts were women.[136] The first of the present authors was one of the experts. He also served as rapporteur of the process, responsible for proposing various formulations and capturing various expert views in a single agreed text. The drafting process took place over a period of some 12 months during 2006–07. While much of the drafting was done by means of electronic communications, many of the experts met at an international seminar that took place in Yogyakarta, Indonesia at Gadjah Mada University from 6 to 9 November 2006 to review and finalise the text. All of the text was agreed by consensus.

Although initially some participants envisioned a very concise statement of legal principles, expressed in general terms, the seminar eventually reached the view that the complexity of circumstances of victims of human rights violations required a highly elaborated approach. They also considered that the text should be expressed in a manner that reflected the formulations in the international human rights treaties, whereby its authority as a statement of the legal standards would be reinforced.

There are 29 principles. Each of these comprises a statement of international human rights law, its application to a given situation and an indication of the nature of the State's duty to implement the legal obligation. There is some order to the Principles. Principles 1 to 3 set out the principles of the universality of human rights and their application to all persons without discrimination, as well as the right of all people to recognition before the law. The experts placed these elements at the beginning of the text in order to recall the primordial significance of the universality of human rights and the scale and extent of discrimination targeted against people of diverse sexual orientations and gender identities, as well as the manner in which they are commonly rendered invisible within a society and its legal structures. Principles 4 to 11 address fundamental rights to life, freedom from violence and torture, privacy, access to justice and freedom from arbitrary detention. Principles 12 to 18 set out the importance of non-discrimination in the enjoyment of economic, social and cultural rights, including employment, accommodation, social security, education and health. Principles 19 to 21 emphasise the importance of the freedom to express oneself, one's identity and one's sexuality, without State interference based on sexual orientation or gender identity, including the rights to participate peaceably in public assemblies and events and otherwise associate in community with others. Principles 22 and 23 highlight the rights of persons to seek asylum from persecution based on sexual orientation or gender identity. Principles 24 to 26 address the rights of persons to participate in family life, public affairs and the cultural life of their community, without discrimination based on sexual orientation or gender identity. Principle 27 recognises the right to defend and promote human rights without discrimination based on sexual orientation and gender identity, and the obligation of States to ensure the protection of human rights defenders working in these areas. Principles 28 and 29 affirm the importance

of holding rights violators accountable, and ensuring appropriate redress for those who face rights violations.

Most of the principles are titled in a manner that directly reflects the provisions of human rights treaties: right to education, highest attainable standard of health, etc. Those that differ are so phrased either to more specifically address a problematic situation (Principle 18, Protection from Medical Abuse), or to better reflect an accepted legal standard that does not derive from any one specific treaty provision (the principles on promotion of human rights—27, effective remedies—28 and accountability—29).

The content of each Principle reflects the particular human rights challenges that the experts identified as well as the precise application of the law for that situation. As such, they vary widely in style and category of contents. However, a general typology for the legal obligations of States can be observed: (i) all necessary legislative, administrative and other measures to eradicate impugned practices; (ii) protection measures for those at risk; (iii) accountability of perpetrators and redress for victims; and, (iv) promotion of a human rights culture by means of education, training and public awareness-raising. It may thus be observed that the Principles take account of the manner in which UN human rights treaty bodies in their General Comments, as well as the theory of rights-based approaches, as discussed earlier, are informing contemporary understanding of the State's implementation obligation.[137]

As has already been noted, the experts sought to capture the existing state of international law. The present authors, based on a review of the consistency of the Principles with their understanding of the law (as presented in the present chapter), suggest that this goal was achieved. It may be argued, however, that in some cases, the Principles could have gone further in identifying the application of the law for certain situations. For instance, Principle 19, on the right to freedom of opinion and expression, where identifying the duty of the State to regulate the media to avoid discrimination, only refers to media that is 'State-regulated'. While it is surely correct that such media should be prohibited from discriminatory practices and outputs it is not evident that the duty should not also be extended to non-state regulated media. In cases such as this we may observe the experts taking account of legal uncertainties regarding the reach of non-discrimination law into the private sphere, as discussed earlier. In a small number of other instances, the Principles are somewhat vague and non-prescriptive, perhaps again reflecting the uncertain state of law or its application. This may explain the provision at Principle 21(b) that 'expression, practice and promotion of different opinions, convictions and beliefs with regard to sexual orientation or gender identity is not undertaken in a manner incompatible with human rights'. Thus expressed it is unclear, for instance, whether a faith community could exclude someone from membership on grounds of sexual orientation, albeit the Principle, at a minimum, would require reflection as to the legitimacy in law of such an exclusion. Another criticism that may be directed to the Principles is that, notwithstanding a concerted effort to address specific fact circumstances, they are not comprehensive in this regard. For instance, it has been suggested that they could usefully have referred to issues of access to medicines in least-developed countries[138] and to the phenomenon of domestic violence in same-sex households.[139] Undoubtedly, as the Principles generate further commentary, additional omissions will be identified.

The desire for consistency with the existing law resulted in the deliberate omission from the final text of a number of elements that had been considered during the drafting phase. For instance, there is no expression of a right to non-heterosexual marriage. Instead, Principle 24 on the right to found a family, at paragraph (e) only speaks of a right to non-discriminatory treatment of same-sex marriage in those States which already recognise it.

It is noteworthy that the Principles are expressed in exclusively gender-neutral terms. The approach was deliberately adopted in order to ensure the application of all aspects of the Principles with regard to the life experience of people regardless of and with full respect for whatever gender identity they may have, while also avoiding binary constructions of gender. This achievement came at the price of the invisibility in the text of any reference to the particular situation and issues of women. It may be considered that this omission detracts from the capacity of the document to forcefully address the problems confronting lesbians in numerous countries.

The experts added a short 9-paragraph preamble to the Principles, but only after some debate, focussing on such matters as the avoidance of additional text that might detract from the Principles themselves. The preamble provides a context for the document, referring to the experiences of suffering and discrimination faced by people because of their actual or perceived sexual orientation or gender identity, the extent to which international human rights law already addresses these situations and the 'significant value in articulating [this law] in a systematic manner'. Notably, the preamble contains definitions of 'sexual orientation' and 'gender identity'. These formulations, drawing on those definitions widely in use within advocacy communities, establish a personal scope of application for the Principles. The preface also includes references that acknowledge the imperfections of the text and the need to keep its contents under review with a view to future reformulations that would take account of legal changes as well as developing understandings of the situation of people of diverse sexual orientations and gender identities.

While the Principles are addressed to States, as the duty-bearers in international human rights law, the experts considered that they should also make recommendations to other actors with relevance for the promotion and protection of human rights of people of diverse sexual orientations and gender identities. There are 16 such recommendations directed to international intergovernmental and nongovernmental bodies, international judicial and other human rights treaty bodies, national human rights institutions, commercial organisations, and others.

ASSESSMENT OF DISSEMINATION AND IMPACT OF THE PRINCIPLES

The Yogyakarta Principles were launched on 26 March 2007, at a public event timed to coincide with the main session of the United Nations Human Rights Council in Geneva. Attended by Ambassadors, other State delegates, a former UN High Commissioner for Human Rights, UN Special Procedures, members of treaty bodies, participating experts and NGO representatives, the launch served as a focal point to move the Yogyakarta Principles onto the international agenda. Immediate discussion of the Principles at the Human Rights Council was encouraged by means of the convening of a Council side-event panel discussion. There have been numerous other launch-related events since, including a presentation of the Principles at an event in UN Headquarters in New York on 7 November 2007, co-hosted by the Governments of Brazil, Argentina and Uruguay, in conjunction with the Third Committee of the General Assembly, and attended by diplomatic representatives of some 20

States.[140] The Principles are available on-line,[141] and have been published in the six official languages of the United Nations: English, French, Spanish, Russian, Chinese and Arabic. In addition to the official translations, NGOs have prepared translations of the Principles in Nepali, Indonesian, German and Portuguese, an annotated version of the Principles has recently been completed to identify the jurisprudential basis for each of the Principles, an international Youth Coalition is preparing a 'youth-friendly' version of the Principles, and work has begun on an Activists' Guide to strengthen the use of the Principles as a tool for advocacy.

A preliminary assessment of the impact of the Yogyakarta Principles can be undertaken by means of an evaluation of the impact they have had since their launch. In this regard, it is of interest to identify the extent to which their addressees, primarily States, but also such actors as international organisations, Special Procedures, treaty bodies and civil society, have reacted. Given the ongoing process of dissemination and the extent to which many initiatives are not reported internationally, it is not possible for such a review to be exhaustive. Instead, the present authors closely examine reactions within the context of the various UN fora and take note of the more significant of the other reported reactions.

Reaction by States and Other Actors within United Nations Fora

This is not a propitious time at which to launch major human rights initiatives at the UN. That organisation is in a phase of reform and, in the context of the Human Rights Council, pre-occupied with institutional development, sometimes detracting from its ability to focus on substantive human rights.[142] Taking account of this, as well as of the relatively short period of time since the launch of the Principles and the generally slow pace of change within international mechanisms, one may conclude that the dissemination of the Principles has met with a surprising degree of success. A number of member and observer States have already cited them in Council proceedings. Within days of the Geneva launch, more than 30 States made positive interventions on sexual orientation and gender identity issues, with seven States specifically referring to the Yogyakarta Principles,[143] describing them as 'groundbreaking', as articulating 'legally-binding international standards that all States must respect' and commending them to the attention of the UN Human Rights Council, the High Commissioner for Human Rights, Special Procedures and treaty bodies. The Principles recommend that the Human Rights Council 'endorse' them and 'give substantive consideration to human rights violations based on sexual orientation or gender identity, with a view to promoting State compliance with these Principles'.[144] Although endorsement by the Council as a body may be seen as ambitious, at least in the short term, it may be recalled that the Norwegian joint statement on sexual orientation, gender identity and human rights called for the President of the Council to allocate time at an appropriate future session of the Council 'for a discussion of sexual orientation and gender identity issues'.[145] The 'substantive consideration' envisaged by the Principles may therefore be expected to take place during 2008–09, in which case the Principles themselves are likely to be referenced by many States in order to frame the debate.

In addition to joint and separate interventions by States, there are a number of other mechanisms available to the Council through which the Principles may be engaged with, with some of these mechanisms subject of specific recommendations in the Principles themselves. The Principles recommend, for example, that the Special Procedures 'pay due attention to human rights violations based on sexual orientation or gender identity, and integrate these Principles into the implementation of their respective mandates'. The Principles were presented by NGOs to the system of Special Procedures at their 2007 annual meeting. The Czech Republic made favourable reference to the Principles during a Council dialogue with the Special Rapporteur on freedom of expression.[146] Egypt raised them in dialogue with the Special Rapporteur on the right to health,[147] citing the definition of 'sexual orientation' and challenging the Special Rapporteur for signing the Principles 'in his capacity as UN Representative'. In his reply, the Special Rapporteur noted that his position on 'the illegality of discrimination on the grounds of sexual orientation' was consistent with that taken by the High Commissioner for Human Rights and a number of Special Procedures, eight of whom had endorsed the Yogyakarta Principles in their official capacity. Highlighting the role that the Principles may come to play in standard-setting, the Special Rapporteur further pointed out to Egypt during an informal briefing that 10 years ago female genital mutilation was considered by many States to be a matter of 'cultural sensitivity', but is now widely regarded as incompatible with the right to health, and that in the future there may well be similar changes with regard to perceptions of homosexuality. In challenging the Special Rapporteur, it is noteworthy that Egypt took no exception to the content of the Principles themselves, or to their endorsement by a number of Special Procedures, only to the fact that the Special Rapporteur had signed them in an official capacity. It further noted that 'we understand that these values are acceptable in many societies, and we have no objection to this. What we have objection to is the persistent attempts to streamline those values at the UN while they are objectionable by the majority of the countries'.[148]

Interesting possibilities for engagement around the Principles are offered by the Universal Periodic Review, a new mechanism of the Council designed to address criticisms of politicisation and selectivity levelled at the former Commission on Human Rights,[149] by ensuring that the human rights records of all 192 United Nations Member States will be reviewed on a periodic four-year cycle.[150] The review is intended to be a co-operative mechanism, to assist States in fulfilling their international commitments and improving their human rights situation. During the first cycle of review, NGOs addressing sexual orientation, gender identity and broader sexual rights issues have made submissions on 13 of the 16 countries under review.[151] Many of these submissions explicitly referenced the Yogyakarta Principles, both to articulate the nature and scope of State obligations under international human rights law, and to identify detailed recommendations for measures that States can take to fulfil these obligations at the national level. The Universal Periodic Review is described as a process, providing multiple opportunities for engagement.[152] Future evaluation of the impact of the Principles may therefore additionally take into account the extent to which they are referenced in the Office of the High Commissioner for Human Rights (OHCHR) compilations of relevant materials, during national consultations by the State under review, in the State report itself, during the Interactive Dialogue conducted in a Working Group between Human Rights Council members and the State under review, in the outcome report and recommendations arising from the Working Group dialogue, during adoption of the report by the Human Rights Council, and in follow-up activities to implement the ensuing recommendations at the national level.[153]

The Principles recommend that the UN High Commissioner for Human Rights endorse them, 'promote their implementation worldwide' and integrate them into the work of OHCHR, 'including at the field level'.[154] In a written statement to the New York launch event, the High Commissioner described the 60th anniversary of the UDHR as an 'ideal opportunity to recall the core human rights principles of equality, universality and non-discrimination'. Describing it as 'unthinkable' to exclude persons from these protections because of their race, religion or social status, she asserted that we must similarly 'reject any attempt to do so on the basis of sexual orientation or gender identity', and described the Yogyakarta Principles as a 'timely reminder' of these basic tenets.[155] While falling short of the recommendation that she 'endorse' the Principles, her statement does affirm their value and it may be observed that she chose their launch event at which to express the 'firm commitment' of her Office to promote and protect the human rights of all persons, regardless of sexual orientation or gender identity.

Whatever restraint may be observed in the High Commissioner's personal statements, at the field level her Office may have some flexibility in integrating the Principles into their work. At annual meetings between the heads of the OHCHR field offices and Geneva-based NGOs, the Yogyakarta Principles were introduced. The field office heads, acknowledging that attention to these concerns has often been sporadic and inconsistent, welcomed the Principles as a useful tool for bringing greater coherence to their efforts.[156] Such previous efforts had included interventions on behalf of victims of sexual orientation and gender identity-related attacks in Nepal and NGOs under threat in Uganda.[157] The first specific citation of the Principles by a field office was in Nepal, in August 2007, where a senior officer delivered a statement at a ceremony 'to inaugurate the Yogyakarta Principles translated into Nepali'.[158] He described the Principles as an 'important document to focus international attention on the need for a more systematic approach to protection'. He went on to situate the Principles within the context of the Nepali peace process and Interim Constitution, acknowledging that the voices of Métis are amongst the most marginalised in society, and concluded that 'the Yogyakarta Principles provide an essential tool for creating awareness, for debate, advocacy and action to develop a proper protective legal framework, and to end abuses against individuals on account of their sexual orientation and gender identity in Nepal'. Similar sentiments were expressed by another senior official in South Africa in December 2007.[159] While such developments are of interest, it must be observed that they occurred in response to civil society invitations rather than on the basis of any policy-level positioning on the part of OHCHR.

Other UN mechanisms to which the Yogyakarta Principles address recommendations include the treaty bodies, the UN ECOSOC and UN agencies. Initial awareness-raising work has begun, with the distribution of the Principles to all treaty-body members, a presentation of the Principles to the annual meeting of Chairpersons of Treaty Bodies, and a briefing to members of the UN HRC.[160] While this preliminary engagement may assist in advancing the recommendation in the Principles that the treaty bodies integrate the Principles into the implementation of their mandates, including their case law and examination of State reports,[161] the recommendation that they adopt relevant 'General Comments or other interpretive texts'[162] is likely to be a significantly longer-term objective.

Recommendation D of the Principles calls upon the UN ECOSOC to accredit NGOs working to promote and protect the human rights of persons of diverse sexual orientations and gender identities. Despite initial rejections, a number of such NGOs have now received ECOSOC accreditation, and the Yogyakarta Principles were cited in advocacy materials when the matter arose for consideration,[163] although it is difficult to measure the extent to which the Principles themselves may have influenced the outcome. The ECOSOC NGO Committee receives accreditation applications from an increasingly diverse range of NGOs, and the issue is likely to remain a lively one for many years. Regarding Recommendations F and G, there has been modest engagement around the Principles with UN agencies. Copies of the Principles have been sent to the Office of the UN High Commissioner for Refugees, which is considering developing clearer guidelines on refugee issues relating to sexual orientation and gender identity. Also, a senior UNAIDS official addressed the New York launch event,[164] observing that the criminalisation of homosexual activities is not an effective method of addressing HIV/AIDS, referencing the non-binding UN International Guidelines on HIV/AIDS,[165] and expressing the support of UNAIDS for the Principles. In addition, the UN Office on Drugs and Crime, in developing a draft Handbook on 'Prisoners with Special Needs', including sexual minorities, drew extensively on the Yogyakarta Principles, including Principle 9 dealing with the Right to Treatment with Humanity while in Detention.[166]

Other Responses by States to the Principles

A number of States have expressed a willingness to draw upon the Principles as a guide to policy-making. The Dutch Minister of Foreign Affairs has developed a new human rights strategy to be debated in Parliament, which affirms that 'the Yogyakarta Principles are seen by the government as a guideline for its policy',[167] and outlines a number of specific initiatives, including capacity-building for international and local NGOs working on these issues. The Canadian government has described the Principles as 'useful blueprints' to measure progress on human rights related to sexual orientation and gender identity around the world,[168] and the Uruguayan government referred to the Principles as an 'important document to assist (it)' in overcoming discrimination based on sexual orientation and gender identity.[169] The Brazilian government intends to publish the Principles in a Portuguese translation and to feature them at an event in 2008 to promote its 'Brazil without homophobia' program.[170] The Argentinean government has stated that many of the issues addressed by the Yogyakarta Principles are also the focus of a National Action Plan for non-discrimination adopted by the government in 2004.[171] Some States are citing the Principles in bilateral relations. Part of the Dutch strategy involves raising the issue of decriminalisation of homosexual conduct with relevant States.

At the regional level, the European Parliament's Intergroup on Gay and Lesbian Rights has endorsed the Principles and a recently appointed Advisor to the Council of Europe's Human Rights Commissioner has indicated that the Yogyakarta Principles will serve as an important tool in advancing one of the Office's core priorities, namely country and thematic monitoring related to discrimination and human rights violations based on sexual orientation and gender identity.[172] Within Latin America, where issues of sexual orientation and gender identity have increasingly been discussed as part of the agenda at Mercosur meetings,[173] the support for the Principles expressed by founding members Brazil, Argentina and Uruguay may be expected to result in increased support from other full and associate members.

Interestingly, while many States have yet to embrace the responsibilities set out in the Yogyakarta Principles, there are early indications that municipal authorities and national human rights institutions may be more ready to engage. For instance, in South Africa, where government representatives declined to attend a conference on Gender, Sexuality, HIV/AIDS and Human Rights, the Speaker of the Johannesburg Municipal Council chose that event to express criticism of a 'collective amnesia' in public life concerning the constitutional prohibition of discrimination on the ground of sexual orientation and to commend the Yogyakarta Principles. He called on conference participants to ensure that 'both the Constitution and the Yogyakarta Principles become accepted by all members of our increasingly diverse communities in Johannesburg and internationally'.[174]

Civil Society Responses

Notwithstanding Recommendation J, the non (or at least limited)-participatory approach inherent in an expert-led process of drafting the Principles raised a risk that the process or text might be rejected as elitist by the very communities whose situation it was intended to address and the support of whom is of crucial significance.[175] Notwithstanding such concerns, preliminary indications of civil society response are encouraging. The Principles have been presented and discussed at regional conferences in Africa,[176] Latin America,[177] Eastern Europe[178] and Asia,[179] and requests for copies for distribution have been received from NGOs in a diverse range of countries around the world.[180] The Principles were referenced by civil society in statements addressed to the 2007 Africa-European Union summit.[181] NGOs are also drawing upon the Principles in negotiations with governments. In Northern Ireland, for example, civil society representatives have introduced the Principles for debate at the Bill of Rights Forum of Northern Ireland, constituted to advise on elements for a Bill of Rights.[182] In Kyrgyzstan, a group is using the Principles in meetings with the government to establish procedures for recognising the right of transgender people to official documentation that reflects their gender identity,[183] and activists in Nicaragua invoked the Principles in meetings with the government to advocate successfully for the decriminalisation of homosexuality.[184] In one particularly well publicised instance, a campaigning group in South Africa launched an anti-hate crimes campaign in response to the murders of lesbian women in Soweto[185] citing Principle 5 of the Principles, on the right to security of the person, and calling upon the government to implement the associated recommendations. Other instances of use of the Principles include NGO actions in South Korea, Belize and the UK.[186] The first known citation in domestic law of the Principles is contained in a brief submitted to the Nepal Supreme Court by the International Commission of Jurists. The brief invokes the Principles' definition of 'gender identity'.[187] The Principles are being used as teaching tools in university-level and other courses in China, Argentina, UK, USA, Brazil and the Philippines. Civil society has also engaged the media. For instance, a Kenyan group is reportedly using the Principles 'to involve the media in our mission through sexual health and rights policy visibility'.[188]

Although it is difficult to speculate as to the reasons for such vigorous civil society activism, informal discussions of the present authors with NGO leaders, suggest a variety of factors.[189] One such is the extent to which the expert drafters of the Principles were representative of so wide a range of competencies and skills relevant both to international law and issues of sexual orientation and gender identity. This representation ensured a balance of expertise contributing to a text that, to be effective, needed to be both jurisprudential and reflective of the 'lives and experiences of persons of diverse sexual orientations and gender identities'.[190] The Preamble to the Principles, for example, explicitly recognises the 'violence, harassment, discrimination, exclusion, stigmatisation and prejudice' directed against persons because of their sexual orientation or gender identity, as well as the resulting concealment of identity, fear and invisibility,[191] factors which resonate with the communities affected. As one online commentator noted at the time of the launch of the Principles, 'I am now, under International Human Rights Law, officially human. And yesterday, I wasn't'.[192] It has also been suggested to the present authors that the use of the widely encompassing grounds of 'sexual orientation' and 'gender identity', rather than attempting to define an exhaustive catalogue of specific identities avoids some of the hazards of identity politics, and ensures a more inclusive approach. There have been favourable comments regarding the manner in which the Principles place gender identity on an equal footing with sexual orientation rather than treating it as an addendum issue. Finally, commentators have referred to the utility for advocacy purposes of the combination of statements of principle with detailed recommendations for State action.

Not all the responses to the Principles have been positive: a faith-based group, the Catholic Family and Human Rights Institute, corresponded with all Permanent Missions to the UN in New York regarding the 'dangerous document' and provided them with briefing materials entitled 'Six Problems with the Yogyakarta Principles', which express concerns that the Principles 'undermine parental and familial authority', 'undermine freedom of speech', 'undermine religious freedom', 'undermine national sovereignty/national democratic institutions', 'encourage (physically, psychologically and morally) unhealthy choices' and 'fail to provide objective standards for evaluating sexual behaviour'.[193] A group called 'The State of America' has also condemned the Principles as 'an affront to all human and especially natural rights' and a 'farce of justice'.[194] Even these critiques, however, reflect the extent to which the Principles have attracted international attention, and are perceived by opponents and supporters alike as a significant step forward in the recognition of human rights for people of diverse sexual orientations and gender identities.

CONCLUSION

The Yogyakarta Principles appear to pass the crucial tests of being relevant to the actual situation of affected communities and being a faithful and coherent reflection of the existing international legal standards. It is not then surprising to consider the impact the Principles have already had, albeit dissemination is only beginning and will require the sustained attention from a global collaboration of lawyers, academics and activists. Equally, and as the Principles themselves attest, they are an imperfect work—set in a moment of time and reliant on the limited available information and understanding. As such, the Principles should be understood as a work-in-progress that must countenance an ongoing and frank consideration of how they might be improved and adjusted. In this way, the Yogyakarta Principles are most likely to contribute to the realisation of their own promise of 'a different future where all people born free and equal in dignity and rights can fulfil that precious birthright'.[195]

REFERENCES

1. Those states are Iran, Mauritania, Saudi Arabia, Sudan, United Arab Emirates, Yemen and Nigeria (the death penalty applies in 12 Northern provinces).
2. See Amnesty International, 'Crimes of Hate, Conspiracy of Silence. Torture and Ill-Treatment Based on Sexual Identity', AI Index ACT 40/016/2001, August 2001 at 21.
3. Statement by the Special Rapporteur on extrajudicial, summary or arbitrary executions, Human Rights Council, 19 September 2006.
4. Amnesty International, 'Stonewalled: Police Abuse and Misconduct against Lesbian, Gay, Bisexual and Transgender People in the US', AI Index AMR 51/122/2005, September 2005.
5. Transgender Day of Remembrance, 'About the Day of Remembrance'.
6. Report of the Special Rapporteur on torture and other cruel, inhuman or degrading treatment or punishment, 'Summary of Information, Including Individual Cases, Transmitted to Governments and Replies Received', Commission on Human Rights, 21 March 2006, E/CN.4/2006/6/Add.1 at paras 180 and 183.
7. Report of the Special Rapporteur on the question of torture and other cruel, inhuman or degrading treatment or punishment, UN General Assembly, 3 July 2001, A/56/156 at para. 17.
8. Report of the Special Rapporteur on the sale of children, child prostitution and child pornography, Commission on Human Rights, 5 January 2004, E/CN.4/2004/9 at para. 123.
9. Findlay, as cited in Egale Canada Human Rights Trust, 'Outlaws & In-laws: Your Guide to LGBT Rights, Same-Sex Relationships and Canadian Law' (2003) at 46.
10. See generally, Rothschild, 'Written Out: How Sexuality Is Used to Attack Women's Organizing', International Gay and Lesbian Human Rights Commission and the Center for Women's Global Leadership (2005).
11. Report of the Special Rapporteur on violence against women, its causes and consequences, Commission on Human Rights, 31 January 2002, E/CN.4/2002/83 at para. 102.
12. Graham and Kiguwa, 'Experiences of Black LGBTI Youth in Peri-Urban Communities in South Africa', Community Media for Development (CMFD) and the Institute for Democracy in South Africa (IDASA), 2004, at 15.
13. Ibid. at 5.
14. Tuite, 'Teen Attacked Couple He Had Mistaken for Two Gay Men', Irish Independent, 10 January 2008.

15. Ottoson, supra n. 1.

16. Amnesty International, 'Morocco/Western Sahara: Drop Charges of Homosexuality against Six Men and Ensure Their Safety', Press Release, 16 January 2008.

17. Johnson, 'Arbitrary Arrests and Detention of Men in Cameroon on Charges Related to Sexual Orientation and Gender Identity', International Gay and Lesbian Human Rights Commission (IGLHRC), 11 September 2007.

18. See, for example, Human Rights Watch, 'Kuwait: Repressive Dress-Code Law Encourages Police Abuse. Arrests Target Transgender People', Press Release, 17 January 2008.

19. Voices against 377, 'Rights for All: Ending Discrimination against Queer Desire under Section 377', 2004.

20. Report by the Special Rapporteur on contemporary forms of racism, racial discrimination, xenophobia and related intolerance, Commission on Human Rights, 27 March 2006.

21. ILGA-Europe, 'Prides against Prejudice. A Toolkit for Pride Organising in a Hostile Environment', September 2006, at 9.

22. Report by the Special Rapporteur on contemporary forms of racism, racial discrimination, xenophobia and related intolerance, supra n. 20 at paras 72–3.

23. See, for example, Abramowicz, 'Situation of Bisexual and Homosexual Persons in Poland', Campaign against Homophobia and Lambda Warsaw Association, Warsaw, 2007, at 20.

24. Report by the Special Rapporteur on adequate housing as a component of the right to an adequate standard of living, and on the right to non-discrimination, Commission on Human Rights, 27 February 2006, E/CN.4/2006/118 at para. 30; and Human Rights Watch, supra n. 2 at 52–5.

25. Amnesty International, supra n. 4 at 113.

26. Human Rights Watch, 'More Than a Name', supra n. 2 at 107.

27. See, for example, Connolly, 'Poland to Ban Schools from Discussing Homosexuality', The Guardian, 20 March 2007. See also former section 28 of the UK Local Government Act 1988 which prohibited the promotion of homosexuality in schools.

28. See Amnesty International, supra n. 2 at 21. Human Rights Watch, 'Hated to Death', supra n. 2; Human Rights Watch, 'More Than a Name', supra n. 2.

29. Toonen v Australia (488/1992), CCPR/C/50/D/488/1992 (1994); 1–3 IHRR 97 (1994) at para. 8.5.

30. See, for example, Coalition for Lesbian and Gay Rights in Ontario, 'Systems Failure: A Report on the Experiences of Sexual Minorities in Ontario's Health-Care and Social-Services Systems' (1997) at 48.

31. See Cabral, Statement to UN Commission on Human Rights, 61st session, Item 13: Rights of the Child, 14 March to 22 April 2005.

32. See, for example, Human Rights and Equal Opportunities Commission, 'Same-Sex: Same Entitlements, National Inquiry into Discrimination against People in Same-Sex Relationships', Australia, 2007.

33. Report of the Special Representative of the Secretary-General on human rights defenders, Human Rights Council, 24 January 2007, A/HRC/4/37 at paras 93–7.

34. See, for example, Report of the Special Rapporteur on the right of everyone to the enjoyment of the highest attainable standard of physical and mental health, supra n. 29 at para. 38; and Narrain, supra n. 29 at 148–50.

35. As cited in Human Rights Watch, 'In a Time of Torture', supra n. 2.

36. Human Rights Watch, 'More Than a Name', supra n. 2 at 172–5.

37. Committee on Economic, Social and Cultural Rights, General Comment No. 18: The right to work, E/C.12/GC/18, 24 November 2005.

38. Committee on Economic, Social and Cultural Rights, General Comment No. 15: The right to water, E/C.12/2002/11, 26 November 2002.

39. Committee on Economic, Social and Cultural Rights, General Comment No. 14: The right to the highest attainable standard of health, E/C.12/2000/4, 11 August 2000.

40. Committee on the Rights of the Child, General Comment No. 4: Adolescent health and development in the context of the Convention on the Rights of the Child, 1 July 2003, CRC/GC/2003/4.

41. O'Flaherty, 'The Concluding Observations of United Nations Human Rights Treaty Bodies', (2006) 6 Human Rights Law Review 27.

42. Concluding Observations of the Committee on Economic, Social and Cultural Rights regarding the People's Republic of China (including Hong Kong and Macau), 13 May 2005, E/C.12/1/Add.107 at para. 78.

43. Concluding Observations of the Committee on Economic, Social and Cultural Rights regarding Kyrgyzstan, 1 September 2000, E/C.12/1/Add.49 at para. 17.

44. Concluding Observations of the Committee on the Elimination of Discrimination Against Women regarding Kyrgyzstan, 5 February 1999, A/54/38 at para. 128.

45. Report of the Special Rapporteur on contemporary forms of racism, racial discrimination, xenophobia and related intolerance, Commission on Human Rights, 28 February 2006, E/CN.4/2006/16/Add.3 at para. 40.

46. Toonen v Australia, supra n. 29 at para. 8.7.

47. Young v Australia (941/2000), CCPR/C/78/D/941/2000 (2003) at para. 10.4.

48. Joslin v New Zealand (902/1999), CCPR/C/75/D/902/1999 (2003); 10 IHRR 40 (2003).

49. Grant v South West Trains Ltd C-249/96 [1998] ECR I-621; (1998) 1 CMLR 993.

50. See discussion in the above Situational Analysis section of this chapter on the linkages between violations based on sex, sexual orientation, gender identity and gender expression.

51. Donnelly, 'Non-Discrimination and Sexual Orientation: Making a Place for Sexual Minorities in the Global Human Rights Regime' in Baehr et al. (eds), Innovation and Inspiration: Fifty Years of the Universal Declaration of Human Rights (Amsterdam: Royal Netherlands Academy of Arts and Sciences, 1999).

52. Young v Australia, supra n. 47.

53. X v Colombia (1361/2005), CCPR/C/89/D/1361/2005 (2007).

54. Joslin v New Zealand, supra n. 48.

55. See, for example, Concluding Observations of the Human Rights Committee regarding Egypt, 28 November 2002, CCPR/CO/76/EGY at para. 19; and Concluding Observations of the Human Rights Committee regarding Kenya, CCPR/CO/83/KEN, 29 April 2005 at para. 27.

56. Concluding Observations of the Human Rights Committee regarding the United States of America, 18 December 2006, CCPR/C/USA/CO/3/Rev.1 at para. 25.

57. See, for example, Concluding Observations of the Human Rights Committee regarding Trinidad and Tobago, 3 November 2000, CCPR/CO/70/TTO at para. 11.

58. Concluding Observations of the Human Rights Committee regarding the Philippines, ibid. at para. 18.

59. Concluding Observations of the Human Rights Committee regarding Austria, 19 November 1998, CCPR/C/79/Add.103 at para. 13.

60. See case relating to certain aspects of the laws on the use of languages in education in Belgium (Belgian Linguistics case) (No. 2) A 6 (1968); (1979–80) 1 EHRR 252 at para. 9.

61. Karner v Austria 2003-IX 199; (2003) 38 EHRR 24.

62. Sutherland v United Kingdom Application No. 25186/94, Report of 1 July 1997 at para. 50.

63. Salgueiro da Silva Mouta v Portugal 1999-IX 309; (1999) 31 EHRR 1055.

64. Karner v Austria, supra n. 61 at paras 39–41.

65. L. and V. v Austria 2003-I 29; (2003) 36 EHRR 55.

66. S.L. v Austria 2003-I 71; (2003) 37 EHRR 39.

67. L. and V. v Austria, supra n. 65; and S.L. v Austria, ibid. at para. 44.

68. Fretté v France 2002-I 345; (2004) 38 EHRR 21.

69. E.B. v France Application No. 43546/02, Judgment of 22 January 2008 at para. 96.

70. Donnelly, supra n. 51.

71. Dudgeon v UK A 45 (1981); (1982) 4 EHRR 149.

72. Norris v Ireland A 142 (1988); (1988) 13 EHRR 186.

73. Modinos v Cyprus A 259 (1993); (1993) 16 EHRR 485.

74. Smith and Grady v United Kingdom 1999-VI 45; (1999) 29 EHRR 493.

75. Lustig-Prean and Beckett v United Kingdom (1999) 29 EHRR 548.

76. Goodwin v United Kingdom (2002) 35 EHRR 18.

77. I. v United Kingdom (2003) 36 EHRR 53.

78. Van Kück v Germany 2003-VII 1; (2003) 37 EHRR

79. Ibid. at para. 69.

80. L. v Lithuania Application No. 27527/03, Judgment of 11 September 2007.

81. Toonen v Australia, supra n. 29 at para. 8.2.

82. Joslin v New Zealand, supra n. 48 at paras 8.1–8.3.

83. The question had been put by the first author of the present chapter.

84. Concluding Observations of the Human Rights Committee regarding the United States of America, supra n. 56.

85. Concluding Observations of the Human Rights Committee regarding Poland, supra n. 57 at para. 18.

86. Concluding Observations of the Human Rights Committee regarding El Salvador, supra n. 57 at para. 16.

87. Concluding Observations of the Committee on the Rights of the Child regarding the United Kingdom, 9 October 2002, CRC/C/15/Add.188 at para. 43.

88. Concluding Observations of the Committee against Torture regarding Argentina, 10 December 2004, CAT/C/CR/33/1 at para. 6(g).

89. Concluding Observations of the Committee against Torture regarding Egypt, 23 December 2002, CAT/C/CR/29/4 at para. 5(e).

90. Concluding Observations of the Committee against Torture regarding Venezuela, 23 December 2002, CAT/C/CR/29/2 at para. 10(d).

91. Report of the Special Representative of the Secretary-General on human rights defenders, Commission on Human Rights, 22 March 2006, E/CN.4/2006/95/Add.1 at para. 290.

92. Report of the Special Representative of the Secretary-General on human rights defenders, Commission on Human Rights, 27 February 2002, E/CN.4/2002/106 at para. 83.

93. Report of the independent expert on minority issues, Commission on Human Rights, 6 January 2006, E/CN.4/2006/74 at paras 28 and 42.

94. Report of the Special Rapporteur on contemporary forms of racism, racial discrimination, xenophobia and related intolerance, supra n. 45 at para. 40.

95. Report of the Special Rapporteur on the right of everyone to the enjoyment of the highest attainable standard of physical and mental health, supra n. 34 at para. 54.

96. Annual report of the Inter-American Commission on Human Rights 2006, Chapter III C (1), OEA/Ser.L/V/II.127, Doc. 4 rev. 1, 3 March 2007, at para. 29.

97. Memorandum to the Polish Government, Council of Europe Commissioner for Human Rights, CommDH(2007)13, 20 June 2007.

98. Joslin v New Zealand, supra n. 48 at para. 8.2.

99. Human Rights Committee, General Comment No. 19: Protection of the family, the right to marriage and equality of the spouses, HRI/GEN/1/Rev.1, 27 June 1990.

100. X v Colombia, supra n. 53.

101. See, for example, Sheffield and Horsham v United Kingdom (1999) 27 EHRR 163.

102. Goodwin v United Kingdom, supra n. 76 at para. 100.

103. See the citations and discussion in Walker, 'Moving Gaily Forward? Lesbian, Gay and Transgender Human Rights in Europe' (2001) 2 Melbourne Journal of International Law 122.

104. Salgueiro da Silva Mouta v Portugal, supra n. 63.

105. Goodwin v United Kingdom, supra n. 76 at paras 98–104.

106. See, for example, Committee on the Rights of the Child, Day of General Discussion on 'Children without Parental Care', 40th session, Geneva, 12–30 September 2005, CRC/C/153 at para. 644.

107. See GA Res. 44/82, International Year of the Family, 8 December 1989, A/RES/44/82.

108. Human Rights Committee, General Comment No. 31: Nature of the general legal obligation imposed on States Parties to the Covenant, CCPR/C/21/Rev.1/Add.13, 26 May 2004.

109. Report of the Second Interagency Workshop on Implementing a Human Rights-Based Approach in the Context of UN Reform, Stamford, Connecticut, 5–7 May 2003.

110. See O'Flaherty, 'Keynote address' to Our Rights, Our Future: Human Rights Based Approaches in Ireland, Amnesty International Conference, Dublin, 27 September 2005.

111. Ibid.

112. Report of the Special Representative of the Secretary-General on human rights defenders, supra n. 33 at para. 95.

113. Presentation of the United Nations High Commissioner for Human Rights Ms Louise Arbour to the International Conference on Lesbian, Gay, Bisexual and Transgender Rights, Montreal, 26 July 2006.

114. Letter from the Ambassador and Permanent Representative of the Permanent Mission of Pakistan, Geneva, 26 February 2004.

115. ARC International, 'Recognizing Human Rights Violations Based on Sexual Orientation and Gender Identity at the Human Rights Council, Session 2', 18 September–6 October 2006.

116. Ibid.

117. See notes of meeting, ECOSOC, July 2006, on file with the second author of the present chapter. See also: United Nations Information Service. 'Economic and Social Council Takes Action on Texts Concerning Consultative Status of Non-Governmental Organizations', Press Release, ECOSOC/6231, 25 July 2006.

118. Rothschild, supra n. 10 at 111–12; and Sanders, 'Human Rights and Sexual Orientation in International Law', 23 November 2004 at 23–5.

119. Sanders, ibid. at 25.

120. ECOSOC Res. 1996/31, 25 July 1996 at preambulatory para. 4. See also GA Res. 60/251, 3 April 2006, establishing the Human Rights Council, which affirms the importance of NGO involvement in the work of the Council.

121. In 2006, the ECOSOC agreed to reject the application of the International Lesbian and Gay Association (ILGA), but overturned the denial of status to three other NGOs.

122. Report on the 59th session, Commission on Human Rights, 17 March–24 April 2003, E/CN.4/2003/135 at paras 575–85.

123. Press Release, Permanent Mission of Brazil to the United Nations, Geneva, 29 March 2004.

124. See, for instance, ILGA, 'ICFTU, The International Confederation of Free Trade Unions Supports the Brazilian Resolution', Press Release, 2 June 2004.

125. Statement made by New Zealand on behalf of 32 States under agenda Item 17.

126. Norwegian joint statement on human rights violations based on sexual orientation and gender identity, Human Rights Council, 3rd session, Geneva, 1 December 2006.

127. CHR Resolution, 20 April 2005, E/CN.4/RES/2005/34 at para. 5.

128. CHR Resolution, 20 April 2005, E/CN.4/RES/2005/59 at para. 7(f).

129. See International Commission of Jurists, supra n. 2 at 48–156.

130. Statement of the Special Rapporteur on the promotion and protection of the right to freedom of opinion and expression, Interactive Dialogue, Human Rights Council, 2nd session, 8 September–6 October 2006.

131. Presentation of the United Nations High Commissioner for Human Rights Ms Louise Arbour to the International Conference on Lesbian, Gay, Bisexual, and Transgender Rights, Montreal, 26 July 2006.

132. ARC International, 'A Place at the Table: Global Advocacy on Sexual Orientation and Gender Identity—And the International Response', November 2006.

133. See ARC International, 'Out at the UN: Advancing Human Rights Based on Sexual Orientation and Gender Identity at the 61st Session of the UN Commission on Human Rights', March–April 2005.

134. See also International Commission of Jurists, supra n. 2.

135. Address of the Rapporteur at the launch event of the Principles, Geneva, March 2007.

136. [The list appears in the original chapter]

137. See supra n. 108.

138. Comment made to the present authors by an activist in sub-Saharan Africa.

139. Comment made to the present authors by an activist who addresses issues of domestic violence.

140. See International Service for Human Rights, Human Rights Watch and International Gay and Lesbian Human Rights Commission, 'Launching the Yogyakarta Principles in New York. Summary of the Panel Discussion on the Yogyakarta Principles on the Application of International Law in Relation to Issues of Sexual Orientation and Gender Identity', New York, 7 November 2007.

141. Supra n. 134.

142. See Hicks and Gillioz, 'The Challenges Facing Non-Governmental Organisations' in Müller (ed.), The First 365 Days of the United Nations Human Rights Council (Bern: Federal Department of Foreign Affairs of Switzerland, 2007) 199 at 202.

143. The Czech Republic, Switzerland and the Nordic Countries Denmark, Finland, Iceland, Sweden and Norway, cited in ARC International, 'Recognising Human Rights Violations Based on Sexual Orientation and Gender Identity at the Human Rights Council, Session 4', April 2007;

and ARC International, 'Report on Launch of Yogyakarta Principles', June 2007.

144. Yogyakarta Principles, supra n. 134 at Additional Recommendation B.

145. Norwegian joint statement, supra n. 126.

146. Statement of the Czech Republic, Interactive Dialogue on the report of the Special Rapporteur on right to freedom of opinion and expression, Human Rights Council, 4th session, Geneva, 12–30 March 2007.

147. Statement of Egypt on the Review, rationalisation and improvement the mandate of the Special Rapporteur on the right of everyone to the enjoyment of the highest attainable standard of physical and mental health, Human Rights Council, 6th session (resumed), Geneva, 10–14 December 2007.

148. Ibid.

149. See Ambassador de Alba, 'Reviewing the Process: Challenges in the Creation of the Human Rights Council', in Müller, supra n. 142, 48 at 49; and Tistounet, 'Facts and Figures: Human Rights Council in Brief,' in Müller, supra n. 142, 57.

150. See HRC Res. 5/1, 'Institution-building of the United Nations Human Rights Council', Human Rights Council, 5th session, A/HRC/RES/5/1, Geneva, 18 June 2007.

151. Bahrain, Ecuador, Tunisia, Morocco, Indonesia, Finland, India, Brazil, Algeria, Poland, South Africa, the Czech Republic and Argentina: ARC International, 'Summary of NGO Submissions addressing Sexual Orientation and Gender Identity in First Cycle of UPR', 2008. A complete copy of the submissions is on file with the second author of the present chapter.

152. OHCHR, 'Information Note for NGOs Regarding the Universal Periodic Review Mechanism', Geneva, 8 January 2008.

153. See HRC Res. 5/1, supra n. 150; OHCHR, ibid.; and ARC International, 'A Guide to the UPR for Sexual Orientation and Gender Identity Advocates', December 2007.

154. Yogyakarta Principles, supra n. 134 at Additional Recommendation A.

155. Statement of Louise Arbour, UN High Commissioner for Human Rights, Launch of the Yogyakarta Principles, New York, 7 November 2007.

156. ARC International, 'Report of Annual Meeting with OHCHR Field Presences', 7 November 2007.

157. Ibid.

158. Statement by Johan Olhagen, Head of Katmandu Field Office, Office of the High Commissioner for Human Rights in Nepal, delivered at a 'Ceremony to Inaugurate the Yogyakarta

Principles translated into Nepali', Blue Diamond Society, Katmandu, 11 August 2007.

159. International Dialogue on Gender, Sexuality, and HIV/AIDS, 'Strengthening Human Rights Responses in Africa and Around the Globe', Johannesburg, 6–10 December 2007.

160. Joint briefing for members of the Human Rights Committee, International Service for Human Rights and ARC International, Geneva, 23 October 2007.

161. Yogyakarta Principles, supra n. 134 at Additional Recommendations E.

162. Ibid.

163. ARC International, Fact Sheet: ECOSOC Accreditation of NGOs addressing Issues of Sexual Orientation & Gender Identity: The Importance of Non-Discriminatory Access and Participation, July 2007.

164. See International Service for Human Rights, Human Rights Watch and International Gay and Lesbian Human Rights Commission, supra n. 140.

165. CHR Res. 1997/33, The protection of human rights in the context of human immunodeficiency virus (HIV) and acquired immunodeficiency syndrome (AIDS), 11 April 1997, E/CN.4/1997/33.

166. UN Office on Drugs and Crime (Criminal Justice Reform Unit), Prisoners with Special Needs (draft), 2007.

167. Dutch Ministry of Foreign Affairs, 'A life of human dignity for all, A human rights strategy for foreign policy', 6 November 2007, at para. 2.7 (pp. 47 and 48) (unauthorised translation).

168. Government of Canada, Response to Petition, Petition No. 391-1634, 6 June 2007.

169. International Service for Human Rights, Human Rights Watch and International Gay and Lesbian Human Rights Commission, supra n. 140.

170. Ibid.

171. Ibid.

172. Dittrich, 'Yogyakarta Principles in New Dutch Human Rights Strategy', 21 November 2007 (unofficial translation); and e-mail communications with Advisor, Office of the Commissioner for Human Rights Council of Europe, January 2008.

173. At the 9th High Level MERCOSUR meeting that was held in Montevideo in August 2007, the first regional seminar on sexual diversity, identity and gender was held with the participation of government representatives and representatives of civil society from the whole region.

174. Speaker of Council, Councillor Nkele Ntingane, City of Johannesburg Metropolitan Municipal Councill, Opening Ceremony for International Dialogue on Gender, Sexuality and HIV/AIDS, Johannesburg, 6 December 2007.

175. In this regard, the Yogyakarta process may be distinguished from the highly participatory manner in which other more aspirational texts have been developed.

176. ILGA Conference, Johannesburg, May 2007; International Dialogue on Gender, Sexuality, HIV/ AIDS and Human Rights, ARC International and Coalition of African Lesbians, Johannesburg, December 2007.

177. International Association for the Study of the Sexuality, Culture and Society (IASSCS) Conference, Peru, June 2007; 4 encuentro de ILGA en América Latina y el Caribe, Peru, September 2007.

178. ILGA Europe Conference, Lithuania, 25–28 October 2007.

179. ILGA Asia-Regional Conference, Thailand, 24–27 January 2008.

180. Requests for copies and supportive comments have been received from NGOs in countries including Andorra, Argentina, Australia, Belarus, Belize, Brazil, Cameroon, Canada, Chile, China, Denmark, Ecuador, France, Germany, Guyana, Hong Kong, India, Indonesia, Ireland, Japan, Kenya, Kyrgyzstan, Latvia, Lithuania, Mexico, Nicaragua, Nigeria, Peru, the Philippines, Romania, Russia, Senegal, South Korea, Thailand, Tonga, Uganda, United Kingdom, Uruguay, the United States of America and Zimbabwe.

181. ILGA, ILGA-Europe, Pan-Africa ILGA, 'African and European LGBT Organisations Call on all States to Fight Homophobia and to Adopt the Yogyakarta Principles', joint media release, Portugal, 7 December 2007.

182. Agreement between the Government of the United Kingdom of Great Britain and Northern Ireland and the Government of Ireland, 10 April, 1998, Strand Three (Rights, Safeguards and Equality of Opportunity) at para. 4.

183. E-mail communications on file with authors, cited in ARC International, supra n. 143.

184. E-mail communications on file with authors, cited in supra n. 143.

185. The Alliance for Campaign 07-07-07, 'Call to Action', Johannesburg, 10 December 2007, at para. 1.3.

186. Immigration Law Practitioners' Association (ILPA) and the UK Lesbian and Gay Immigration Group (UKLGIG), 'Sexual and Gender Identity Guidelines for the Determination of Asylum Claims in the UK', July 2007 at para. 3.2.3.

187. International Commission of Jurists, 'Submissions to the Supreme Court of The State

of Nepal, Providing the Basis in International Human Rights Law for the Prohibition of Discrimination Based on Sexual Orientation and Gender Identity, and Other Connected Matters', 2007.

188. As cited in: O'Flaherty, 'New Principles on Sexual Orientation, Gender Equality and Human Rights', Rights News, Irish Council for Civil Liberties, Summer 2007, at 4.

189. The speculative elements in this paragraph are supported by notes of such discussions on file with the present authors.

190. Yogyakarta Principles, supra n. 134 at Preamble, paras 8 and 9.

191. Ibid. at Preamble at para. 2.

192. 'Victory in Yogyakarta', 26 March 2007.

193. Catholic Family and Human Rights Institute, 'Six Problems with the Yogyakarta Principles', 13 April 2007.

194. Downs, State of America, e-mail communication on file with second author of the present article, 9 November 2007.

195. Supra n. 134 at 'About the Principles'.

QUESTIONS

1. Not explicitly considered within the chapter is the progression of the Lesbian, Gay, Bisexual and Transgender (LGBT) human rights movement worldwide. Using historical evidence, suggest an appropriate timeline for the global LGBT human rights movement. In general, does evidence suggest a recent improvement in LGBT rights throughout the world?

2. The authors state, "The notion that there are two and only two genders is one of the most basic ideas in our binary Western way of thinking. Transgender people challenge our very understanding of the world. And we make them pay the cost of our confusion by their suffering." Defend or refute this statement.

3. Propose an agenda or campaign that could be used to promote the Yogyakarta Principles. What modes of communication and types of media would you implement? Who will be your allies? Who will be your opponents? What aspects of your campaign will be universal? What aspects will vary by country?

FURTHER READING

1. International Commission of Jurists (ICJ), *Yogyakarta Principles—Principles on the application of international human rights law in relation to sexual orientation and gender identity* (2007), http://www.yogyakartaprinciples. org/principles_en.html

2. Saiz, I., Bracketing Sexuality: Human Rights and Sexual Orientation: A Decade of Development and Denial at the UN. *Health and Human Rights,* 2004; 7: 48–80 http://www.idahomophobia.net/IMG/pdf/Ignacio_Saiz_-_Bracketing_ Sexuality_at_the_UN.pdf

3. Johnson, P., An Essentially Private Manifestation of Human Personality: Constructions of Homosexuality in the European Court of Human Rights. *Human Rights Law Review,* 2010, 10:67.

POINT OF VIEW

Men Who Have Sex with Men, HIV, and Human Rights: A Call to Action

Chris Beyrer

MSM AND HIV

Gay, bisexual, and other men who have sex with men (MSM) have been a core population affected by the HIV/AIDS epidemic since the syndrome we now know as AIDS was first identified among previously healthy homosexual men in the United States in 1981. The fact that HIV was first identified among gay men indelibly marked the global response, stigmatized those living with the virus, limited effective public health responses in some cases, and drove coercive and punitive ones in others. In the fourth decade of HIV, it is unconscionable that these men and their communities should continue to suffer stigma, discrimination, and lack of access to HIV services and that homophobia should continue to potentiate the epidemic. Yet in too many countries and for too many communities, this remains the case.

The newfound optimism in the HIV field, that early anti-retrovial treatment is an effective prevention tool, and that other new prevention tools such as oral pre-exposure prophylaxis are also effective for MSM, opens up real possibilities for eventually achieving control of HIV for these men and their communities. These advances, coupled with the provision of culturally competent care, provide pathways forward toward the realization of the right to health. None of these goals can be achieved, however, if MSM continue to be denied access and use of health care services. In too many settings today, MSM still do not have access to the most basic of HIV services and technologies including affordable and accessible condoms, appropriate lubricants, and access to safe HIV testing and counseling.

The global AIDS community is now at a crossroads. Research advances suggest pathways to reach what U.S. Secretary of State Hillary Clinton has called "an AIDS-free generation." Many argue that we now have the tools in hand to achieve this goal—unimaginable only a few years ago. But the evidence is now clear that achieving an AIDS-free generation will not happen unless new and effective approaches are developed and implemented at scale for MSM. And that will not happen if these men are excluded from health care, and from full social recognition and political engagement. No population can be excluded if we are to achieve control of global AIDS.

How might a human rights framework assist in the goal of achieving services for MSM, particularly where they are stigmatized, face discrimination, or where same sex behavior between consenting adults remains a crime?

THE YOGYAKARTA PRINCIPLES

Human rights abuses are important social determinants of vulnerability to HIV, while rights *protections* can enhance uptake, utilization, and impact of HIV interventions. Human rights principles, language, and frameworks have helped in the advocacy for ending discriminatory practices in health care, the push for antiviral drug access, and in mitigating daily struggles for human dignity and social justice. For sexual minority populations, human rights abrogation or protection have had particularly profound impacts. LGBT persons continue to be criminalized for their sexual orientation in more than 80 countries; in many others, they face discrimination in education, housing, employment, family life, and health care. Men in several countries still face the death penalty for same sex relations between consenting adults.

The use of human rights laws and rights-based approaches has in some settings been limited by criminalization—by the argument that sexual minorities are excluded from universal human rights by virtue of engaging in criminal behavior. A clear articulation of the universality of human rights for all persons, including sexual and gender minorities, is contained in the *Yogyakarta Principles* (YP) of 2006. The YP use the language of sexual orientation (the common relevant western terms would be homosexual, bisexual, and heterosexual orientations) and gender identity (male, female, and transgender identities) but have full relevance to MSM. When considering sexual activity between men, the public health and HIV communities have most commonly used the term men who have sex with men (MSM) to avoid artificially imposing sexual orientation or gender identity categorizations on men who engage in sex with other men. The legal sanctions against same sex behavior are largely, though not exclusively, colonial era statutes and so use archaic terms (sodomy, buggery, acts against nature) which have imprecise meaning in our time. There is a public health consensus to use the term MSM despite its limitations, even as legal and human rights discourses will largely use other terms.

Four of the YP principles arguably have particular relevance for MSM and HIV.

Principle 1 articulates entitlement to full human rights, freedom, equality, and dignity, and has been invoked in recent court decisions decriminalizing homosexuality in Nepal and India. In the Indian case, the repeal of colonial era sodomy laws was explicitly argued from the position that these laws were impeding HIV responses for MSM, as well as Transgender persons.

Principle 17 reaffirms existing human rights conventions on the right to health care access and its implications for access to services for MSM are clear.

Principle 18, the right to the highest attainable standard of health, is of critical import to MSM globally, because approaches to changing sexual orientation (sometimes called reparative therapy or conversion therapy) are common and are not evidence-based. Indeed, the scientific evidence suggests that these approaches, while having little or no effect on sexual orientation, can have potent impacts on increasing depression, suicidal ideation, suicide attempts, and substance use.

Principle 18 is particularly important for LGBT adolescents, who are vulnerable to family, and institutional attempts to alter sexual orientation or gender identity and for whom such approaches may be particularly harmful.

Principle 24, the right to found a family, also has relevance to HIV prevention for MSM. In many settings it is virtually impossible for male same-sex couples to found families, to live together, find housing, or enjoy privacy rights. These realities undermine stable relationships, and can increase the likelihood of anonymous and unsafe sexual encounters.

CONCLUSIONS

It is clear that prejudice and discrimination have helped maintain HIV burdens among MSM. It is equally clear that the current global generation of young people is changing the world we live in. Sexual minority communities are communicating, engaging in political life, and demanding the right to participate in decisions which affect their lives, including those which relate to HIV programs and policies. These are welcome changes, but this will not be a simple effort nor can it be a short-lived one. The struggle for equity in HIV services is likely to be inseparably linked to the struggle for sexual minority rights—and hence to be both a human rights struggle, and in many countries, a civil rights one. The history of AIDS is rich with examples of how affected communities pushed for inclusion—and of how their inclusion improved responses. For MSM this has been a many decades struggle. And it is not over by any means. Indeed, for many communities, countries, and regions, it has just begun.

Adapted from Beyrer, C., Sullivan, P., Sanchez, J., Dowdy, D., Altman, D., Trapence, G., Collins, C., Katabira, E., Kazatchkine, M., Sidibe, S., and Mayer, K.H. "A Call to Action for Comprehensive HIV Services for Men Who Have Sex with Men," *The Lancet* MSM and HIV Series. *The Lancet* 2012; 380:424–438.

Chris Beyrer is the Director of the Johns Hopkins Fogarty AIDS International Training and Research Program and Johns Hopkins Center for Public Health and Human Rights, Johns Hopkins Center for Global Health, Johns Hopkins University, Baltimore, MD, USA.

CHAPTER 25

Reproductive Health as a Human Right: A Matter of Access or Provision?

Sara E. Davies

The enjoyment of the highest attainable standard of health is one of the fundamental rights of every human being without distinction of race, religion, political belief, economic or social condition. WHO Constitution 1946 (World Health Assembly [WHA] 1946, Article 1)

What does the highest attainable standard of health for a woman look like? Globally, women continue to bear the brunt of health inequalities, which in turn affects their ability to seek financial independence, education, and freedom from social mores. For instance, the one demographic that shows a continuing upward trend for HIV infection between 1990 and 2007 is women (UNAIDS 2007: 8–9). Less than half of all women in Asia and Africa are assisted by health care personnel during birth (United Nations General Assembly [UNGA] 2008: 4–5).[1] Women in sub-Saharan Africa and South Asia have a lifetime risk of maternal death that is 1,000 times greater than that in industrialized regions (UNGA 2008). The likelihood of achieving the fifth Millennium Development Goal (MDG), which calls for a three-quarters reduction in maternal related deaths by 2015, is remote. Indeed, between 1990 and 2005, there were approximately 535,900 maternal deaths per year and the numbers in sub-Saharan Africa and South Asia have shown little, if any, sign of any improvement (Hill et al., 2007: 1311–1319). Between 1995 and 2003, 48% of all abortions were unsafe, causing at least 68,000 deaths each year (Glasier et al., 2006: 1598; Sedghet al. 2007: 1344). In 2008, the Global Campaign for Health Millennium Development Goals High Level Task Force was established by the Norwegian government. Announcing the Task Force, Prime Minister Jens Stoltenberg stated that "the fact that we have not made any significant progress at all in reducing the number of women who die in pregnancy or childbirth is appalling. There can only be one reason for this awful situation—and that is persistent neglect of women in a world dominated by men" (United Nations Department of Public Information [UNDPI] 2008a).

Stoltenberg's point reflects a renewed interest in the impact on women who endure such health inequalities, but the question is why—despite a protracted campaign by international and nongovernmental organizations to establish women's reproductive health as a human right (Beaglehole and Bonita 2008)—has the number of women dying from lack of reproductive health care continued to remain a "silent emergency" (UNDPI 2008b)? Global commitment to improving women's health has been promoted through a variety of international declarations, which have established putative obligations that have been increasingly referred to as "rights." Yet the persistent inequalities identified earlier remain. This chapter argues that the limits to improving women's health as a human right are due to a lack of political will at the domestic and international levels. As long as the process upon which realizing human rights requires—political engagement and resources—are lacking, so too will women's access to reproductive health care and sexual self-determination. Any advancement in human rights at the local level benefits the most when states provide the means and measures by which these rights can be accessed. There are currently no incentive structures for developing states, which primarily bear the burden of reproductive health inequalities (Glasier et al., 2006: 1598–1599), to change this situation when it comes to advancing women's reproductive health. As a result most states that have poor health indicators for women will continue to ignore the cultural and capacity obstacles that prevent women from securing reproductive health care. As long as women's poor health care has no political or economical consequences for a state, women's health will be neglected. The key, this chapter will suggest, is to enumerate the precise rights essential for advancing women's reproductive health through developing a framework of indicators and then link this framework to an incentive structure that encourages political will to change this situation. For the purposes of this chapter, I define reproductive health care according to the 1994 United Nations International Conference on Population and Development (ICPD) definition:

> [A] state of complete physical, mental and social well-being and not merely the absence of disease or infirmity, in all matters relating to the reproductive system and to its functions and processes. Reproductive health therefore implies that people are able to have a satisfactory and safe sex life and that they have the capability to reproduce and the freedom to decide if, when and how often to do so. Implicitly in this last condition are the right of men and women to be informed and to have access to safe, effective, affordable and acceptable methods of family planning of their choice, as well as other methods of their choice for the regulation of fertility which are not against the law, and the right of access to appropriate health care services that will enable women to go safely through pregnancy and childbirth and provide couples with the best chance of having a healthy infant.
>
> (International Conference on Population and Development [ICPD] 1994: para. 7.2)

This chapter will proceed in four parts. In the first section, I will trace the development of the health and human rights movement. This movement developed as a strategy to win the hearts and minds of developing states, donor states, and international organizations (who were often also involved in the movement) by referring to health care and treatment as a right that individuals could claim and that states had a duty to respect, to protect, and to fulfill. As the second section argues, the process of turning a declared human right into a public good accessible to all, ultimately requires states to make the necessary improvements to health care systems. However, the focus has remained on the right to access health care and the capacity of states to fulfill rights, rather than the instrumental question of how rights advocates ensure that states meet their positive duties. These problems are most pronounced in the area of women's reproductive health, which is discussed in depth in the third section of the chapter. The fourth and final section looks at proposed strategies to advance reproductive health outcomes, based on identifying the specific rights that require satisfaction and tracing the fulfillment by states of their health-as-a-human-right obligations. Monitoring frameworks, such as the ones examined in the fourth section, may serve as a prelude to the construction of an evaluation system that could be used to fund aid projects and to attract states with the attachment of incentives for gender responsive reproductive health care policies (Behlhadj and Touré 2008). Furthermore, monitoring human rights obligations may be the start to identifying the precise scope of individual state responsibility to fulfill their reproductive rights obligations and to generate the necessary political will to ensure further devotion of political and financial resources to save women's lives. Together, these initiatives may help establish an incentive structure that encourages reluctant states to deliver on their responsibilities in this area. In this chapter, I argue that at present, the largest obstacle to be overcome in establishing health as a human right beyond declaratory status in the case of reproductive rights is to create the political means and motivation that will force states to live up to the human rights declarations that they have ratified.

HEALTH AS A HUMAN RIGHT

The World Health Organization (WHO) Constitution (1946) states that health is a universal right. In so doing, it defined health as "a state of complete physical, mental and social well-being" (WHA 1946: 1). The association between health and human rights has been reaffirmed several times since the establishment of WHO. It was enshrined, for instance, in the 1948 Universal Declaration of Human Rights which stated that

1. Everyone has the right to a standard of living adequate for the health and well-being of himself and of his family, including food, clothing, housing and medical care and necessary social services, and the right to security in the event of unemployment, sickness, disability, widowhood, old age or other lack of livelihood in circumstances beyond his control.

2. Motherhood and childhood are entitled to special care and assistance. All children, whether born in or out of wedlock, shall enjoy the same social protection. (UNGA 1948: Article 25)

Moreover, the 1966 International Covenant on Economic, Social and Cultural Rights (ICESCR), which came into force in 1976, expressed the right to health in the following way:

1. The State Parties to the present Covenant recognize the right of everyone to the enjoyment of the highest attainable standard of physical and mental health.

2. The steps to be taken by the State Parties to the present Covenant to achieve the full realization of this right shall include those necessary for:

   a. The provision for the reduction of the stillbirth-rate and of infant mortality and for the health development of the child;

   b. The improvement of all aspects of environmental and industrial hygiene;

   c. The prevention, treatment and control of epidemic, endemic, occupational and other diseases;

   d. The creation of conditions which would assure to all medical service and medical attention in the event of sickness. (UNGA 1966: Article 12)

Importantly, no government argued that health should not constitute a right during the drafting of the WHO Constitution, the Universal Declaration of Human Rights, or the International Covenant on Economic, Social and Cultural Rights (ICESCR; Toebes 1999). However, neither was it clear *whose* responsibility it was to realize this right, *how* the right would be realized, and *when* the right to health had been satisfied (Taylor 1992: 327). As Tomasevski argued, "public health spelled out individual obligations rather than rights" (2005: 3). Emphasis was placed mostly on what the individual should do to improve one's health. According to Paul Hunt, the UN's Special Rapporteur on the Right to Health, the "right to health" remained "little more than a slogan for more than 50 years" (Hunt 2007: 369). It was not, he maintained, until the UN Economic and Social Council adopted General Comment 14 in 2000 that it became clear what the right to health encompassed. The General Comment confirmed that

> [T]he express wording of article 12.2 acknowledges that the right to health embraces a wide range of socio-economic factors that promote conditions in which people can lead a healthy life, and extends to the underlying determinants of health, such as food and nutrition, housing, access to safe and potable water and adequate sanitation, safe and healthy working conditions, and a healthy environment . . . [5]. The Committee is aware that, for millions of people throughout the world, the full enjoyment of the right to health still remains a distant goal. Moreover, in many cases, especially for those living in poverty, this goal is becoming increasingly remote. The Committee recognizes the formidable structural and other obstacles resulting from international and other factors beyond the control of States that impede the full realization of article 12 in many States parties. [6] With a view to assisting States parties' implementation of the Covenant and the fulfilment of their reporting obligations, this General Comment focuses on the normative content of article 12 (Part I), States parties' obligations (Part II), violations (Part III) and implementation at the national level (Part IV), while the obligations of actors other than States parties are addressed in Part V.
>
> (UNSEC 2000: paras. 4–6)

The problem that remained even after General Comment 14 was the understanding which aspects of the right to health required simple access—for example, freedom from discrimination—and which aspects required the positive provision of goods by a specific duty bearer. The emphasis remains on the capacity of the state to meet these rights, rather than their nonderrogable responsibility to fulfill these rights. States have also been reluctant to develop empirical indicators that might measure progress towards attaining these rights. Therefore, it is worth noting that while these articles indicate that a state is responsible for the health of its citizens, the Covenant does not provide thresholds or indicators for when the right to health has been fulfilled (Toebes 1999). Critics argue that this is because a "right to health" cannot be realized because it either implies that there is such a thing as perfect health or that individuals need no more than the right conditions for good health to prevail. This denies, of course, an individual's genetic predisposition to disease, disability and infirmity, and an individual's own lifestyle choices that are also important factors (Aginam 2005: 5). It also ignores the extent to which the provision of other sorts of rights, such as social and economical freedoms, is then essential to improve individual health (Mann et al. 1999). Therefore, whilst the right to health is a well-established aspiration, there remains little clarity about what is required "on the ground" to satisfy it. In order to fully develop the right to health, former Special Rapporteur on the Right to Health Paul Hunt argued that key indicators and national benchmarks were essential for holding states, even aid agencies, to be "held accountable for their failures" (Palmer et al. 2009: 1990).

Access and Provision

At the heart of the debate about health and human rights is a tension between access and provision that mirrors the philosophical distinction between negative and positive rights. Simply put, negative rights require that actors refrain from certain types of activities that infringe on the rights of others. For instance, the right to life, the right to be free from torture, and the right to choose one's religion only require that actors desist from killing people, torturing them, and inhibiting their freedom to choose their religion. In their simplest form, they do not require positive action to ensure their fulfillment. By contrast, positive rights require that actors take positive steps. For instance, they may require that the state make social, economical, and legislative provisions to accommodate and provide these rights. The right to education, the right to shelter, and the right to clean water are positive rights because they require duty-bearers to make material provisions to provide them, rather than simply refrain from certain courses of action. Put another way, Jack Donnelly suggests that negative rights only require the "forbearance on the part of others," whilst positive rights require "others to provide goods, services, or opportunities" (Donnelly 2003: 30). However, critics contend that the bifurcation of rights into negative and positive is of little moral significance because even negative rights entail positive duties for their fulfillment (Shue 1980). For instance, all the "negative rights" noted above require significant positive steps by the government to take action to ensure these rights are fulfilled—the right to be free from torture requires a number of legislative, judicial, and policing checks and balances to ensure this right is respected. Likewise, Donnelly argues that "all human rights required both

positive action and restraint on the part of the state" (Donnelly 2003: 30). Philosophically therefore, the idea that any right could require no material change to the behavior of actors has been largely debunked. However, in practice, there is a significant difference between a negative and positive approach to health rights.

The distinction between negative and positive rights has been important in the debate about health as a human right. There is a big difference between the insistence that "all I have to do is not prevent people seeking the best health care they can afford," which is a negative right based on the "do no harm principle," and a claim that "I have a duty to ensure that every person is able to access the best health care possible," which is implied by the positive rights approach. The distinction in understanding what a human right to health means, is one between *access* (the right to seek care and not be prevented from doing so with no specific duty-bearer assuming responsibility for the provision of care) and *provision* (the right to be provided with the best care possible with a duty-bearer having an obligation to ensure that such a provision is made available). This distinction is vitally important for understanding the "empirical circumstances" (Donnelly 2003: 31) surrounding how the right to health is claimed and fulfilled as well as the scope of the right itself.

In the area of health, the tension between access—the obligation not to deny access to basic health care—and provision—the obligation to provide basic health care to all—pivots around two key questions. First, what is the scope of the right and responsibility to fulfill this right in relation to access and provision? Second, on whom does the obligation fall? To some extent, the relatively recent General Comment 14 on the ICE-SCR has gone a long way to answering these questions. But a third question remains: How can states be compelled to move from acknowledging a right exists to feeling obligated to fulfill this right? The health and human rights movement has argued that the responsibility is shared between those seeking better health (i.e., the individual), those who have the power to deny or permit access (i.e., the state), and those who see inequality in the provision of the right as it is at present and seek to plug the gaps (i.e., the international donor community, including NGOs; Gruskin et al. 2005; Hunt 2003). However, in practice the scope and focus of responsibility remains largely located in the state—as we will see next in the case of reproductive health. Therefore, the tension between access and provision is often rooted in the fact that there are no thresholds or series of indicators attached to the human rights articles that are to hold states to account for their fulfillment. The best measure thus far has been to trace domestic legal proceedings when individuals or groups of individuals claim that the state should fulfill their right obligation under the ICESCR. However, this relies upon effective, independent judicial systems, governments willing to implement the courts' findings, and, in addition, it does not resolve the degree of social and political freedom required for individuals to feel able to claim such rights from their state in the first place. Therefore, legal proceedings alone are only one facet of ethical, practical, and moral capacity of rights language to deliver tangible improvements in the provision of health care, particularly in the case of women's health needs. What is required is to enumerate the precise rights essential for advancing women's reproductive health and link this to an incentive structure that encourages political will to change the situation.

CLAIMING WOMEN'S HEALTH AS A HUMAN RIGHT

Thus far I have argued that to realize a human right to health we must keep in mind that there are at least two distinct needs—access and provision. There must be an obligation on behalf of a duty-bearer to not deny access to basic health care and, at the same time, an obligation upon a duty-bearer to provide the best care possible. What consideration has been given, then, to how access and provision of the right to health can be best realized for the specific reproductive health needs of women? As this section will argue, women's right to reproductive health has taken a journey similar to the health as a human rights movement more generally. Though there has been much effort to establish women's right to access gender-responsive health care policies, there has been little attention given to thinking about how specific rights can be fulfilled to ensure that women experience measurable change in reproductive health care.

The problem of provision and building political pressure on states to fulfill women's health needs is partly related to the broader failure to articulate the political responsibilities of states and to create incentive structures for their fulfillment. As identified earlier, while the ICESCR and General Comment 14 in 2000 have been essential for identifying the responsibility of the state with respect to human rights, moving from commitment to action remains the key obstacle to achieving health as a human right, especially in the case of women's reproductive rights (UNESC 2009). Reproductive health is particularly harder because it is often the states that are responsible for violating women's rights in general (UNGA 2008: 18). In addition, forced early marriage, access to contraceptives, choice surrounding unwanted pregnancies, and female genital mutilation are core rights-related issues that must be dealt with by the state through legal, economical, and social reform in order to provide women with the best provision of health care. However, as will be discussed, these issues are politically and culturally controversial, stymieing any efforts to advance women's health. Moreover, the lack of consistent international funding to improve women's access to health care and to demand recalcitrant states to meet their obligations further hinders efforts to satisfy women's health needs. In essence, the greatest cause for women's right to reproductive health remaining a "silent emergency" is that there is a disconnect between what is being declared at the international level and what is being enforced at the national-local level. This disconnect exists because there has been no precise political thresholds or repercussions attached to realizing reproductive health as a human right. The failure to attach political force to the lip service paid by states to women's reproductive needs has enabled states to continually evade their responsibility and the silent emergency to continue.

We can see the effects of this in the statistics set out at the beginning of the chapter. Today, those fighting for improvements to women's reproductive health refer to such statistics as proof that women's right to decide matters relating to their sexual health—and access to health treatment in general—is pivotal but is still lacking progress in political engagement (Glasier et al. 2006; Hudson 2005; Low et al. 2005; Wellings et al. 2006). However, in line with the general health as a human rights movement, I would argue that the reproductive health movement has not always agreed on how the provision versus access tension in human rights can best deliver the advances that women need in order to control and improve their reproductive health. *Right to reproductive self-determination* advocates generally argue that women do not need just family planning services, they also need the autonomy to decide when they should have sex and with whom, and a choice of reproductive health care options (Asal, Brown, and Gis-

bson Figueroa 2008; Cook, Dickens, and Schrecker 2003; Kelly and Cook 2007). The self-determination movement maintains that the right to refuse sex and the right to contraceptive choice has to be a major part of a woman's right to health (Tomasevski 2005). By contrast, *right to reproductive health care* advocates generally argue that women need to enjoy access to safe, high-quality reproductive and sexual health care (Yamin 2005). In particular, they argue that the right of self-determination is more an "end product" that comes after the fulfillment of essential health care rights (Cottingham and Myntti 2002; Menken and Rahman 2006). The right to reproductive health care movement argues that the provision of services such as access to basic health care and reproductive care is what leads to the right to sexual and reproductive self-determination. Sociopolitical rights such as the right to choose contraceptive devices and access to particular services, the right to refuse sex, and the right to public sex education are all important, but they will follow once health care is promoted as the first and foremost priority (Fathalla et al. 2006; Low et al. 2005). The difference in the academic literature between the two camps on reproductive rights may be heuristic, but it *is* reflected in how states and international organizations take different positions and prioritize domestic programs according to these views. While neither "camp" has wavered on the need for women's health to be expressed as a *right* (Buse et al. 2006; Cleland et al. 2006; Yamin 2005), the variance in what is being sought to achieve reproductive health progress has enabled political exploitation—as will be discussed next.

The subordination of women's health has a long history. Women's lack of education has long been associated with the premature death of their children (Knudsen 2006; Starr 2007), and their reproductive health has been dominated by myth, superstition, and trivialization, resulting in the widespread use of local remedies, forced circumcision, and social exclusion (Doyal 1995). To understand how the language of rights has been used to address some of these problems, I will briefly recount some of the international efforts. The 1979 Convention on the Elimination of Discrimination against Women (CEDAW) demanded women's right to health and was seen as a breakthrough because it "explicitly addresses human rights regarding family planning services, care and nutrition during pregnancy, information, and, for instance, education to decide the number and spacing of one's children" (Cook et al. 2003: 153–154). However, its reference to health was limited to one article, Article 12, and largely discussed women's health in the context of family planning:

1. States Parties shall take all appropriate measures to eliminate discrimination against women in the field of health care in order to ensure, on a basis of equality of men and women, access to health care services, including those related to family planning.
2. Notwithstanding the provisions of paragraph I of this article, States Parties shall ensure to women appropriate services in connection with pregnancy, confinement and the post-natal period, granting free services where necessary, as well as adequate nutrition during pregnancy and lactation. (UNGA 1979: Article 12)

Similar to the ICESCR, the CEDAW required signatory states to establish the capacity to deliver on women's right to health but provided no political or funding incentives on how this might be achieved. Nor has there been consensus amongst the international women's movement that the Convention's focus on contraception best expresses the diverse health needs

and lack of inequity that afflicts women of all age groups; reflecting an early division between those emphasizing reproductive health care versus reproductive self-determination (Lush and Campbell 2001: 185).

The next element of the campaign to establish reproductive health as a human right focused on promoting maternal rights through the global Safe Motherhood Initiative. The initiative was launched in 1987 by a group of NGOs, international organizations, and governments and it sought to address the health needs of mothers. The intention of the initiative was to "generate political will, identify effective interventions, and mobilize resources that would" prevent the death of half a million women each year dying from pregnancy and childbirth (99% of the deaths were in developing countries) (Starr 2007: 1285). A recent study of the initiative found that between 1990 and 2005 there was an overall decrease of 2.5% per year in the maternal mortality ratio, but there were still 535,900 maternal deaths each year and sub-Saharan Africa and South Asia—where the highest number of maternal deaths occur—showed little, if any, improvement (Hill et al. 2007). Furthermore, the initiative, though crucial for raising awareness on maternal mortality, drew attention to the reproductive health needs of women but not to the reproductive health choices that women also had the right to claim.

Around the same time as the HIV/AIDS health human rights movement appeared on the international scene, a third important step came for those advocating reproductive self-determination at the 1994 United Nations International Conference on Population and Development (ICPD) in Cairo, Egypt (Cottingham and Myntti 2002; Lush and Campbell 2001). The ICPD recognized a Program of Action to protect reproductive health *and* sexual health as a matter of social justice best realized through human rights claims (Cook et al.

2003: 148–149). One hundred seventy-nine states agreed that the definition of reproductive health—ostensibly the health care that women would have a right to claim in these countries—was:

> [A] state of complete physical, mental and social well-being and not merely the absence of disease or infirmity, in all matters relating to the reproductive system and to its functions and processes. Reproductive health therefore implies that people are able to have a satisfactory and safe sex life and that they have the capability to reproduce and the freedom to decide if, when and how often to do so. Implicitly in this last condition are the right of men and women to be informed and to have access to safe, effective, affordable and acceptable methods of family planning of their choice, as well as other methods of their choice for the regulation of fertility which are not against the law, and the right of access to appropriate health care services that will enable women to go safely through pregnancy and childbirth and provide couples with the best chance of having a healthy infant.
>
> (ICPD 1994: Paragraph 7.2)

It is important to note that the ICPD outcome, as with the Safe Motherhood Initiative, placed primary emphasis on reproductive health care. But unlike previous international agreements, it focused on the sexual rights of women (and men) (e.g., the right to have sex that is not exploitative; Higer 1999; Richey 2005). Resources were to be dedicated towards family planning, emergency obstetric care, and diagnosis and treatment of sexually transmitted diseases, including HIV/AIDS (Fathalla et al. 2006: 2098). The program was in marked contrast to earlier reproductive health initiatives that focused more on the need to control population size than on women's abilities and right to control their own fertility (Freedman 1999b: 238). However, the ICPD Program still encountered resistance when the Catholic and Islamic participants joined forces to denounce the conference and the Program of Action on religious grounds (Freedman 1999a: 164).

The commitments made at the ICPD have not been translated into action. There were significant shortfalls in both financial contributions and in finding the political will within individual states to introduce the legislative and public health provisions that would allow women to access greater reproductive health care and choices (Glasier et al. 2006; Ngwena 2004). The cost of implementing the Program of Action was estimated to be $17 billion by 2000 and $22 billion by 2015, which was the year the Program of Action was to come to a close (Senanayake and Hamm 2004: 70). National governments were to contribute two-thirds of their health budget to meet this investment in women's health needs, and donor states would provide the remaining one-third. In 1997, the United Nations Fund for Population Activities announced that annual expenditure was already well below the ICPD estimated amount required to roll out the Program of Action by 2000. Economic distress for developing countries at the time was exacerbated by currency devaluations and rapid inflation, affecting their capacity to invest. This meant that "80% of the investment by less developed countries comes from China, India, Indonesia, Mexico, and Iran. The remainder of the less-developed countries will, therefore, have only a few tens of cents per person from domestic budgets to support the whole of reproductive health and family planning" (Potts and Walsh 1999: 315). The roll out of the ICPD Program has been hampered not only by developing countries' financial inability to meet their obligations but also by developed states not meeting theirs; by the end of the first call for funding, the United States had invested $64 million (despite a target of $2.2 billion), the United Kingdom invested $100 million (target $380 million), and Japan invested only $100 million (target of $1.4 billion) (Lush and Campbell 2001: 188). These funding shortfalls have persisted. For instance, it was estimated that it would cost $3.8 billion over ten years for sub-Saharan Africa to meet the MDGs relating to family-planning programs. However, projected donations total approximately $113 million (Cleland et al. 2006: 1823). Glasier et al. (2006: 1605) argue that one key reason for this shortfall has been the success of the HIV/AIDS campaign. Money for family planning and reproductive health once accounted for 70% of expenditure on AIDS and population control, but funding priorities have shifted to the control and treatment of HIV/AIDS and STDs. Another reason is sociocultural opposition within both donor and recipient programs to sexual and reproductive health programs that promote the freedom and empowerment of women.

Cultural and religious resistance to women's right to reproductive self-determination remains a key obstacle to implementing vital reproductive health care initiatives in many countries (UNGA 2008: 18). The ICPD revealed that that there was a wide gap between global aspirations and the political and cultural interests of many states and their societies. Consider, for example, the Program of Action's likelihood of success in Egypt when, in 1992, the WHO Regional Office in Cairo published a report stating that "to safeguard young people against sexual misbehavior, early marriages must be encouraged" (cited in Tomasevki 2005: 7). In addition, the right to access reproductive health care was limited under the ICPD to cases only where the state was willing to make it available and providing that none of the measures violated domestic law (i.e., abortion). This meant that states were under no obligation to grant access to abortion, for instance, if it remained illegal within the country. However, this cultural resistance to the reproductive freedoms thought

necessary to advance women's reproductive health did not just affect the rights of women in states with poor reproductive health care indicators. It has also created obstacles for the political advancement of this issue at the international level (UNGA 2008). Donor states also played a role in delaying the progress of the ICPD due to their own domestic political considerations. Under the administration of President George W. Bush (2001–2009) the United States, which accounts for 50% of all population health funding, reintroduced the "global gag rule" that prevented funding to health clinics that provided abortive services or information on abortion. This policy had global ramifications, forcing women in countries dependent on US aid to seek dangerous and illegal abortions and undermining local arguments by civil society organizations in favor of legalizing the procedure (British Broadcasting Commission [BBC] 2003; Senanayake and Hamm 2004: 70).[6]

As a result, there was some debate amongst reproductive rights advocates as to whether the ICPD had gone far enough. While some argued that the gains for women were significant, others pointed out that the constraints would limit their positive impact (Higer 1999). Nonetheless, the ICPD was considered an important step for reproductive health because it reoriented "family planning away from meeting demographic targets and towards a primary level service designed to meet the needs of individual women" (Lush and Campbell 2001: 187).

What was lacking in the aftermath of the adoption of the ICPD Program of Action was a series of benchmarks that would measure states' political commitment to deliver on these newly proclaimed rights. For the ICPD to work, women required education and access to health care to ensure safe sex, to prevent sexually transmitted diseases, to allow access to, and a choice of, family planning measures (including safe abortions), as well as clear laws prohibiting sexual violence and setting out a minimum marriage age (Billson 2006). The implementation of the ICPD in individual countries also required the political will to overcome cultural and religious resistance. But even where political will existed in low- to middle-income countries, significant investment by the international community has not been forthcoming (Cleland et al. 2006: 1811; Fathalla et al. 2006: 2095). For example, between 1995 and 2003, donor support for family-planning commodities and service delivery *fell* from US$560 million to $460 million (Cleland et al. 2006: 1811). While there has been an increase in maternal and newborn health funding since then, up to US$1.2 billion in 2006, roughly half of the total continues to be apportioned to child health. Fluctuating aid income and tied-aid complicates "efforts for effective planning for strategic priorities in developing countries" (UNICEF 2008: 101). UN Secretary-General Ban Ki-moon noted in October 2009 that funding still remains a problem for advancing reproductive health and maternal care:

> We have a clear plan to address these problems: the ICPD Program of Action. The Program is critical to achieving the Millennium Development Goals. It is especially important for goal number 5: to cut maternal mortality and achieve universal access to reproductive health care. Progress on reaching that target has been slower than on any other. Maternal health is linked directly to a country's health system. When we improve maternal health, all people will benefit. To fully carry out the [ICPD] Cairo Program of Action means providing women with reproductive health services, including family planning. It means backing poverty-eradication initiatives. And it means preventing rape during wartime and ending the culture of impunity. All of these actions require funding.
>
> (UNDPI 2009)

Margaret Chan, Director General of WHO, has argued that the persistent failure by the international community to invest in health systems over the past two decades explains why there has been no progress in maternal health (UNDPI 2008a). The UN Secretary-General's report on obstetric fistula also noted that, particularly in sub-Saharan Africa and South Asia, women in poor and rural regions, particularly adolescent girls, were not being included in national plans to address the "underlying social, cultural and economic determinants of maternal death and disability" (UNGA 2008: 18). In sum, neglect at *both* the international and domestic level has contributed to women's health continuing to be a "silent emergency" (UNDP/UNFPA/WHO/World Bank 2004: 11; UNDPI 2008b).

The need to address reproductive self-determination was again addressed in a 1999 review of the program's progress. It was reaffirmed that reproductive health for all was an important goal, but, a year later, the Millennium Declaration did not mention the need for a universal right to sexual and reproductive health, leading to a subsequent failure to adopt specific benchmarks in the area of sexual and reproductive health as a Millennium Development Goal (MDG) in 2000. All of this added to concerns that states had backtracked on the reproductive health agenda (Glasier and Gülmezoglu 2007: 1550). The MDGs fifth goal—to reduce maternal mortality by three quarters by 2015—further raised concerns that reproductive health was again being reduced to a health care issue that attempts to gain wider reproductive freedom of choice for women had been abandoned. However, a broader analysis of the UN's effort reveals that in the same year the Committee for the ICESCR included in General Comment 14 specific references to sexual and reproductive health in paragraphs 8, 14, 20, 21, and 34. In fact, paragraph 34 stated that "[S]tates should refrain from limiting access to contraceptives and other means of maintaining sexual and reproductive health, from censoring, withholding or intentionally misrepresenting health-related information, including sexual education and information, as well as from preventing people's participation in health-related matters" (UNSEC 2000).

Furthermore, to readdress the MDGs' neglect of reproductive health care, at the 2005 UN World Summit member states attached a second target to the MDG fifth goal, known as Target B, which sought to achieve universal access to reproductive health by 2015 through monitoring progress in the following areas:

> Contraceptive prevalence rate—Percentage of women aged 15–49 in union currently using contraception.
> Adolescent birth rate—Annual number of births to women aged 15–19 per 1,000 women in that age group. Alternatively, it is referred to as the age-specific fertility rate for women aged 15–19.
> Antenatal care coverage—Percentage of women aged 15–49 attended at least once during pregnancy by skilled health personnel (doctors, nurses or midwives) and the percentage attended by any provider at least four times.
> Unmet need for family planning—Refers to women who are fecund and sexually active but are not using any method of contraception and report not wanting any more children or wanting to delay the birth of the next child.
>
> (UNICEF 2008: 20)

Both the General Comment and the World Summit document allayed these concerns somewhat, but there remains cause for little more than cautious optimism. First, as noted above, only 62 countries have actually ratified the ICESCR and therefore, their obligation to fulfill paragraph 34 in the General Comment depends on whether the state has provided

legal, social, and economical means allowing women freedom of choice. Second, the World Summit's paragraph was a declaratory reference to sexual and reproductive health—there are no specific targets to be met (i.e., beyond those made under the 1994 ICPD)—and some critics argue that its inclusion was more a cynical ploy to keep voices quiet than a commitment to actually deliver tangible results on a women's right to reproductive health (Glasier et al. 2006: 1597).

Therefore, in relation to the state's level of obligation in the field of reproductive health, we see the stark contrast between access and provision (Senanayake and Hamm 2004: 70). The right to contraception and maternal health care depends not just on women having the right to seek these goods but also on these goods being available without restraint. For example, while the ICPD included abortion in its Program of Action, it was conditional on the state legalizing the procedure. However, we know that "unsafe and safe abortions correspond in large part with illegal and legal abortions, respectively" (Sedgh et al. 2007: 1343). Between 1995 and 2003, the proportion of all abortions that were unsafe increased from approximately 44% to 48%, primarily in countries where seeking and performing an abortion is illegal, heightening women's risk of death and long-term health consequences (Sedgh et al. 2007: 1344). The disjuncture between claiming the right and having it met, to some extent, reveals that while the distinction between negative and positive rights distinction may be untenable philosophically, in practice it can literally be the difference between a woman dying or living.

Jack Donnelly argues that to claim "something" as a human right is a claim to this "thing" as being "'needed' for a life worthy of a human being" (Donnelly 2003: 14). From this perspective, the health and human rights movement in the area of reproductive health has been successful. Governments may have argued about the substance, but there have been few—if any—arguments against the *need* for reproductive/sexual health care. It is generally accepted that an adequate response to reproductive health is vital for the well-being of women as well as communities, and that states have responsibility in this area, as demonstrated in the 2005 World Summit document. Even if this has not resulted in better health outcomes for women, this is an important advancement in clarifying the responsibility of states. Of course, accepting that women have a right to claim sexual and reproductive health care is not the same as actually realizing or providing the means to seek that right. It is in this disconnect between the right to access and the duty to provide that women's health becomes imperiled. As I noted earlier, one of the keys lies in the absence of an incentive structure. In the final section, I will briefly illustrate how state responsibilities could be clearly identified and earmarked against specific benchmarks required for women's reproductive health to be realized, as a basis for a system of incentives that could be implemented by individual donor states, international organizations, or collectively.

TRANSLATING RIGHTS FROM RHETORIC TO REALITY

Thomas Risse and Kathryn Sikkink argue that "agents of change" are crucial for human rights mobilization at the national level. Failure occurs when there is ready acceptance by international institutions and some states of declaratory prescriptions without support among donors or at the local level (Risse and Sikkink 1999: 33–35). I argue that this is what has occurred in the case of reproductive health. There has yet to be a clear agreement by states about how to measure compliance with the

ICESCR, its General Comment 14, and CEDAW and no system of incentives for compliance. Given this, it is not hard to see why many states may be reluctant to tackle the political, cultural, and religious obstacles to reform, not to mention the economic costs involved in reform.

Andrew Cooper, John Kirton, and Ted Schrecker thus may be right to argue that the "recurrent claim that health is a human right ... still has little appeal beyond the human rights community. It has almost none for the many major power governments that do not domestically recognise a national right to health" (Cooper, Kirton, and Schrecker 2007: 232). While there is little normative argument against the right of individuals to make their own health choices in order to have a life of dignity, this has not led to significant progress in women's health outcomes in the area of reproductive and sexual health. Thus, it is estimated that "if contraception were provided to the 137 million women estimated to want contraception, but who lack access, maternal mortality could fall by an additional 25–35%" (*The Lancet* 2007: 231). Approximately 97% of the estimated 20 million annual unsafe abortions are carried out in the developing world. In Kenya, for example, abortion is only legal to save a mother's life, which means that 300,000 unsafe abortions are carried out every year, which accounts for 50% of the country's maternal mortality (*The Lancet* 2007). The question then becomes how, for instance, can an international statement declaring the right and medical benefits of legal abortion be realized in a country that refuses to recognize its health benefits for women? Furthermore, how can the needs of women be satisfied in cooperation with the sovereign right of the state to determine its own laws? A proposed solution here includes two steps. First, precisely identifying what is required to deliver on the right and, second, establishing a system of incentives that enables and rewards reform and compliance.

Part of the solution sought by the Office of the United Nations High Commissioner for Human Rights (OHCHR) has been to identify and compile the essential indicators entailed in the right to health from data on states' performance in this area (OHCHR 2006: paras. 10–13; OHCHR/WHO 2008: 60). The indicator framework, agreed to in 2006, uses data compiled from participating states as well as nongovernment sources to ensure validity and transparency (see Table 25.1). Reproductive health is one of the five areas that the framework

identifies as essential for the enjoyment of the "highest attainable standard" of health. This framework targets the indicators according to a structure-outcome-process formula, which focuses on the implementation of relevant human rights treaties (structure), coverage of reproductive needs and maternal care (process), and infant/perinatal/maternal mortality rate (outcome) (OHCHR 2008: 25).

In contrast to the OHCHR study, another recent study on "national health systems equity" published in *The Lancet*, proposed that a concept of "equity" should be measured in addition to legal treaty

Table 25.1 Sexual and reproductive health (OHCHR 2008: 25)

Structural	• International human rights treaties, relevant to the right to enjoyment of the highest attainable standard of physical and mental health (right to health), ratified by the State. • Date of entry into force and coverage of the right to health in the Constitution or other forms of superior law. • Date of entry into force and coverage of domestic laws for implementing the right to health, including a law prohibiting female genital mutilation. • Number of registered and/or active nongovernmental organizations (per 100,000 persons) involved in the promotion and protection of the right to health. • Estimated proportions of births, deaths, and marriages recorded through vital registration system. • Time frame and coverage of national policy on sexual and reproductive health. • Time frame and coverage of national policy on abortion and fetal sex determination.
Process	• Proportion of received complaints on the right to health investigated and adjudicated by the national human rights institution, human rights ombudsperson, or other mechanisms and the proportion of these responded to effectively by the government. • Net official development assistance (ODA) for the promotion of health sector received or provided as a proportion of public expenditure on health or Gross National Income.* • Proportion of births attended by skilled health personnel.* • Antenatal care coverage (at least one visit and at least four visits).* • Increase in proportion of women of reproductive age using, or whose partner is using, contraception (CPR).* • Unmet need for family planning.* • Medical terminations of pregnancy as a proportion of live births. • Proportion of reported cases of genital mutilation, rape, and other violence restricting women's sexual and reproductive freedom responded to effectively by the government.
Outcome	• Proportion of live births with low birth weight. • Perinatal mortality rate. • Maternal mortality ratio.*

 All indicators should be disaggregated by prohibited grounds of discrimination, as applicable and reflected in metasheets.

* MDG-related indicators.

implementation (Backman et al. 2008). Rights fulfillment is not just about the ratification of treaties and the number of women surviving childbirth but also about states having a health system that allows equitable access to health care services that is available for all women (regardless of ethnic, religious, or economic background). The study develops its measurement criteria for 194 states from the right-to-health criteria developed from Article 12 and General Comment 14 of the ICESCR. The study traced the extent to which having the legal right to health provided claimants (patients) with the opportunity to further claim equitable health care and treatment. The study developed 72 indicators to ascertain the degree to which the right to health featured within national health systems through health care delivery, access to treatment, and compilation of health data—demonstrating that the state is conducting its own evaluations to ensure public health services are being delivered and directed according to greatest public need (Backman et al. 2008: 2048). The objective of the study was to create a framework of analysis that included indicators and benchmarks that would allow governments to measure their progress in fulfilling both the access and provision components of the right to health. Within the study, there are a number of indicators that seek to trace each state's performance in meeting reproductive health needs from maternal mortality statistics, to freedom from discrimination and sexual health education for young girls and boys. Backman et al. identify "key health system" features that are required for states to meet the most basic health rights of populations: "[A] comprehensive national health plan, a published national list of essential medicines, a national health workforce strategy, or government expenditure on health per person above the minimum required for a basic effective public health system" (2008: 2077).

There are two vital differences between the OHCHR (2008) framework and Backman et al.'s (2008) framework. First, Backman et al.'s framework dedicates a whole section to measuring the role of international donors in assisting states to meet their health as human right obligations. By contrast, the OHCHR (2008) study focuses solely on the measures that states need to take to meet their own core health care commitments. In the OHCHR framework, data gathered on external actors is limited to illustrating the level of nonstate actor engagement and filling in gaps in the data provided by states. Second, the OHCHR framework dedicates specific structure-process-outcome indicators to the five areas of health identified as essential for the enjoyment of the "highest attainable standard" of health, whereas the Backman et al. study is more of a panoramic study that does not pay attention to specific right-to-health areas (Backman et al. 2008: 2056). Under the "Structural" heading, the OHCHR lists the legal instruments that should be ratified and implemented, a registration system for births, deaths, and marriages, and notes the timeframe for implementation if these elements have not yet been implemented. Under the "Process" heading, the OHCHR framework asks for data on proportion of births attended by a health care professional, provision of antenatal coverage, women of reproductive age using contraception, proportion of population with unmet need for family planning, medical termination data, proportion of cases reported involving rape, female genital mutilation, and other violence restricting women's sexual and reproductive freedom responded to by the government (OHCHR 2008: 24). Finally, the "Outcome" section analyzes the country's maternal and perinatal morality rates, and the proportion of live births, as the best measures of a country's performance in fulfilling the right to sexual and reproductive health.

The OHCHR is certainly one of the most comprehensive attempts to measure implementation of the right to sexual and reproductive health. However, there remain significant shortcomings in relation to access. An additional indicator that would undoubtedly affect the outcome indicators is the provision of compulsory sexual and reproductive health education. Interestingly, Backman et al. (2008: 2058) list compulsory sexual and reproductive health education as one of their indicators, but the OHCHR study does not. In the poorest countries, the second most important risk factor for disease is unsafe sex. Education in safe sex and provision of safe, affordable contraceptives could easily prevent 340 million people becoming infected each year with STDs, 5 million HIV infections, and 80 million women from having unwanted and unplanned pregnancies (Glasier et al. 2006: 1597). In the UNESC General Comment 14, from 2000, access to impartial sexual and reproductive health education is listed as necessary to fulfilling the right to sexual and reproductive health and is vital for improving both the welfare of the woman and the children that she may have (UNESC 2000: Article 12, 14; Perkins 2010: 45).

Advancing these indicators as being vital for tracing the progress states are (or are not) making in realizing specific rights that improve the lives of women, in the case of reproductive rights, is essential and long overdue. But by itself it cannot overcome the inertia that states have been allowed to adopt in the area of rights due to the "fatal loophole" that states are allowed to appeal to under the ICESCR and General Comment 14: the lack of administrative or financial capacity to meet rights obligations. Therefore, in addition to indicators tracing states fulfillment of human rights indicators, there needs to be an incentive structure that encour-

ages states to fulfill these rights. While a framework of indicators will highlight the attempts that states have made to meet their health as a human right obligation, we still have the problem of political and financial will, particularly in the case of reproductive rights wherein women most affected by a lack of reproductive health care also tend to reside in states where women have the least amount of political, social, and economical rights, and where there are powerful cultural barriers to the attainment of those rights. Clearly more work is required to test which incentives may work in encouraging states to improve their performance in the areas of maternal mortality data, perinatal care, access to contraceptives, and sexual and reproductive health education. However, at this stage I would like to canvass three core reasons why any serious attempt to realize reproductive health rights requires an incentive structure to be attached to a framework of indicators.

First, a framework of indicators supported by the Human Rights Council, as the OHCHR framework requires, helps relieve the political inertia that had plagued earlier efforts to compel states to accept their responsibility to respect, to protect, and to fulfill human rights. Such a framework advances General Comment 14 of the ICESCR to not only outline where states' obligations in the area of human right to health exist but through a data-gathering exercise, indicating which specific benchmarks must be met. When states are unable to compile this data, or when their data is not supported by independent data gathering and analysis, such as allowed under the OCHCR framework, it elevates health issues such as reproductive rights to a political forum (in this case the Human Rights Council) in which a country's performance (such as access to free/affordable health care, government bureaucracy and transparency, regional distribution of clinics and prioritization of women's health care) would have to be openly discussed.

Second, the selection of reproductive health as one of the five attributes for physical and mental health under the OCHCR framework highlights the political momentum for advancing women's rights that exists in this area. The key to maintaining this focus and ensuring actual progress for women's health, as the "national health systems equity" study suggests, is to focus not just on indicators that reveal states' performance in implementing the legal provisions of human rights but also by devoting indicators to identify what targets states should be striving to reach in order to fulfill the right to reproductive health. This does mean then that the OCHCR framework must consider expanding its framework to include, as former UN Special Rapporteur on the Right to Health Paul Hunt has recommended, an assessment framework that traces not just states legal ratification of rights but also their efforts to ensure—in this case—what policy initiatives the government is putting in place to ensure women can freely access and be provided with care that suits their reproductive and sexual health needs (without fear of punishment, judgment, or discrimination).

Third, political momentum will not be achieved without the dedication of resources. Therefore, the "national health systems equity" study is right to insist that evaluations of donor investment in specific areas of health systems should be adopted under any rights-indicator framework analysis. Commitments made by donor states to assist poor countries in strengthening reproductive health care have been repeatedly left unfulfilled. Therefore, a measurement framework needs to also measure the performance of donor states. Even the most concerted efforts of developing countries to address reproductive health needs are likely to fall short of the mark unless they receive adequate external funding

support and technical assistance. If there is no continued evaluation of donor states' performance in meeting their financial obligations to such projects, developing states and international agencies are constrained in their ability to force the issue. The value of linking an incentive structure to a framework of indicators is that it measures not just the efforts being made at the domestic level to improve reproductive rights but evaluates donor state performance and would establish whether international reproductive aid programs are meeting their obligations under human rights treaties. However, financial incentives are not the only type of incentive that would be required.

There are also the political incentives that come from a framework of indicators. A framework on reproductive health would inevitably reveal performance—and as the "national health systems equity" study suggests—states that invest in health have better health outcomes. Such states are revealed to have better performances in child and maternal mortality statistics and, generally, to have stronger public health systems. Therefore, this linked scheme would not only encourage shared political responsibility between donors and aid recipients but would provide a benchmark against which it would be hard for states still resistant to improving women's reproductive health care—for cultural and religious reasons—to avoid the link between reproductive health care reform and improved health outcomes. In addition, the two-stage approach—indictors and incentives—places public pressure on donor states to invest political and financial capital into health. Aid-recipient states are still overwhelmingly dependent on external aid and assistance in the delivery of their basic health care programs. Raising the profile of primary health care strengthening through specific and vital areas such as reproductive health through an indicator and incentive scheme will serve to enhance the political importance of health at the global level. As Margaret Chan argues, addressing inequities in health outcomes is vital for greater security in the health sector—differences in life expectancy contributes to broader political vulnerabilities (Chan 2009).

Of course, both developing and developed states will resist such an in-depth framework that is publicly available; however, the groundwork has already been laid by the Human Rights Council agreeing to the OHCHR health data framework. Furthermore, such an approach is not the only solution to this problem, but one of the many measures that need to be considered in advancing reproductive rights (Palmer et al. 2009). The benefit that a framework brings is that it addresses targets and indicators, aid-recipient states and donor states, and the legal as well as substantive health measures required to advance—in this case—women's health. Everyone shares the blame and the solution to the "silent emergency" that faces too many women.

CONCLUSION

The purpose of this chapter has not been to criticize the utility in claiming health as a human right, nor the advances made by the reproductive health rights movement, but to better identify ways of translating its promise into practical action. The movement has secured some important achievements, but there remains a considerable lack of scrutiny on what states are individually doing to address the reproductive needs of women (Risse and Sikkink 1999: 35). The key issue now is not to further refine existing legal treaties on health as a human right, in this case, women's reproductive rights—we have 30 years of establishing that the right does exist. Instead, the challenge is to identify ways of implementing these rights. I have sug-

gested a two-stage process: (1) developing a framework of indicators on states performance in reforming their health care systems to better reflect the reproductive health care needs of women and (2) attaching an incentive structure to this framework that measures the performance of states, donors, and international organizations in meeting their collective obligation to improve women's reproductive health.

REFERENCES

Aginam, Obijiofor. (2005) *Global Health Governance* (Toronto, Canada: University of Toronto Press).

Asal, Victor, Brown, Mitchell, and Gibson Figueroa, Renee. (2008) Structure, empowerment and the liberalization of cross-national abortion rights. *Politics and Gender*, 4(2), 265–284.

Backman, Gillian, et al. (2008) Health systems and the right to health: An assessment of 194 countries. *The Lancet*, 372, 2047–2085.

Beaglehole, Robert, and Bonita, Ruth. (2008) Good public health: A scorecard. *The Lancet*, 372, 1988–1996.

Belhadj, Hedia, and Touré, Aminata. (2008) Gender equality and the right to health. *The Lancet*, 372(13), 2008–2009.

Billson, Janet Mancini. (2006) The complexities of defining female well-being. In *Female Well-Being: Toward a Global Theory of Social Change*, Janet Mancini Billson and Carolyn Fluehr-Lobban (eds.) (London, UK: Zed Books).

British Broadcasting Commission (BBC). (2003) *US abortion rule "hits Africa women,"* 26 September.

Buse, Kent, et al. (2006) Management of the politics of evidence-based sexual and reproductive health policy. *The Lancet*, 368, 2101–2103.

Chan, Margaret. (2009) Primary health care as a route to health security. *The Lancet*, 373, 1586–1587.

Cleland, John, et al. (2006) Family planning: The unfinished agenda. *The Lancet*, 368, 1810–1827.

Cook, Rebecca J., Dickens, Bernard M., and Fathalla, Mahmoud F. (2003) *Reproductive Health and Human Rights: Integrating Medicine, Ethics and Law* (Oxford: Clarendon Press).

Cooper, Andrew F., Kirton, John J. and Schrecker, Ted. (2007) Toward innovation in global health governance. In *Governing Global Health: Challenge, Response, Innovation*, Andrew F. Cooper, John J. Kirton, and Ted Schrecker (eds.) (Aldershot, UK: Ashgate).

Cottingham, Jane, and Myntti, Cynthia. (2002) Reproductive health: Conceptual mapping and evidence. In *Engendering International Health*, Gita Sen, Asha George, and Piroska Ostlin (eds.) (Cambridge, MA: The MIT Press).

Donnelly, Jack. (2003) *Universal Human Rights in Theory and Practice*, 2nd ed. (Ithaca, NY: Cornell University Press).

Doyal, Lesley. (1995) *What Makes Women Sick: Gender and the Political Economy of Health* (Basingstoke: Macmillan Press).

Fathalla, Mahmoud F., et al. (2006) Sexual and reproductive health for all: A call for action. *The Lancet*, 368, 2095–2100.

Freedman, Lynn P. (1999a) Censorship and manipulation of family planning information: An issue of human rights and women's health. In *Health and Human Rights: A Reader*, Jonathan M. Mann, Sofia Gruskin, Michael A. Grodin, and George J. Annas (eds.) (New York, NY: Routledge).

Freedman, Lynn P. (1999b) Reflections on emerging frameworks of health and human rights. In *Health and Human Rights: A Reader*, Jonathan M. Mann, Sofia Gruskin, Michael A. Grodin, and George J. Annas (eds.) (New York, NY: Routledge).

Glasier, Anna, and Metin Gülmezoglu, A. (2006) Putting sexual and reproductive health on the agenda. *The Lancet*, 368, 1550–1551.

Glasier, Anna, et al. (2006) Sexual and reproductive health: a matter of life and death. *The Lancet*, 368, 1595–1607.

Gruskin, Sofia, et al. (2005) The links between health and human rights. In *Perspective on Health and Human Rights*, Sofia Gruskin, Michael A. Grodin, George J. Annas, and Stephen P. Marks (eds.) (New York, NY: Routledge).

Higer, Amy J. (1999) International women's activism and the 1994 Cairo Population Conference. In *Gender Politics in Global Governance*, Mary K. Meyer And Elisabeth Prugl (eds.) (Lanham, MD: Rowman and Littlefield Publishers).

Hill, Kenneth, et al. (2007) Estimates of maternal mortality worldwide between 1990 and 2005: An assessment of available data. *The Lancet*, 370, 1311–1319.

Hudson, Heidi. (2005) "Live and let die"—A decade of contestation over HIV/AIDS, human security and gender in South Africa. *Journal for Contemporary History*, 29(3), 86–106.

Hunt, Paul. (2003) Neglected diseases, social justice and human rights: Some preliminary observations. *Health and Human Rights Working Paper Series No. 4* (Geneva: World Health Organization).

Hunt, Paul. (2007) Right to the highest attainable standard of health. *The Lancet*, 370, 369.

International Conference on Population and Development (ICPD). (1994) *Program of Action of the International Conference on Population and Development*. United Nations Population Fund.

Kelly, Lisa M., and Cook, Rebecca J. (2007) Book review: Learning to dance: Advancing women's reproductive health and well being from the perspectives of public health and human rights. *Global Public Health: An International Journal for Research, Policy and Practice*, 2(1), 99–102.

Knudsen, Lara M. (2006) *Reproductive Rights in a Global Context: South Africa, Uganda, Peru, Denmark, United States, Vietnam, Jordan* (Nashville, TN: Vanderbilt University Press).

The Lancet. (2007) Making abortion legal, safe and rare. *The Lancet*, 370, 291.

Low, Nicola, et al. (2005) Global control of sexuality transmitted infections. *The Lancet*, 368, 2001–2016.

Lush, Louisiana, and Campbell, Oona. (2001) International co-operation for reproductive health: too much ideology? In *International Co-operation in Health*, Martin McKee, Paul Garner, and Robin Stott (eds.) (Oxford: Oxford University Press).

Macklin, Audrey. (2006) The double-edged sword: Using the criminal law against female genital mutilation in Canada. In *Female Circumcision: Multicultural Perspectives*, Rogaia Mustafa Abusharaf (ed.) (Philadelphia, PA: University of Pennsylvania Press).

Mann, Jonathan M., et al. (1999) Health and human rights. In *Health and Human Rights: A Reader*, Jonathan M. Mann, Sofia Gruskin, Michael A. Grodin, and George J. Annas (eds.) (New York, NY: Routledge).

Menken, Jane, and M. Omar Rahman. (2006) Reproductive Health. In *International Public Health: Diseases, Programs, Systems and Policies*, 2nd ed., Michael H. Merson, Robert E. Black, and Anne J. Mills (eds.) (Boston, MA: Jones and Bartlett Publishers).

Ngwena, Charles. (2004) An appraisal of abortion laws in Southern Africa from a reproductive health rights perspective. *The Journal of Law, Medicine and ethics*, 32(4), 708–717.

Office of the High Commissioner For Human Rights (Ohchr). (2006) *Principles and Guidelines for a Human Rights Approach to Poverty Reduction Strategies*. HR/PUB/06/12 (Geneva, Switzerland: OHCHR).

Office of the High Commissioner For Human Rights (Ohchr). (2008) *Report on Indicators for Promoting and Monitoring the Implementation of Human Rights*. International Human Rights Instruments, HRI/MC/2008/3, 6 June, (Geneva, Switzerland: OHCHR).

OHCHR and World Health Organization (Who). (2008) Human rights, health and poverty reduction strategies. *Health and Human Rights Publication Series*, 5, (Geneva, Switzerland: OHCHR).

Palmer, Alexis, et al. (2009) Does ratification of human-rights treaties have effects on population health? *The Lancet*, 373, 1987–1992.

Perkins, Anne. (2010). Is Africa underpopulated? *The Guardian Weekly*, 2 April, p. 45. POTTS, Malcolm, and WALSH, Julia. (1999) Making Cairo work. *The Lancet*, 353, 315–318.

Potts, Malcolm, and Walsh, Julia (1999) Making Cairo work. *The Lancet*, 353, 315–318.

Richey, Lisa Ann. (2005) Uganda: HIV/AIDS and reproductive health. In *Where Human Rights Begin: Health, Sexuality and Women in the New Millennium*, Wendy Chavkin and Ellen Chesler (eds.) (New Brunswick, NJ: Rutgers University Press).

Risse, Thomas, and SIKKINK, Kathryn. (1999) The socialization of international human rights norms into domestic practices: Introduction. In *The Power of Human Rights: International Norms and Domestic Change*, Thomas Risse, Stephen C. Ropp, and Kathryn Sikkink (eds.) (Cambridge, UK: Cambridge University Press).

Sedgh, Gilda, et al. (2007) Induced abortion: Estimated rates and trends worldwide. *The Lancet*, 370, 1338–1345.

Senanayake, Pramilla, and Hamm, Susanne. (2004) Sexual and reproductive health funding: Donors and restrictions. *The Lancet*, 363, 70.

Shue, Henry. (1980) *Basic Rights: Subsistence, Affluence, and US Foreign Policy* (Princeton, NJ: Princeton University Press).

Starr, Ann M. (2007) Delivering for women. *Lancet*, 370, 1285.

Taylor, Allyn Lise. (1992) Making the World Health Organization work: A legal framework for universal access to the conditions for health. *American Journal of Law and Medicine*, 18(4), 301–346.

Toebes, Brigit. (1999) Towards an improved understanding of the international human right to health. *Human Rights Quarterly*, 21(3), 661–679.

Tomasevski, Katarina. (2005) Why a human rights approach to HIV/AIDS makes all the difference. *Human Rights and Poverty Reduction Paper, February*. London: Overseas Development Institute.

UN Economic and Social Council (UNESC). (2000) *The Right to the Highest Attainable Standard of Health*. E/C.12/2000/4 (General Comments), 11 August.

UNAIDS. (2007) *AIDS Epidemic Update: December 2007*. Geneva: UNAIDS and World Health Organization.

UNDP/UNFPA/WHO/World Bank Special Program of Research, Development and Research Training in Human Reproduction. (2004) *Research on Reproductive Health at WHO—Pushing the Frontiers of Knowledge* (Geneva, Switzerland: World Health Organization).

United Nations Department of Public Information (UNDPI). (2008a) Press Conference on Global Campaign for Health Millennium Development Goals. News and Media Division, 25 September.

United Nations Department of Public Information (UNDPI). (2008b) *Secretary-General Calls Recordon Maternal Health a Silent Emergency*. United-Nations Radio, 25 September.

United Nations Department of Public Information (UNDPI). (2009), "*All People Benefit" When Maternal Health Care Is Improved, Secretary-General Says, Marking Fifteenth Anniversary of Population and Development Conference*. 12 October.

United Nations Economic and Social Council (UNESC). (2009) Background Note. Moving from commitment to action—Meeting the internationally agreed goals and commitments in regard to global public health, *Global Preparatory Meeting for the 2009 Annual Ministerial Review, 31 March* (New York, NY: United Nations).

United Nations General Assembly (UNGA). (1948) *Universal Declaration of Human Rights*. New York, NY: United Nations.

United Nations General Assembly (UNGA). (1966) *International Covenant on Economic, Social and Cultural Rights*. New York, NY: United Nations.

United Nations General Assembly (UNGA). (1979) *Convention on the Elimination of All Forms of Discrimination against Women (CEDAW)*, Resolution 34/180, 18 December.

United Nations General Assembly (UNGA). (2008) Supporting efforts to end obstetric fistula. *Report of the Secretary-General, Sixty-third session*, Item 59 of the provisional agenda, A/63/222, 6 August.

UNICEF. (2008) *The State of the World's Children 2009: Maternal and Newborn Health* (New York, NY: United Nations Children's Fund).

Wellings, Kaye, et al. (2006) Sexual behaviour in context: A global perspective. *The Lancet*, 368, 1706–1728.

World Health Assembly. (1946) *Constitution of the World Health Assembly*. Geneva: World Health Organization.

Yamin, Alicia Ely. (2005) Learning to dance: Bringing the fields of human rights and public health together to promote women's well-being. In *Learning to Dance: Case Studies on Advancing Women's Reproductive Health and Well-Being from the Perspectives of Public Health and Human Rights*, Alicia Ely Yamin (ed.) (Cambridge, MA: Harvard University Press).

QUESTIONS

1. "The fact that we have not made any significant progress at all in reducing the number of women who die in pregnancy and childbirth is appalling. There can only be one reason for this awful situation—and that is persistent neglect for women in a world dominated by men" (United Nations Department of Public Information 2008). Comment on this statement from the perspective of the UN Secretary-General.

2. In the chapter, it is stated that extremist Catholic and Islamic forces denounced the International Convention on Population and Development (ICPD) Program of Action on religious grounds. To what extent are reproductive rights universal? To what extent should women's reproductive rights be tailored to be consistent with religious or cultural mores?

3. Consider Table 25.1. Pretend you are asked to provide a formal review of this list before it is presented to the High Commissioner for Human Rights. Do you foresee any problems with assessment of any of these indicators in health and human rights terms? Do you feel any valuable indicators are missing?

FURTHER READING

1. Asal, V., Brown, M., & Gibson Figueroa, R., Structure, Empowerment and the Liberalization of Cross-national Abortion Rights. *Politics and Gender*, 4:, 2654–284 http://journals.cambridge.org/action/displayFulltext?type=1&fid=1890820&jid=PAG&volumeId=4&issueId=02&aid=1890812

2. Cottingham, J., Kismodi, E., Hillber A.M., Lincetto, O., Stahlhofer, M. & Gruskin, S., Using Human Rights for Sexual and Reproductive Health: Improving Legal and Regulatory Frameworks. *Bulletin of the World Health Organization*, 2010; 88.

3. Backman, G. et al., Health Systems and the Right to Health: An Assessment of 194 Countries. *Lancet*, 2008, 372: 2047–2085, http://www.thelancet.com/journals/lancet/article/PIIS0140-6736(08)61781-X/abstract

CHAPTER 26

Use of Human Rights to Meet the Unmet Need for Family Planning

Jane Cottingham, Adrienne Germain and Paul Hunt

INTRODUCTION

Others have outlined the many benefits of investment in family planning, including acceleration of progress towards achieving the Millennium Development Goals. We explain how measures to respect, protect, and fulfil human rights[1] enable people to use contraceptive information and services and help achieve the full benefits of such investments.

Many people think of human rights in terms of violations. This aspect is important, and the history of family planning policies and programmes—particularly some undertaken for population control—includes instances of people being coerced to accept contraceptive implants or intrauterine devices and being subjected to forced abortion or sterilisation.[2–9] Human rights mechanisms, such as treaty monitoring bodies, regional human rights tribunals, and national courts, enable individuals and communities to seek redress for such violations.[6, 7] Human rights law can also be used to prevent violations occurring in the first place. For example, consideration of human rights standards can ensure that health services do not discriminate against particular groups such as people younger than 18 years, ethnic minorities, or people with HIV infection, and can also require improvements in the quality of services.

When human rights are integrated into policy-making processes, they can help to ensure that health facilities and services are non-discriminatory and of good quality from the outset. The application of human rights law and standards to programme design and monitoring, and use of human rights mechanisms to hold governments accountable, are essential devices to ensure health for all.

Internationally agreed human rights that are particularly relevant to contraceptive information and services include the rights to: non-discrimination, information and education, the highest attainable standard of health, privacy, and life.[10–12] These rights are inextricably linked. For example, the right to the highest attainable standard of health, which includes access to health services and health-related information, cannot be fulfilled without promotion and protection of the rights to education and information because people must know about services to use them. In this report we give special attention to the right to contraceptive information and services, which is grounded in these internationally recognised human rights,[13, 14] and we suggest that the promotion and protection of these rights should be part of a multidimensional strategy to satisfy the unmet need for family planning.

Over the past four decades, international human rights law has established and expanded standards for sexual and reproductive health, including family planning. For example, states have affirmed the right to the highest attainable standard of health,[10] authoritatively interpreted to encompass "sexual and reproductive health services, including access to family planning".[15] They have also agreed to "eliminate discrimination against women in the field of health care in order to ensure, on a basis of equality of men and women, access to health care services, including those related to family planning".[11]

These agreements are legally binding for all the countries that have ratified the relevant covenants and conventions, such as the International Covenant on Economic, Social and Cultural Rights, the Convention on the Rights of the Child (CRC), and the Convention on the Elimination of All Forms of Discrimination against Women (CEDAW). All states in the world have ratified at least one of the core international human rights treaties and most have ratified many more.[16] Many have translated these standards into their national laws and regulations, and many national constitutions guarantee rights such as the right to non-discrimination. These standards place legal obligations on governments to make high quality contraceptive information and services accessible for everyone, and to enable people to demand access to such services.

Human rights treaties are supported and amplified by intergovernmental consensus documents such as the Programme of Action of the International Conference on Population and Development.[17] Such agreements can be used by various groups to hold accountable the governments that are party to them, and they also guide the policies and programmes of UN agencies, donor governments, and nongovernmental organisations.

Because this series focuses on family planning, defined as contraceptive information and services, we do not discuss access to other essential sexual and reproductive health services such as prevention, diagnosis, and treatment of sexually transmitted infections, and provision of safe abortion, although access to safe abortion is also central to women's ability to regulate their fertility. International human rights law requires that governments provide a comprehensive legal and policy framework to ensure that abortion services allowable by law are safe and accessible in practice.[18-20] This obligation requires that health providers be trained and equipped, and that other measures be taken to protect women's health. Other issues crucial to the health and human rights of women are outside the scope of this report, such as early and forced marriage and female genital mutilation, both of which breach international human rights law.[12, 21-23]

WHOSE UNMET NEED?

The human rights principle of non-discrimination leads us to examine who is included in prevailing definitions of unmet need by policy makers, programme managers, service providers, and demographers. The sources used to estimate unmet need generally include only married or cohabiting women of reproductive age who do not want to become pregnant, but who are not currently using a modern method of contraception. However, as data have become available from some countries for sexually active unmarried women, the most recent unmet need estimates include unmarried women. About 215 million women in developing countries are estimated to have an unmet need for family planning.[24] Still left out of the estimate are women who are using a modern method that is unsatisfactory to them and who, without the necessary programme support, are at risk of unwanted pregnancy or of stopping contraceptive use or both. Boys and men are not explicitly addressed in estimates of unmet need because the woman who reports contraceptive use is asked to include use by her husband or partner.

About half all sexually active adolescent women (aged 15–19 years) in sub-Saharan Africa and Latin America and the Caribbean who want to prevent pregnancy are unmarried.[25] Of those, only 41% in sub-Saharan Africa and 50% in Latin America and the Caribbean are using a modern method of contraception. No equivalent data for sexually active adolescent men are available. Yet, there are 1.4 billion adolescents aged 10–19 years, many of whom are, or soon will be, sexually active. About 90% of them live in low-income and middle-income countries, have limited access to schooling and health services, and are likely to engage in sexual activity before or outside, as well as within, marriage.

The decisions of these young people about beginning sexual activity, marriage, sexual expression, and use (or not) of contraception will have a great effect on their lives and determine a major portion of future population growth. Whether married or not, they have particular needs in family planning because they are more likely to have unprotected and non-consensual sex, and commonly lack the information and services needed to protect themselves.[26] Nor are these young people drawn to services that are designed to meet adults' needs. Many young people can be interested in contraception to prevent unwanted pregnancy and to protect against sexually transmitted infections, but conventional messages about planning their families are irrelevant. Addressing their needs requires trained and supportive staff, privacy and confidentiality, emphasis on both contraception and disease prevention, and comprehensive sexuality education which is grounded in human rights, including gender equality and non-discrimination, sexual attitudes, and behaviour.[27–30]

The many women who are using a method that they do not like are not currently considered to have an unmet need. In some countries, more than four women in ten discontinue their contraceptive method within the first year of use.[31] Yet these women, before they discontinue, are not included in the estimates of unmet need, which is indicative of the long-standing failure of many programmes to recognise the importance of provision of suficient information about side-effects, and support for women to tolerate them or switch methods.

In all regions, entire categories of women have little or no access to contraceptive services; these groups include refugees and internally displaced women, those in stigmatised occupations such as sex work, those who are otherwise stigmatised, such as rape victims, women with disabilities, HIV infection, or AIDS, and those from religious or ethnic minorities.[32–35] The human rights principle of non-discrimination requires that contraceptive information and services are available and accessible to all these groups. Special outreach, training, and other investments that are needed, will affect cost estimates of both global and national resources required to address the unmet need. In many countries, meeting these unmet needs will also require changes in laws, policies, strategies, and programmes, consistent with national and international human rights standards.

USE OF HUMAN RIGHTS TO OVERCOME BARRIERS TO ACCESS

The right to the highest attainable standard of health requires that everyone can access health information and services without restrictions, including specific services related to family planning[15] that are both affordable and delivered in a timely fashion.[33] Nonetheless, many barriers impede women's access to contraception, including: conditions that do not allow them to make free and informed decisions (such as lack of intelligible information or counselling); lack of confidentiality; the requirement for authorisation by spouse, parent, or hospital authorities; high fees for services; distance from health facilities and the absence of affordable public transport; lack of choice of a wide range of contraceptive methods;[36–40] and inadequate training, insufficient numbers, and poor supervision of health-care providers.[17, 41]

Laws that restrict access to services for particular population groups, or that ban the display of materials about, or sale of contraceptives, have been identified as serious barriers to women's access to family planning services.[40–44] Each of these barriers could be the focus of a report, but we describe below four examples where human rights standards have been used to remove barriers, thus contributing to reduction of unmet need.

Inadequate Supplies of Safe and Effective Commodities

Reports from the past 3 years show that, in some African countries, stock-outs of contraceptives are a chronic problem.[45–47] In Kenya, for instance, 24% of women who do not want another child within the next 2 years are not using contraception because many methods, particularly implants and injectables, are not available.[45] Such shortages are likely to contribute to maternal morbidity and mortality.[45] In some instances, substandard contraceptives are available at low prices, but pose a serious threat to people's lives and health.[47] The human rights and public health obligations of governments require them to establish strict quality controls for manufacture and import of contraceptives, and effective surveillance of other sources such as the internet.

Human rights standards require that a wide range of approved contraceptive supplies be continuously available.[11, 15, 36–39] Approved contraceptives are those, at a minimum, that are on the WHO Model List of Essential Medicines[48] and its companion Essential Medicines for Reproductive Health.[49] These lists include emergency contraception, a method that is often not available even when other methods are, and a range of contraceptives including condoms and other barrier methods, hormonal contraceptives (oral, injectable, implants, rings), intrauterine devices, and contraceptive sterilisation. An example of how human rights standards have been used is a decision by the Colombian Council of state, which ruled that access to emergency contraception is in accordance with the right to life as established in the Colombian Constitution, thus rejecting efforts by some groups to ban such contraceptives.[44] Another problem is that the ability of states to ensure continuous supplies has been, and in many cases remains, dependent on donor funding, which has been reduced over the past decade, and on free supplies from international agencies, which can be erratic.[45–46]

Poor Quality Services

In the early 1990s, poor quality of care in contraceptive services was identified as a major problem, and a user-centred quality of care framework was designed that is implicitly grounded in human rights.[50] Its elements are: choice among contraceptive methods; accurate information about the effectiveness, risks, and benefits of different methods; technical competence of providers; provider–user relationships based on respect for informed choice, privacy, and confidentiality; follow-up; and the appropriate constellation of services.[50] The framework has been variously adapted to include additional elements such as cost, proximity of services, and consideration of gender relations. Studies in Bangladesh, the Philippines, Senegal, and Tanzania have shown that improvement of care quality according to these standards increases women's contraceptive use; where women felt they were receiving good care, rates of contraceptive use were higher than in regions with lower quality provision of health care.[51–54] In addition to the public health imperative, the right to the highest attainable standard of health obligates governments to ensure that health facilities, goods, and services, including contraceptive services, are of good quality.[15] The framework provides guidance for this requirement and experience shows that it helps address unmet need by improving women's satisfaction with and effective use of contraceptives and can increase the numbers of women and young people accessing services.

Conscientious Objection

An apparently increasing number of health-care providers refuse to provide various sexual and reproductive health services including contraception on grounds of conscience, because they disagree, for personal or religious reasons, with the use of contraception. Human rights law is clear: providers' exercise of their rights to freedom of thought, conscience, and religion must not jeopardise their patients' health.[33, 55] The European Court of Human Rights elaborated this standard in a case in which two pharmacists in France were found liable for refusing to provide doctorprescribed contraceptives to several women on religious grounds.[55] The court explained that as long as the sale of contraceptives is legal and occurs by medical prescription only in pharmacies, pharmacists "cannot impose their religious beliefs on others as a justification for their refusal to sell such products, . . . [They] can manifest those beliefs in many ways outside the professional sphere".[55] The pharmacists were subsequently also found guilty of violating France's Consumer Code, which prohibits refusal to sell a product or provide a service to a customer for no legitimate reason.[55, 56] These decisions are consistent with the Ethical Guidelines of the International Federation of Gynecology and Obstetrics.[57] Individuals who object on grounds of conscience to providing contraceptives must refer patients to willing providers, and provide services where they have a monopoly and in emergency situations.

Lack of Community Engagement

Participation in the decision-making process by the people who are affected is a core human rights principle. In family planning, if communities are not engaged in processes of contraceptive introduction, the result is likely to be less effective.[58] In recognition of this, WHO has outlined a participatory approach to contraceptive introduction explicitly grounded in human rights, which has been effectively used in nearly 20 countries.[58]

Engaging not only the Ministry of Health, but also representatives of women's health advocacy and other community groups, health-care providers, and researchers, this strategic approach culminates in changes to improve people's access to contraceptive services. In Romania, for example, the process drew attention to free family planning services in one part of the country, by contrast with fees charged to users in a much poorer region; consequently contraceptive methods became available free of charge throughout the country.

LAWS AND POLICIES IN LINE WITH HUMAN RIGHTS COMMITMENTS

Making human rights explicit in a country's laws, policies, and programmes can help to ensure positive health outcomes for all. For example, for more than a decade, Brazil has put in place various strategies aimed at improving women's health, particularly sexual and reproductive health, explicitly shaped by human rights.[59] In 1996, the National Congress approved a law on family planning according to which family planning is a right of every citizen.[60] Thereafter, two successive national policies were implemented to broaden the provision of reversible birth-control methods by the public health system, and to provide free contraception to women and men of reproductive age. Use of contraception by sexually active women in Brazil increased from 55% in 1996 to 68% in 2006, and access to oral contraceptives through the public health system more than doubled during the same period, including among some disadvantaged populations.[61] Problems remain, especially with regard to ensuring access to all disadvantaged and remote communities. Nonetheless, overall progress is impressive, and although many factors contributed to the development and implementation of these strategies, the explicit use of human rights in the design of the policy and strategies seems very likely to have contributed to their success.

Since 1994, many intergovernmental negotiations have affirmed the right of adolescents and young people to contraceptive information and services and comprehensive sexuality education, in line with the human rights standard that adolescents must be treated according to their evolving capacities for decision making, not according to any arbitrary age limitation.[17, 29] Evidence available from a range of countries shows that comprehensive sexuality education improves sexual health outcomes, including reduction of unintended pregnancies, delay of sexual debut, and reduction of high-risk sexual behaviour.[62–66] In 2006 and 2008 respectively, African Ministers of Health[67] and Latin American Ministers of Health and Education[68] each adopted declarations, framed by human rights, that commit their governments to concrete actions to provide sexuality education. Many countries are in various stages of taking such concrete actions, inspired by, and based on, these declarations. The provision of comprehensive sexuality education is a public health imperative backed by international human rights standards that place legally binding obligations on governments to take steps to ensure that adolescents have access to such education, including information about contraception.[29, 30]

Although many developed countries provide outstanding sexuality education to adolescents, the USA has struggled to do so. Between 1998 and 2009, the American federal government invested more than US$1.5 billion in promotion of abstinence-only-until-marriage programmes, which prohibited distribution of information about contraception. Under President George W Bush, such programmes became the leading federal government strategy for dealing with adolescent sexuality—both domestically and internationally. In 2009, during President Obama's administration, most federal support for domestic abstinence-only programmes ended and funding shifted to science-based approaches, although some funding for abstinence-only programmes was revived by Congress in 2010.

Human rights and health arguments contributed to the Obama administration's decisions. For example, the influential 2006 Society for Adolescent Medicine report concludes: "Current U.S. federal law and guidelines regarding abstinence-only funding are ethically flawed and interfere with fundamental human rights".[69] Opposition to American domestic abstinence-only programmes also came from constitutional litigation brought by the American Civil Liberties Union. In the opinion of Santelli and colleagues:[70] "Documentation of the scientific and rights-based problems was instrumental in reducing . . . federal support for [abstinence-only-until-marriage] AOUM programs in the USA".

LEGAL OBLIGATIONS AND MECHANISMS FOR ACCOUNTABILITY

Because international and national human rights give rise to legally binding obligations on states, they demand accountability of states for their performance. Accountability can be achieved through many different mechanisms and procedures that vary from country to country, and also include the UN and other mechanisms with global responsibility. A few examples include national courts, national human rights institutions, international human rights treaty bodies, democratically elected local health councils, patients' committees, professional disciplinary proceedings, and other civil society organisations.[71]

Some countries enshrine human rights in their national constitutions and provide effective judicial remedies when these rights are violated. For example, the South African Constitutional Court, relying on the right to the highest attainable standard of health and other constitutional protections, ordered the government to provide the antiretroviral drug nevirapine in public hospitals and clinics when medically indicated.[72] In Argentina, a court relied upon CEDAW and CRC to uphold the constitutionality of a law requiring the provision of sexual and reproductive health services to all fertile people, including adolescent girls.[73] National courts are increasingly relying on international human rights law to uphold access to emergency contraception,[74–77] in the same way that national organisations and individuals are using international and regional human rights tribunals to uphold access to lawful abortion.[78, 79]

Established by national law, national human rights institutions, such as the Kenyan National Commission on Human Rights, are not judicial, but can receive and investigate complaints and undertake public enquiries. The Kenyan commission received a major report[80] from civil society drawing attention to profound problems in the country's health-care sector, including with family planning, in light of which the commission launched a public enquiry into reproductive health services for women. The enquiry took written and oral evidence from all interested groups across the country. Its report and recommendations will be submitted to the President and Parliament.[81] Such processes are likely to lead to improvements in women's access to reproductive health services including family planning.

International human rights accountability mechanisms, such as the CEDAW Committee, can be used to good effect. In the case of a Roma woman who was forcibly sterilised, the committee ruled that Hungary had failed to provide appropriate information and advice on family planning, and had not ensured that the woman had given her fully informed consent to be sterilised. It ordered the government to take specific measures to ensure the occurrence was not repeated.[7] The CEDAW Committee can also undertake inquiries in situations that are deemed to be grave or systematic. In 2008, and 2009, a coalition of nongovernmental organisations requested that the committee investigate Manila City's ban on the sale of modern contraceptives in the public health system, to support the lawsuit they filed against the Office of the Mayor of Manila. At the time of writing, the case is still pending.[82] International human rights tribunals are increasingly elaborating on their understanding of certain rights and principles, such as privacy and confidentiality, free and informed decision making, autonomy and self-determination, and the freedom to give and receive information,[83–85] all of which are essential to improve access to contraceptive information and services. Such elaboration enhances the possibility of judicial application of these human rights principles to family planning.

Some international human rights demand immediate action. For example, the prohibition against discrimination requires that, if a policy discriminates against women, the government must take immediate remedial action, whatever its resource capacity. Various elements of the right to health, including the right to contraceptive information and services, require immediate action, such as ensuring that services are not discriminatory, providing access to essential medicines, and putting in place a national health strategy based on epidemiological evidence.[15] However, international human rights, including the right to contraceptive information and services, also have elements that are subject to progressive realisation and resource availability,[10] such as the obligation to construct an effective health system. Progressive realisation means that countries have to improve their performance steadily, consistent with their available resources. If indicators and benchmarks suggest inadequate progress, a government has to provide a rational and objective explanation, otherwise an accountability mechanism could find that the government is in breach of its legally binding human rights obligations.

Millennium Development Goal target 5B—universal access to reproductive health by 2015—strongly corresponds to the right to contraceptive information and services. One of the indicators for this target is unmet need for family planning. Thus, if unmet need is not decreasing in a country, the government is neither on track to achieve Millennium Development Goal 5, nor in conformity with its binding obligations to fulfil the right to contraceptive information and services, unless the authorities can provide a compelling explanation for the country's performance.

Of particular importance are commitments made by wealthy countries and international agencies to provide resource-poor countries with financial support and contraceptives and other reproductive health commodities. Mechanisms to hold donors accountable for these commitments are very weak.[86] In a new development, all stakeholders, including donors and businesses will be held accountable by a global independent Expert Review Group, and national accountability mechanisms, for their commitments to the UN Secretary-General's Global Strategy for Women's and Children's Health, which encompasses contraceptive information and services.[86]

CONCLUSIONS: LEGALLY REQUIRED PRIORITIES

We have shown that taking a human rights perspective of unmet need for family planning results in a broader definition than that conventionally used of who has a need and right to contraceptive information and services, of what kind, under what conditions. The right to contraceptive information and services, like other human rights, requires translation into many practical actions that will meet the needs of diverse groups living in diverse circumstances. Thus priorities and plans must be determined primarily at country level, buttressed by local, national, and international accountability mechanisms, and donor support for low-resource countries. Priority setting and planning must take into account three crucial considerations.

First, contraceptive information and services are necessary but not sufficient to reduce the unmet need for family planning. As agreed in the International Conference on Population and Development Programme of Action, they are most effectively delivered as a key element of a package of mutually reinforcing sexual and reproductive health services,[17] which must be a priority in health systems strengthening,[87] and must be provided with full respect for the human rights of the user.

Second, states have human rights obligations to protect people from discrimination. They must therefore ensure that policies, programmes, and accountability mechanisms for contraceptive information and services are designed to enable all, especially vulnerable and disadvantaged groups, to exercise their right to information and services free of discrimination, coercion, and violence. Who is vulnerable or disadvantaged varies between country and within countries and needs to be explicitly assessed in each case for policy and programme development and monitoring.

Third, progressive realisation and resource constraints cannot be used as a reason for failure to make required progress.[88–93] These principles and other human rights considerations, including consideration of epidemiological evidence, must be used to establish priority among the many necessary measures needed to implement the right to contraceptive information and services, and to protect against abuses. Concrete ways to finance the priority measures are available even for low-income countries.[94]

Taking into account these three considerations, and recognising that countries are at different stages of meeting their sexual and reproductive health and rights obligations, we emphasise in the panel seven priority measures that are required by human rights standards and principles for governments to eliminate unmet need for family planning and achieve universal access to contraceptive information and services.

Governments have a legal obligation to do all they reasonably can to put these measures in place as a matter of urgent priority. If they fail to do so without compelling justification, they are in breach of their legally binding international human rights commitments in relation to health, contraceptive information and services, and women's equality. For this reason, human rights are a strong device that could be more widely used by governments to shape, and secure support for, effective and inclusive policies, but also by health-care providers and advocates to improve the quality of services and achieve universal access to reproductive health including family planning. Guidance and other assistance are available to help countries meet their human rights obligations. For example, WHO has developed an instrument[95] that helps governments and other stake-holders to identify inconsistencies between national laws and human rights obligations (e.g., denying unmarried women contraceptive services although CEDAW has been adopted into law) and agree on actions to remove such barriers to people's access to, and the provision of, good quality sexual and reproductive health services including family planning. Such processes can contribute much to fulfilment of the unmet need for family planning.

REFERENCES

1. UN. General Comment no. 14: the right to the highest attainable standard of health. Geneva: United Nations Committee on Economic, Social and Cultural Rights, 2000: paras 33–37. (E/C.12/2000/4).

2. Bland A. Chinese state holds parents hostage in sterilisation drive. The Independent (London). April 17, 2010.

3. Greenhalgh S, Winckler EA. Governing China's population: from Leninist to neoliberal biopolitics. Stanford: Stanford University Press, 2009.

4. Dhanraj D (director). Something like a war. VHS/DVD. India/ England, 1991.

5. Schmidt B. Forced sterilization in Peru. Political Environ 1998.

6. María Mamérita Mestanza Chávez, Perú. Inter-

American commission on human rights, friendly settlement, report no 71/03, petition 12.191. Oct 22, 2003.

7. AS vs Hungary. UN Committee on the Elimination of Discrimination against Women (CEDAW), communication No 4/2004. Aug 14, 2006. (CEDAW/C/36/D/4/2004).

8. Center for Reproductive Rights. Dignity denied: violations of the rights of HIV-positive women in Chilean health facilities. New York, NY: Center for Reproductive Rights, 2010.

9. Namibia: women take legal action over alleged sterilisations. Irin PlusNews. June 25, 2009.

10. International covenant on economic, social and cultural rights. New York: United Nations, 1966.

11. Convention on the elimination of all forms of discrimination against women. New York: United Nations, 1979.

12. Convention on the rights of the child. New York: United Nations, 1989.

13. Center for Reproductive Rights, UNFPA. Brieng paper: The right to contraceptive information and services for women and adolescents. New York: Center for Reproductive Rights and United Nations Population Fund, 2010. http://reproductiverights.org/sites/crr.civicactions.net/les/documents/BP_unfpa_12.10.pdf (accessed Aug 25, 2011).

14. IPPF. Charter on sexual and reproductive rights. London: International Planned Parenthood Federation, 2003.

15. UN Committee on Economic, Social and Cultural Rights. General comment no. 14: the right to the highest attainable standard of health. Geneva: United Nations, 2000. (E/C.12/2000/4).

16. Office of the United Nations High Commissioner for Human Rights. International law.

17. Programme of action adopted at the International Conference on Population and Development, Cairo. Sept 5–13, 1994. New York: United Nations Population Fund, 1994.

18. Tysiac vs Poland. European Court of Human Rights, application no. 5410/03. March 20, 2007.

19. Paulina del Carmen Ramírez Jacinto, Mexico. Inter-American commission on human rights, friendly settlement, report No. 21/07, Petition 161–01. March 9, 2007.

20. WHO. Safe abortion: technical and policy guidance for health systems. Geneva: World Health Organization, 2003.

21. UN Committee on the Elimination of Discrimination against Women. General recommendation No. 21: equality in marriage and family relations. New York: United Nations, 1994.

22. Silva-de-Alwis R. Child marriage and the law. New York: UNICEF, 2008.

23. WHO. Eliminating female genital mutilation: an interagency statement. Geneva: World Health Organization, 2008.

24. Singh S, Darroch JE, Ashford LS, Vlasso M. Adding it up: the costs and benets of investing in family planning and maternal and newborn health. New York: Guttmacher Institute and United Nations Population Fund, 2009.

25. Guttmacher Institute, IPPF. Facts on the sexual and reproductive health of adolescent women in the developing world. New York and London: Guttmacher Institute and International Planned Parenthood Federation, 2010.

26. WHO. Why is giving special attention to adolescents important for achieving Millennium Development Goal 5? Factsheet. Geneva: World Health Organization, 2008.

27. UNESCO. International technical guidance on sexuality education. Paris: United Nations Educational, Scientic and Cultural Organization, 2009. (ED-2009/WS-36).

28. Muñoz V. UN Special Rapporteur on the right to education—sexual education. A/65/162. Geneva: United Nations, July 23, 2010.

29. UN Committee on the Rights of the Child. General comment no. 4: adolescent health and development in the context of the Convention on the Rights of the Child. Geneva: United Nations, 2003. (CRC/GC/2003/4).

30. UN Committee on the Rights of the Child. General comment no. 3: HIV/AIDS and the rights of the child. Geneva: United Nations, 2003: paras 15–21. (CRC/GC/2003/1).

31. Curtis S, Evens E, Sambisa W. Contraceptive discontinuation and unintended pregnancy: an imperfect relationship. Int Perspect Sex Reprod Health 2011; 37: 58–66.

32. UN Committee on the Elimination of Discrimination against Women. Concluding comments: Azerbaijan. New York: United Nations, 2007: paras. 31–32. (CEDAW/C/AZE/CO/3).

33. UN Committee on the Elimination of Discrimination against Women. General recommendation no. 24: women and health. New York: United Nations, 1999.

34. UN Committee on the Elimination of Discrimination against Women. Concluding observations: Myanmar. New York: United Nations, 2008. (CEDAW/C/MMR/CO/3).

35. UN Committee on the Elimination of Discrimination against Women. Concluding observations: Slovenia. New York: United Nations, 2008: paras. 35–36. (CEDAW/C/SVN/CO/4).

36. UN Committee on the Elimination of Discrimination against Women. Concluding com-

ments: Kazakhstan. New York: United Nations, 2007: paras. 25–26. (CEDAW/C/KAZ/CO/2).

37. UN Committee on the Elimination of Discrimination against Women. Concluding comments: Chile. New York: United Nations, 2006: para. 19. (CEDAW/C/CHI/CO/4).

38. UN Committee on the Elimination of Discrimination against Women. Concluding comments: Serbia. New York: United Nations, 2007: para. 33. (CEDAW/C/SCG/CO/1).

39. UN Committee on the Elimination of Discrimination against Women. Concluding comments: the former Yugoslav Republic of Macedonia. New York: United Nations, 2006: para. 32. (CEDAW/C/ MKD/CO/3).

40. UN Committee on the Elimination of Discrimination against Women. Concluding comments: Azerbaijan. New York: United Nations, 2007: paras. 25–26. (CEDAW/C/AZE/CO/3).

41. UN Committee on the Elimination of Discrimination against Women. Concluding comments: Suriname. New York: United Nations, 2007: paras. 31–32. (CEDAW/C/SUR/CO/3).

42. UN Special Rapporteur on the right of everyone to the enjoyment of the highest attainable standard of physical and mental health (Hunt P). (The rights to sexual and reproductive health) Geneva: United Nations, 16 February 2004. (E/CN.4/2004/49).

43. Grover A. UN Special Rapporteur on the right of everyone to the enjoyment of the highest attainable standard of physical and mental health—criminalisation of sexual and reproductive health. Geneva: United Nations, Aug 3, 2011. (A/66/254).

44. Center for Reproductive Rights. In re access to emergency contraception in Colombia (amicus brief) (Colombian Council of State).

45. Mulama J. Contraceptives: stock-outs threaten family planning. Inter Press Service. May 15, 2009.

46. Nigeria: contraceptive stock-out puts more women on the brink. Daily Independent (Lagos). Nov 24, 2010.

47. Gathura G. Substandard drugs fast becoming threat to Kenyans. Daily Nation. Sept 27, 2009.

48. WHO. WHO model list of essential medicines: 17th list. Geneva: World Health Organization, 2011.

49. PATH, WHO, UNFPA. The interagency list of essential medicines for reproductive health. Geneva: World Health Organization, International Planned Parenthood Federation, John Snow, PATH, Population Services International, United Nations Population Fund, World Bank, 2006.

50. Bruce J. Fundamental elements of the quality of care: a simple framework. Stud Fam Plann 1990; 21: 61–91.

51. Koenig MA. The impact of quality of care on contraceptive use: evidence from longitudinal data from rural Bangladesh. Baltimore: Johns Hopkins University, 2003.

52. Arends-Kuenning M, Kessy FL. The impact of demand factors, quality of care and access to facilities on contraceptive use in Tanzania. J Biosoc Sci 2007; 39: 1–26.

53. RamaRao S, Lacuesta M, Costello M, Pangolibay B, Jones H. The link between quality of care and contraceptive use. Int Fam Plan Perspec 2003; 29: 76–83.

54. Sanogo D, RamaRao S, Jones H, N'diaye P, M'bow B, Diop CB. Improving quality of care and use of contraceptives in Senegal. Afr J Reprod Health 2003; 7: 57–73.

55. Pichon and Sajous vs France. European Court of Human Rights, application no. 49853/99. Admissibility decision. Oct 2, 2001.

56. Westeson J. Sexual health and human rights: European region. Geneva: International Council on Human Rights Policy, 2010.

57. FIGO Committee for the Ethical Aspects of Human Reproduction and Women's Health. Ethical guidelines on conscientious objection. Int J Gynaecol Obstet 2006; 92: 333–34.

58. WHO. Making decisions about contraceptive introduction: a guide for conducting assessments to broaden contraceptive choice and improve quality of care. Geneva: World Health Organization, 2002.

59. Alves JED. The context of family planning in Brazil. In: Cavenaghi S ed. Demographic transformations and inequalities in Latin America. Rio de Janeiro: Latin American Population Association, 2009: 297–302.

60. The family planning law of Brazil (no 9263), Art. 1.

61. WHO. Universal access to reproductive health: accelerated actions to enhance progress on Millennium Development Goal 5 through advancing Target 5B. Geneva: World Health Organization, 2011.

62. Oringanje C, Meremikwu MM, Eko H, Esu E, Meremikwu A, Ehiri JE. Interventions for preventing unintended pregnancies among adolescents. Cochrane Database Syst Rev 2009; 4: CD005215.

63. Robin L, Dittus P, Whitaker D, et al. Behavioral interventions to reduce incidence of HIV, STD, and pregnancy among adolescents: a decade in review. J Adolesc Health 2004; 34: 3–26.

64. Kirby D. The impact of schools and school

programs on adolescent sexual behaviour. J Sex Res 2002; 39: 2733.

65. Lazarus JV, Sihvonen-Riemenschneider H, Laukamm-Josten U, Wong F, Liljestrand J. Systematic review of interventions to prevent the spread of sexually transmitted infections, including HIV, among young people in Europe. Croat Med J 2010; 51: 74–84.

66. Michielsen K, Chersich MF, Luchters S, De Koker P, Van Rossem R, Temmerman M. Eectiveness of HIV prevention for youth in sub-Saharan Africa: systematic review and meta-analysis of randomized and nonrandomized trials. AIDS 2010; 24: 1193–202.

67. African Union, Maputo plan of action for the operationalisation of the continental policy framework for sexual and reproductive health and rights 2007–2010. Sp/MIN/CAMH/5(I). Addis Ababa: African Union, 2006.

68. Ministers of Health and Education in Latin America and the Caribbean. Ministerial declaration: preventing through education. First meeting of Ministers of Health and Education to stop HIV and STIs in Latin America and the Caribbean; Mexico City, Mexico; Aug 1, 2008.

69. Santelli J, Ott MA, Lyon M, Rogers J, Summers D. Abstinence-only education policies and programs: a position paper of the Society for Adolescent Medicine. J Adolesc Health 2006; 38: 83–87.

70. Santelli J, Ott MA, Csete J, Samant S, Czuczka D. Abstinence only until marriage programs in the United States of America (USA): science and human rights. In: O'Dea J ed. Current issues and controversies in school and community health, sport and physical education. New York: Nova Science Publishers, 2012.

71. Potts H. Accountability and the right to the highest attainable standard of health. Colchester: University of Essex, 2008.

72. Minister of Heath vs Treatment Action Campaign. South Africa Constitutional Court, case CCT 9/02. July 5, 2002.

73. Tribunal Superior de Justicia de la Ciudad Autónoma de Buenos Aires, Argentina, Liga de Amas de Casa, Consumidores y Usuarios de la República Argentina y otros c/CGBA s/acción declarativa de inconstitucionalidad. Oct 14, 2003.

74. Constitutional Tribunal of Peru. Decision 7435-2006-PC/TC. Nov 13, 2006.

75. Council State of Colombia. Decision 11001-03-24-000-2002-00251-01. June 5, 2008.

76. Supreme Court of Mexico. Decision CC 54/2009. May 26, 2010.

77. Smeaton vs Secretary of State for Health. England and Wales Supreme Court of Justice. April 18, 2002.

78. K L vs Peru. UN Human Rights Committee, communication no 1153/2003. Nov 22, 2005. (CCPR/C/85/D/1153/2003).

79. A,B, and C vs Ireland. European Court of Human Rights, application no 25579/05. Dec 16, 2010.

80. Center for Reproductive Rights, Federation of Women Lawyers— Kenya (FIDA). Failure to deliver: violations of women's human rights in Kenyan health facilities. New York: Center for Reproductive Rights, 2007.

81. Lichuma W. The role of national human rights institutions in reduction of maternal mortality: a case study of the Kenya National Commission on Human Rights. Sept 2, 2010. http://righttomaternalhealth.org/roundtable-presentations (accessed Aug 18, 2011).

82. EnGendeRights. Advancing reproductive rights using the inquiry procedure of the OP CEDAW and the UN special procedures: the Philippine experience. Manila: EnGendeRights, 2009.

83. De La Cruz-Florez vs Peru. Inter-American Court of Human Rights (merits, reparations and costs). Nov 18, e2004.

84. Open Door Counselling Ltd and Dublin Well Women Centre Ltd and others vs Ireland. European Court of Human Rights, application no. 14234/88. Oct 29, 1992.

85. Women on Waves and others vs Portugal. European Court of Human Rights, application no. 31276/05. Feb 3, 2009.

86. UN Commission on Information and Accountability for Women's and Children's Health. Keeping promises, measuring results. Geneva: UN, 2011: recommendations 7 and 10.

87. Backman, G, Hunt P, Khosla R, et al. Health systems and the right to health: an assessment of 194 countries. Lancet 2008; 372: 2047–85.

88. UN Committee on Economic, Social and Cultural Rights (CESCR). General comment no. 3: the nature of States parties obligations (art 2, par 1). Dec 14, 1990. Geneva: United Nations, 2000.

89. UN Office of the High Commissioner for Human Rights. Human rights and poverty reduction: a conceptual framework. New York and Geneva: United Nations, 2004: 22–26.

90. UN Office of the High Commissioner for Human Rights. Principles and guidelines for a human rights approach to poverty reduction strategies, Geneva: United Nations, 2006: guideline 4.

91. UN Office of the High Commissioner for Human Rights and WHO. Human rights, health and poverty reduction strategies. Geneva: World Health Organization, 2008.

92. Hunt P. UN Special Rapporteur on the right

of everyone to the enjoyment of the highest attainable standard of physical and mental health. Mission to India. Geneva: United Nations, 2010. (A/HRC/14/20/Add.2).

93. UN Special Rapporteur on the right of everyone to the enjoyment of the highest attainable standard of physical and mental health (Hunt P). Supplementary note on the UN Special Rapporteur's Report on maternal mortality in India. Geneva: United Nations, 2010: section III.

94. WHO. The world health report—health systems nancing: the path to universal coverage. Geneva: World Health Organization, 2010

95. Cottingham JC, Kismodi E, Martin Hilber A, Lincetto O, Stahlhofer M, Gruskin S. Using human rights for sexual and reproductive health: improving legal and regulatory frameworks. Bull World Health Organ 2010; 88: 551–55.

QUESTIONS

1. The chapter argues that to meet the unmet need for family planning will require changes in laws, policies and programs that are consistent with human rights standards. What other factors are important in ensuring access to adequate contraception information and services? What role do human rights norms and standards have to play in ensuring these additional factors are adequately addressed?

2. The chapter discusses how specific groups of women, including displaced women, women working in stigmatized occupations such as sex work, women living with HIV, etc. have little to no access to contraceptive services. Consider examples of restrictive laws, policies or programs that you are aware of that inhibit specific groups from accessing contraceptive information and services. What can be done to ensure access for these specific groups? How can human rights be helpful?

3. Examine the seven priority measures suggested by the authors to eliminate the unmet need for family planning. In a situation of limited resources, would implementation of these seven measures be realistic? How would you prioritize? Is there anything missing from the list? How can public health and human rights goals support actions in these areas?

FURTHER READING

1. Santelli, J., Ott, M.A., Lyon, M., Rogers, J. & Summers, D., Abstinence-only until Marriage Programs: A Position Paper of the Society for Adolescent Medicine, *Journal of Adolescent Health*, 2006; 38: 83–87. http://www.adolescenthealth.org/AM/Template.cfm?Section=Position_Papers&Template=/CM/Content-Display.cfm&ContentID=1461.

2. Lazdane, G., The Role of Policies in the Area of Sexual and Reproductive Health in Accelerating Progress in Improving Access and Quality of Services. *European Journal of Contraception & Reproductive Health Care*, 2012; 17, S14. http://0-search.proquest.com.oasys.lib.oxy.edu/docview/1017547984/13863BAE4A94119B81C/13?accountid=12935

3. Tripathy, P. et al., Effect of a Participatory Intervention with Women's Groups on Birth Outcomes and Maternal Depression, in Jharkhand and Orissa, India: A Cluster-Randomized Controlled Trial. *Lancet*, 2010; 375: 1182–92.

Assisted Reproduction: Canada's Supreme Court and the "Global Baby"

George J. Annas

The debate in the U.S. Supreme Court about whether it is legitimate for the justices to consider the opinions of courts in other countries is ongoing. There is no parallel debate about the relevance of medical findings from other countries, because human anatomy and physiology are universal. Law is jurisdictional. There are, nonetheless, lessons that U.S. Supreme Court justices, health care regulators, and physicians can learn from legal controversies in foreign courts. The recent decision of the Canadian Supreme Court on the regulation of reproductive medicine is a prime example, especially because it divided the court in a five-to-four decision, giving both sides the opportunity to express strongly held views.[1]

Because it centers on babies and pregnancy and is fostered by the creation of extracorporeal embryos and the private recruitment of "surrogate mothers," reproductive medicine has proved impossible to regulate at the federal level in the United States and formidable to regulate at the state level.[2] More recently, the Internet, Facebook, and Twitter have helped to promote an international trade in reproductive medicine that could ultimately make even national regulation ineffective. A *Wall Street Journal* article, subtitled "Assembling the Global Baby," concisely described the current state of disarray in reproductive medicine: "With an international network of surrogate mothers and egg and sperm donors, a new industry is emerging to produce children on the cheap and outside the reach of restrictive laws."[3]

International norms themselves are unlikely to be followed because of the lack of national laws to give them teeth. Thus, human-rights advocates who think that only international standards can prevent reproductive medicine from becoming a branch of international trafficking in women and children are greatly concerned that the two major national regulatory agencies in reproductive medicine—the United Kingdom's Human Fertilisation and Embryology Authority and Canada's Assisted Human Reproduction Agency—are both under attack. The United Kingdom's agency may survive, but it was slated by the government to be discontinued for budgetary reasons.[4] Canada's agency has been gutted by Canada's Supreme Court, primarily on the basis that reproductive medicine, like all other medical practice, should be regulated at the provincial level, not at the national level.[1] Of course, the question of what should be regulated (and what should be outlawed altogether) is a much more important substantive question than the jurisdictional one of what level of government should be responsible for regulation.

CANADA'S ASSISTED HUMAN REPRODUCTION ACT

Canada established the Royal Commission on New Reproductive Technologies (the Baird Commission), chaired by pediatrician Patricia Baird, in 1989. In 1993, the commission issued what is still the most comprehensive public-policy document on the subject, its two-volume report, *Proceed with Care*.[5] The report made a series of recommendations, including recommendations that some practices be outlawed and that many others be subject to regulatory oversight, including special licensing. Legislative proposals were put before Parliament, and in 2004 Canada enacted the Assisted Human Reproduction Act.[6] The province of Quebec, never entirely comfortable with federal rules, sought judicial review of major parts of the act on the basis that it exceeded the authority of the federal government.[7] The Supreme Court of Canada issued its decision at the end of 2010.

On the basis of the federal government's powers to enact criminal laws, Canada's act outlaws specific acts countrywide (prohibited activities) and sets up a national oversight panel to regulate reproductive medicine through licensing and regulatory standards (controlled activities).[6] The province of Quebec, which only recently enacted its own law on the subject,[7] brought suit against the federal government challenging most of the provisions of the law as trespassing on provincial jurisdiction over health and social services. Only two sections of the act's criminal prohibitions, both involving consent, were challenged. Section 8 requires written consent for a number of procedures, including posthumous use of gametes, embryo creation, and embryo research. Section 9 prohibits obtaining sperm or ova from anyone younger than 18 years of age for any purpose other than to preserve the gametes for the person's future procreation.[6]

The unchallenged criminal prohibitions include acts that were once thought to be so universally condemned that prohibitions against them could be incorporated in an international treaty.[8] These prohibitions include the knowing creation of a human clone, the creation of an embryo from the cell of a human fetus or from another embryo, the maintenance of an embryo ex utero for more than 14 days after fertilization, the use of sex-selection techniques for a reason other than the diagnosis of a sex-linked disorder, the performance of germline genetic engineering, the use of nonhuman life forms with human gametes, the creation of chimeras for any purpose, and the creation of hybrids for reproduction. The other major prohibitions explicitly reject the U.S. market model by outlawing the commercialization of human reproduction—including banning the purchase and sale of human sperm, ova, and embryos—and payment for the "services" of "surrogate mothers."[6]

The major issue in the case is whether and to what extent Canada's federal government has the constitutional authority to regulate the practice of reproductive medicine and medical research. The act placed this authority in the hands of the federal government by establishing a new federal regulatory agency with licensing and inspection powers, the Assisted Human Reproduction Agency. Four justices concluded that the federal government could lawfully establish the Assisted Human Reproduction Agency to regulate the entire area (as proposed by the Baird Commission), four justices concluded that the federal government could regulate none of it, and one justice concluded that it could regulate some of it (and he provided the fifth and deciding vote in the case).

THE ARGUMENT IN FAVOR OF FEDERAL REGULATION

Chief Justice Beverley McLachlin wrote the opinion of the four justices who concluded that all the provisions of the act were constitutional as valid exercises of federal power over criminal law (unlike criminal law in the United States, criminal law in Canada is a federal power). The first paragraph of her opinion summarizes it well:

> Among the most important moral issues faced by this generation are questions arising from technologically assisted reproduction—the artificial creation of human life.... The question on appeal is whether this [new criminal] law represents a proper exercise of Parliament's criminal law power. I conclude that it does.[1]

According to the chief justice, whether the act is constitutional depends on whether its dominant purpose is to prohibit "practices that would undercut moral values, produce public health evils, and threaten the security of donors, donees, and persons conceived by assisted reproduction."[1] She concluded, contrary to the Quebec Court of Appeal, that even though jurisdiction over medical practice and research is provincial, there is a realm of "overlapping" jurisdiction broad enough to encompass federal use of criminal law to regulate reproductive medicine.

For the chief justice, the critical issue was whether the dominant matter (usually referred to in Canada as the "pith and substance") of the entire statute was criminal in nature, and therefore within federal jurisdiction. In her opinion, the act was fundamentally a series of criminal prohibitions followed by a "set of subsidiary provisions for their administration" that only "incidentally permits beneficial practices through regulations."[1] She addressed two questions to arrive at this conclusion: Is the act within the scope of federal criminal power? And does the act serve a valid criminal-law purpose?

The central issue regarding federal powers involves the extent to which the act seeks to regulate the practice of medicine and

medical research, because these are areas of provincial authority. This is a crucial question because the "doctrine of paramountcy" (what is called "supremacy" in the United States) holds that federal law would prevail over provincial law in areas in which they conflict such that federal law "would effectively oust provincial power over health." The chief justice concluded that the regulations are only "carve-outs" for specific practices that Parliament does not wish to prohibit, and the act specifically permits provinces to adopt regulations that are as strict as or stricter than those of the federal government. She also concluded that the act is valid as an exercise to uphold central moral issues, to combat a "legitimate public health evil," and to protect personal security. In this context, she noted that evil simply involves "any injurious or undesirable effect" of a procedure or product. Having determined that the act as a whole is constitutional, she then reviewed each of the contested provisions in the act and determined that each either itself constitutes a valid criminal law or is a "legitimate ancillary provision" designed to supplement rather than exclude provincial legislation."[1]

It is worth underlining that the only issue in this case is federal jurisdiction; this case is not about whether any provision in the act infringes on individual liberties in an unconstitutional manner. This is a central question that is left to another day—and has not been decided by any supreme court in the world to date.

ARGUMENTS THAT THE CHALLENGED PROVISIONS OF THE ACT ARE UNCONSTITUTIONAL

In an opinion written by Justices Louis LeBel and Marie Deschamps, four other justices found that all of the challenged provisions were beyond the constitutional power of the federal government because they "belong to the jurisdiction of the provinces over hospitals, civil rights and local matters." To determine whether the act was a justified use of federal criminal-law power, these justices found it necessary to delve more deeply into the legislative history of the act, most importantly into the Baird Commission report. This report divided the new reproductive medicine into two categories: those that should be prohibited by the criminal law and those that should be overseen by a national regulatory body.[5] In determining which procedures should be in each category, Parliament set forth a statement of principles at the beginning of the act, including that "the health and well-being of children born through the application of assisted reproductive technologies must be given priority in all decisions respecting their use, and the health and well-being of women must be protected."[6]

On the basis of the recommendations of the Baird Commission, the principles set forth by Parliament, and the language of the act itself, the four justices concluded that, other than the criminal prohibitions that were not challenged, the statutory scheme to regulate or "control" assisted reproduction did not involve the regulation of an "evil" but rather of a "good." Therefore, its dominant characteristic could not reasonably be seen as within the authority of federal criminal law.[1] Conceding that federal licensing would not necessarily conflict with provincial regulation, the justices nonetheless argued that federal requirements could "at the very least, result in extensive duplication in the requirements of the two levels of government ... with all its potential for red tape," and would "have a significant impact on the practice of medicine."[1]

The justices agreed that the prohibited activities are a reasonable exercise of federal criminal jurisdiction, but they found that the controlled activities correspond to regulation of the practice of medicine, a

provincial jurisdiction. As the justices conclude, "the purpose and the effects of the provisions [on the controlled activities] ... relate to the regulation of a specific type of health services provided in health-care institutions by health-care professionals to individuals who for pathological or physiological reasons need help to reproduce. Their pith and substance must be characterized as the regulation of assisted human reproduction as a health service."[1] This purpose is to be contrasted with criminal law that is designed to "suppress an evil," including permitting the federal government "to deal with and make laws with regard to new realities, such as pollution, and genetic manipulations that are considered undesirable ... [or] reprehensible."[1]

Because it is designed to "create" children and often uses genetically unrelated women to aid in this goal, reproductive medicine can properly be treated as uniquely deserving additional regulatory oversight. Nonetheless, as these four justices saw it, Parliament's "true objective was ... to establish national standards [of medical practice in reproductive medicine] ... which is unacceptable under the constitutional principles that ground Canadian federalism."[1]

THE DECISION OF THE TIE BREAKING JUSTICE

Justice Thomas Cromwell cast the deciding vote in this otherwise four-to-four opinion, and he split his own decision between the two in a frustratingly brief opinion. In his view, the central issue was whether its federal criminal-law power permitted Parliament "to regulate virtually all aspects of research and clinical practice in relation to assisted human reproduction."[1] He concluded that the answer to his question is no, but he nonetheless found that the "controlled" activities contain some provisions that are within federal criminal-law authority. These include the provisions on consent, including the age of consent, because consent falls "within the traditional boundaries of criminal law."[1, 6] Similarly, Cromwell upheld section 12, which prohibits any payment, other than reimbursement of expenses for sperm or ovum donations, or for "surrogate mother" services unless they are in accordance with regulations. The licensing and enforcement provisions of the act, however, are constitutional only as they relate to the issues of consent and expense reimbursement, and not to the practice of medicine, including the practice of reproductive medicine.[1, 6] This limitation, of course, guts the Assisted Human Reproduction Agency's oversight authority.

THE CANADIAN BOTTOM LINE

The heart of the majority opinion (and of the Baird Commission report) is that reproductive medicine is a branch of the practice of medicine, and since regulation of the practice of medicine is a provincial power, regulation of reproductive medicine is not constitutional when conducted by the federal government (unless it involves the prohibition of an activity that is inherently "evil"). Once the justices reached the conclusion that practices (and potential practices) in the field of reproductive medicine could be separated into "evil" ones, such as cloning, germline genetic engineering, and commercialization of human gametes and pregnancy, and legitimate or "good" ones, such as in vitro fertilization and noncommercial gamete donation and surrogacy, it was a logical step, at least for five of the justices, to divide federal and provincial jurisdiction along these lines.

The core criminal-law prohibitions of the federal act were upheld, as well as the national regulatory scheme needed to enforce them. However, the author-ity of the new federal regulatory agency is now limited to enforcing these criminal prohibitions, and it cannot require a special license for physicians or health care institutions to carry out other research or medical practices in assisted reproduction. If specifically regulated at all, research and treatment activities involving assisted reproduction must be done on the provincial level. It seems likely that many of the provinces will now take steps to regulate them. To the extent that there are major differences among the provinces, however, patients may travel from one province to another to avoid what they see as overly strict regulation. Far from settling the law in Canada, in my opinion the Canadian Supreme Court has managed to make it more fragmented and confusing.

U.S. AND GLOBAL IMPLICATIONS

The implications for the United States are reasonably straightforward. In the United States, there are no federal criminal prohibitions such as those in Canada's act. The federal government in the United States does not have direct criminal-law authority. Rather, to enact a criminal law, the U.S. federal government must derive its power from another specific power granted to it in the Constitution. In research-related activities, the most likely source is the commerce clause, and the federal government could, for example, prohibit all of the acts prohibited in Canada under this clause.[9] Likewise, the practice of medicine has traditionally been seen as a state power in the United States, and the Supreme Court would probably conclude, as did Canada's, that it should continue to be regulated at the state level (at least unless Congress made a specific finding that uniform regulation of assisted reproduction was required under a national health care program that was itself grounded in commerce-clause authority).[10]

Unless and until the United States restricts commercialism in this area, Canadians seeking reproductive assistance involving the purchase of sperm or ova, payment to surrogate mothers, or all of these, will come to the United States to seek these services. In addition, because reproductive services are so expensive, many Canadians will probably seek them in other countries. India, for example, has a growing market in reproductive tourism, with only tangential involvement of physicians.[11] Just as multiple and diverse regulations affecting reproductive medicine on the state level in the United States have led to growing businesses in states that have little or no regulation, so will national laws encourage people to cross national boundaries to seek the services they want that are illegal or overly expensive in their own country. Only the development of international norms, adopted and followed by the medical profession itself, is likely to ever produce uniformity in global practices.[12]

The Canadian case focused on federalism, and it did not assess the human rights of the people using assisted reproductive services, the ovum donors, the surrogate mothers, or the resulting children. Thus, for example, the questions of whether the children who have resulted from the use of assisted reproductive techniques have a right to know the identity of their genetic parents, and whether surrogate mothers have the right to change their minds and retain custody of the children they give birth to, remain unresolved.[12–16] Medical commercialization is commonplace around the world, but the vast majority of countries in the world reject commercialism involving human reproduction and the gametes and women used to make babies, as well as the babies themselves. Therefore, it seems plausible to add women and children in the reproductive medicine marketplace to current treaties that prohibit trafficking in humans "for sex and labor."[17, 18]

Canadian novelist Margaret Atwood has, for example, written eloquently of how easy it is to dehumanize women whose only use to others is to bear children. In the words of the narrator of her novel *The Handmaid's Tale*, "We are two-legged wombs, that's all: sacred vessels, ambulatory chalices."[19]

The Canadian experience illustrates the multifaceted barriers to regulating assisted human reproduction. Perhaps existing legal regulatory mechanisms, rather than medical ethics and professional standards, are incapable of performing this task. Currently, however, international ethical norms are inadequate to set practice standards for reproductive tourism or to keep pace with the reach of modern communications. Trafficking in babies can (and probably will) get worse.[20] Governments should consistently categorize assisted reproduction as the practice of medicine, and physicians should set and follow high ethical standards to protect the health and welfare of women and children. If the medical community cannot control assisted reproductive procedures that require the application of medical skills, an unregulated market will determine the price, place, and manner in which human sperm, ova, embryos, and services of surrogate mothers will be made available as well as how family relationships with the resulting babies will be structured. The "global baby" has arrived in practice, but neither legal theory nor medical ethics has kept pace with the globalization of human reproduction.

REFERENCES

1. Attorney General of Canada v. Attorney General of Quebec, 410 N.R. 199, 2010 SCC 61 (2010).
2. Assisted reproductive technologies: analysis and recommendations for public policy. New York: New York State Task Force on Life and the Law, 1998.
3. Audi T, Chang A. Assembling the global baby. Wall Street Journal. December 10, 2010:D1-D2.

4. Human Fertilisation and Embryology Authority, Human Tissue Authority, House of Lords Proceedings. February 1, 2011.

5. Proceed with care: final report of the Royal Commission on new reproductive technologies. Ottawa: Canada Communications Group, 1993.

6. Assisted Human Reproduction Act (Canada), S.C. 2004, c. 2.

7. Attorney General of Quebec v. Attorney General of Canada, 2008 QCCA 1167, 298 D.L.R. 1551 (2008).

8. Annas GJ, Andrews LB, Isasi RM. Protecting the endangered human: toward an international treaty prohibiting cloning and inheritable alterations. Am J Law Med 2002;28:151–78.

9. Reproduction and responsibility: the regulation of new biotechnologies. Washington, DC: President's Council on Bioethics, 2004.

10. Gonzales v. Oregon, 546 U.S. 243 (2006).

11. Carney S. The red market: on the trail of the world's organ brokers, bone thieves, blood farmers, and child traffickers. New York: William Morrow, 2011:135–51.

12. Annas GJ. The changing face of family law: global consequences of embedding physicians and biotechnology in the parent-child relationship. Fam Law Q 2008;42:511–28.

13. Robertson JR. Reproductive rights and reproductive technology in 2030. Washington, DC: Governance Studies at Brookings, January 21, 2011.

14. Fukuyama F, Furger F. Beyond bioethics: a proposal for modernizing regulation of human biotechnologies. Washington, DC: Paul H. Nitze School of Advanced International Studies, 2007.

15. Somerville M. Children's rights and unlinking child–parent biological bonds with adoption, same-sex marriage and new reproductive technologies. J Family Studies 2007;13: 179–201.

16. Coeytaux F, Darnovsky M, Fogel SB. Assisted reproduction and choice in the biotech age: recommendations for a way forward. Contraception 2011;83:1–4.

17. Joint Council of Europe/United Nations Study. Trafficking in organs, tissues and cells and trafficking in human beings for the purpose of the removal of organs. Strasbourg, France: Council of Europe, 2009.

18. Todres J. Moving upstream: the merits of a public health approach to human trafficking. North Carol Law Rev 2011;89:447–506.

19. Atwood M. The handmaid's tale. Boston: Houghton Mifflin, 1986:176.

20. Chayutworakan S. Pregnant Vietnamese sent home: police hunt for Taiwanese suspect in surrogacy gang. Bangkok Post. May 31, 2011.

QUESTIONS

1. As described in the chapter, how does human trafficking relate to laws governing assisted reproduction?

2. The author discusses Canadian law which bans the "commercialization of human reproduction" including banning the purchase and sale of human sperm, ova and embryos—and payment for 'services' of 'surrogate mothers.'" Make a principled argument for or against the commercialization of human reproduction. The Canadian government believes that commercialization almost necessarily would lead to exploitation of women. Do you agree?

3. The author remarks that the Canadian Supreme Court leaves to another day the question of whether there is a human right to reproduce that is broad enough to include the right to use a "surrogatge mother" if necessary. Discuss the relevant human rights of the infertile woman who wants to rear a child, and of the fertile woman who wants to carry a child for the infertile woman and give it to the infertile woman to raise after birth. Does it make any sense to say that the child has rights in this situation as well? Is it helpful to consider how the right to family planning might affect recognition of a right to assisted reproduction?

FURTHER READING

1. Ehrenreich, Nancy, *The Reproductive Rights Reader.* New York: New York University Press, 2008.
2. Cook, Rebecca J., Dickens, Bernard M., & Fathalla, Mahmoud F., *Reproductive Health and Human Rights: Integrating Medicine, Ethics, and Law.* Oxford: Clarendon Press, 2003.
3. Robertson, John, *Children of Choice.* Princeton: Princeton University Press, 1994.
4. Harris, John, *Enhancing Evolution: The Ethical Case for Making Better People.* Princeton: Princeton University Press, 2007.

POINT OF VIEW

Enhancing the Role of Men for Gender Equality and Reproductive Rights

Aminata Touré

If men are to play a critical role in women's realization of their reproductive rights, it has to be a win-win game. The potential gain for men needs to be clearly articulated, particularly in societies where men's power and social hegemony remains largely uncontested or in places where the day-to-day privileges that men enjoy, far surpass those of women. In such contexts, men's role in achieving women's reproductive rights cannot be treated only as a vehicle to improve women's situation, the fulfillment of men's specific needs and rights, especially those who are marginalized by poverty, deserve greater attention. The first step, however, is to overcome the resistance of men.

Where resistance by men to positive involvement in women's free enjoyment of reproductive rights exists, this stems from the unequal power relations between women and men. The realization of reproductive rights for both men and women requires gender equality, which ultimately means redefining and balancing power dynamics between men and women. Certain men resist gender equality in active, hostile and sometimes organized ways. But for others, resistance is more insidious. To address men's resistance where it does exist, it is useful to understand men's relations to power in personal life, professional life, politics, economics and policy-making. Resistance comes for a wide variety of reasons: patriarchal practices, sexism, maintenance of power, perception of gender

equality as "women's business," and the belief that gender issues are not the main or most important concerns in Development are only some of the myriad reasons cited. Therefore, changing men's relations to women entails changing men's relations to power, and there are good examples of how this can be done. In Niger, for example, the United Nations Population Fund (UNFPA) experimented with engaging men in supporting women's safe delivery and family planning. The project selected respected men whose wives were of reproductive age and sensitized them about safe pregnancy, the positive advantages of family planning and the nefarious effects of girls' early marriage and denial of schooling, as well as violence against women. In eight years, there was a significant drop in maternal mortality in the areas covered by the programme and evaluations showed men to have much more positive attitudes towards women, and women's reproductive health.

Men, however, are not the only ones resisting their participation in gender quality programmes. There has been much resistance on the part of women activists against the involvement of men in gender and development work as well. Fears about dilution of the feminist agenda and anxieties over the diversion of limited resources, away, for example, from women's empowerment initiatives and back into the hands of men, keep some women activists opposing the idea. Yet at the level of institutions and states, budget allocations for gender equality programmes, are a valuable measurement tool that can be used to gauge commitment beyond political window-dressing.

The significant gains to be had in involving men and boys in gender equality efforts, especially for the longer-term, deserves greater attention. This will contribute to rearing the next generation of boys and girls in a culture of equality as well as respect for human rights. Shifting the attitudes and behaviours of men and boys should also improve the lives of women and girls in the home, the workplace, and the community. Involving men may help to create wider consensus and support on issues which have previously been marginalized or seen as "of interest to women only" (e.g., violence in the family, sexual and reproductive health).

What are the specific areas where partnership with men is possible and desirable? Involving men can be a prominent part of ensuring attention not only to family planning but to a broader reproductive health agenda. Efforts to involve men in ways that transform gender relations and promote gender equality can contribute to a broader development and rights agenda.

Another critical area where strengthening men's involvement will help promote gender equality and reproductive rights is gender-based violence. Gender-based violence is related to the construction of masculinities informed by belief systems, cultural norms and socialization processes. In many societies, men are central to most acts of violence. The social pressures to perform as males can encourage them to compete, resort to violence or take sexual risks to demonstrate their "manliness." Although gender norms are often rigid and limiting, they are not static. Positive alternatives can be cultivated. The notion of strength, for example, can lead to violent behaviour, but can also find expression in resisting peer pressure or in protecting oneself and loved ones. This idea was successfully taken up by the "real men" campaign in Brazil supported by the NGO Promundo. The campaign aimed to shift masculinity paradigms among youngsters caught in the culture of violence in poor neighbourhoods of Rio de Janeiro so as to reshape the vision of a real man as someone who would respect and protect his girlfriend instead of abusing her. Engaging men in preventive strategies is a critical component of ending gender-based violence.

Sometimes the way the message is framed can make all the difference. In some countries, telling young men that they have the right to be involved in their children's lives has had a positive impact, while framing their involvement as a duty or obligation—proved to have the opposite effect. Research shows that men in all parts of the world express an interest in supporting and becoming more involved in the reproductive health of their partners. But negative feedback from other men, family members and employers, as well as resistance by health providers, may prevent men from putting any such interest into practice. They may be uncomfortable with rigid gender norms, but at the same time, unable to challenge them without the support of peers and a conducive social environment.

Connecting with boys and young men may offer the greatest opportunity for the future by instilling gender equitable values early on. Most school curricula do not provide for young people to learn relationship skills, discuss norms and peer pressures, or raise questions. School might seem a strategic place to target adolescent boys, but consideration has to be given also to impoverished or marginalized adolescents boys who are not in school. Boys who grow up around positive male, and female, role models are more likely to question gender inequities and harmful stereotypes. It is high time for more systematic engagement of men and boys in reproductive health programming. Only through such efforts can we build a culture of gender equality which would, in turn, advance women's reproductive rights.

Aminata Touré is the Minister of Justice of the Government of the Republic of Senegal, and former senior staff of the United Nations Population Programme.

CHAPTER 28

On the "Rights" Track: The Importance of a Rights-Based Approach to Reducing Maternal Deaths

Helen de Pinho

The Millennium Development Goals (MDGs), in particular MDG 5, have sharpened the world's focus on the critical need to reduce maternal mortality. Commitments have been made. One hundred and eighty nine countries signed on to the MDGs, committing their governments to achieving a 75% reduction in maternal mortality (based on the 1990 figure) by the year 2015. International development partners have committed significant resources towards decreasing the number of women and newborns dying as a result of obstetric complications. NGOs have committed to advocating for action globally and locally to reduce maternal deaths. And at national levels in most developing countries there exists a strategic plan, a Road Map, a programme of work, even a budget—all geared towards reducing maternal mortality. But there has been little action. There is a huge gap between the plans and the actions, the rhetoric and the reality. It is generally recognized that of all the MDGs, progress towards meeting MDG 5 is deemed to have stalled.[1]

And yet the causes of maternal deaths are known, the interventions have been clearly articulated and the WHO estimates that 88–98% of maternal deaths are preventable.[2] Direct obstetric causes, which make up about 80% of all maternal deaths, are due to haemorrhage, pregnancy related hypertension and eclampsia, sepsis, complications secondary to unsafe abortions and obstructed labour. Increasingly in some countries, women are also dying of causes related to HIV or malaria.

There is general consensus that a three-pronged strategy is necessary to reduce these maternal deaths: All women must have access to contraception to avoid unintended pregnancies; all pregnant women must have access to skilled care at the time of birth; and all women who experience complications in pregnancy and childbirth must have timely access to quality emergency obstetric care.[3] This in turn requires a functioning and sustainable health system that engages communities and facilities[4] and that makes sure that health services are accessible to all women where the notion of accessibility encompasses principles of affordability, acceptability and availability.

The task is enormous. In many developing countries, the capacity of health systems to respond to the quiet tsunami of maternal deaths is questionable. In these countries, health systems have deteriorated over the past three decades, some as a result of conflict, others because of a systematic undermining of government health systems and, in a handful of countries, as a result of inadequate governance.

Strengthening health systems will take more than simply tinkering around the edges. It will require a fundamental reframing of how governments perceive health systems, the health care they deliver, and specifically how they take action to reduce maternal deaths. As Lynn Freedman indicates, it is no longer about "business as usual".

Why the need to reframe the way in which governments and development partners think about health systems? In short—history matters.

In 1985, at the end of the UN Decade for Women, the World Health Organization (WHO) reported that over 500,000 women per year were dying as a result of obstetric complications. In the same year, Allan Rosenfield and Deborah Maine published their seminal article, "Maternal Mortality—A Neglected Tragedy: Where is the M in MCH [Maternal and Child Health]?",[5] challenging public health specialists to explain why most of the interventions traditionally bundled into maternal health care packages benefited the child and failed to address the key causes of maternal deaths. These two critical events galvanized the international community to focus on this previously disregarded and hidden crisis and led to the 1987 Safe Motherhood Conference in Kenya.[6]

The Nairobi Safe Motherhood Conference launched the Safe Motherhood Initiative which, in turn, saw the formation of the Safe Motherhood Inter-Agency Group and a series of regional and national conferences that sought to entrench safe motherhood as an "accepted and understood term in the public-health realm" and core component of reproductive health.[7] In her paper, "Safe Motherhood Initiative: 20 Years and Counting",[8] Starrs describes how public health specialists and women's health advocates worked together to develop a comprehensive approach to reducing maternal deaths. This broad approach required action within the health systems—expanding the core elements of maternal health including antenatal care, clean, safe delivery, essential obstetric care and postnatal care from within the community through to the referral levels, as well as action to increase women's status, provide good nutrition to young girls, educate communities and provide family planning.

And yet, more than twenty years later, the WHO continues to report that over 500,000 women per year die as a result of obstetric complications.[9] The overall picture has barely changed. WHO reports that 99% of these deaths occur in developing countries, 13 countries account for 67% of the deaths.[10] Further analysis of these numbers reveals huge inequities in the maternal mortality ratios (MMRs) between developed and developing countries, and similar orders of difference within countries—urban to rural. Whereas women in the developed world face MMRs of less than 20 deaths per 100,000 live births, translating into a lifetime risk of death of less than 1 in 7,300, this risk of dying increases exponentially to higher than 1 in 22, with MMRs soaring over 1,000 maternal deaths per 100,000 live births for women in many developing countries, especially parts of Africa and Asia.[11] Where there has been a small decrease in the maternal mortality ratio over the past 10 years—an average of 1% decline per year, this decline is amongst countries that already have relatively low levels of maternal deaths.[12]

WHAT WENT WRONG?

Maine and Rosenfield argue that the Safe Motherhood Initiative lacked strategic focus,[13] especially if compared to the successful Child Survival Initiative. The Child Survival Initiative provided government and international agencies with a compact set of interventions that stopped children from dying, interventions captured under the acronym GOBI—growth monitoring, oral rehydration, breast-feeding and immunization—all of which could be delivered, if necessary, in the community and outside of a health facility. In comparison, the Safe Motherhood initiative was much broader, each action "clearly worthy and important goals, (but) only one, essential obstetric care, includes actions that can substantially reduce maternal deaths."[14]

Without a strategic focus, the Safe Motherhood Initiative was carved up into a menu of separate interventions from which donors, international agencies and governments could select, usually according to their resource levels, political expedience and, perceived cost-efficient "quick wins" and short cuts. Often excluded from the menu selection were the more "controversial" interventions, including access to family planning and provision of safe abortion care. Anti-abortionists came to regard safe motherhood as the Trojan horse for the introduction of legal abortion, and donors and international agencies became wary of providing support to the Safe Motherhood Initiatives.[15]

Selected Safe Motherhood interventions were generally implemented vertically through programmes outside of the national health system, with a lot of duplication and with little cohesion between them. Moreover, they were seldom evaluated with regard to their impact on reducing maternal deaths and the interventions were often fuelled by misconceptions.

Two key misconceptions resulted in widespread adoption of interventions that forced efforts to reduce maternal deaths down the wrong track. The first was that complications in pregnancy or childbirth in women most at risk could be prevented or predicted. Adopting a risk approach would identify some "high risk" women and could indeed reduce deaths amongst these women. But, such a focus on high-risk prediction would also create a false sense of security, generating the belief that it is possible to identify all women who will develop complications and require emergency care. This is not actually possible. In absolute numbers, more "low risk" women develop complications unexpectedly. Unfortunately, amongst these "low risk" women complications tend to be recognized late, there are inadequate systems to ensure timely referral to emergency care, and upon reaching these health services, appropriate care may not be available.

The second misconception was that training scores of traditional birth attendants (TBAs) in developing countries to assist women delivering at home would reduce maternal deaths. As a result, governments and international agencies invested lots of energy and millions of dollars in training TBAs to work in the community—regarded as a high coverage, cost-efficient approach.[16] Unfortunately, while TBAs may improve the routine delivery care that mothers and newborns receive, and have some impact on reducing newborn deaths, research has shown that they have proved ineffective in significantly reducing the maternal mortality ratio.[17] The TBAs are seldom supported by health services, many are unable or unwilling to refer a woman requiring emergency care, and they lack the infrastructure and life-saving skills necessary to manage complications effectively.

It is not by chance that Safe Motherhood programmes initiated in the 1990s favoured low cost interventions that could be delivered outside of a health system, nor was it accidental that these programmes were characterized by selective interventions and vertical programmes oftentimes associated with user fees. The failure to reduce maternal deaths over the past thirty years, or to reverse significant inequity in access to lifesaving health care, cannot be divorced from a political context shaped by a broader set of neo-liberal macro-economic policies that framed the associated health sector reforms underfoot in the

1990s. These reforms argued for: Decreased government spending on social services including health services; a shrinking role for government as service provider while at the same time expanding the role for the private sector and markets; changes in priority-setting mechanisms, with a focus on cost-efficiency analyses; the introduction of user fees masked as community participation; and the development of "essential packages of care".[18] In essence, these policies represented a technical response that embraced the commodification of health care as a product to be bought and sold, benefiting those "consumers" with resources.[19]

An approach which suggests "more of the same" is just not acceptable. If we are serious about making sure that even the most vulnerable woman in the most rural part of a country has access to family planning, skilled attendance at birth and, access to emergency obstetric care without delays, then we need to do more than deliver a set of technical interventions.

HOW WOULD A RIGHTS-BASED APPROACH REDUCE MATERNAL MORTALITY?

The fundamental right to the highest attainable standard of health is enshrined in the International Covenant on Economic, Social and Cultural Rights,[20] as well as other international human rights treaties including the Convention on the Elimination of All Forms of Discrimination Against Women.[21] As a consequence of these treaties, every woman's life is given equal value, and thus every woman has the right to a safe pregnancy, delivery and post-natal outcome, and access to emergency obstetric care should she develop complications.

Securing the right to health is a necessary step towards maternal mortality reduction, but is not sufficient to ensure action. We know that rights embedded in treaties do not automatically translate into services on the ground,[22] but a rights-based approach does shape how governments respond to the crisis of maternal deaths in a manner that is fundamentally different to the efficiency driven neo-liberal approach experienced over the past four decades. This is important.

A rights-based approach demands that states reject the notion of health and the delivery of health care as a commodity to be bought and sold in an open market. A rights-based approach requires that states understand the dynamics of power at work in structuring health outcomes, in this instance maternal death, and make visible the connections between poverty, discrimination, inequality and health.[23] A rights-based approach is ultimately about how communities, governments, development partners and other key stakeholders identify these workings of power and then employ a set of practices to demand, implement, and ensure the rearrangements of power necessary for change,[24] offering a counter to the decades of systematic undermining of health services.

The strength of using a rights-based approach to improve maternal health and reduce maternal mortality is that it provides both the formal mechanisms to hold governments accountable and expose rights violations, as well as defining a developmental approach based on a set of principles and values that guide the progressive realization of these rights. These principles of equity, transparency, accountability, participation and nondiscrimination,[25] provide a lens that guides how maternal health policy should be made, priorities set, budgets made relevant, and programmes implemented.[26] In the context of resource strapped health services, a rights-based approach promotes systemic long term health system planning centred around a functioning health system necessary for sustained maternal mortality reduction.

WHAT DOES A RIGHTS-BASED APPROACH LOOK LIKE ON THE GROUND?

A rights-based approach should be evident in the coherent workings of government, development partners, international agencies and civil society. Examples of such actions include:

- An integrated approach to implementation—as seen in Malawi's implementation of their national Road Map to Reduce Maternal Mortality. This includes scaling-up access to basic emergency obstetric care through an overall strengthening of the health system—aligning health worker training, infrastructure development, procurement of drugs and supplies and attention to improved referral and communication systems.
- Health information systems that incorporate indicators to monitor both progress towards realizing access to emergency obstetric care and skilled attendance at birth, disaggregated according to social class, geographical regions, age and ethnicity.
- A willingness to seek innovative solutions to the human resource crisis through the use of non-physician clinicians to expand access to comprehensive emergency obstetric care even in the most remote districts—a strategy successfully deployed over the past three decades in Malawi, Mozambique and Tanzania.[27]
- Development of constructive accountability mechanisms that create an effective dynamic of entitlement and obligation between people and their government.[28] This requires not only the creation of spaces, both internal and external to government, for participation and engagement to occur, but also requires government to make more transparent its planning processes and priority setting criteria, and civil society to work together to translate available data into information that communities can use to hold government accountable.

We know that progress towards meeting MDG 5 is possible—countries such as Mozambique and Sri Lanka appear to be on track to meeting MDG 5. Hard experience tells us that technical interventions, while critical, are never enough. If the world is serious about reducing maternal deaths, that vision must be framed by a rights-based approach that guides hard political choices, setting priorities, confronting entrenched power interests, and a steadfast commitment to accountability.

REFERENCES

1. O. M. R. Campbell and W. J. Graham, 'Strategies for reducing maternal mortality: getting on with what works' 368(9543) *The Lancet* (2006), at 1284–99.
2. World Health Organization (WHO) *The World Health Report 2005: Make Every Mother and Child Count* (Geneva: World Health Organization, 2005).
3. UNFPA, 'Stepping Up Efforts to Save Mothers' Lives 2007', available at http://www.unfpa.org/mothers/index.htm.
4. L. P. Freedman, W. J. Graham, E. Brazier et al., 'Practical Lessons from Global Safe Motherhood Initiatives: Time for a New Focus on Implementation' 370(9595) *The Lancet* (2007), at 1383–91.
5. A. Rosenfield, D. Maine, 'Maternal Mortality—A Neglected Tragedy: Where's the M in MCH?' 2 (8446) *The Lancet* (1985), at 83–5.
6. A. M. Starrs 'Safe Motherhood Initiative: 20 Years and Counting' 368(9542) *The Lancet* (2006) 1130–2.
7. United Nations, 'Report of the International Conference on Population and Development', 18 October 1994, UN Doc. A/CONF.171/13.
8. A. M. Starrs, *supra* note 6.
9. United Nations, *The Millennium Development Goals Report 2008* (New York: United Nations, 2008).

10. WHO, UNICEF, UNFPA, *Maternal Mortality in 2000: Estimates Developed by WHO, UNICEF and UNFPA* (Geneva: World Health Organization, 2004).

11. United Nations, *supra* note 9.

12. 'Maternal Mortality Ratio Falling Too Slowly to Meet Goal', Joint News Release WHO/UNICEF/ UNFPA/World Bank, available at http://www. who.int/mediacentre/news/releases/2007/ pr56/en/print.html.

13. D. Maine and A. Rosenfield 'The Safe Motherhood Initiative: Why Has it Stalled?' 89(4) *American Journal of Public Health* (1999), at 480–2.

14. Ibid.

15. C. AbouZahr, 'Safe Motherhood: A Brief History of the Global Movement 1947–2002' 67 *British Medical Bulletin* (2003), at 13–25.

16. M. Koblinsky, 'Indonesia: 1990–1999', in M. Koblinsky (ed.) *Reducing Maternal Mortality: Learning From Bolivia, China, Egypt, Honduras, Indonesia, Jamaica and Zimbabwe* (Washington, DC: The World Bank, 2003).

17. Rosenfield and Maine, *supra* note 5.

18. H. de Pinho, 'Towards The "Right" Reforms: The Impact of Health Sector Reforms on Sexual and Reproductive Health' 48(4) *Development* (2005), at 61–8.

19. H. de Pinho, 'Conclusion: Towards the "Right" Reforms' in T. S. Ravindran and H. de Pinho (eds.) *The Right Reforms? Health Sector Reform and Sexual and Reproductive Health* (Johannesburg: Women's Health Project, School of Public Health, University of the Witwatersrand, 2005); L. P. Freedman, R. J. Waldman, H. de Pinho, M. E. Wirth, A. M. R. Chowdhury, A. Rosenfield, *Who's Got The Power? Transforming Health Systems For Women and Children* (New York: United Nations Development Programme, 2005).

20. Committee on Economic, Social and Cultural Rights (CESCR), *General Comment No. 14 on the right to the highest attainable standard of health*, 11 August 2000, UN Doc. E/C.12/2000/4.

21. Convention on the Elimination of All Forms of Discrimination Against Women (1979).

22. L. P. Freedman et al., *supra* note 19; A. E. Yamin, 'Will We Take Suffering Seriously? Ref lections on What Applying a Human Rights Framework to Health Means and Why We Should Care' 10(1) *Health and Human Rights* (2008).

23. Yamin, *supra* note 22.

24. L. P. Freedman et al., *supra* note 19.

25. A. E. Yamin, *supra* note 22; L. London 'What Is A Human Rights-Based Approach to Health and Does It Matter?' 10(1) *Health and Human Rights* (2008).

26. L. P. Freedman, 'Using Human Rights in Maternal Mortality Programs: From Analysis to Strategy' 75 *International Journal of Gynecology and Obstetrics* (2001) 51–60; P. Hunt, J. Bueno de Mesquita, 'Reducing Maternal Mortality: The Contribution of the Right to the Highest Attainable Standard Of Health' (New York: United Nations Population Fund and Human Rights Centre, University of Essex, 2007).

27. G. C hilopora, C. Pereira, F. Kamwendo et al., 'Postoperative Outcome of Caesarean Sections and Other Major Emergency Obstetric Surgery by Clinical Officers and Medical Officers in Malawi', *Human Resources for Health* (2007); C. Pereira, A. Cumbi, R. Malalane et al. 'Meeting The Need For Emergency Obstetrical Care in Mozambique: Work Performance and Work Histories of Medical Doctors and Assistant Medical Officers Trained For Surgery' 114 *British Journal Obstetrics Gynaecology* (2007), at 1253–1260.

28. L. P. Freedman, R. J. Waldman, H. de Pinho, M. E. Wirth, A. M. R. Chowdhury, A. Rosenfield, *Who's Got The Power? Transforming Health Systems for Women and Children* (New York: United Nations Development Programme, 2005).

QUESTIONS

1. Of all the Millennium Development Goals (MDG), why has MDG 5 in particular "stalled"?

2. The author proposes that the reforms to reduce maternal deaths were shaped by "broader" policies that were "underfoot" in the 1990s. These broader policies were characterized by "decreased government spending on social services including health services; a shrinking role of government as service provider while at the same time expanding the role of the private sector and markets . . ." Comment on this point as it applies to MDG 5. What inherent problems do you foresee in using this to frame the MDGs in general?

3. The author notes three countries as having facets of a rights-based approach to MDG 5 "on the ground." These countries are Malawi, Mozambique and Sri Lanka. Research one of these countries. Are there any indicators which suggest recent reductions in maternal deaths in these countries?

FURTHER READING

1. Kuruvilla, S., Bustreo, F., Hunt, P., Singh, A., et al., The Millennium Development Goals and Human Rights: Realizing Shared Commitments. *Human Rights Quarterly,* 2012; 34: 141–177.
2. Dixon-Mueller, R., & Germain, A., Fertility Regulation and Reproductive Health in the Millennium Development Goals: The Search for a Perfect Indicator. *American Journal of Public Health,* 2007; 97: 45–5.
3. Koblinsky, M., Anwar, I., Mridha, M. K., Chowdhury, M. E., & Botlero, R. Reducing Maternal Mortality and Improving Maternal Health: Bangladesh and MDG 5. *Journal of Health, Population and Nutrition,* 2008; 26: 280–94.

CHAPTER 29

Protection of Sexual and Reproductive Health Rights: Addressing Violence Against Women

Claudia García-Moreno and Heidi Stöckl

INTRODUCTION

Violence against women is one of the most widespread human rights violations as well as a public health problem in need of urgent attention. It is sometimes called gender-based violence as it is both maintained by, and in turn perpetuates, gender inequality that puts women and girls in subordinate positions. This violence has many devastating consequences for women's lives and their health, including their sexual and reproductive health, and their human rights.

Violence against women can take many forms: physical, sexual, and emotional. It can take place in the home, the community, and state institutions, and be perpetrated by intimate male partners, acquaintances, or strangers. In certain settings, such as those in conflict or involving displacement or in prisons, women may be at increased risk, particularly of sexual violence by both State and non-State actors.

Most of the data on the impact of violence on health comes from studies of either intimate partner violence or sexual violence. While recognizing that other forms of violence are important also, this chapter predominantly addresses these two forms. It provides an overview of the prevalence of this violence, its impact on women's sexual and reproductive health, and on their human rights. It considers the implications of this for health care provision and makes some recommendations for action.

VIOLENCE AGAINST WOMEN: PREVALENCE, RISK FACTORS, AND HEALTH CONSEQUENCES

The World Health Organization defines violence as: "The intentional use of physical force or power, threatened or actual ... that results in or has a high likelihood of resulting in injury, death, psychological harm, maldevelopment or deprivation." The inclusion of the word "power" broadens "the conventional understanding of violence to include those acts that result from a power relationship, including threats and intimidation."[1]

Intimate male partners are most often the main perpetrators of violence against women, a form of violence known as intimate partner violence, "domestic" violence or "spousal (or wife) abuse." Intimate partner violence and sexual violence, whether by partners, acquaintances or strangers, are common worldwide and disproportionately affect women, although are not exclusive to them. Other forms of violence such as trafficking also affect women and children more often. In situations of conflict, sexual violence against civilians, including men, is increasingly being documented.

Globally, studies have shown that:

- between 10% and 69% of women report that an intimate partner has physically abused them at least once in their lifetime;[2, 3]
- between 6% and 59% of women report attempted or completed forced sex by an intimate partner in their lifetime;[2]
- between 1% and 28% of women report they have been physically abused during pregnancy by an intimate partner;[2, 4]
- between 7% and 48% of adolescent girls and between 0.2% and 32% of adolescent boys report that their first experience of sexual intercourse was forced;[1]
- approximately 20% of women and 5%–10% of men report having been sexually abused as children;[5]
- between 0.3% and 12% of women report sexual violence by a non-partner,[2]
- it is estimated that 2.5 million people are trafficked every year,[6] the majority of them women and children.

Risk Factors for Intimate Partner Violence (and Sexual Violence)

Violence against women is a complex phenomenon driven by factors at the level of the individual woman, the perpetrator, the relationship and family, the community, and the society. Research has identified the following as common "risk factors" for intimate partner violence:[7] being young; witnessing or suffering family violence as a child; suffering sexual abuse as a child; alcohol and substance abuse; relationships characterized by inequality and power imbalance; poverty, economic stress, and unemployment; gender inequality; lack of institutional support or sanctions; and

social norms that support traditional gender norms, condone violence, or promote models of masculinity based on abuse of power and aggressiveness.

The majority of research on risk and protective factors has until recently been conducted in high-income countries and therefore needs to be tested for its relevance to middle- and low-income countries. Some factors may operate differently in different contexts, as has been shown for example with women's education levels and status disparities within couples.[8] In high-income settings women's education is usually protective, whereas in low-income settings it may be a risk factor, particularly when it is the exception and there are disparities of education status within the couple.

Health Consequences

Violence is associated with a wide range of negative health outcomes for women. These range from mild to severe injuries including fractures and permanent damage to ears and eyes,[9] chronic pain syndromes including chronic pelvic pain,[10] depression, anxiety disorders, eating disorders and many other mental health problems,[11] and sexual and reproductive health problems. Whether directly increasing the risk of sexually transmitted infections (STIs) including HIV/AIDS, and unwanted or mistimed pregnancies through rape and sexual assault, or indirectly through inability to request or negotiate the use of condoms because of actual violence, coercion/intimidation or fear of violence (Figure 29.1), violence contributes to women's increased risk of unwanted pregnancies—which may lead to unsafe abortion and gynecological problems.[12] This association has been documented in many countries.[13]

Intimate partner violence during pregnancy is not uncommon. In the WHO multi-country study between 1% and 28% of women reported being physically abused by a partner in at least one of their pregnancies, with between 4% and 12% reporting this in the majority of the sites.[2] This frequently involved blows or kicks to the abdomen. This is consistent with findings in other studies where the range in low-income countries was between 4% and 32%.[4] It must be noted however that the studies in this review use different measures of violence and some also include sexual and emotional violence. There is clearly some cultural variation in the level of protection to violence that pregnancy may confer to women and in most places violence appears to reduce during pregnancy, but there is a group of women for whom the pregnancy may be what triggers the violence or for whom the violence gets worse during pregnancy.[14]

Violence during pregnancy has been found to be associated with pre-term labor,[15] miscarriage, stillbirth,[16] abortion,[17] low birth weight,[18] lower levels of breastfeeding,[19] and higher rates of smoking and drinking during pregnancy.[20] Recent studies also document an association of intimate partner violence with infant and child mortality.[21]

Half to two-thirds of femicide or the murder of women is perpetrated by an intimate partner.[22] In situations of conflict, such as we have seen recently in many countries in Africa and elsewhere, sexual violence against women has increasingly become part of war tactics and has taken egregious forms.[23] While precise numbers are hard to come by, estimates range in the hundreds of thousands.[23]

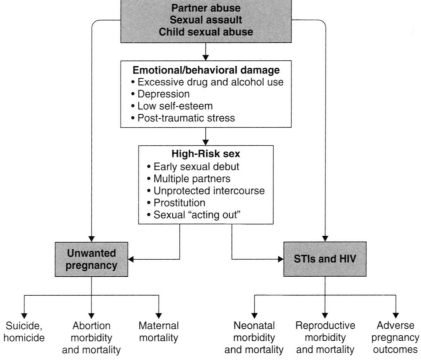

Figure 29.1 Violence against women: Direct and indirect pathways to unwanted pregnancy and sexually transmitted infections. Source: Heise L, Ellsberg M, Gottemoeller M. Ending Violence Against Women. Population Reports, Series L. No. 11. Baltimore: Population Information Program, Johns Hopkins University School of Public Health (JHUSPH); Takoma Park: Center for Health and Gender Equity (CHANGE). Vol. XXVII, No. 4, December; 1999.

VIOLENCE AGAINST WOMEN IN THE INTERNATIONAL AGENDA: RIGHT TO A LIFE FREE OF VIOLENCE

Long recognized by women's health and rights advocates as a critical issue in the lives of many women, violence against women was firmly placed on the international agenda in the early 1990s; the Human Rights Conference in Vienna (1993), the International Conference on Population and Development in Cairo (1994), and the Fourth World Conference on Women in Beijing (1995) all recognized and highlighted violence against women and made specific recommendations for governments to respond to it. In 1996, the World Health Assembly recognized the prevention of violence, including violence against women, as a public health priority requiring urgent action with resolution 49.25, and in 2002 the WHO published the first ever world report on violence and health,[1] which included chapters on intimate partner violence and sexual violence. In 1997, the International Federation of Gynecology Obstetrics (FIGO) initiated a pre-congress workshop and a declaration on violence against women, outlining the role that FIGO and its country affiliates could play to address violence against women.

More recently, the United Nations Security Council passed resolution SCR 1820 and thereby recognized rape during war as a crime against humanity and a threat to global security. The resolution demands that all parties to armed conflict immediately take appropriate measures to protect civilians from all forms of sexual violence. It also calls on governments to ensure that all victims of sexual violence, particularly women and girls, have equal protection and access to justice, and it requires governments to strengthen services to respond to the needs of women who have been raped.

The Right to the Highest Attainable Standard of Health

Violence against women is a serious public health problem, as noted above. It clearly impacts people's ability to achieve the highest attainable standard of physical and mental health.[24] It also impinges on many other human rights, not least women's reproductive rights as defined at the International Conference on Population and Development.[25] These include the right of women to make decisions about reproduction, free of discrimination, coercion or violence. Specifically, sexual violence and intimate partner violence against women, whether physical, sexual or emotional, impinge on women's ability to decide freely if and when to get pregnant and to protect themselves from STIs, including HIV/AIDS. Other human rights that are potentially affected are the right to life, the right to bodily integrity, and the right to nondiscrimination, among others.

Right to Non-Discrimination

Much of the violence that women experience is condoned and at times exacerbated by gender inequality. Laws that discriminate against women with regard to age of marriage, divorce, right to own property and to inherit, for example, can contribute to violence and make it difficult for women to leave abusive relationships. In addition, the violence itself can be considered a form of discrimination. Some have gone further and argued that extreme forms of domestic violence constitute private torture and invoke the Convention Against Torture as a form of protection states' responsibilities.[26]

Human Rights and Healthcare Provision

All individuals are entitled to the protection of, and respect for, their human rights by healthcare providers. In terms of service provision, survivors of domestic violence, rape, and other forms of sexual abuse have a right to receive good quality health services, including reproductive health care to manage the physical and psychological consequences of the violence and to prevent and manage pregnancy and STIs. Health providers should ensure they do not in any way "revictimize" women, force them to have any examination against their will, or take away their agency and decision-making. All patients need to be treated with respect, be given the information they need to make decisions, and have their privacy and the confidentiality of their health records guaranteed.

Governments have a legal obligation to take all appropriate measures to prevent violence against women and to ensure that quality health services are available that can respond to the needs of survivors. The Convention on the Elimination of All forms of Discrimination against Women (CEDAW) and other human rights treaties can be used to invoke states' responsibilities to ensure women's protection and access to services.[27, 28]

ACTION

Both public health and international human rights law provide tools for responding in a more systematic way to women's right to be free from violence and its consequences. Governments and non government actors, including the international community, have a responsibility and must be accountable to do what is within their sphere.

Addressing violence requires action at multiple levels. Countries must abide by the human rights agreements and treaties that they have signed and ratified and ensure they are translated into national law and that these laws are implemented. For example, they need to ensure that laws do not discriminate against women, by providing them the same right as men to divorce, own and inherit property, and to ensure that laws are in place that recognize marital rape as a crime. Laws need to be enforced and prosecution and conviction should be commensurate to the crime and not place the burden of proof on women. In terms of protection it is important to train police, prosecutors, and judges to implement the law in nondiscriminatory ways, ensure the protection of victims from further abuse, and to guarantee the availability of a female officer at police stations, special family courts, or other special measures as appropriate.

In terms of service provision, it is important that women living with abuse are able to access the services they need: medical, psychological, legal, housing, and other support services as needed. As regards health care, providers should as a minimum be informed and aware of the possibility of violence as an underlying factor in women's ill health. This is particularly important in relation to obstetric and gynecologic care as this is one of the most common points of contact with the health service for women. This is particularly the case in resource-poor settings, where women are most likely to use family planning, prenatal care, delivery, and at times postnatal care. All of these offer potential opportunities for identification of women experiencing abuse, providing appropriate interventions and, if necessary, referral to other services. Equally, if not more important, are interventions to prevent violence against women from happening in the first place through increased awareness among the general public and actions targeted at specific groups. Campaigns that break the silence and shroud of privacy about these issues and advocate for no tolerance have been shown to be effective in modifying social norms around the acceptability of violence, as has work with men and young boys to challenge notions of masculinity[7] and interventions to empower women economically and otherwise.[29] Programs that focus on prevention of childhood abuse and neglect, including sexual abuse, and those that target children who witness partner violence, are also important for prevention of violence later in life.[30]

Policies and programs for sexual and reproductive health, maternal and new-born health, adolescent health, and HIV/AIDS prevention should include issues of violence, sexuality, and power dynamics in gender relations as key elements.

CONCLUSION

Violence against women operates as a risk factor for a wide range of women's health problems, as well as being a potential cause of neonatal, infant, and child health problems. It affects women's well-being, their productivity, and their ability to support their children and families. The human and economic costs of this makes it imperative that both public health and healthcare providers educate themselves on the problem and implement relevant prevention and response strategies.

Violence is also a violation of women's human rights and a human rights framework is essential in guiding public health policy and action. Fifteen years after ICPD, while we have made some progress, particularly in recognizing the need to address violence as a key element to achieve sexual and reproductive health rights, there is still a long way to go. Health policies and healthcare delivery, particularly those related to sexual and reproductive health, need to address violence more systematically. This will also allow us to achieve the Millennium Development Goal (MDG) 5 targets of universal access to reproductive health and reduction of maternal mortality, as well as contributing to achieving all of the MDGs.

REFERENCES

1. Krug E, Dahlberg LL, Mercy JA, Zwi AB, Lozano R. World report on violence and health. Geneva: WHO; 2002.
2. García-Moreno C, Jansen HA, Ellsberg M, Heise L, Watts C. WHO multi-country study on women's health and domestic violence against women: initial results on prevalence, health outcomes and women's responses. Geneva: WHO; 2005.
3. Heise L, Ellsberg M, Gottemuller M. Ending violence against women. Baltimore, MD: Johns Hopkins University School of Public Health, Population Information Program; 1999.
4. Campbell J, Garcia-Moreno C, Sharps P. Abuse during pregnancy in industrialized and developing countries. Violence Against Women 2004; 10(7): 770–89.
5. World Health Organization. Preventing child maltreatment. A guide to taking action and generating evidence. Geneva: WHO and ISPCAN; 2006.
6. International Labour Organization. A Global Alliance against Forced Labour. Geneva: International Labour Office; 2005.
7. Harvey A, Garcia-Moreno C, Butchart A. Primary prevention of intimate-partner violence and sexual violence: Background paper for WHO expert meeting. World Health Organization; 2007.
8. Kishor S, Johnson K. Domestic violence in nine developing countries: a comparative study. Calverton, MD: ORC MACRO; 2004.
9. El-Mouelhy M. Violence Against Women. A Public Health Problem. J Prim Prev 2004; 25(2): 289–303.
10. Coker A, Smith P, Bethea L, King M, McKeown R. Physical health consequences of physical and psychological intimate partner violence. Arch Fam Med 2000; 9(5): 451–7.
11. Loxton D, Schoeld M, Hussain R. Psychological health in midlife among women who have ever lived with a violent partner or spouse. J Interpers Violence 2006; 21(8): 1092–107.
12. Rodrigues T, Rocha L, Barros H. Physical abuse during pregnancy and preterm delivery. Am J Obstet Gynecol 2008; 198(2): 171.e1–6.
13. Kaye DK, Mirembe FM, Bantebya G, Johansson A, Ekstrom AM. Domestic violence during pregnancy and risk of low birthweight and maternal complications: a prospective cohort study at Mulago Hospital, Uganda. Trop Med Int Health 2006; 11(10): 1576–84.
14. Castro R, Peek-Asa C, Ruiz A. Violence against women in Mexico: a study of abuse before and during pregnancy. Am J Public Health 2003;93(70): 1110–6.

15. Shumway J, O'Campo P, Gielen A, Witter FR, Khouzami AN, Blakemore KJ. Preterm labor, placental abruption, and premature rupture of membranes in relation to maternal violence or verbal abuse. J Matern Fetal Med 1999; 8(3): 76–80.

16. Morland LA, Leskin GA, Block CR, Campbell JC, Friedman MJ. Intimate Partner Violence and Miscarriage Examination of the Role of Physical and Psychological Abuse and Posttraumatic Stress Disorder. J Interpers Violence 2008; 23(5): 652–69.

17. Glander SS, Moore ML, Michielutte R, Parsons LH. The prevalence of domestic violence among women seeking abortion. Obstet Gynecol 1998; 91(6): 1002–6.

18. Murphy CC, Schei B, Myhr TL, Du Mont J. Abuse: a risk factor for low birth weight? A systematic review and meta-analysis. CMAJ 2001; 164(11): 1567–72.

19. Lau Y, Chan KS. Inuence of intimate partner violence during pregnancy and early postpartum depressive symptoms on breastfeeding among Chinese women in Hong Kong. J Midwifery Women's Health 2007; 52(2): e15–20.

20. Bailey BA, Daugherty RA. Intimate Partner Violence During Pregnancy: Incidence and Associated Health Behaviors in a Rural Population. Matern Child Health J 2008; 11(5): 495–503.

21. Ahmed S, Koenig MA, Stephenson R. Effects of Domestic Violence on Perinatal and Early-Childhood Mortality: Evidence from North India. Am J Public Health 2006; 96(8): 1423–8.

22. Campbell J, Jones AS, Dienemann J, Kub J, Schollenberger J, O'Campo P, et al. Intimate partner violence and physical health consequences. Arch Intern Med 2002; 162(10): 1157–63.

23. Watts C, Zimmerman C. Violence against women: global scope and magnitude. Lancet 2002; 359(9313): 1232–7.

24. United Nations Economic and Social Council. The right to the highest attainable standard of health. E/C12/2000/4 (General Comments). Geneva: United Nations Economic and Social Council; 2000.

25. United Nations, International Conference on Population and Development: Cairo Programme of Action. United Nations International Conference on Population and Development (ICPD). Cairo, Egypt. 1994.

26. Meyersfeld BC. Reconceptualizing Domestic Violence in International Law. Albany Law Rev 2003; 67: 371–426.

27. Culliton KM. Finding a Mechanism to Enforce Women's Right to State Protection from Domestic Violence in the Americas. Harvard Int Law J 1993;34:507–61.

28. Engle Merry S. Constructing a Global Law—Violence Against Women and the Human Rights System. Law Soc Inq 2003; 28: 941–74.

29. Pronyk PM, Hargreaves JR, Kim JC, Morison LA, Phetla G, Watts C, et al. Effect of a structural intervention for the prevention of intimate-partner violence and HIV in rural South Africa: a cluster randomised trial. Lancet 2006; 368(9551): 1973–83.

30. Olds D, Henderson CR, Cole R, Eckenrode J, Kitzman H, Luckey D, et al. Long-term Effects of Nurse Home Visitation on Children's Criminal and Antisocial Behavior: 15-Year Follow-up of a Randomized Controlled Trial. JAMA 1998; 280(14): 1238–44.

QUESTIONS

1. The authors list numerous risk factors related to the prevalence of sexual violence. In light of these risk factors, how might sexual violence be framed within a broader human rights context?

2. The authors state that "between 10% and 69% of women report that an intimate partner has physically abused them at least once in their lifetime, and between 6% and 59% of women report . . . forced sex by an intimate partner in their lifetime." What do you deduce about the state of sexual violence around the world from statistics such as these? How are such statistics gathered? What might be challenges to accurately assessing the prevalence of sexual violence against women? What challenges exist in determining the prevalence of sexual violence against men and transgender populations?

3. Consider the section entitled "action." According to the authors, what additional measures are needed to significantly reduce sexual violence? Why were the commitments made at the Human Rights Conference in Vienna (1993), the International Conference on Population and Development in Cairo (1994), and the Fourth World Conference on Women in Beijing (1995) insufficient to significantly reduce sexual violence?

FURTHER READING

1. Londono, P., Developing Human Rights Principals in Cases of Gender-based Violence: Opuz v Turkey in the European Court of Human Rights. *Human Rights Law Review*, 9: 657–667, http://hrlr.oxfordjournals.org/content/9/4/657.
2. Miller, A., Sexuality, Violence against Women, and Human Rights: Women Make Demands and Ladies Get Protection, *Health and Human Rights*, 2004, 7: 16–47.
3. Montes, S. G., Challenging Custom: Domestic Violence and Women's Struggles for Sexual and Reproductive Rights in a Mexican Indian Region. *Sexuality Research & Social Policy*, 2007; 4(3): 50–61, http://0-search.proquest.com.oasys.lib.oxy.edu/socscijournals/docview/858941409/abstract/138633C2DE5741186A0/10?accountid=12935

Mental Health and Inequity: A Human Rights Approach to Inequality, Discrimination and Mental Disability

Jonathan Kenneth Burns

INTRODUCTION

On October 3, 2008, The Paul Wellstone and Pete Domenici Mental Health Parity and Addiction Equity Act was signed into law in the United States. This legislation introduced parity for mental health coverage for the first time in large group health insurance plans.[1] Theoretically, this brought an end to a system in which it was legal for insurers to limit care for mental health and substance abuse conditions and to require patients to pay more out-of-pocket costs than are required for other medical conditions.[2] The Act has been hailed as a progressive step toward removing inequities in access to and affordability of mental health care. At a political and public level, this may reassure those who live with serious mental disabilities and those who campaign for equality. The reality, however, is that the significant array of parity provisions at both the state and national levels constitute a major barrier for service users and clinicians in realizing real equality as an outcome of this legislation. The Act allows health insurers to determine which mental health and substance use conditions they will cover, to define for what conditions coverage is "medically necessary," and to gain exemption from the law if providing mental health and substance use coverage increases their costs by 2% or more in the first year or by 1% or more in subsequent years. Furthermore, as Richard G. Frank, a health economist at Harvard Medical School, has observed, people with serious mental disabilities such as schizophrenia require many services, including psychosocial and occupational rehabilitation services, which are crucial to their recovery but are not provided for by the Act.[3]

Thus, legislation may be enacted to reduce or eradicate inequalities in health care, but statutes on their own often introduce only "formal equality"—that is, the law treats all individuals or health conditions alike. This is a superficial and deceptive form of equality, however, as there are many social, economic, and political factors at play that obstruct the translation of a law into the real, individual experience of equality. Formal equality alone gives an illusion that all are equal and that fairness exists, without addressing underlying inequalities in power, access, and socioeconomic and political circumstances.[4] In this way, formal equality alone tends to perpetuate discrimination and inequality because it often fails to address real inequality in circumstances. Under a seemingly progressive veneer of respectability, disparities grow unchecked as public advocacy groups relax their activist efforts.

Thus, far from bringing about progressive change, the introduction of equality legislation can have reactionary effects, exacerbating existing disparities in health access and care.

Within the human rights framework, it is imperative that we strive to achieve "substantive equality," defined here as equality of opportunity, within the context of structural inequalities present in society. This means that circumstances that prevent the individual from achieving equality of opportunity must be addressed and that barriers to access and empowerment must be removed. Within health care, substantive equality does not guarantee equality of treatment outcomes, but it does guarantee equality of opportunity in trying to achieve those best outcomes.[5]

Mental disability and mental health care are surprisingly overlooked within the global discourse on health equality, and mental health has always appeared to be a side issue in both the public and academic health debate.[6] There appears to be social distaste for issues pertaining to mental health and disability.

A significant exception to this attitude was the adoption of the United Nations Convention on the Rights of Persons with Disabilities on December 13, 2006.[7] The Convention was negotiated during eight sessions of an Ad Hoc Committee of the General Assembly from 2002 to 2006. To date, there have been 140 signatories to the Convention (with 59 ratifications) and 83 signatories to the Optional Protocol (with 37 ratifications). The Convention is intended as a human rights instrument with an explicit social development dimension:

> It marks a "paradigm shift" in attitudes and approaches ... from viewing persons with disabilities as "objects" of charity, medical treatment and social protection towards viewing [them] as "subjects" with rights, who are capable of claiming those rights and making decisions for their lives based on their free and informed consent as well as being active members of society.[8]

The Convention is broadly inclusive in terms of what is defined as disability, stating that "[p]ersons with disabilities include those who have long-term physical, mental, intellectual or sensory impairments which in interaction with various barriers may hinder their full and effective participation in society on an equal basis with others."[9] Thus, the Convention constitutes a significant global commitment to a human rights framework in which issues of achieving substantive equality and the full and unfettered rights of persons with disabilities are placed at center-stage.

The importance of this Convention (as well as that of other recent regional declarations on mental disability) cannot be underestimated; mental disabilities are pervasive, common, and responsible for a significant proportion of disability, suffering, mortality, and lost productivity in human society. The social and economic "burden" borne by individuals, their families, their communities, and nations due to mental disability is enormous.[10] Co-morbidity with physical illness and substance abuse is considerable.[11] The relationship between mental disability and poverty, income inequality, social dislocation and alienation, and homelessness is well supported by growing evidence.[12] Mental disability impacts education, social behavior, economic productivity, and cultural norms. Moreover, in the treatment of such conditions as HIV/AIDS and drug-resistant tuberculosis, mental disability is associated with high-risk behavior, poor treatment adherence, and inability to access care. In short, mental disability is a protean phenomenon whose often hidden tentacles extend into multiple areas of human experience and functioning. And yet, in both high-income countries (HICs) and low- and middle-income countries (LMICs) throughout the world, mental health care is a low priority, receiving stunted budgets, inadequate resources, and little attention from government.[13] Globally, the integration of mental health into primary care is still in its infancy, while the skills, knowledge, and confidence of generalist health practitioners in managing mental disability are pitiful.[14] In most countries, the level of mental health and substance use education and knowledge within the general public is minimal, if not negligible. Inequalities in mental health service development, provision, and access exist at all levels and in different contexts.[15]

The care, treatment, rehabilitation, and full integration of persons with mental disabilities is a complex challenge that cannot be met through the narrow confines of a purely biomedical or even public health model. The social, economic, cultural, and political factors that interact with innate and acquired biological processes in the genesis, course, and outcome of mental disabilities cannot be ignored in striving for equality. Efforts to improve global mental health will fail dismally if they are limited to the development of new drugs and therapeutic interventions. Likewise, attaining full human rights for persons with mental disabilities will never be achieved through a reliance on public health system reform alone.

Importantly, a human rights approach to mental disability requires a paradigm shift, as the Convention articulates, away from a public health approach in its conventional sense. A public health approach is inadequate, as it serves to reinforce paternalism and charity in identifying mental disability as a medical issue necessitating a medical "solution." It views mental disability as a health issue only, requiring a health services response. In contrast, a rights-based approach to mental disability means

acknowledging the social, economic, and political forces that result in the disability experienced by people with impairments. It also means ensuring that the principle of participation, as well as leadership by persons with disability in advocacy for substantive equality, is key to any international or domestic efforts to redress the inequalities and discrimination that exist in society. For health professionals involved in efforts to achieve real equality, a clinical role alone is ineffective. Instead, clinical expertise must be complemented by a commitment to an activist agenda in partnership with persons with mental disabilities—an agenda focused on bringing about change to the structural inequalities within social, economic, and political life that prejudice mental health, promote social exclusion, and retard recovery from mental disability.

TERMINOLOGY AND MODELS OF MENTAL DISABILITY

The institutionalized medical language of mental disability is, at best, pejorative and situates mental conditions squarely within an individual disease framework. Terms such as "mental disease" and "mental disorder" construct psychological, emotional, and behavioral conditions as innate, biological, pathological states independent of socioeconomic, cultural, and political context. Likewise, the prevailing medical model of mental disability—which defines disability as an individual's "restriction in the ability to perform tasks" and handicap as "the social disadvantage that could be associated with either impairment and/ or disability"—serves to establish a direct causal relationship between individual impairment and disability.[16] In contrast, the social model of disability, theorized by disabled activist and scholar Michael Oliver, views disability as something imposed upon persons by an oppressive and discriminating social and institutional structure and that is over and above their impairment.[17]

While the social model has characterized the disability movement and has been adopted as a basis for a human rights approach to disability, it is not beyond critique. For example, the British medical sociologist, Michael Bury, adheres to what he calls a sociomedical model of disability in which he reaffirms the reality of impairment in contributing to disability.[18] In addressing the "causality" of mental disability, I am inclined to agree with Bury. Research has largely discredited a strict social model view of the causality of serious mental disability associated with such conditions as schizophrenia and bipolar illness to instead support a significant role for genetic and other biological factors in conferring vulnerability to these conditions. Importantly, this integrated, or multifactorial, view of the genesis of mental disability does not support the traditional medical or individual model either. In other words, a critique of the social model does not imply a return to the strict medical model that it superseded. Instead, what is consistent with current evidence from both the biological and sociological fields of research is a model of mental disability that integrates biological and social (as well as cultural and political) factors in establishing cause for these conditions.

The concept of "impairment" is not straightforward here. In terms of mental disabilities, impairment cannot be understood as a fixed structural or mechanical "abnormality" or "departure from human normality," as Lorella Terzi expresses it.[19] Innate or acquired genetic or biological factors associated with the origins of serious mental disabilities are not fixed impairments in the sense that blindness and spinal paralysis are. Rather, these factors exist as "vulnerability factors"—rendering the individual susceptible to psycho-

social and environmental factors within society. Structural environmental forces act in concert with innate or acquired vulnerability factors over time to give rise to illness and disability. Complex reciprocal gene–environment interactions throughout neurodevelopment, involving both environmental mediation of gene expression and genetic influence over individual responses to environmental stressors, lie at the heart of most mental disabilities.[20]

MULTIPLE LEVELS OF INEQUALITY AND DISCRIMINATION

A rights-based approach to mental disability needs to be informed by a clear analysis of the multiple levels of inequality and discrimination that exist in relation to individuals with mental disabilities both within and outside the health system. In a sense then, a "situation analysis" is required to illustrate the clear links that exist among social, economic, political, and cultural aspects of the environment and the origin, personal experience, and outcome of mental disabilities. The following discussion details how substantive inequality and discrimination characterize the manifestation and experience of mental disability in society as well as the provision of mental health care. While this analysis is intended to have global relevance, it contains an overrepresentation of data from the United States. This is not because that nation is alone in experiencing the inequalities cited, but rather, it is a reflection of the fact that significant research has been conducted in this field within the US, while there is a relative paucity of evidence available from other countries.

Unequal Prevalence Due to Structural Inequalities

In recent years it has become apparent that the prevalence of a number of mental disabilities varies in relation to social and economic disparities within societies. For example, systematic reviews show differences in both the prevalence and incidence of schizophrenia in relation to variables including urban versus rural status, social class, migration, unemployment, homelessness, and income inequality.[21] In the case of schizophrenia, social and economic factors mediate expression of the condition in biologically vulnerable individuals.[22] Such is the extent to which these factors impact negatively upon both the onset and outcome of schizophrenia that Brendan Kelly has invoked Paul Farmer's concept of "structural violence" in relation to this illness.[23] Kelly argues that social, economic, and political factors such as poverty and income inequality "shape both the landscape of risk for developing [schizophrenia] and the context in which health-care is provided."[24] He maintains that these forces constitute a form of "structural violence" that impacts the development and course of schizophrenic illness. Common mental disabilities such as anxiety, depression, and substance abuse also show an increased prevalence in relation to social class, unemployment, low income, homelessness, poverty, and income inequality.[25] This means that individuals, families, and communities that occupy lower social classes, that are experiencing high levels of unemployment, and that are living in poverty also bear the burden of increased risk for mental disability along with all of its associated consequences. With respect to income inequality, it appears that health depends not just on personal income but also on the incomes of others in the society.[26] While individual rank within the income distribution is undoubtedly important, it is clear that a large rich–poor gap within a community is bad for everyone in that community regardless of rank, not just for those at the bottom.

Unequal Service Access Due to Structural Inequalities

Social and economic factors may serve as barriers to accessing mental health services in high-income countries as well as low- and middle-income countries. A community survey in the US (a high-income country), for example, reported that low-income individuals cited financial barriers to accessing care. However, this was not the case in the Netherlands or in Canada, both HICs, where economic disparities and income inequality are lower.[27] Also in the US, a household survey of adolescents found that those of low-income status reported far more structural barriers to accessing mental health services than did their middle- and high-income counterparts.[28] In LMICs, the impact of socioeconomic factors is likely to be greater.

The "treatment gap" (that is, the absolute difference between prevalence and percentage treated) for mental disabilities is significant worldwide and is due to a number of factors, including lack of knowledge about mental disabilities, stigma, lack of service availability, and socioeconomic barriers to accessing available services.[29] An earlier study in Belize, for example, reported that 63% of individuals with schizophrenia, 89% of individuals with affective conditions, and 99% of individuals with anxiety conditions were untreated.[30] The World Health Organization Mental Health Survey conducted in 14 countries found that 76–85% of individuals with serious mental disabilities in LMICs received no treatment, while 35–50% of those in HICs received treatment.[31] Clearly, lack of treatment cannot be attributed solely to socioeconomic barriers to access—other likely reasons have already been mentioned. However, within LMICs like South Africa, it is patently obvious that poverty, disempowerment, and inadequate health education impede access to care. In such countries with high poverty and unemployment rates, those in need often cannot afford medical fees, the medicines prescribed, or the transport to convey them to clinics and hospitals. In such contexts, it is glaringly apparent how social and economic inequities lead to inequalities in access to care.

Unequal Service Access Due to Race, Ethnicity, and Gender

Racial and ethnic minorities in the United States are discriminated against in terms of their access to mental health services and appropriate treatments.[32] Margarita Alegría and colleagues reported that of those who had depressive disorder in the previous year, more African Americans (59%), Latinos (64%), and Asians (69%) received no mental health treatment for depression compared with non-Latino whites (40%), while Daniel Rosen and colleagues found that nearly a quarter of white women (23%) with a mental disability received treatment as opposed to only 9% of African American women.[33] In a sample of patients with schizophrenia living in the community, Richard Van Dorn and colleagues reported that significantly fewer African American patients had received atypical antipsychotics (the preferred therapy) than their white counterparts.[34] Disparities in access to mental health services also exist with regard to gender. Women of low socioeconomic status have been shown to be at particular disadvantage in accessing mental health care, and there are clear barriers to accessing alcohol and substance abuse services for women compared with men.[35] Furthermore, women diagnosed with borderline personality disorder encounter significant stigma and denial of access to optimal mental health care in comparison with women with other psychiatric diagnoses.[36] There is a significant body of literature exploring the prejudices and discrimination that underlie the apparent gender bias in the diagnosis of this stigmatized "disorder."

Unequal Service Access Due to a Diagnosis of Mental Disability

In many contexts in both HICs and LMICs, the diagnosis of mental disability itself creates a barrier for individuals in terms of future access to health care. Both real and perceived prejudice against the mentally disabled within the health sector is a potent barrier to accessing care. Graham Thornicroft argues that factors increasing the likelihood of treatment avoidance or delay before presenting for care include lack of knowledge about the features and treatability of mental disabilities, ignorance about how to access services, prejudice against people who have mental disability, and expectations of discrimination against people who have a diagnosis of mental disability.[37] There is good evidence that real prejudices do exist within the health sector toward providing care for those with mental disabilities.[38] Within some countries, the mentally disabled are still treated in abusive health care environments.[39] There is also evidence that the mentally disabled receive unequal treatment for co-morbid physical disorders in comparison to their mentally well counterparts—meaning that a diagnosis of mental disability increases an individual's risk of a poor outcome for co-morbid physical illness.[40] Real and perceived discrimination contribute significantly to non-treatment, delays in accessing treatment, treatment non-adherence, and, ultimately, poorer outcomes.

Unequal Funding and Resource Provision for Mental Versus Physical Disabilities

Globally, government funding for mental health services is disproportionately low compared with the burden of mental disability. Despite the fact that mental and substance use disabilities account for 12% of the global "burden" of disease, more than two-thirds of the world's population lives in countries that spend less than 1% of their total public sector health budget on mental health services.[41] Similarly, in many regions of the world, human resources for mental health care are severely limited in comparison with human resources for physical health care. Many countries, in both high-income and low- and middle-income contexts, report serious shortages of psychiatrists, psychologists, psychiatric nurses, and other mental health care professionals. This inequality in funding and service provision, in the face of the major burden of mental disability, represents global discrimination against mental disability and its care at the level of policy makers, health planners, and governments. Discriminating against those with mental disabilities by failing to pay for and provide care is particularly shortsighted as there are many effective and cheap interventions available that can be highly cost-effective in preventing co-morbidity, reducing disability, and returning mentally ill individuals to productive employment and social reintegration.

Unequal Funding, Resource Provision, and Protection from Abuse Across Nations

Low- and middle-income countries, which arguably support the bulk of the burden of mental disability, tend to spend less on mental health services than HICs. For example, of the 19 African countries for which data are available, 15 spend less than 1% of their health budgets on mental health.[42] An additional inequality is the fact that it is very often the poorest people in the poorest countries who are required to make out-of-pocket payments for mental health care as their governments have made little or no provision for public funding of mental health services.[43] Table 30.1 presents a comparison of the proportion of health budgets spent as well as the main method of funding for mental health among high-, upper middle-, lower middle-, and low-income countries. With respect to human resources, LMICs experience far greater shortages of mental health professionals than HICs. The average number of psychiatrists in HICs, for example, is 10.5 per 100,000 population, as opposed to low-income countries (LICs), where the average number is 0.05 per 100,000.[44] The vast majority of HICs have established community mental health services, but only

Table 30.1 A comparison of the proportion of health budgets spent on mental health as well as the main method of funding for mental health between high-, upper middle-, lower middle-, and low-income countries. Calculated from data in World Health Organization, *Atlas: Country profiles on mental health resources* (Geneva: WHO, 2005). Available at http://www.who.int/mental_health/evidence/atlas/.

Income Group	Mean percentage of the health budget spent on mental health (%)	Primary method of financing mental health care (% countries)	
		Tax-based/Social Insurance	Out-of-pocket/Private Insurance
High Income	7.0	96	4
Upper Middle Income	3.8	100	0
Lower Middle Income	2.4	78	22
Low Income	2.1	48	52

half of LMICs have this critical resource for mental health care.[45] Furthermore, 20% of countries (all in the "developing world") do not have basic antidepressant and antipsychotic medications available within their public health services, while the majority of LICs do not provide basic psychological therapeutic services for their citizens. Finally, whereas almost all high- and upper middle-income countries have legislated against abuse of the mentally disabled (both within and outside health care facilities), there are a significant number of lower middle- and low-income countries in which no such legislation has been passed. While it is conceded that legislation does not necessarily equate to an absence of abuse of the mentally disabled, it is nevertheless likely that a complete absence of legal protection is associated with more frequent occurrences of abuse. Certainly this has been the case in a number of LMICs without adequate mental health care legislation.[46]

A HUMAN RIGHTS APPROACH TO INEQUALITY AND DISCRIMINATION IN RELATION TO MENTAL DISABILITY

The UN Convention sets out a framework for a rights-based approach to disability and in doing so "calls for changes that go beyond quality of care to include both legal and services reforms" and "demands that we develop policies and take actions to end discrimination in the overall society that has a direct effect on the health and well-being of the [mentally] disabled."[47] The Convention sets out a number of guiding principles:

- Respect for inherent dignity, individual autonomy including the freedom to make one's own choices, and independence of persons;
- Non-discrimination;
- Full and effective participation and inclusion in society;
- Respect for differences and acceptance of persons with disabilities as part of human diversity and humanity;
- Equality of opportunity;
- Accessibility;
- Equality between men and women;
- Respect for the evolving capacities of children with disabilities and respect for the right of children with disabilities to preserve their identities.[48]

In addition to these principles, the Convention highlights the importance of a number of related rights. These include the following:

- Equal recognition before the law, access to justice, and legislative reform to abolish discrimination in society;
- Awareness-raising to educate society, combat prejudices, and promote awareness of the capabilities of persons with disabilities;
- The right to life, liberty, and security of person including freedom from degrading treatment, abuse, exploitation, and violence;
- The right to movement, mobility, independent living, and full inclusion within the community including full access to and participation in cultural life, recreation, leisure, and sport;
- Freedom of expression and opinion, access to information, and full participation in political and public life;
- Respect for privacy, for the home and the family, including the freedom to make decisions related to marriage and parenthood;
- The right to equal education, work, and employment including the full accommodation of individual requirements;
- The right to health, habilitation, and rehabilitation;
- The right to an adequate standard of

living, suitable accommodation, and social protection.[49]

With respect to mental disability, how does this framework inform our response to the inequities and discrimination present at multiple levels of society and mental health care? Specifically, if we take these principles and rights and apply them to the global "situation analysis" presented in the previous section, what actions are required to transform our societies so that persons with mental disabilities experience full equality, an end to discrimination, and full recognition of their personhood? I would propose that such an action plan at national as well as local levels include the following components:

1. *The development of a strong advocacy movement, led by persons with mental disabilities.* Repeatedly it has been shown that "user-led" advocacy around issues of legal reform, services development, and societal transformation has been most effective in ending discrimination and stigmatization and achieving human rights for specific minority communities.[50]

2. *Legislative reform to abolish discrimination, to outlaw abuse and exploitation, and to protect personal freedom, dignity, and autonomy.* Civil commitment laws that deprive individuals of their freedom "must provide for minimum substantive and procedural protections that protect mentally ill individuals' fundamental agency."[51] In addition, such laws should guarantee the rights to counsel, appeal, and review in relation to involuntary commitment as well as redress for violations. As mentally disabled persons may not be in a position to safeguard their personal rights while unwell, there should be a mechanism for active monitoring and enforcement of such rights. In

South Africa, for example, the Mental Health Care Act (2002) legislated for the establishment of independent regional "review boards" that are tasked with Ombuds office functions.[52]

3. *Legislative reform to enforce equality of opportunity, access, and participation in all aspects of life.* While health-related legislative reform is important, this must be accompanied by legal measures aimed at rectifying inequalities and discrimination that exist with respect to the mentally disabled in social, economic, and political facets of society. Substantive equality requires attention to the social context that contributes to the origin of mental disabilities as well as to the use of mental health services by individuals.

4. *Inclusion of mental disability on the agenda of development programs and targets such as the Millennium Development Goals.* At international, national, and regional levels, mental disability rights and "needs" must be included in programs aimed at achieving development targets and alleviating poverty and inequality—especially within LMICs.

5. *Mental health and social services reform with equitable funding for resources, infrastructure, and program development.* Governments should be pressured to heed growing calls for the scaling up of health and social services relevant to mental disability as well as increased budget allocations for mental health.[53] Signatories to the UN Convention and its Optional Protocol must be held accountable in terms of their domestic planning. The establishment of the Committee on the Rights of Persons with Disabilities as a monitoring organ means that citizens of States party to the Convention have a means of reporting local violations of the Convention and obtaining redress.[54]

6. *Removal of barriers to health services access encountered by persons with mental disabilities.* Legal reforms such as The Paul Wellstone and Pete Domenici Mental Health Parity and Addiction Equity Act are required within most nations to remove financial barriers to accessing services for those with mental disabilities.[55] Legislation is also required to enforce equality and outlaw discrimination based on ethnicity, race, gender, and age within health services. Finally, education campaigns and programs on mental disability and the rights of mentally disabled persons should be conducted on an ongoing basis within all health services.

7. *Removal of barriers to accessing social, family-related, accommodation, educational, occupational, and recreational opportunities and to full participation for persons with mental disabilities.* Legislative reforms, as well as public and institutional education campaigns and programs, should be implemented at national and local levels to remove these barriers to access, to eradicate stigma, and to ensure the full participation of persons with mental disabilities. Suitable accommodation is a fundamental right as enshrined in the Convention, and domestic policies, planning, and legal reform need to be informed by an acknowledgement of this right.

8. *Service systems reform to move away from institutional care toward providing treatment, care, rehabilitation, and reintegration within the community.* As Alicia Ely Yamin and Eric Rosenthal state, "From a human rights perspective, people are entitled to live in and receive care in the community not because it is more efficient, but because all human beings develop their identities within social contexts, and have rights to work and study, as well as be with family and friends."[56] Furthermore, planning and decision-making power related to care in the community needs to be transferred to "the individuals and communities that the health system is supposed to serve."[57] This means the integration of "users" and family members into both national and local decision-making structures.

CONCLUSION

Mental disability and mental health care have been neglected in the global debate on health, human rights, and equality. Within the mental health field itself, much of the debate has been at a theoretical level, with a focus on stigma concepts and attitudes rather than on acts of discrimination and on strategies to change behavior.[58] Graham Thornicroft and Aliya Kassam argue that stigma research in this field is, to some extent, "beside the point" as it tends to have focused on "hypothetical rather than real situations, shorn of emotions and feelings, divorced from context, indirectly rather than directly experienced, and without clear implications for how to intervene to reduce social rejection."[59] They call for a shift of focus from stigma to discrimination as this would place the mentally disabled in a position of parity with respect to anti-discrimination legislation and the human rights agenda.

The development of mental health policy and legislation within countries that have not established formal equality for mental disability is indeed a priority, and there are a number of global institutions actively engaged in this task.[60] While highly necessary and laudable, these efforts to achieve formal equality should not stand alone, without similar advocacy focused on the achievement of substantive equality for persons with mental disabilities. Real life factors such as poverty; illiteracy; income inequality; homelessness; war and displacement; discrimination based on ethnicity, race, and gender; social exclusion; stigma; and abuse all impact the mentally ill individual's ability to access services and realize full personhood within their communities. These factors also play a role in enhancing individual risk for mental disabilities, and so, too, they act to hinder recovery and reintegration into social and occupational life.

A rights-based approach to mental disability means domesticating treaties such as the United Nations Convention on the Rights of Persons with Disabilities. Using the framework of this convention and others like it, it is possible to formulate an active plan of response to the multiple inequalities and discrimination that exist in relation to mental disability within our communities. While health care professionals arguably have a role to play as advocates for equality, non-discrimination, and justice, it is persons with mental disabilities themselves who have the right to exercise agency in their own lives and who, consequently, should be at the center of advocacy movements and the setting of the advocacy agenda. In support of this agenda, health care professionals need to become activists for the social and economic transformation of society into an environment in which those with mental disabilities can experience substantive equality.[61]

REFERENCES

1. For an excellent summary of the Act and its implications, see Harvard Medical School, "Benefiting from mental health parity," *Harvard Mental Health Letter* (January 2009). For an overview of the historical background of this legislation, see C. L. Barry, "The political evolution of mental health parity," *Harvard Review of Psychiatry* 14 (2006), pp. 185–194.

2. With respect to mental health, substance abuse conditions include a spectrum ranging from problematic abuse of alcohol and drugs to addiction to so-called "dual diagnosis" conditions (co-incidental substance abuse and mental disability where each compounds the negative impact of the other.)

3. Harvard Medical School (see note 1).

4. See S. Day and G. Brodsky, "Women's equality: The normative commitment," in S. Day and G. Brodsky (eds), *Women and the equality deficit: The impact of restructuring Canada's social programs* (Ottawa: Status of Women Canada, 1998), pp. 43–78.

5. See *Factum of the intervenor, Canadian Council of Disabilities,* Part III.

6. For example, mental health is notably absent from the Millennium Development Goals (MDGs). For a critique, see J. J. Miranda and V. Patel, "Achieving the millennium development goals: Does mental health play a role?" *PLoS Medicine* 2/10 (2005), pp. 962–965

7. The UN Enable website was established to report all aspects of the treaty and contains information on the guiding principles, entry into force, signatories, and monitoring of the Convention, as well as full-text versions of the Convention and its Optional Protocol in a number of languages.

8. Ibid.

9. From the United Nations Convention on the Rights of Persons with Disabilities, Article 1, (2006), p. 4.

10. The use of the term "burden" here requires clarification. The term is not used in the sense of individuals being "burdensome" or a cause of hardship for others.

11. See M. Prince, V. Patel, S. Saxena, et al., "No health without mental health," *Lancet* 370 (2007), pp. 859–877. For discussion of co-morbid mental disability and substance abuse, with particular emphasis on developing LMICs, see R. Srinivasa Murthy, "Psychiatric comorbidity presents special challenges in developing countries," *World Psychiatry* 3/1 (2004), pp. 28–30.

12. For a discussion of socioeconomic factors such as poverty and inequality and their effects on mental health, especially in LMICs, see V. Patel and A. Kleinman, "Poverty and common mental disorders in developing countries," *Bulletin of the World Health Organization* 81/8 (2003), pp. 609–615.

13. The 2001 World Health Report was dedicated to mental health, documenting many of the inequalities that exist. For more information, see World Health Organization, *World health report 2001. Mental health: New understanding, new hope* (Geneva: WHO, 2001).

14. See World Health Organization and World Organization of Family Doctors, *Integrating mental health into primary care: A global perspective* (Geneva: WHO, 2008).

15. A September 2007 volume of *The Lancet* contained a series of six papers documenting the current evidence related to global mental health, with a focus on LMICs.

16. See M. Bury, "Defining and researching disability: Challenges and responses," in C. Barnes and G. Mercer (eds), *Exploring the divide: Illness and disability* (Leeds: The Disability Press, 1996), pp. 17–38. Also see World Health Organization, *The international classification of impairments, activities and participation (ICDH-2)* (Geneva: WHO, 1980) for the prevailing medical model of disability.

17. See M. Oliver, *Understanding disability: From theory to practice* (Basingstoke: Palgrave, 1996), p. 32. According to Oliver, the social model "does not deny the problem of disability but locates it

18. See M. Bury, "On chronic illness and disability," in C. E. Bird, P. Conrad, and A. M. Fremont (eds), *Handbook of medical sociology* (5th edition) (New Jersey, PA: Prentice Hall, 2000), p. 179.

19. Terzi (see note 18).

20. For good reviews of the literature on geneenvironment interactions during neurodevelopment and in relation to the causation of mental disabilities, see J. Van Os and P. Sham, "Gene-environment correlation and interaction in schizophrenia," in R. M. Murray, P. B. Jones, E. Susser, et al. (eds), *The epidemiology of schizophrenia* (Cambridge, UK: Cambridge University Press, 2003.)

21. For systematic reviews of the prevalence and incidence of schizophrenia, see E. M. Goldner, L. Hsu, P. Waraich, et al., "Prevalence and incidence studies of schizophrenic disorders: A systematic review of the literature," *Canadian Journal of Psychiatry* 47 (2002), pp. 833–843; and S. Saha, D. Chant, J. Welham, et al., "A systematic review of the prevalence of schizophrenia," *PLoS Medicine* 2 (2005), p. e141

22. For example, see S. Wicks, A. Hjern, D. Gunnell, et al., "Social adversity in childhood and the risk of developing psychosis: A national cohort study," *American Journal of Psychiatry* 162 (2005), pp. 1652–1657.

23. Paul Farmer introduced the term "structural violence" to public health literature in relation to infectious diseases (in particular) and their relationship to social, political, and economic forces; see P. Farmer, *Pathologies of power: Health, human rights and the new war on the poor* (Berkeley, CA: University of California Press, Berkeley, 2005), pp. 40–50. Brendan Kelly applied the concept of "structural violence" to schizophrenia; see B. D. Kelly, "Structural violence and schizophrenia," *Social Science and Medicine* 61 (2005), pp. 721–730.

24. Kelly (see note 23).

25. See A. B. Ludermir and G. Lewis, "Links between social class and common mental disorders in Northeast Brazil," *Social Psychiatry and Psychiatric Epidemiology* 36/3 (2001), pp. 101–107; T. Fryers, D. Melzer, and R. Jenkins, "Social inequalities and the common mental disorders: A systematic review of the evidence," *Social Psychiatry and Psychiatric Epidemiology* 38/5 (2003), pp. 229–237; S. Weich and G. Lewis, "Material standard of living, social class, and the prevalence of common mental disorders in Great Britain," *Journal of Epidemiology and Community Health* 52/1 (1998), pp. 8–14; S. Fazel, V. Khosla, H. Doll, et al., "The prevalence of mental disorders among the homeless in western countries: Systematic review and meta-regression analysis," *PLoS Medicine* 5/12 (2008), p. e225; S. Weich, G. Lewis, and S. P. Jenkins, "Income inequality and the prevalence of common mental disorders in Britain," *British Journal of Psychiatry* 179 (2001), pp. 222–227; R. S. Kahn, P. H. Wise, B. P. Kennedy, et al., "State income inequality, household income, and maternal mental and physical health: Cross sectional national survey," *British Medical Journal* 321 (2000), pp. 1311–1315; and Patel and Kleinman (see note 12).

26. See I. Kawachi, S. V. Subramanian, and N. Almeida-Filho, "A glossary for health inequalities," *Journal of Epidemiology and Community Health* 56 (2002), pp. 647–652.

27. See J. Sareen, A. Jaqdeo, B. J. Cox, et al., "Perceived barriers to mental health service utilization in the United States, Ontario and the Netherlands," *Psychiatric Services* 58/3 (2007), pp. 357–364.

28. See P. W. Newacheck, Y. Y. Hung, M. J. Park, et al., "Disparities in adolescent health and health care: Does socioeconomic status matter?" *Health Services Research* 38/5 (2003), pp. 1229–1233.

29. See, for example, R. Kohn, S. Saxena, I. Levav, et al., "The treatment gap in mental health care," *Bulletin of the World Health Organization* 82/11 (2004), pp. 858–866.

30. See J. Bonander, R. Kohn, B. Arana, et al., "An anthropological and epidemiological overview of mental health in Belize," *Transcultural Psychiatry* 37 (2000), pp. 57–72.

31. The World Health Organization Mental Health Survey was conducted by a consortium from many countries throughout the world, yielding much valuable data. See WHO World Mental Health Survey Consortium, "Prevalence, severity, and unmet need for treatment of mental disorders in World Health Organization World Mental Health Surveys," *Journal of the American Medical Association* 291/21 (2004), pp. 2581–2590.

32. For evidence on racial and ethnic discrimination in mental health care, see M. Alegría, P. Chatterji, K. Wells, et al., "Disparity in depression treatment among racial and ethnic minority populations in the United States," *Psychiatric Services* 59/11 (2008), pp. 1264–1272; and D. Rosen, R. M. Tolman, L. A. Warner, et al., "Racial differences in mental health service utilization among low-income women," *Social Work and Public Health* 23/2–3 (2007), pp. 89–105.

33. Ibid.

34. See, for example, R. A. Van Dorn, J. W. Swanson, M. S. Swartz, et al., "The effects of race and criminal justice involvement on access to atypical antipsychotic medications among persons with schizophrenia," *Mental Health Services Research* 7/2 (2005), pp. 123–134.

35. For evidence that women are disadvantaged in accessing alcohol treatment services, see C. Weisner and L. Schmidt, "Gender disparities in treatment for alcohol problems," *Journal of the American Medical Association* 268/14 (1992), pp. 1872–1876.

36. For an excellent discussion of gender issues underlying the borderline personality disorder diagnosis, see N. Nehls, "Borderline personality disorder: Gender stereotypes, stigma, and limited system of care," *Issues in Mental Health Nursing* 19/2 (1998), pp. 97–112.

37. See G. Thornicroft, "Stigma and discrimination limit access to mental health care," *Epidemiologia e Psichiatria Sociale* 17/1 (2008), pp. 1–9.

38. D. Lawrence and R. Coghlan, "Health inequalities and the health needs of people with mental illness," *NSW Public Health Bulletin* 13/7 (2002), pp. 155–158.

39. See, for example, D. L. Mkize, "Human rights abuses at a psychiatric hospital in KwaZulu-Natal," *South African Journal of Psychiatry* 13/4 (2007), pp. 137–142.

40. For discussion of differential care of co-morbid physical illness in those with mental disabilities within HICs, see A. Bahm and C. Forchuk, "Interlocking oppressions: The effect of a comorbid physical disability on perceived stigma and discrimination among mental health consumers in Canada," *Health and Social Care in the Community* 17/1 (2009), pp. 63–70; and M. M. Desai, R. A. Rosenheck, B. G. Druss, et al., "Mental disorders and quality of diabetes care in the veterans health administration," *American Journal of Psychiatry* 159/9 (2002), pp. 1584–1590. For similar discussion and evidence from LMICs, see A. Cohen, V. Patel, R. Thara, et al., "Questioning an axiom: Better prognosis for schizophrenia in the developing world?" *Schizophrenia Bulletin* 34/2 (2008), pp. 229–244.

41. See World Health Organization, *Mental health fact sheet* (2009). Available at http://www.who.int/mental_health/en/index.html; and A. A. Shah and R. H. Beinecke, "Global mental health needs, services, barriers and challenges," *International Journal of Mental Health* 38/1 (2009), pp. 14–29. For an excellent interactive database on the WHO website containing a range of data on mental health systems in over 100 countries, see World Health Organization, *Atlas: Country profiles on mental health resources* (2005). Available at http://www.who.int/mental_health/evidence/atlas/.

42. Shah and Bienecke (see note 40).

43. World Health Organization (2005, see note 40).

44. Shah and Bienecke (see note 40).

45. For a review, see G. Thornicroft and M. Tansella, "Components of a modern mental health service: A pragmatic balance of community and hospital care. Overview of systematic evidence," *British Journal of Psychiatry* 185/4 (2004), pp. 283–290.

46. Mkize (see note 38).

47. See A. E. Yamin and E. Rosenthal, "Out of the shadows: Using human rights approaches to secure dignity and well-being for people with mental disabilities," *PLoS Medicine* 2/4 (2005), pp. 296–298.

48. UN Enable (see note 7).

49. Ibid.

50. See D. Goodley, "Empowerment, self-advocacy and resilience," *Journal of Intellectual Disability* 9/4 (2005), pp. 333–343.

51. Yamin and Rosenthal (see note 46).

52. For an online version of the South African Mental Health Care Act (2002), see http://www.acts.co.za/mental_health_care_act_2002.htm.

53. See Lancet Global Mental Health Group, "Scale up services for mental disorders: A call for action," *Lancet* 370/9594 (2007), pp. 1241–1252.

54. UN Enable (see note 7).

55. Harvard Medical School (see note 1).

56. Yamin and Rosenthal (see note 46).

57. Ibid.

58. See G. Thornicroft and A. Kassam, "Public attitudes, stigma and discrimination against people with mental illness," in C. Morgan, K. McKenzie, and P. Fearon (eds), *Society and psychosis* (Cambridge, UK: Cambridge University Press, 2008), pp. 179–197.

59. Ibid.

60. For a discussion of policy development within Africa, see O. Gureje and A. Alem, "Mental health policy development in Africa," *Bulletin of the World Health Organization* 78/4 (2000), pp. 475–482. WHO is actively engaged in projects to promote the development of mental health

policy and legislation around the globe (with an emphasis on LMICs.) For an excellent WHO resource, see World Health Organization, *WHO resource book on mental health, human rights and legislation* (2005).

61. M. Donohoe, "Roles and responsibilities of health care professionals in combating environmental degradation and social injustice: Education and activism," *Monash Bioethics Review* 27/1–2 (2008), pp. 65–82.

QUESTIONS

1. The author suggests a movement away from a public health approach and towards a human rights approach in treating persons with mental disabilities. Why? What is the difference Burns posits between the two approaches? Do you see them as similar or distinct? Why or why not?

2. What does equality mean in this context? How does this relate to the definition of disability, as presented in the United Nations Convention on the Rights of Persons with Disabilities (2006)?

3. The author states, "the institutionalized medical language of mental disability is, at best, pejorative and situates mental conditions squarely within an individual disease framework." What does this mean? Why is this language non-conducive to the total care of persons with mental disabilities? Does it threaten or violate human rights?

FURTHER READING

1. Perlin, Michael L., *International Human Rights and Mental Disability Law: When the Silenced Are Heard.* Oxford: Oxford University Press, 2012.
2. Kanter, Arlene S., Treuthart, Mary Pat, Szeli, Eva, Gledhill, Kris, & Perlin, Michael L., *International Human Rights and Comparative Mental Disability Law: Cases and Materials.* Carolina Academic Press, 2006. http://www.amazon.com/s/ref=ntt_athr_dp_sr_1?_encoding=UTF8&field-author=Arlene%20S.%20Kanter&ie=UTF8&search-alias=books&sort=relevancerank
3. Dimopoulos, Andreas, *Issues in Human Rights Protection of Intellectually Disabled Persons.* Aldershot: Ashgate, 2010.

POINT OF VIEW

The Human Right to Water and Sanitation

Pablo Solón

Around two thirds of our organism is comprised of water. Some 75% of our brain is made up of water, and water is the principal vehicle for the electrochemical transmissions of our body. Our blood flows like a network of rivers in our body. Blood helps transport nutrients and energy to our organism. Water also carries from our cells waste products for excretion. Water helps to regulate the temperature of our body. The loss of 20% of body water can cause death. It is possible to survive for various weeks without food, but it is not possible to survive more than a few days without water. Water is life.

The right to health was originally recognized by the World Health Organization in 1946. In 1948, the Universal Declaration of Human Rights declared "the right to life," "the right to education," and "the right to work," among others. In 1966, these were furthered in the International Covenant on Economic, Social and Cultural Rights with the recognition of "the right to social security," and "the right to an adequate standard of living," including adequate food, clothing and shelter.

However, the human right to water has, for a long time, continued to fail to be fully recognized, despite clear references in various international legal instruments, such as: the Convention on the Elimination of All Forms of Racial Discrimination, the Convention on the Elimination of All Forms of Discrimination Against Women, the Convention on the Rights of the Child, and the Convention on the Rights of Persons with Disabilities.

Every year, 3.5 million people die of waterborne illness: illness caused by lack of drinking water and sanitation causes more deaths than does war. Diarrhea is the second largest cause of death among children under five. Lack of access to potable water kills more children than AIDS, malaria and smallpox combined. Worldwide, approximately 1 in 8 people lack potable water. In just one day, more than 200 million hours of women's time is consumed by collecting and transporting water for domestic use. The situation of lack of sanitation is far worse, for it affects 2.6 billion people, or 40% of the global population.

According to the report on sanitation by the Independent expert on the Right to Water: "Sanitation, more than many other human rights issue, evokes the concept of human dignity; consider the vulnerability and shame that so many people experience every day when, again, they are forced to defecate in the open, in a bucket or a plastic bag. It is the indignity of this situation that causes the embarrassment." The vast majority of illnesses around the world are caused by fecal matter. It is estimated that sanitation could reduce child death due to diarrhea by more than one third. On any given day, half of the world's hospital beds are occupied by patients suffering from illnesses associated with lack of access to safe water and lack of sanitation.

Human rights were not born as fully developed concepts, but are built on reality and experience. For example, the human rights to education and work included in the Universal Declaration on Human Rights were constructed and specified over time, with the International Covenant on Economic, Social and Cultural Rights and other international legal instruments such as the Declaration on the Rights of Indigenous Peoples. The same will occur with the human right to water and sanitation.

The Millennium Development Goals is approaching its 2015 milestone, and it is necessary to give a clear signal to the world that drinking water and sanitation are a human right, and that we will do everything possible to reach this goal, which we have only a few more years to achieve. The right to drinking water and sanitation is a human right that is essential for the full enjoyment of life. Drinking water and sanitation are not only elements or principal components of other rights such as "the right to an adequate standard of living." The right to drinking water and sanitation are independent rights that should be recognized as such.

As a step in the right direction, a new resolution passed by the UN Human Rights Council at its 18th session calls on states to ensure enough financing for sustainable delivery of water and sanitation services. Passed by consensus on 28 September 2011, resolution (A/HRC/RES/18/1 http://www2. ohchr.org/english/bodies/hrcouncil/ docs/18session/A.HRC.RES.18.1_English. pdf) has taken a step further the 2009 Council's landmark decision by recognising the right to water and sanitation as legally binding under international law. The resolution emphasises universal service provision, giving priority to realizing a basic level of service for everyone before improving service levels for those already served. It also calls on states to: (a) consider wastewater management, including treatment and reuse; (b) include disaggregated data in monitoring indicators; and (c) ensure that national standards are applied in decentralised services.

It is not sufficient to urge States to comply with their human rights obligations relative to access to drinking water and sanitation. Instead, it is now possible and necessary to call on states to promote and protect the human right to drinking water and sanitation.

As my people say, "Now is the time."

Edited excerpts from a speech delivered by Ambassador Pablo Solón of the Plurinational State of Bolivia before the General Assembly of the United Nations on 28 July, 2010.

Pablo Solón, former Ambassador of the Plurinational State of Bolivia, Executive Director of Focus on the Global South.

CHAPTER 31

Governments in Times of Crisis: Neglecting to Uphold the Human Right to Nutrition?

Claudio Schuftan

Let's face it, elites are not really interested in the development of rural infrastructures that can and will eventually lead not only to local and national food security, but even less to food sovereignty. Expressing such an inconvenient truth may be unpopular, but it is indispensable if there is to be a call for change. The sense of urgency over the growing hunger and malnutrition situation has to sink into the heads of still unwilling leaders. The time for declarations of intent is over. Ultimately, what we have to tackle is the lack of democratic structures, a fact that is putting both remedial and preventive actions on hold. Considering the dire consequences, the question is not whether the needed solutions are too expensive, but whether it will be too expensive not to do anything. Governments have to respect, protect and fulfill the human right to nutrition[1] of their own citizens—and they are not going to do so without putting in place mechanisms to hold them accountable.

THE ROOTS OF THE CRISIS

The latest and ongoing concomitant financial and food (and other) crises are the result of an economic and political system that favors economic growth over equitable social and economic development. These crises highlight some of the most shameful contradictions of our time: The year 2008 saw more than 854 million poor people living in hunger at a time of record global harvests and profits for the world's major agribusiness corporations. To date, more than a billion people do not have enough to eat.[2]

The still lingering global food crisis is not being caused by actual food shortages, but is more a crisis of food-price inflation that has exacerbated already existing hunger and poverty and has created new vulnerabilities. The soaring prices of staple foods hit not only the urban poor, but also the numerous poor farmers who are net food buyers. Contrary to what one might think, higher prices have not benefited small farmers. They are in no position to respond to market signals and will, additionally, face new challenges as the value of land rises and competition increases. Further investments in agriculture have perennially been asked for, but purely speculative investments in land are hardly what the development community had in mind. Several causes of this ongoing trend can be identified: the protectionist strategy imposed in Europe and the United States that affords massive subsidy payments to their agribusiness corporations, the emergence of a middle class in India and China, which has led to a significant change in diets, including more meat consumption, on a large scale. Other causes include: the increase in oil prices, which are passed on to consumers and make agricultural inputs and production more expensive, the growing demand for agrofuels, water scarcity and the loss of arable land. But all these are really eclipsed as causes by the ludicrous speculation we see in food commodity markets.

IMPACT ON THE LIVES OF POOR FAMILIES

The food crisis is generating reallocations in household spending, which are having a cascading effect, especially, on the lives of poor families. Vulnerable groups like children, women and minorities are particularly affected. Their access to food, health services and education is compromised. Some other probable consequences involve damage to the very social fabric due to the effect of the crisis on family support systems, increased domestic violence, child neglect, as well as abandonment of children by families no longer able to cope.[3] Rising food prices lead to a lowering of household food purchasing power and to a reduced dietary diversity of households very likely resulting in increased micronutrient malnutrition. Consumers are forced to spend a much larger share of their income on food. The same is true for the numerous developing countries that import a sizable part of their grain needs. This higher expenditure affects their national budget and consequently the supply of services to the poor segments of the population. These countries' options are restricted by their limited access to foreign financing, low reserve cushions and high external or public debt burdens. However, only insignificant external financing, which could help them adjust, has been made available to them. This is further exacerbated by the cuts in funding of food aid agencies which

has forced them to reduce their activities. This has had very serious nutrition and public health implications and is clearly a threat to the right to nutrition. In short, the food crisis has had widespread detrimental effects on the health of many individuals worldwide. Reduced micronutrient and calorie intake have resulted in well-known problems, such as iron deficiency anemia, low birth weights, stunted growth of children and their respective consequences on wellbeing. The consequences are strongest for breastfeeding mothers since they result in declines in maternal nutrition. It is important to note here that the adequacy of nutrition of young children cannot be separated from the adequacy of their mother's diet.

THE CRISIS SEEN THROUGH A HUMAN RIGHTS PERSPECTIVE

The global food crisis must be treated, not as a natural disaster, but as a threat to the right to nutrition for millions of individuals. It is thus essential to focus on the root causes underlying the lack of access to food and inadequate nutrition, as well as pay more attention to the negative repercussions of the current situation on specific groups, not only children, but the elderly, the marginalized, minorities, and people living with disabilities. The human rights framework compels us to identify the most vulnerable groups in society by studying patterns of discrimination, as well as the relevant actors (rights holders and duty bearers—including those in the private sector) and the gaps in their capacity, their authority and the resources at their disposal. It also requires us to analize the underlying social determinants of vulnerability also called social determinants of nutrition (exclusion from policy formulation, no access to land, to property and to inheritance; lack of productive and economic resources; unemployment; no access to credit; gross social protection gaps, etc.). Moreover, the analysis of the programs in place that either enable or constrain the realization of the human right to food need to be scrutinized. Using the human rights framework, on top of calling on all of us to help empower and ultimately mobilize rights holders to claim their rights, also calls on us to strengthen the capacity of duty bearers, so that they can fulfill their obligations to respect, protect and fulfill the right to nutrition of citizens. This makes it a must for us to monitor progress being made on the implementation of related interventions using clear, targeted process indicators and benchmarks that ensure the accountability of all duty bearers, as well as access to remedial actions for victims of violations of this right.

To address the looming crisis, governments must be made responsible for their citizens. They cannot act on the basis of handouts or isolated interventions since these do not really fulfill their ultimate obligations. National governments have a major role to play and should not pass the responsibility on to foreign aid. They need to increase their investments in the food and nutrition system, not only to raise agricultural productivity (by improving rural infrastructures and market access for small farmers), but also to act on the economic and social determinants of urban and rural poverty and malnutrition. They can do this by expanding social protection interventions, especially in relation to maternal and child nutrition, as well as to health and to care. Seeking international loans and grants can seem attractive in the current situation, but it will ultimately increase the debt burden, which will prevent governments from providing social protection in the future.

THE TIME TO ACT IS NOW

A myriad of concrete responses for preventing hunger and malnutrition can be found in the literature. For example: supporting the poorest income groups via cash transfers or vouchers, risk mitigation and insurance schemes to help farmers dealing with unpredictable price drops, reviewing the debts of food importing countries so as to provide them with budget support, scrapping food and medicines import tariffs, targeting food price subsidies, facilitating access to credit, and creating employment. Furthermore, some measures specifically designed to improve nutrition, for example are: food supplementation during the last trimester of pregnancy and during lactation, promotion of breastfeeding to 24 months (exclusively, for the first six months), complementary feeding for the age group 6–24 months, a higher number of daycare centers with child feeding capacity, universal access to primary health care and to clean water, public awareness campaigns (especially on immunizations and sanitation issues), mechanisms to reduce existing gender imbalances especially in intra-household access to food, kitchen gardens, vitamin and mineral supplements and food fortification (support for the distribution systems of iodine, iron, vitamin A and zinc), and school feeding programs.

These measures should be embedded in a human rights framework. For example:

- School feeding programs should rely more on locally produced foods, building on the strengths of local farmers;
- Fortified products should be produced and distributed locally, contributing to local economic development;
- Day care centers should be set up to address the specific needs of women and should be properly monitored;
- Women should be able to enjoy the right to breastfeed their babies in the work place.

The ultimate question here is, which of these strategies are politically feasible in each country? There is no quick fix to these problems, but it is no longer tolerable, and it is even criminal, to simply carry on in the same old way, tackling only the immediate crises, when in fact, these feed on chronic, well known situations of macro and micro nutrition deficiencies. Therefore, to safeguard the principle of concomitantly acting on food, health and care, and to reestablish the rights of family members, which have now been further violated by the current crisis, governments must urgently implement the following—keeping in mind that each country's situation is unique:

1. Increase the funding for public health care to help alleviate the impact of the crisis on mothers, children and minorities.
2. Restore commensurate family income flows—especially the income of female household members, which is more directly linked to better nutrition.
3. Ensure that private investments neither displace communities from their land nor degrade natural resources, but instead support the livelihoods of small-scale farmers, pastoralists and fisherfolks, promote sustainable and agro-ecological production systems, and develop effective accountability systems at national and international level in order to curtail the growing corporate control over the food system.
4. Develop food markets in a way that rewards sustainable practices by applying special safeguard measures to protect consumers from price volatility, as well as in ways that favor the adoption of healthy dietary patterns instead of falling into monotonous and fast food diets of high energy, high fat and low nutrient density.
5. Revise local and national policies to protect customary land tenure, women's access to land, communal use of land and peasant-based production.

6. Focus investments on food, health and care interventions following local priorities identified through participatory and transparent processes; the communities themselves are best able to identify the most vulnerable among them and the best workable help to address their needs.
7. Continued monitoring and analysis of the evolving global food security and local nutrition situation so as to preempt any deterioration in the same.
8. Seek partnerships with local and foreign actors, as well as NGOs in the implementation and monitoring of food, health and care programs.
9. Provide information and adequate institutional mechanisms to strengthen the ability of civil society organizations to effectively participate in nutrition related policy decision making and to challenge decisions that threaten their rights.
10. Implement recourse mechanisms to which people can resort in cases where their right to nutrition is being violated or is not being guaranteed.
11. Set up needed support mechanisms for children without family support (orphanages, safe houses for refugees), and other general social supports (e.g., for domestic violence mitigation) and supports for overall child protection (e.g., programs against child exploitation).[4]
12. Implement the key recommendations made in the World Health Organization (WHO) Report on the Social Determinants of Health.[5]

A growing literature is validating the duty bearer status also of non-state actors, importantly those in the private sector. Herein fall, among other, international NGOs, private foundations, transnational corporations. Moreover, extraterritorial human rights obligations have recently been codified making it clear that states are not only responsible for the fulfillment of human rights in their own countries, but also in other countries. Finally, be reminded that an Optional Protocol for economic, social and cultural rights is in the process of being globally ratified. The same spells out recourse mechanisms claimants can use to have their rights fulfilled. A growing literature is validating the duty bearer status also of non-state actors, importantly those in the private sector.[6] Herein fall, among other, international NGOs, private foundations, and transnational corporations. Moreover, extraterritorial human rights obligations have recently been codified making it clear that states are not only responsible for the fulfillment of human rights in their own countries, but also have obligations when certain human rights are violated in other countries.[7] Finally, an Optional Protocol for Economic, Social and Cultural rights was adopted by the United Nations General Assembly in 2008 and is being globally ratified. It provides for individuals whose Economic, Social and Cultural (ESC) rights have been violated to seek redress at the international level by filing complaints before the United nations Committee on Economic, Social and Cultural Rights and will also stimulate States to comply with their ESC obligations. The adoption of the new Optional Protocol should be largely credited to the advocacy of NGOs[8] who have relentlessly campaigned for the recognition that ESC and Civil and Political rights should be regarded as universal, indivisibile and interdependent of all human rights, and thus should receive similar treatment under international human rights law. Taken together, once the Optional Protocol enters into force, the above three instruments are invaluable in our work on the right to water and sanitation and also on the rights to food and nutrition, and on all other human rights. They encompass principles, norms and processes framing the relationship between State and non-State actors, in particular trans-national corporations, and create grievance and redress mechanisms that people can use when their ESC rights have been violated both within and outside the country where they live.

CONCLUSIONS

All levels of government have legally binding obligations to fulfill the right to nutrition of their citizens and to implement policies that respond to needs while, at the same time, protecting the environment. It is also the duty of the rights holders (citizens) to demand accountability and enforcement of their right to nutrition. This is the only way we can ensure that governments live up to their responsibilities. Only strong popular pressure will enable the changes needed to eradicate hunger, malnutrition and poverty. Growing mobilization efforts and strong pressure from civil society, including labor unions, farmer and fisherfolk organizations, indigenous people, and women, as well as other broad-based social movements, are indispensable for changing the prevailing power structures and policies that dominate today's decision making.[9]

REFERENCES

1. Convention on the Rights of the Child, Art. 24; CEDAW, Art 12.
2. FAO, Economic crises—impacts and lessons learned, The State of the Food Insecurity in the World, Rome, 2009.
3. Gordon, J., and al. (Center for International Economics), Impact of the Asia crisis on children: Issues for social safety nets, A report sponsored by the Australian Government for Asia-Pacific Economic Cooperation (APEC), Australia, August 1999.
4. *Ibid.*
5. Commission on Social Determinants of Health (CSDH), Closing the gap in a generation: Health

equity through action on the social determinants of health, Final report, WHO, August 2008, available at: whqlibdoc.who.int/publications/2008/9789241563703_eng.pdf.

6. John Ruggie, Protect, Respect and Remedy: a Framework for Business and Human Rights Report of the Special Representative of the Secretary-General on the issue of human rights and transnational corporations and other business enterprises, Human Rights Council, Eighth session Agenda item 3 A/HRC/8/5, 2008.

7. King H., The Extraterritorial Human Rights Obligations of States, Human Rights Law Review, Oxford Journals, vol. 9, Issue 4, pp. 521–556 (2009)

8. See, for example, the Dec. 10, 2009 Statement of the International Coalition of NGO on the First Anniversary of the Adoption of the Optional Protocol to the International Covenant on Economic, Social and Cultural Rights and other background documents on the ESCR Optional Protocol.

9. For more information on the civil society initiatives, see the collaborative report, Policies and actions to eradicate hunger and malnutrition, Working Document, November 2009.

QUESTIONS

1. The author of this chapter provides a solid list of "concrete responses for preventing hunger and malnutrition." Why and through what processes would you prioritize these responses? Which of the responses recommended by the author are, in your view, likely to achieve their desirable impacts in the short term (i.e. within the next 1–2 years of their implementation)? Which other responses will require sustained actions over a longer period before they become feasible?

2. The author calls on readers to "monitor progress being made on the implementation of related interventions using clear, targeted process indicators and benchmarks that ensure the accountability of all duty bearers . . ." Please suggest 3–4 indicators and benchmarks for monitoring progress? Who should be accountable for progress (or lack thereof), and to whom?

3. A UNDP document *Applying a Human Rights-Based Approach to Development Cooperation and Programming*, UNDP, September 2006 http://www.hurilink.org/tools/Applying_a_HR_approach_to_UNDP_Technical_Cooperation--unr_revision.pdf (see p. 4 in particular), recognizes that reactive and protective approaches to the protection and promotion of human rights are complementary and mutually reinforcing. Which of the action points suggested by the author of the above article would fall in each of these categories? Who are/should be key actors with regards to the human right to food and nutrition and in what ways can they influence the shaping and implementation of national agendas?

4. An Open Letter titled "Commitments to water and sanitation must come with real commitments to human rights" was addressed to States negotiating the Outcome Document of the Rio+20 Earth Summit by Catarina de Albuquerque, United Nations Special Rapporteur on the human right to safe drinking water and sanitation, prior to the Summit. http://www.righttowater.info/commitments-to-water-and-sanitation-must-come-with-real-commitments-to-human-rights/. Please access and review the outcome report of the Rio+20 Earth Summit: to what extent did it respond to the Special Rapporteur's call? What reasons could be invoked to explain any variance between her call and the reported Summit outcome? What do you intend to do about it?

FURTHER READINGS

1. Ruggie, J., Business and Human Rights: The Evolving International Agenda, John F. Kennedy School of Government - Harvard University, *Faculty Research Working Papers Series*, RWP07-029 (June 2007). http://web.hks.harvard.edu/publications/workingpapers/citation.aspx?PubId=4875. See also, for a dissenting view: Alejandro Teitelbaum, A., Observations on the Final Report of the Special Representative of the UN Secretary General on the issue of human rights and transnational corporations and other business enterprises, John Ruggie, *The Jus Semper Global Alliance* (May 2011).South http://www.jussemper.org/Resources/Corporate%20Activity/Resources/Observations_to%20Ruggies_final-2011.pdf.

2. Kinley, D. & Joseph, S. Multinational Corporations and Human Rights: Questions about their Relationship, *Alternative Law Journal* (2002), www.law.monsah.ed.au/castancentre/projects/arc_kinley.pdf

3. Ziegler, J., Golay, C., Mahon, C. & Way, S., *The Fight for the Right to Food: Lessons Learned.* New York: Palgrave Macmillan, 2011.

4. Kent, G., *Freedom from Want: The Human Right to Adequate Food.* Washington DC: Georgetown U. Press, 2005.

CHAPTER 32

Human Rights-Based Approach to Tobacco Control

Carolyn Dresler, Harry Lando, Nick Schneider and Hitakshi Sehgal

HUMAN RIGHTS-BASED APPROACH TO TOBACCO CONTROL

Human rights rhetoric became universally defined with the Universal Declaration of Human Rights in 1948, specifically related to health with: 'the right to a standard of living adequate for health and well-being of himself and his family, including food, clothing, housing and medical care and necessary social service'.[1] Since then, nine core international human rights treaties have been adopted and brought into force (Table 32.1). Of particular relevance to the rights relative to health and well-being, under which tobacco control would be pertinent are: the International Covenant on Civil and Political Rights (ICCPR, 1966), the International Covenant on Economic, Social and Cultural Rights (ICESCR, 1966), the Convention on the Elimination on Discrimination Against Women (CEDAW, 1979) and the Convention on the Rights of the Child (CRC, 1989). To ensure that the agreed rights are also enjoyed in practice, each of these treaties has clear and independent mechanisms to monitor the implementation of the respective treaty provisions.

Unlike the WHO Framework Convention on Tobacco Control (FCTC),[2] the core human rights treaties rely on periodic reporting by the state parties and additionally have international committees of independent experts (treaty bodies) to regularly monitor national implementation and report back to the UN system. These treaty bodies consist of 10 to 23 internationally recognized independent experts who are nominated and elected by state parties. The committees receive reports from state parties as well as additional information on the human rights situation in the respective country, examine them in a dialogue with government representatives and publish their concerns and recommendations as 'concluding observations/comments'. Some treaty bodies introduced further monitoring mechanisms including an enquiry procedure, the examination of interstate complaints and the examination of individual complaints (Table 32.1). The treaties complement each other, are interdependent and mutually reinforcing. That said, many countries have derogated from important portions of treaties, have ignored implementation or adherence because of lack of will or ability to do so. Often the ability to adhere or progress on treaty implementation is hampered by financial constraints. If there are not financial resources to allow full implementation of a treaty requirement, then progressive realisation of the right is to be expected as finances allow.

Table 32.1 Monitoring instruments and complaints procedures contained in the UN Human Rights Treaties vis à vis the WHO Framework Convention on Tobacco Control

Multilateral treaty (acronym, year of adoption); optional protocols	State reporting obligations (in years after acceding)	Expert committee		Additional complaints procedures			
		Monitoring by expert committee	Number and lengths of sessions	Individual complaints/ communications	Interstate complaints	Enquiries (by the committee)	Other
UN human rights treaties							
International Convention on the Elimination of all forms of Racial Discrimination (ICERD, 1965)	One or more every 2 years	Yes	Two per year, 3 weeks each	Yes	Yes	—	Early warnings
International Covenant on Civil and Political Rights (ICCPR, 1966) and two optional protocols	One year after acceding then upon request, usually every 4 years	Yes	Three per year, 3 weeks each	Yes	Yes	—	—
International Covenant on Economic, Social and Cultural Rights (ICESCR, 1966) and one optional protocol	Two or more every 5 years	Yes	Two per year, 3 weeks plenary and 1 week working group prior to session	Yes	—	—	—
Convention on the Elimination of all forms of Discrimination Against Women (CEDAW, 1979)	One or more upon request (at least every 4 years)	Yes	One per year, maximum 2 weeks	Yes	—	Yes	—
Convention Against Torture and Other Cruel, Inhuman or Degrading Treatment or Punishment (CAT, 1984) and one optional protocol	One or more every 4 years	Yes	Two per year, 3 weeks each	Yes	Yes	Yes	Inspections
Convention on the Rights of the Child (CRC, 1989) and two optional protocols	Two years after acceding, then every 5 years	Yes	Three per year, 3 weeks plenary and 1	—	Yes	—	—

Table 32.1 (Continued)

Multilateral treaty (acronym, year of adoption); optional protocols	State reporting obligations (in years after acceding)	Expert committee		Additional complaints procedures			
		Monitoring by expert committee	Number and lengths of sessions	Individual complaints/ communications	Interstate complaints	Enquiries (by the committee)	Other
			week working group prior to session				
International Convention on the Protection of the Rights of all Migrant Workers and Members of their Families (ICPMW, 1990)	One or more every 5 years	Yes	Two per year, 1 week each	Yes	—	—	—
International Convention for the Protection of all Persons from Enforced Disappearance (CPED, 2006)	Two or more upon request	Yes	Two per year	Yes	—	—	—
Convention on the Rights of Persons with Disabilities (CRPD, 2006), one optional protocol	Two or more every 4 years	Yes	Two per year, 1 week each	Yes	—	—	—
Multilateral public health treaties (WHO)							
WHO framework convention on tobacco Control (FCTC, 2003)	Two years after acceding, then every 5 years until 2012, then every 2 years	—	—	—	—	—	—

A key principle underpinning human rights is the recognition of states' obligations to respect, protect and fulfil these international rights. Most states in the world are party to most of the human rights conventions, the USA unfortunately being a notable exception. An excellent example is Uruguay, which is party to the nine core human rights treaties, but significantly the ICESCR, CEDAW, CRC and the FCTC, and works diligently to respect, protect and fulfil fundamental human rights—pertinently, as they apply to tobacco control.[3] Uruguay has established comprehensive smoke-free laws, dedicated a portion of its tobacco tax to health related purposes, has required pictorial warnings on cigarettes packs, has banned electronic cigarettes and has established evidence-based tobacco cessation guidelines that include support for nicotine replacement and bupropion.

FROM THE RIGHT TO HEALTH TO THE RIGHT TO TOBACCO CONTROL?

By tightly adhering to the principles that have been delineated for interpreting human rights, one can construct legal claims to rights related to tobacco control.[4] These would include human rights more broadly than just the right to health. All human rights are interrelated, interdependent and indivisible. States have a duty (see http://plato.stanford.edu/entries/rights-human/ for discussion of rights and duties) to provide all human rights to the best of their economic and political ability. In many poorly resourced countries this can be difficult as the tobacco industry, with its unlimited resources, can overwhelm states' best intentions to comply with health-based rights by using those resources strategically in ways that undermine tobacco control progress. States and their citizens must be empowered with knowledge, resources and ability to claim their rights and resist the tobacco industry's 'corporate social responsibility', 'corporate social investment' or outright bribery that can inhibit realisations of such rights. An example of tobacco industry corporate social responsibility is the establishment by the tobacco industry of Eliminating Child Labour in Tobacco Growing, while hundreds of thousands of children are still working in tobacco production (including bidi rolling).[5] Educated and empowered citizens give the human rights-based approach to tobacco control its utility. The right to health, or the right to the highest attainable standard of health, is claimed within Article 12 of the ICESCR. This right is then further elucidated and defined within a structure that is called a General Comment (see Box 32.1). The key axioms that underpin a human rights-based approach to tobacco control are derived from Article 12 of the ICESCR, General Comment 14:

1. The States Parties to the present Covenant recognise the right of everyone to the enjoyment of the highest attainable standard of physical and mental health.
2. The improvement of all aspects of environmental and industrial hygiene; (c) The prevention, treatment and control of epidemic, endemic, occupational and other diseases; . . .

Protection from secondhand smoke, tobacco production regulation, marketing restrictions and efforts to decrease tobacco consumption are clearly covered by General Comment 14 (see Box 32.1).

Besides the right to health, however, there are several other human rights equally important to respect, protect and fulfil. For example, the right to a healthy environment (consider secondhand smoke or protection from nicotine from green tobacco sickness, or exposure to pesticides during tobacco agriculture);

BOX 32.1 TECHNICAL EXPLANATIONS OF GENERAL COMMENT (GC) AND PERTINENT LANGUAGE WITHIN THE INTERNATIONAL COVENANT ON ECONOMIC, SOCIAL AND CULTURAL RIGHTS (ICESCR) RELATIVE TO TOBACCO CONTROL

A 'General Comment' (GC) is an elucidation and expansion of the intent of the phrasing within a Convention. In this instance, GC 14 further defines the intent of the right to health proscribed within Article 12 of the ICESCR.

Pertinent to tobacco control, General Comment 14 maintains: Violations of the obligation to protect follow from the failure of a state to take all necessary measures to safeguard persons within their jurisdiction from infringements of the right to health by third parties. This category includes such omissions as the failure to regulate the activities of individuals, groups or corporations so as to prevent them from violating the right to health of others; the failure to protect consumers and workers from practices detrimental to health, for example by employers and manufacturers of medicines or food; the failure to discourage production, marketing and consumption of tobacco, narcotics and other harmful substances.

Sources: http://www.ohchr.org; http://www.who.int/fctc.

---

right to information (consider knowledge relative to risks of nicotine addiction, risks from tobacco use such as lung cancer or vascular disease, risk from exposure to secondhand smoke, risk from exposure to tobacco agriculture: nicotine, fertilizers, pesticides etc.); right to education (consider children kept from school for tobacco agriculture); right to a sustainable income (consider indentured servitude or 'company store'); right to a standard of living adequate for the child's physical, mental, spiritual, moral and social development (consider use of limited family income to purchase tobacco rather than food). A human rights approach can readily work within the Articles of the FCTC, along with other international conventions and treaties to help enforce their intent.

FROM THEORY TO ACTION: THE USE OF SHADOW REPORTS

Several methodologies are being explored to use the human rights-based approach to tobacco control. Claims can be brought to appropriate courts that oversee regional human rights conventions. For example, the European Convention on Human Rights, the African Commission on Human and People's Rights and the Inter-American Commission have respective Courts to enforce their conventions. These courts are available to individuals, such as the successful appeal of a non-smoker in a Russian prison to the European Court, which found a violation of the European Convention and awarded damages.[4]

'Shadow reports' are another established method for providing information to the different treaty-reviewing committees to assist in their assessments of official state reports. Parties to the different conventions are required to submit state reports on their fulfilment of the requirements of the treaty. Shadow reports are submitted by interested non-state parties; for example, non-governmental organisations within the country, that help provide evidence on the progress of the state in implementation of the treaty. These shadow reports can more clearly and explicitly address progress or the lack of progress that the state is achieving in tobacco control. Reviewing committees can then recommend improvements/remedies for the country to pursue; for example, the treaty-body Committee with oversight for the ICESCR or CESCR recommended 'that the state party take measures to ban the promotion of tobacco products and enact legislation to ensure that all enclosed public environments are completely free of tobacco'.[3] In addition, the CESCR had recommendations for Brazil concerning child labour, slavery and deforestation (although not specifically in reference to tobacco agriculture).[6]

ACTIVITIES SO FAR: THE HUMAN RIGHTS AND TOBACCO CONTROL NETWORK (HRTCN)

To develop action plans for using a human rights-based approach in tobacco control, a small cadre of tobacco control advocates from multidisciplinary backgrounds met in Lausanne, Switzerland in 2008 and established the HRTCN (http://www.hrtcn.net). Two other meetings followed, one in conjunction with the World Conference on Tobacco or Health in Mumbai in 2009 and a working group meeting with the WHO human rights and tobacco control units in Geneva in 2010. HRTCN networks with partners around the world to connect and educate about the power of the human rights approach to advance tobacco control. These partners come from diverse backgrounds, including medicine and nursing, social scientists, faith communities, legal experts, tobacco control advocates and others; this provides for diverse perspectives. For example, many tobacco control advocates are firmly opposed to any negotiations with the tobacco industry, whereas others

have vigorously engaged in such negotiations in order to advance goals such as labour rights. A pilot project is to develop an approach to inform the Committees of pertinent Conventions, such as the CESCR, by using 'short' reports. Global HRTCN partners are piloting a review of each of the country reports to the CESCR and are preparing one-page summary documents. These elucidate key tobacco control issues and progress or lack of progress by individual countries. For example, it might be noted that a country has ratified the FCTC, but has no comprehensive secondhand smoke exposure law, or continues to tolerate use of child labour in tobacco agriculture. Such information should be useful for the committees, specifically for the ICESCR, CEDAW and the CRC, as they formulate their country specific recommendations; Figure 32.1.

THE FUTURE: INTEGRATION OF A TOBACCO CONTROL BASED APPROACH IN HUMAN RIGHTS MONITORING?

The WHO FCTC reporting instrument includes an extensive set of indicators for monitoring its implementation on national levels. WHO and the FCTC Secretariat could provide relevant input to the respective treaty bodies, for example by sharing the FCTC implementation reports or by presenting findings at committee sessions. The UN Ad Hoc Interagency Task Force on Tobacco Control meets every 2 years and, at the last meeting, the first author presented on the human rights-based approach to tobacco control. The WHO's health and human rights Team is active and supportive of a human rights-based approach to tobacco control, and hosted a meeting in 2010 where relevant treaty representatives (CEDAW, CRC, ICESCR) were actively engaged. The UN Task Force on Tobacco Control

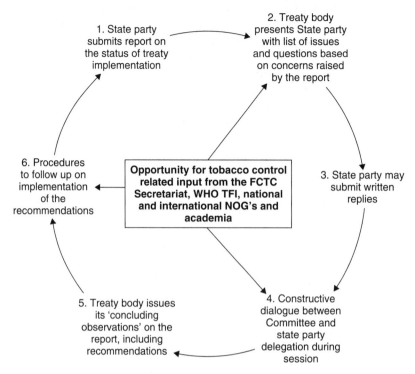

Figure 32.1 The reporting cycle under the human rights treaties and opportunities for input related to tobacco control (adapted from the Office of the United Nations High Commissioner for Human Rights, The United Nations Human Rights Treaty System, Factsheet 30).[7] FCTC, WHO Framework Convention on Tobacco Control; NGO, non-governmental organisation; TFI, WHO Tobacco-Free Initiative.

offers an ideal platform to provide collaboration and exchange of information regarding common areas of interest, such as the right to a healthy environment (secondhand smoke or green tobacco sickness) or the right to education (knowledge of the harm of tobacco use) and other rights covered in different legal instruments. Incorporation of tobacco-related indicators in the monitoring mechanisms of human rights treaties appears to be a feasible option to support implementation of the FCTC in the absence of an independent monitoring mechanism. Additional input could be provided by academia and civil society involved in tobacco control,

as well as other entities involved in human rights advocacy and research. In order to facilitate this process, national and international training and capacity building should be supported, for example in writing shadow reports and participation in hearings during committee sessions.

The complaint procedures contained in some of the treaties could be used to communicate tobacco control related human rights violations to the respective committees. Under particular circumstances, CEDAW and CRC may consider complaints from individuals or from third parties representing individuals whose rights have been violated. As discussed above, individuals can bring a claim to one of the regional courts, or, if their country is party to the ICESCR, an individual could petition his/her own country for a legal remedy. Another opportunity is to engage the Special Rapporteur on the right of everyone to the highest attainable standard of physical and mental health in helping to expose human rights violations promulgated by the tobacco industry, including agricultural and manufacturing abuses. In addition, calling for a General Day of Discussion on Tobacco Control at the United Nations could lead to a General Comment for Article 12 of the ICESCR on the right to tobacco control and could further spur compliance and implementation of the FCTC. In the interim, tobacco control with implementation of the Framework Convention should be included in the upcoming high level meeting on 20–21 September 2011 on non-communicable diseases, particularly as they relate to developing countries.

REFERENCES

1. The Universal Declaration of Human Rights; United Nations website.
2. *The Framework Convention on Tobacco Control; World Health Organization website.*http://www.who.int/fctc/en/
3. Cabrera OA, Madrazo A. Human rights as a tool for tobacco control in Latin America. *Salud Publica de México* 2010;52(Suppl 2): 228e97.
4. Dresler CM, Marks S. The emerging human right to tobacco control. *Hum Right Q* 2006;28: 599e651.
5. http://www.independent.co.uk/life-style/health-and-families/health-news/the-unstoppable-march-of-the-tobacco-giants-2290583.html
6. *Office of United Nations High Commissioner on Human Rights; Committee on Economic, Social and Cultural Rights review of Brazil Country Report.* http://www2.ohchr.org/english/bodies/cescr/cescrs42.htm
7. *Office of the United Nations High Commissioner for Human Rights. The United Nations Human Rights Treaty System: An Introduction to the Core Human Rights Treaties and the Treaty Bodies. Fact Sheet No.30.*Geneva, 2005. http://www.ohchr.org/Documents/Publications/FactSheet30en.pdf

QUESTIONS

1. The connection between tobacco control and health is clear, but what is the connection between tobacco control and human rights?

2. What should the "monitoring report," discussed in the chapter, monitor? How should this be carried out?

3. Discuss specific strategies by which the right to health could be used to ensure a right to a tobacco free environment.

FURTHER READING

1. Reynolds, L. A., & Tansey, E. M. *WHO Framework Convention on Tobacco Control: The Transcript of a Witness Seminar.* London: University of London, 2012.
2. De Beyer, Joy, & Waverley Brigden, Linda, *Tobacco Control Policy: Strategies, Successes, and Setbacks.* Washington, DC: World Bank, 2003.
3. Proctor, Robert, *Cancer Wars: How Politics Shapes What We Know and Don't Know About Cancer.* New York: Basic Books, 1995.

PART V

Changing World

Introduction

Health and human rights do not operate in a vacuum, and major changes in the world directly affect human rights, human health and their interactions across the globe. Perhaps the major changes of the past decade are related to post-9/11 fears of terrorism and increased emphasis on national security which lead directly to wars in Iraq and Afghanistan, and heightened security across Europe and North America. But other trends may turn out to be even more important in the longer term, including climate change, sustainable development and depleting energy resources. These trends are emerging in the context of an international economic recession which carried in its trail a drastic move towards deficit reduction, decreased public sector spending, crackdowns on immigration and shrinking funds for global health initiatives. All of this impacts the willingness and capacity of governments to deliver on their human rights obligations, both domestically and globally. And this is occurring simultaneously with the widespread growth and power of transnational corporations that have been reluctant to accept responsibilities in the human rights realm. All of these changes underscore not only the interconnectedness between health and human rights, but as importantly, the interconnectedness of human life and human dignity with changes in economics, climate and national security.

Major global health trends include the increasing recognition of the magnitude of the disease burden attributable to chronic diseases (moving away from communicable diseases, like HIV/AIDS and TB, that dominated health and human rights during its formative years), population growth and urbanization around the world, dramatically increasing economic disparities, the continuing "war on drugs," and tentative attempts to merge medicine with public health, and to merge bioethics with human rights. The growth of the internet and the increasing use of electronic media, especially personal computers and smart phones, around the world means that events anywhere can have an impact on everyone. New uses, such as Facebook, both enable easy communication among groups of individuals, and pose major privacy challenges.

At the birth and early development of the field of health and human rights it seemed almost natural to describe them as "inextricably linked," like a chain. This metaphor worked well in the beginning of the HIV pandemic, where human rights and human dignity were understood to be much more important than access to ineffective medicines which, at that time, could do little good in terms of treatment or cure. With the advent of antiretroviral therapy, access to effective treatment has been properly framed as a fundamental human right. In the context of building a healthcare system, however, it has also been recognized that just dealing with HIV (with or without TB and malaria—together the world's biggest killers), or any single disease, is insufficient, as is choosing between prevention and treatment strategies. A holistic approach requires attention to medical care and public health, as well as to its close relatives, education, employment, housing, and sanitation. This broad-based approach is not new in itself, but the political, economic, and terrorism-infused context for meeting the reasonable goals of promoting human rights and improving human health has changed. It is easier, for example, to get global support to attempt to prevent and respond to worldwide pandemics, such as SARS or H5N1 and H1N1 flu, than to get such support for more local diseases, like cholera, which are less likely to affect people living in high-income countries.

The readings in this part have been chosen to highlight many of the current challenges in our changing world as they pertain to health and human rights, especially the implementation and design of public policies and programs to promote human rights in ways that improve health, and vice-versa.

Benatar and his colleagues open this part with a description of how global health has been directly and adversely affected by the global economic crisis. They seem correct to emphasize the utter failure of market economics to promote global health, as well as the threat that rapid privatization of public health poses to global health. They challenge all of us to develop constructive and effective responses to our "dysfunctional global economic system" that is "geared primarily to the pursuit of profit at the expense of human flourishing and human rights." It is worth considering that in the triad of health, human rights and money, money has historically taken priority. This observation also implies that private actors, including transnational corporations, philanthropic organizations and NGOs, will be as important as governments in anticipating and responding to global health problems.

At Rio+20, the UN climate change conference held in 2012, the world began preparations to follow the Millennium Development Goals (2000–2015) with a set of Sustainable Development Goals (2015–2030) that would put much more emphasis on economic development and environmental sustainability, but hopefully not at the expense of the health of the poor and people living in low-income countries. It is in this context that the chapter by Humphreys on climate change and human rights fits. As he highlights, the worst effects of climate change are likely to be felt most by those groups whose rights and health are already precarious. He provides a "rough" (and useful) guide as to how human rights activists can help ensure that a bad situation for already marginalized populations is not made even worse by state and private responses to climate change. Robinson's Point of View is a call to arms.

Elliott and his colleagues address the question of how the international community and individual governments can act at cross-purposes in addressing global problems. They suggest that the global "war on drugs," which they term the "global drug control regime," has to be rethought in the context of the HIV epidemic. A recognition that injection drug use has driven a large part of the epidemic leads to a recognition that both harm reduction and human rights support public health interventions like syringe exchange programs and safer injection facilities.

Hurtig and colleagues also show us how a human rights framework can improve the effectiveness of treatment programs for tuberculosis. This is counterintuitive for many, if not most, public health officials who see mandatory and monitored treatment as the gold standard. But public health effectiveness and human rights are not mutually exclusive;

they can and should be complementary. When the human rights of people are respected, public health can concentrate on eliminating the barriers to effective prevention and treatment of disease, rather than on stigmatizing and restricting the rights of individuals who are sick.

HIV/AIDS and TB are in a sense "old" communicable disease problems. SARS was a "new" one. Burci and Koskenmaki describe the reaction of the World Health Organization (WHO) to SARS, and consider the amendments of the International Health Regulations in the wake of the SARS pandemic, including what it means for individual states to declare a "public health emergency" and what "right to health" obligations the states necessarily retain during the emergency. It is not an understatement that global health will never be the same after the SARS pandemic and the changes at the WHO it provoked.

Global pandemics, like SARS and the H1N1 and H5N1 flu, provoked widespread fear in the first decade of the 21st century, but even more terrifying has been the post-9/11 fear of a bioterrorist attack with a novel pathogen. Annas explores the reaction (or, as he would say, overreaction) of the US government to the threat of bioterrorism using either an "old" pathogen, such as plague or small pox, and the use of genetic engineering techniques to create a new plague. In this context it is often suggested that we must trade human rights for health and safety, but this is almost always an assertion without an evidentiary basis.

One of the major trends is the growth of global health to encompass a commitment to deal with chronic noncommunicable diseases as well, especially diabetes, cancer and cardiovascular disease. In her chapter, Nygren-Krug applies a health and human rights approach to chronic diseases, the cause of a majority of deaths worldwide. As with a human rights approach to communicable diseases, such as TB, she argues that a human rights approach is not only the "right" way to treat people, it is also the most effective long-term approach, based especially on the right to health, equality, nondiscrimination, and the right to participate. Since many noncommunicable diseases can be promoted or made worse by the products sold by major transnational corporations (e.g., infant formulas, tobacco, alcohol, fast foods) effective health action will require either the cooperation of these corporations, or more effective regulation of them by states. It is a changing world, and health and human rights strategies must adapt to be effective.

The Point of View by Grover uses the right for everyone to the enjoyment of the highest attainable standard of physical and mental health to argue that occupational health is integral to well-being. The state must respect, protect and fulfill its obligations to the workers through law and public policy.

Puhl and Brownell's chapter uses what has become the major focus of public health action in recent years, the obesity epidemic, to illustrate the recurring and multifaceted face of stigmatization and discrimination that can easily follow, as it did with AIDS, the identification of a major public health problem. The remarkable observation in the realm of chronic diseases is that stigma and discrimination seem to follow us wherever we go in public health, and the only effective response is likely to be focused attention on human rights.

Finally, Morgan helps us begin to deal with the rapidly changing age distribution of the population around the globe, which means both a much larger percentage of the population will be retired, and a much larger percentage of the population will be in declining health and will need more healthcare resources and community services to continue to live with dignity.

TOPICS FOR DISCUSSION

1. The field of health and human rights was born in the midst of the HIV pandemic. How is the growth of interest in chronic diseases changing the field, and how might future health challenges change it even more?
2. One of the major changes in the world over the past decade has been increased recognition of growing income inequality around the world. What are the implications of this for global health, and what steps do you think can and should be taken to address income inequality, both in resource rich and developing countries?
3. A theme in this book is that health and human rights are "inextricably linked." Explain what you think is meant to be conveyed by this "link in a chain" metaphor. Can you think of other ways to describe the relationship between health and human rights in a changing world? What are the advantages and disadvantages of using these different descriptions?
4. What change is the world undergoing now that you think will have the most serious impact on health, and how might a human rights approach to it help to mitigate the negative impact?

CHAPTER 33

Global Health and the Global Economic Crisis

Solomon R. Benatar, Stephen Gill and Isabella Bakker

Despite impressive scientific advances and massive economic growth over the past 60 years, disparities in wealth and health have persisted and, in many places, widened. As a result, the hope of achieving significantly improved health for a greater proportion of the world's people—one of the most pressing problems of our time—has become an ever more distant prospect.[1-5] Our failure to make adequate advances in this direction is starkly illustrated by insufficient progress toward achieving the limited Millennium Development Goals for health in the poorest countries,[6] the growing threat of infectious diseases associated with poverty,[7] and the increasing burden of chronic diseases on lifestyle.[8] All of these challenges, now exacerbated by the most severe global economic crisis since the 1930s, are likely to become even more urgent in the years ahead.[9,10]

We describe aspects of an increasingly unstable world and why the market-driven growth paradigm is insufficient to achieve improved global health. We then suggest a number of new ways of thinking that we believe should be adopted to improve global health.

AN UNSTABLE WORLD

The economic crisis is a manifestation of a world made more unstable in large part because of socially unjust and excessive patterns of consumption that are resource depleting and wasteful. There is disjunction between two sets of factors: (1) rapid economic growth (according to World Bank statistics, the real-world annual income, measured in purchasing power parities, increased from $25.096 trillion in 1990 to $71.845 trillion in 2009)[11a] and unprecedented advances in science, technology, and medical care; and (2) the ability to use these advances to improve the lives of more people globally. Moreover, the current global economic and debt crisis[11b] has involved a flawed economic paradigm and policies (based since the 1970s on increasingly deregulated markets) that produced a catastrophe described as "the result of the combination of negligence, hubris and wrong economic theory."[12] Fox,[13] for example, has exploded the myth of the rational market. Many other economists—for example, Stiglitz[14] and Krugman[15]—have also recognized what Galbraith,[16] Gill,[17] and others have long understood as the serious imperfections of the economic theories propagated and linked to justify the free market and present-day finance capitalism that have produced evidently disastrous results.

Modern advances in health care are also now increasingly driven by market forces.[18–20] They have largely benefited only about 20% of the world's population. In the 1990s, 89% of annual world expenditure on health care was spent on 16% of the world's population, who bear 7% of the global burden of disease (in disability-adjusted life years).[21] Annual per capita expenditure on health care ranges from more than $6,000 in the United States (17% of gross domestic product [GDP]) to less than $10 in the poorest countries in Africa (< 3% of GDP). Half the world's population lives in countries that cannot afford annual per capita health expenditures of more than $15, and many people do not have access to even basic drugs. Between 51% and 60% of the world's population (3.2–3.8 billion people) live in miserable conditions, below what has been defined as the "ethical poverty line" of living on $2.80 to $3.00 per person per day,[22] benefiting little from progress in science and medicine.[1,23] Recent large public bailouts for private firms involving trillions of dollars have failed to stem massive job losses; at the same time, rising food prices have resulted in a further decline of living conditions for most of the world's population.[24–27]

Other manifestations of global instability, all in some way connected to excessive and wasteful consumption patterns, include the following: environmental degradation and global warming[28] (much of which results from energy-intensive production and distribution methods); emerging new infectious diseases that cause millions of premature deaths, with the significant possibility of future major pandemics of H1NI or H5N1 flu[29,30] (through closer contact with animals, in part as a result of intensive animal farming, which allows pathogens to cross species barriers); and an increasing global burden of disease from noncommunicable diseases,[8] accidents and trauma,[31] and pervasively adverse social conditions.[32–34]

THE NEED FOR NEW WAYS OF THINKING

We need a new balance of values and new ways of thinking and acting. This new thinking must transcend national and institutional boundaries and recognize that, in a globalizing world, health and disease in the most privileged nations is closely linked to health and disease in impoverished countries.[2,5,23,34] Sustainable improvement in health and well-being is a necessity for all, and the value placed on health should permeate every area of social and economic activity.

Improved population health is achievable but requires a new critical paradigm of what it means for people to flourish. At a basic level, human flourishing could be defined as lives in which essential life needs are met, including a safe and nurturing childhood, adequate nourishment and accommodation, clean water, sewerage facilities, childhood vaccination, education, and safety from easily preventable everyday health, economic, and other social threats within a broadly originated framework of respect for human rights.[35]

To facilitate escape from the current global impasse, in which less than one third of the world's population flourishes amid conditions of relative affluence and more than two thirds do not have their essential needs met, we offer the hypothesis that achieving improved global health will be less dependent on new scientific discoveries or technological advances, or on economic growth alone (both of which are necessary but not sufficient), than on working toward achieving the greater social justice that must lie at the core of public health.[36] This work will entail economic redistribution as well as enhanced democratization of processes associated with economic decision-making and the means of reproducing caring social institutions. The latter include educational facilities, health care services, and social services that could enable new generations of children to achieve their potential. These social services constitute the bedrock of civilized societies and have facilitated massive economic growth and improvement in many lives after World War II. The recent, long-overdue focus by the World Health Organization on the social determinants of health[6] is one of many evaluations supportive of our view.

The health of populations is shaped by systemic interaction between different forms and dimensions of power (such as those of states and constitutions), productive capacity (including markets), and powers that shape the ability effectively to sustain caring social services, such as education and health care, into the future. The persistence of the processes that undermine such institutions and public provisions, particularly through neoliberal economic policies and governance, tends to deepen the already extreme inequalities of income and wealth, and thus will likely further intensify current global health inequalities.[5,10,37]

ARRIVING AT THE CURRENT POSITION

Globalization has had many acknowledged beneficial effects,[38] including advances in knowledge, science, and technology; increased life expectancy for many; enhanced economic growth; greater freedom and prosperity for many; improvements in the speed and cost of communications and transportation; and popularization of the concept of human rights. Although only about 20% of the world's population has benefited maximally from such progress, a lower incidence of child labor has been reported in countries that are more open to trade and receive greater amounts of foreign direct investment.[39] Market-oriented economic policies have

also been linked to lower rates of infant mortality across the world.[40] In addition, new scientific discoveries (e.g., the human papillomavirus vaccine to prevent cervical cancer) offer much to improve health. However, many obstacles remain to ensuring availability of such new vaccines to those most at risk.[41]

The global political economy that has emerged over the past 30 to 40 years is increasingly governed by laws and regulations that are dominated by neoliberal economic ideas of unregulated market freedoms that suit transnational corporations and large investors. Since the 1980s, privatization, de-regulation, and liberalization have opened up world markets for corporations through policies related to the so-called "Washington Consensus" of Wall Street, the International Monetary Fund (IMF), the World Bank, and the US Treasury. The wider context is a free enterprise economic system dominated globally by the firms that control most large industries (e.g., food, pharmaceuticals, software). Whether it is in the form of World Bank structural adjustment policies or IMF stabilization, neoliberalism has become central to defining programs of political and economic reform and responses to the economic crises of ever-increasing severity since the late 1970s.[42]

What the World Bank has called the "locking in" of neoliberal economic policies through laws, regulations, and institutional changes such as independent central banks has therefore resulted in private economic forces gaining greater weight over basic economic policies.[42] For example, the independence of central banks from government interference or popular accountability has allowed financial capitalism to dictate monetary policies (boards of governors of central banks consist mainly of individuals representing financial interests) as well as many of the large bailouts of banks following the 2008 economic meltdown on Wall Street. Before the current financial collapse, central banks tended to pursue legally mandated low-inflation targets (even if this practice resulted in higher unemployment).[17,43] This innovation was coupled to fiscal restraint laws (e.g., to balance budgets), resulting in lower public expenditures on social and health provisions.

All of these policies were elements in the deepening of social inequality and the erosion of public health systems in recent years. More generally, neoliberal discourses of self-help and fiscal austerity underpin the argument that such public expenditures are not affordable—something the IMF emphasized in 2010, calling for 10 to 20 years of fiscal austerity to finance the huge public debts incurred in bailing out the big banks and auto firms.[43,44] More broadly, in a world of highly mobile capital, neoliberal policy must be perceived by the markets (investors) as credible—that is, making trade, fiscal, and monetary policies that favor business and thus inspire business confidence.

Nevertheless, at the heart of the recent financial crisis was not only a collapse in the credibility of regulation and government policy but, more fundamentally, a crisis of confidence of the trustworthiness and solvency of the big banks themselves. At a certain moment, fear and panic took over the markets, and private banks were unwilling to lend to each other or to other firms, causing a credit crunch. Such characteristics of poorly regulated finance capitalism help to explain why the crisis that began in 2008 was predictable. Indeed, some far-sighted political economists long argued that a collapse would ensue from too-rapid economic liberalization, excessive leveraging, and the use of poorly understood financial derivatives in the context of financial regulations that were effectively written by financial interests, providing little real oversight of banks and hedge funds.[17,45]

This free enterprise financial system is dominated by giant corporations on Wall Street and in London and, to a lesser extent, Tokyo, Frankfurt, and Paris. These interests, by controlling the financial markets and particularly the US Treasury and the US Federal Reserve System (particularly under the long stewardship of Alan Greenspan, who is a self-confessed devotee of the libertarian philosopher Ayn Rand[46]), succeeded in institutionalizing a self-regulating market system that allowed them to create new ways of making profits while taking excessive risks with other people's money. These strategies were all justified by the so-called efficient markets hypothesis,[13] which effectively asserts (with no theoretical or empirical evidence to substantiate it) that markets are best left to self-regulate since they have inbuilt incentives to spread risk and act with prudence. This combination of financial power and abstract theorizing proved to be a catastrophic admixture of ideology, interest, and recklessness.

Several insightful economists who have not been encumbered by flawed conventional economic theory have written extensively on such issues, and the US government's inspector general for the Troubled Asset Relief Program has published at least two reports on this topic.[47] Samuelson drew attention to Greenspan's flawed analysis of the financial crisis, for which Greenspan is at last "in part contrite."[48]

Thus, such economic governance frameworks are not simply the technical work of expert economists; they are deeply political, with enormous consequences for democracy and social justice. They have reshaped democratic and social choices at the local or national level (central banks are independent of local political pressures). The policy framework just outlined tends to militate against expenditures for public health or other caring institutions because it mandates policies to sustain confidence in the markets—confidence that the first priority of fiscal policy will be to repay public debts owed to bondholders as a consequence of financing the bailouts. The direct and indirect impact of policies that prioritize such private interests has been to widen disparities in health, access to health care, and life expectancy, within and between countries. This trend is likely to continue if neoliberal policies continue to dictate the fiscal response to financing the bailouts.[1,5,23,37]

The political nature of such choices is therefore now much more obvious than in the past. Policies of "sound finance" designed to curb excessive market freedoms and consequent aberrations have been abandoned, and central banks have been given the independent status that allowed them to access public money for private financial bailouts.[12,43,49] Corporations that engaged in unregulated investment and highly leveraged borrowing strategies, and that have long argued against state ownership of the means of production, now want their losses socialized or, when faced with complete financial ruin, their firms nationalized. Moreover, they claim that such interventions are required to restore the health of the market system.[43,49]

FAILURE OF THE MARKET-DRIVEN PARADIGM AS A MEANS TO GLOBAL HEALTH

Global public policy driven by the ideology of neoliberalism over the past 30 to 40 years has had many adverse effects on health and health policy. These adverse effects are evident in the policies of the World Bank and IMF, institutions that have held the balance of power in much of the global South for several decades in formulating global health policy. Liberalization of economies, reduced subsidies for basic foods, and shifts in agricultural policy that promote export crops to the detriment of homegrown food production have

resulted in the regulation of food prices via the global market—a development that has helped cause devastating malnutrition and starvation, especially in Africa. It is an indictment of the IMF and World Bank's structural adjustment programs that they imposed reduced government expenditure on health care, education, and other social services and encouraged privatization, even within health care. Structural adjustment programs, growing debt repayments, cuts in aid budgets (especially by the United States), discrimination against African trade, increasing malnutrition, and the Cold War activities of the great powers have all played a significant part in sustaining high rates of infectious disease and in fanning the flames of the AIDS pandemic.[2,5,34,50]

There has been an accompanying transformation of social institutions that made it possible (through provision of health care, education, and other social support) for new generations of society to live good lives.[2,17,51] Globally, there has been backtracking from the governing principles that characterized the post-1945 period, during which, to a greater or lesser degree, economics supported human development based on the power of governments to regulate banks and financial flows and to ensure universal access to basic social needs and a reasonable level of health care for the broader population.[50,52]

One of the enduring characteristics of the current global economic order is that it involves systematic transfers of real resources and wealth from the impoverished majorities of the poorer countries both to the wealthy within such countries and to the richer members of wealthier nations.[53] This transfer of resources has the most pronounced effect when market forces are inadequately regulated, as evidenced by the recent crisis that was precipitated by the effects of the deregulation of banks and financial institutions. In response to those who cite average increases in per capita GDP as a sign of poverty alleviation, average increases in country per capita GDP are not the best indicator of progress, as they do not reveal the distributive impact resulting from market liberalization and economic growth and are thus not necessarily associated with poverty reduction.[6]

Direct adverse influences on health include privatization of health care globally (and thus increased inequities of health care access).[54,55] Privatization of public health services is indirectly promoted by the World Trade Organization, with adverse effects on public health care in many countries.[39,56,57]

Increasing costs are associated with unregulated fee-for-service medical practice[20] and laws that protect private intellectual property rights, which prevent the sharing of information and keep prices high. These laws enable the pharmaceutical industry to skew research toward expensive profitable medications and away from diseases that principally afflict the poor. Between 1975 and 2004, with about 90% of medical research expenditure on health problems accounting for only 10% of the global burden of disease, and with 50% of global expenditure on medical research funded by the pharmaceutical industry, global medical research produced 1556 approved drug patents. Of these drugs, only 18 were for use against tropical diseases and 3 against tuberculosis, despite the great need for new drugs for these diseases.[58]

Indirect influences in a neoliberal market include the many powerful forces that sustain poverty, with all its adverse effects on health.[5,14,17,50,51,56,57] These forces include policies that have provided private firms (and capital in general) with legal rights and protections against most local obligations and often responsibilities to pay taxes, while reserving the right to obtain public subsidies and bailout funds if

needed. Firms have become much freer to move titles and funds across borders to offshore tax havens and thus reduce or avoid local taxes.[59] On the one hand, corporations benefit from a globally locked-in set of rights that are designed to provide security to capital; on the other, protections traditionally provided by governments for human security (e.g., against unemployment or ill health caused by a lack of basic needs or access to health care) are being systematically rolled back or removed as impediments to the efficient operation of labor markets and to free flows of trade and investment.[34,40,60] Indeed, as the Group of Eight (G8) nations pumped trillions of dollars into stabilizing financial markets, the World Health Organization offered evidence-based predictions of cuts in social and health expenditures and development assistance in 2009.[24]

Neoliberalism involves protection and socialization of losses for the strong (e.g., big insurance companies, financial houses, auto firms) and market discipline for the weak, who have little to fall back on if they lose their jobs and income flows. Poor people are more at the mercy of market forces if, for example, the cost of food and health care goes up. In a crisis, this vulnerability becomes more acute. As a 2009 Financial Times editorial put it:

> Almost unnoticed behind the economic crisis, a combination of lower growth, rising unemployment and falling remittances together with persistently high food prices has pushed the number of chronically hungry above 1 [billion] for the first time.[61]

This food crisis specifically originated with sharp increases in the price of major food grain prices. The average price of maize increased by more than 50% between 2003 and 2006, and in 2008 rice prices were 100% higher than they were in 2003. The United Nations has estimated that such food price increases—along with the immediate effects of higher energy prices and the financial crisis—are responsible for pushing more than 100 million people back into poverty and ill health.[62]

As in the global financial, food, and energy markets, there is now a shift toward privatization in which health—like food or oil—becomes a commodity that can be bought and sold by the few while the majority is increasingly deprived. Power lies with an emerging new hybrid of public and private health care institutions that are increasingly governed by the forces of the world market.[44,55–57] Costs of health care are deflected to households in which women have traditionally carried a large burden of caring work and have become the principal shock absorbers of this individualized risk.[45,60] Economist Uwe Reinhardt has noted that 9 million US children are uninsured,[63] and physician Deborah Frank has described the extent of food insecurity among children in the United States.[64] These observations have poignantly highlighted the impact of fiscal trends on the value accorded to the health and lives of children in the most privatized health market in the world.

HEALTH AND MEDICAL PRACTICE

The trends described in the previous section have massively distorted the practice of medicine and its research agenda globally, leading us to reflect on the quest for health and what the role of medicine is in achieving this goal.[65] suggest that health be defined as the ability and the opportunity to use one's natural endowments to achieve the potential to live a full and satisfying life. Achievement of health, so defined, requires attention to the social determinants of disease[6,34] and a lifelong supportive environment that includes good prenatal care, safe childbirth, a nurturing childhood, adequate education, prevention of avoidable diseases, and opportunities to flourish physically, socially, and intellectually. Health services in this context should provide access to affordable, effective health care, with recognition of the limits of medicine, particularly at the end of long lives or irremediable prolonged suffering, when at best only marginal benefits can be achieved. Corrective attention is also required to the opportunity costs of the excessive pursuit of profit in medicine, which gives precedence to vast expenditure on some aspects of clinical care that offer minimal improvement in health (or may even cause greater suffering) over more effective forms of treatment that could be more widely applied.[66,67]

Health, illness, and medicine go beyond individuals and their families to involve and affect whole societies, their institutions, and their global interconnections and ramifications.[65] Many countries consider access to basic health care as an essential human right that nation states should be committed to honoring for all. By its nature, the right to basic health care is a collective right—not an individual or exclusionary right, as is the right to private property, or the private ownership of a commodity. Social solidarity in health care implies that governments should provide basic public goods not only as a matter of economic and social efficiency but also as a public duty to their citizens. Because a long history of discrimination against the poor in the United States (who are disproportionately Black and Hispanic) lies behind the reluctance to subsidize the health of the poor, Krugman proposed that universal health care coverage should be at the center of a new, progressive US administration's agenda.[15] Recent progress in health reform in the United States is hopeful.

THREE SCENARIOS FOR HEALTH CARE IN THE FUTURE

We contemplate three potential scenarios for health care to help envisage and thus potentially shape future health care strategies. The first is an increasingly unequal market-governed future in which inequalities in income and health are accentuated, and new advances are applied predominantly for the benefit of the wealthy. This scenario, which is regrettably the most likely (as a continuation of neoliberalism), would be associated with a continued erosion of publicly supported health care systems, even in wealthy countries.

The second scenario would be a system of neoliberal market governance with some additional redistribution that would result in significant improvement in health for many people, but with residual wide disparities still affecting billions. The Millennium Development Goals; the Global Fund to Fight AIDS, Tuberculosis, and Malaria (Global Fund); and many other endeavors fit within this scenario, but regrettably, to date these efforts have been far less successful than anticipated.[67] Regardless, an era of generosity, characterized by a decade of increasing interest in and funding for global health, may be coming to an end.[68] Funding for these projects may be further limited by reprioritization of public expenditure to bail out large corporations.[69]

The third possibility, which we support, is redistribution based on creative new thinking and action within a paradigm of health and social development that could couple economic growth to redistribution of resources and fairer access to effective health care.

AVAILABILITY OF RESOURCES TO IMPROVE HEALTH GLOBALLY

On the basis of existing data on global economics, we believe that there are adequate resources to achieve immediate short-term improvements in global health. For example, health care and health for the 1 billion people in the world who live in countries that cannot afford to spend more than $15 per capita each year on health care could be greatly enhanced if the additional funds required for basic health care services—estimated by the World Health Organization at $35 per capita annually—were provided. A tax of 0.1% (1 cent of each $10) applied to the wealthiest 1 billion people in the world (who enjoy annual per capita expenditures on health of about $3,000) would raise the $35 billion required each year to provide the $50 per person package of health care for the poorest billion people.[70] A sign of relative economic abundance in the world that suggests this tax is achievable is the fact that many trillions of dollars were rapidly injected into collapsing and often corrupt financial institutions. Against this background, it is shameful that even $15 billion cannot be raised annually for efforts such as the Global Fund.

Notably, up to one third of the ownership of total global economic product is now held offshore, and about 50% of all world trade passes through tax havens, allowing for the shifting of profits and losses between locations and avoidance of taxes. For example, Microsoft reported a $12.3 billion profit in 1999, but paid no federal corporate income taxes that year.[59,71] Such practices have been facilitated by the liberalization of money, trade, and investment regulations.

Substantial improvements in global health could therefore be achieved in the short term, although such improvement will be contingent on a significant redistribution of global economic resources. In time, new resources could be mobilized for thoroughly justified and ambitious global health goals—provided that social and political forces can confront the misallocation, waste, and distorted preferences currently characterizing a consumption-driven, energy-intensive, and wasteful neoliberal economic system premised on support for the affluent.[72–74]

Although governments are now paying more attention to tax evasion and the offshore world because of the looming fiscal pressures caused by the global economic crisis, their efforts need to go further. By rectifying tax evasion, eliminating transfer-pricing systems used by corporations, and abolishing offshore tax havens, governments could generate enormous new resources for funding social and health provisions. In addition, a small tax on the massive international financial transactions within a casino economy[75,76] (95% of which are purely speculative and hence unconnected to real economic activity) could yield more than $150 billion a year—more than enough to fund the Millennium Development Goals, which would vastly improve the incomes, health care, and educational facilities of half the world's population. All of these endeavors to achieve basic reforms of the international tax regime[59] should be combined with efforts to fundamentally reform global economic governance, including much stricter prudential regulation of banks to prevent a repeat of past reckless practices.

SHIFTING PARADIGMS

These material questions highlight the need for a more intense focus on basic human needs if we wish to define a civilized world as one characterized by policies and activities capable of sustaining the advancement of decent human lives for all.[17,37,50] A new paradigm to meet such global health challenges calls for a new language and new concepts that could take health care beyond what has been achieved through the narrowly materialist and reductionist approach that characterizes market-driven health under neoliberal governance

(i.e., which seeks to govern all social provisions through market principles). More socially accountable and democratic institutions are needed, and these institutions should be linked to capacity-building for self-sufficiency while promoting local sustainability within an increasingly interdependent world.[6,9,35] These goals will not be easily achieved, and they will require extensive transdisciplinary research programs that embrace integration of various discourses on progress, sustainability, and development and that find ways of promoting public dialogue on these issues as well as visionary political will.

FIVE STEPS TOWARD IMPROVING GLOBAL HEALTH

We suggest several steps to broaden our discourses, which in turn would help develop policies that could have a practical effect.

Extension of the Ethical Discourse

The dominant ethics discourse of our time has been focused on the ethics of interpersonal relationships (e.g., interpersonal morality). This discourse must now be extended to include the ethics of how institutions (e.g., health care institutions) should function (civic morality) and the ethics of interactions between nations (ethics of international relations), as has been articulated in more detail previously.[38,74,77] The language of cosmopolitan justice and of the equal moral worth of all individuals[78] adds to the perspective outlined in that previous work.

Broadening Concern for Human Rights

Similarly, concern for human rights should include consideration of the social, economic, and cultural rights required for more people to have the opportunity to achieve their human potential. To achieve this goal, "rights language" needs to be supplemented with a focus on the human needs that generate rights claims, the identification of duty bearers to ensure the reciprocal duties required for satisfaction of rights, and the development of operational procedures to ensure delivery of sustainable and equitable health policies to enhance human capabilities.[41,79,80]

Immediate Social and Economic Policy Responses

These policies would include the promotion of socially sustainable economic recovery and social cohesion, new financing mechanisms for health to provide more equitable distribution of benefits, and macroeconomic stabilization that could provide greater social protection for the poor.[10,16,35,57] The approximately $17 trillion allocated for "economic emergency funds" by the United States, European Union, and other G8 nations to promote macroeconomic stabilization from 2007 through 2010 is about 22 times as much as that pledged for the Millennium Development Goals. In the United States, more than 90% of the total committed thus far has been to bail out corporate interests, notably large banks, wealthy investors, and the big auto firms, thus socializing their risks. A political economy analysis reveals the opportunity costs of such choices—the possible alternative uses forgone in the decision to spend the funds in this way. Many of these funds could have been spent on job retraining, health care, accessible education, and affordable housing. Moreover, such social expenditures have far more favorable effects on macroeconomic stabilization because they raise aggregate demand in greater measure than do outlays on financial bailouts—because poorer people spend more of their income

than the wealthy. This additional spending is needed to reverse the economic slump and to mitigate rising unemployment. Economic arguments for the general socialization of risk were made by Keynes, in his analysis of the Great Depression of the 1930s, as a means to stabilize and legitimate capitalism. These arguments became a staple of mainstream economic thinking between 1945 and 1975, the era before neoliberal capitalism.[34,35,50]

Medium-Term Social and Economic Policies for a Healthier Society

These policies would include initiatives to

1. Revise the tax base in a more macroeconomically efficient way while ensuring that the future distribution of tax burdens is equitable and sustainable;
2. Develop comprehensive measures to ensure that the economy is regulated effectively and prudently (e.g., preventing financial institutions from excessively risky practices such as using financial derivatives and products that are not properly understood or secure);
3. Develop policies to revitalize public and collective services such as public health systems, as well as infrastructure for public transportation, public information, and communications systems;
4. Deal with demographic shifts (e.g., health issues associated with the aging society in Europe and Japan) and break down the unhelpful dichotomies that govern policies in such areas such as young and old as well as so-called productive and unproductive members of society; and
5. Rethink policies to change the destructive logic of affluent lifestyles and thus minimize over-consumption, waste, and bad (especially meat-based) afflu-

ent diets and to promote healthier ways of living, while preserving toleration and diversity of social choices.[5,14,17,60,81]

Changing Mindsets for Potentially Enduring Long-Term Benefit

Engagement in critique and popular education is needed to counteract the tenacity of a paradigm based on the assumption that continuous economic growth for some, driven by the profit motive, provides necessary and sufficient conditions to protect privileged ways of life. There is a need to develop policies for education and culture to help emancipate creative potentials in new ways. Specifically, knowledge and media systems should promote widespread understanding of how inequality and ill health result from economic governance and geopolitical arrangements that extract resources from the poor and maintain economic growth and profit for the privileged at the expense of others in the short term and of all in the longer term. New mindsets would imply significant changes—not only in the field of economics but also across the social and natural sciences—to produce a more integrated and forward-looking understanding to promote sustainability and justice.[74,78,79,81]

CONCLUSIONS

The dysfunctional global economic system we have described is geared primarily to the pursuit of profit at the expense of human flourishing and human rights.[1,2,51,52,72,79,81] Restructuring this system will require imaginative ideas and proposals—in sum, bold action. Thomas Pogge's innovative Health Impact Fund project, designed to facilitate the development of drugs that have the maximum potential for saving lives, is an example of how such trends could feasibly be reversed on the basis of a new compact between private and public interests,

because it would still reward pharmaceutical companies.[73] Another innovative idea is the call for researching and addressing some alternative grand challenges[82] that would go beyond the Gates Grand Challenges, which are limited to encouraging innovations in science and technology, and speed up reduction in the global burden of disease.[83]

Beyond specific initiatives, the challenges enumerated here call for the development of imaginative international strategic alliances using varied expertise from many academic disciplines and the mobilization of political will within multiple spheres of influence—in the public and private sectors—to force change on unresponsive leaders and the military, economic, and social power that they seek to protect. This moral challenge for the 21st century requires many centers of political action to produce and implement a new perspective on political economy, civic life, human flourishing, and health care. To achieve this goal requires a change in cultural ethos to facilitate the extensive multidisciplinary research needed to show the path ahead. Such enlightenment could enable us to (1) be served by the market system rather than us serving the market[84] and (2) deal constructively with upstream causes of poor health. The challenge of funding and undertaking this research is of the order of magnitude of researching and developing an HIV vaccine. We hope that this brief review will stimulate the discussion, debate, and commitment to research of sufficient depth, breadth, and intensity to achieve ambitious global health goals.

REFERENCES

1. Benatar SR. Global disparities in health and human rights. Am J Public Health. 1998;88(2):295–300.
2. Farmer P. Pathologies of Power: Health, Human Rights, and the New War on the Poor. Berkeley: University of California Press; 2003.

3. Amnesty International. The G8: global arms exporters: failing to prevent irresponsible arms transfers.

4. Birdsall N. Inequality matters. Boston Review. March/April 2007.

5. V. Neoliberalism, Globalization and Inequalities: Consequences for Health and Quality of Life. Amityville, NY: Baywood; 2007.

6. Social Determinants of Health. Geneva, Switzerland: World Health Organization; 2008.

7. Selgelid MJ. Ethics and infectious disease. Bioethics. 2005;19(3):272–289.

8. Yach D, Hawkes C, Gould L, Hofman KJ. The global burden of chronic diseases: overcoming impediments to prevention and control. JAMA. 2004;291(21):2616 2622.

9. Benatar SR. Global health: where to now? Glob Health Gov. 2008/09;2(2).

10. Fidler D. After the revolution: global health politics in a time of economic crisis and threatening future trends. Glob Health Gov. 2008/09;2(2).

11a. World Bank. International Comparison Program database. GNI, PPP (current international $).. Accessed January 30, 2011.

11b. Milner B. The world cup of diplomacy. Toronto Globe and Mail. June 24, 2010.

12. Mueller A. What's behind the financial market crisis? Mises Daily, Ludwig von Mises Institute.

13. Fox J. The Myth of the Rational Market: A History of Risk, Reward, and Delusion on Wall Street. New York, NY: Harper Business/Harper Collins; 2009.

14. Stiglitz JE. Globalization and Its Discontents. New York, NY: W. W. Norton & Co; 2002.

15. Krugman P. The Conscience of a Liberal. New York, NY: W. W. Norton & Co; 2009.

16. Galbraith JK. The Economics of Innocent Fraud: Truth for Our Time. Boston, MA: Houghton Mifflin; 2004.

17. Gill S. Finance, production and panopticism. In: Gill S, ed. Globalization, Democratization and Multilateralism. New York, NY: Macmillan Press; 1997:51–75.

18. Relman AS. A physician's view of Freidson's analysis. J Health Polit Policy Law. 2003;28(1):164–168.

19. Gawande A. The cost conundrum. New Yorker. June 1, 2009.

20. Herzlinger R. Market-Driven Health Care. Reading, MA: Addison Wesley; 1997.

21. Iglehart JK. The American health care system: expenditures. N Engl J Med. 1999;340(1):70–76.

22. Edward P. The Ethical Poverty Line: a moral quantification of absolute poverty. Third World Q. 2006; 27(2):377–393.

23. Growing Unequal? Income Distribution and Poverty in OECD Countries. Paris, France: Organisation for Economic Co-Operation and Development; 2008.

24. World Health Organization. Impact of the global financial and economic crisis on health: statement by WHO Director-General Dr Margaret Chan. November 12, 2008.

25. The consequences of bad economics. Financial Times. March 9, 2009.

26. Leonhardt D. Broader measure of US unemployment stands at 17.5%. New York Times. November 6, 2009.

27. Lewis A. Business ethic slammed. Cape Times. November 11, 2009:1.

28. United Nations Development Program. Global Environment Outlook: GEO 4, Environment for Development.

29. Garrett L. The Coming Plague: Newly Emerging Diseases in a World Out of Balance. New York, NY: Farrar, Strauss and Giroux; 1994.

30. Osterholm MT. Preparing for the next pandemic. N Engl J Med. 2005;352(18):1839–1842.

31. World Health Organization. The Injury Chartbook: a graphical overview of the global burden of injuries.

32. Stonington S, Holmes SM. Social medicine in the 21st century. PLoS Med. 2006;3(10):e445.

33. Goldberg DS. In support of a broad model of public health: disparities, social epidemiology and public health causation. Public Health Ethics. 2009;2(1):70–83.

34. The political economy of health and development. In: Birn A-E, Pillay Y, Holtz TH. Textbook of International Health. 3rd ed. Oxford, UK: Oxford University Press; 2009:132–191.

35. Held D. Global Covenant: The Social Democratic Alternative to the Washington Consensus. Cambridge, UK: Polity Press; 2004.

36. Powers M, Faden R. Social Justice: The Moral Foundations of Public Health and Health Policy. New York, NY: Oxford University Press; 2006.

37. Labonte R, Schrecker T, Sanders D, Meeus W. Fatal Indifference: The G8 and Global Health. Cape Town, South Africa; UCT Press and International Development Research Centre Ottawa; 2004.

38. Benatar SR, Daar AS, Singer PA. Global health ethics: a rationale for mutual caring. Int Aff. 2003;79(1):107–138.

39. Neumayer E, de Soysa I. Trade openness, foreign direct investment and child labour. World Dev. 2005; 33(1):43–63.

40. Gerring J, Thacker SC. Do neoliberal economic policies kill or save lives? Business and Politics. 2009;10(3).

41. Benatar SR. Human rights in the biotechnology era. BMC International Health and Human Rights. 2002;2(3).

42. Gill S, Bakker IC. The global crisis and global health. In: Benatar S, Brock G, eds. Global Health and Global Health Ethics. Cambridge, UK: Cambridge University Press; 2011.

43. Cukierman A. Central bank independence and monetary policymaking institutions: past, present and future. Eur J Polit Econ. 2008;24(4):722–736.

44. Project Uncensored. New trade treaty seeks to privatize global social services.

45. Bakker I, Silvey R. Beyond States and Markets: The Challenges of Social Reproduction. New York, NY: Routledge; 2008.

46. Greenspan A. The Age of Turbulence: Adventures in a New World. New York, NY: Penguin Press; 2007.

47. Krugman P. The big squander. New York Times. November 21, 2009.

48. Samuelson RJ. Alan Greenspan's flawed analysis of the financial crisis. Washington Post. March 22, 2010.

49. Harrison E. The FDIC and the socialization of banking losses. August 26, 2009.

50. Rowden R. The Deadly Ideas of Neoliberalism: How the IMF Has Undermined Public Health and the Fight Against AIDS. London, UK: Zed Books; 2009.

51. Bakker I, Gill S, eds. Power, Production and Social Reproduction. Human In/Security in the Global Political Economy. New York, NY: Palgrave Macmillan; 2003.

52. Fox J. In the long run. New York Times. October 30, 2009. Accessed November 21, 2009.

53. Toye J, Toye R. The UN and Global Political Economy. Indianapolis: Indiana University Press; 2004. UN Intellectual History Project Series.

54. Basu S. The privatization of global health..

55. Stuckler D, King L, McKee M. Mass privatisation and the post-communist mortality crisis: a cross-national analysis. Lancet. 2009;373(9661):399–407.

56. Global Health Watch 2005–2006. London, UK: Zed Books; 2005.

57. Global Health Watch 2: An Alternative World Health Report. London, UK: Zed Books; 2008.

58. Chirac P, Torreele E. Global framework on essential health R&D. Lancet. 2006;367(9522):1560–1561.

59. Brock G. Taxation and global justice: closing the gap between theory and practice. J Soc Philos. 2008;39(2):161–184.

60. Gill S. New constitutionalism, democratisation and global political economy. Pacifica Rev. 1998;10(1):23–38.

61. Blas J. Relentless tide of global hunger engulfs 1bn. Financial Times. April 6, 2009.

62. Digital Journal. UN Conference: Starvation a "world emergency."

63. Reinhardt UE. Seriously, what is a child? New York Times. April 24, 2009.

64. Frank D. Testimony before the Committee on the Budget, US House of Representatives. February 15, 2007.

65. Benatar SR, Fox RC. Meeting threats to global health: a call for American leadership. Perspect Biol Med. 2005;48(3):344–361.

66. Deber RB. Access without appropriateness: Chicken Little in charge? Healthc Policy. 2008;4(1):23–29.

67. Changing course: alternative approaches to achieve the Millennial Development Goals and fight HIV/AIDS. ActionAid International USA. September 2005.

68. Schneider K, Garret LG. The end of the era of generosity? Global health amid economic crisis. Philos Ethics Humanit Med. 2009;4(1).

69. Stiglitz J. Reform is needed. Reform is in the air. We can't afford to fail. Guardian. March 27, 2009.

70. Notes on Canadian Conference on International Health, 2009.

71. Techrights. Summary of Microsoft tax evasion stories. Available at: http://boycottnovell.com/2008/11/16/microsoft-tax-evasion-roundup.

72. Sanders DM, Todd C, Chopra M. Confronting Africa's health crisis: more of the same will not be enough. BMJ. 2005;331(7519):755–758.

73. Pogge T. The Health Impact Fund: making new medicines available to all. Available at: http://www.yale.edu/macmillan/igh/hif_book.pdf.

74. Benatar SR. Moral imagination: the missing component in global health. PLoS Med. 2005;2(12):e400.

75. Ellwood E. No-Nonsense Guide to Globalization. London, UK: Verso Press; 2003.

76. Global Policy Forum. Available at: http://www.globalpolicy.org/socecon/glotax/currtax/index.htm.

77. Benatar SR, Daar AS, Singer PA. Global health ethics: the need for an expanded discourse on bioethics. PloS Med. 2005;2(7):e143.

78. Brock G. Global Justice: A Cosmopolitan Account. Oxford, UK: Oxford University Press; 2009.

79. Benatar SR, Doyal L. Human rights abuses: toward balancing two perspectives. Int J Health Serv. 2009;39(1):139–159.

80. Doyal L, Gough I. A Theory of Human Need. London, UK: Macmillan; 1991.

81. Building a World Community: Globalization and the Common Good. Copenhagen, Denmark:

Royal Danish Ministry of Foreign Affairs; 2000.

82. Birn A-E. Gates' grandest challenge: transcending technology as public health ideology. Lancet. 2005; 366(9484):514–519.

83. Gates Foundation picks 14 grand challenges for global disease research. Bull World Health Organ. 2003;81:915–916.

84. Barber B. A revolution in spirit. The Nation. February 9, 2009.

QUESTIONS

1. What do you think the authors mean by "globalization?" Is it true that the globalization movement is primarily a product of market economics and the growth of transnational corporations? How can transnational corporations be encouraged to promote and protect human rights?

2. What does it mean to say that "healthcare is not a market good?" There is no "right to health" in the US, but after passage of the Affordable Care Act it is moving closer to a "right to healthcare insurance." Why is the right to insurance the best the US has been able to do?

3. The agenda proposed in this chapter can seem overwhelming. Where would you start first?

4. Bill Foege, a leader in global health, has suggested that it is a mistake for global health advocates to rely too much on "the overheads and bureaucracy of superstructures" like WHO and UNICEF, suggesting that corporations (e.g., Merck, river blindness), organizations (e.g., Red Cross, measles), and NGOs (Carter Center, guinea worm) play major roles in global health. Does this observation let the governments (and the UN) off the hook, and undermine their ability to be leaders in global health, leading global health on a perilous and leaderless path? How do you think it would be best to develop global health governance mechanisms?

FURTHER READING

1. Ghemawat, Pankaj, *World 3.0: Global Prosperity and How to Achieve It.* Boston: Harvard Business Review Press, 2011.
2. Kim, Jim, et al., eds., *Dying for Growth: Global Inequality and the Health of the Poor*, Monroe, Maine: Common Courage Press, 2000.
3. Pogge, Thomas, *World Poverty and Human Rights*, 2nd ed. New York: Polity, 2008.
4. Sachs, Jeffrey, *The Price of Civilization: Reawakening American Virtue and Prosperity.* New York: Random House, 2011.

CHAPTER 34

Climate Change and Human Rights: A Rough Guide

Stephen Humphreys

INTRODUCTION: WHY HUMAN RIGHTS?

Two starting points inform this chapter. The first is that, as a matter of simple fact, climate change is already undermining the realisation of a broad range of internationally protected human rights: rights to health and even life; rights to food, water, shelter and property; rights associated with livelihood and culture; with migration and resettlement; and with personal security in the event of conflict.[1] Few dispute that this is the case.

Moreover, the interlinkages are deep and complex. The worst effects of climate change are likely to be felt by those individuals and groups whose rights protections are already precarious.[2] This is partly coincidence. As it happens, the most dramatic impacts of climate change are expected to occur (and are already being experienced) in the world's poorest countries, where rights protections too are often weak. But the effect is also causal and mutually reinforcing. Populations whose rights are poorly protected are likely to be less well-equipped to understand or prepare for climate change effects; less able to lobby effectively for government or international action; and more likely to lack the resources needed to adapt to expected alterations of their environmental and economic situation. A vicious circle links precarious access to natural resources, poor physical infrastructure, weak rights protections, and vulnerability to climate change-related harms.

At another level, the close relation between climate change and human rights vulnerability has a common economic root. Rights protections are inevitably weakest in resource-poor contexts. But resource shortages also limit the capacity (of governments as well as individuals) to respond and adapt to climate change. Worse, where governments are poorly resourced, climate change harms will tend to impact populations unevenly and unequally, in ways that are *de facto* discriminatory because the private capacity of individuals to resist and adapt differs greatly.

The construction of an international climate change regime too has rights implications. Mitigation policies have clear human rights dimensions. On one hand, any strategy (or mix of strategies) that is successful at global level will tend to determine the long-term access that many millions of people will have to basic public goods. On the other, choices made in the shorter-term—such as whether and where to cultivate biofuels or preserve forests—will affect food, water and health security and, by extension, the cultures and livelihoods of numerous particular persons in particular places.

Adaptation policies will raise comparable human rights concerns. Adaptation may be reframed as a compensatory or corrective response to potential or actual climate change-related human rights violations. Adaptive interventions before or during climate change impacts reduce the likelihood that rights violations might result from those impacts; adaptation actions after the fact may provide redress where violations have already taken place. Indeed, discussions of adaptation at international and government level (as opposed to autonomous local measures) already assume a rights basis for policy construction, even if it is rarely articulated in those terms. At the same time, adaptation actions can themselves affect human rights—such as, for example, if communities or individuals are forcibly removed from disaster or flood-prone areas, or, less forcibly, expected to conform to new economic policy imperatives (by adopting different cash crops or energy sources, for example).

Despite the obvious overlaps outlined above, the mainstream climate change literature and debate has, until very recently, given little or no attention to human rights concerns.[3] This has been so even though the reports of the Intergovernmental Panel on Climate Change (IPCC) have steadily examined the social impacts of climate change—in particular on food, water and health—and have progressively expanded their sphere of reference to include the social as well as the physical sciences. Nonetheless, perhaps unavoidably, climate change analyses generally remain aggregated at continental or subregional level: the available information is still not sufficiently nuanced to cover the situation of individuals and communities who experience climate impacts directly as rights infringements. This too reflects the resource asymmetries that everywhere inform climate change discussion and research. Information is far more detailed for those areas likely to experience lesser impacts than for those where the consequences will be most devastating.

The paucity of rights-specific information is not, of course, merely a *cause* of the negligible analysis of the human rights dimensions of climate change, it is also a *consequence*. Given their salience to the main themes discussed in the IPCC's fourth assessment report ("IPCC AR4"), for example, it is remarkable that human rights are scarcely signalled in almost 3,000 pages of analysis.[4]

This would appear to indicate a near complete disciplinary disconnect, an impression borne out by a glance at the 10,000-strong participants' list for the recent (thirteenth) Conference of the Parties of December 2007, among whom no more than a tiny handful hailed from human rights backgrounds. Scanning for human rights "language" is, of course, a poor analytical tool. Similar concerns may be addressed using different terms—and this appears to be at least partly true in this instance. Nevertheless, the choice of language and disciplinary lens will determine to some extent the relevance of certain kinds of information, orientation and response. Since the IPCC reports are essentially literature reviews, the shortage of rights references no doubt indicates a mere vacuum in the literature rather than any conclusion, bias or failing on the part of the IPCC authors. That vacuum says as much about an absence of interest in climate change among human rights professionals to date as vice versa.

WHY THE SILENCE ON HUMAN RIGHTS?

What explains this mutual disinterest? The primary cause appears to be a kind of disciplinary path-dependence. The study of climate change began among meteorologists, became firmly entrenched in the physical sciences, and has only gradually—if inevitably—reached into the social sciences. The basic orientation has remained pre-eminently, though not solely, economic. Climate change negotiations have centred on consensus-driven welfare-based solutions, approaches that have historically thrived independently of and in parallel to human rights. Human rights organisations, for their part, are unlikely, as a matter of professional orientation, to take up issues framed as "hypothetical" or scenario-based, quite aside from the disciplinary boundaries that have long existed between environmental and human rights law. It may be that consideration of "new and additional" *future* harms simply escapes the ordinary purview of human rights analysis. The confluence is consequently marginal: on the few occasions human rights are mentioned in the IPCC reports, it is almost exclusively in connection with harms that have already taken place.[5]

In addition, experts in either discipline might identify plausible reasons for doubting that a "human rights approach" would assist the formation of effective policies to address climate change. Listed below are five such reasons.[6]

The rights at issue are difficult to enforce. Climate change generally (if not exclusively) affects categories of human rights that have notoriously weak enforcement mechanisms under international law—social and economic rights, the rights of migrants, rights protections during conflicts.[7] Even those rights that have strong protections, such as rights to life and to property, are not subject to their normal enforcement procedures, because the harms caused by climate change can be attributed only indirectly to the identified perpetrators. In the absence of strong enforcement institutions, either at national or international level, it is not immediately obvious what human rights can add to a policy discussion that is already notably welfare-conscious, even if focused on the general good rather than on individual complaints.

Extraterritorial responsibility is hard to establish. Under human rights law, a person's government ordinarily has the primary duty to act when rights are violated. In the context of climate change, however, responsibility for impacts in the most vulnerable countries often lies not with the government nearest to hand, but with diffuse actors, both public and private, many of whom are located far away. Human rights law does not easily reach across international borders to impose obligations in matters such as these.[8]

Local accountability is hard to establish. Although countries that lack economic resources and infrastructure are least likely to be major emitters of greenhouse gases, they are most likely to suffer devastating effects of climate change—effects whose human consequences will be worsened by their low capacity to adapt. Resource constraints inevitably impair a state's ability to provide quality public goods to its population. This problem, which underpins the inadequate fulfilment of social and economic rights in some countries, has led to the notion of "progressive realisation" of those rights under international law. Under existing circumstances, however, climate change is likely to lead to a *progressive deterioration* of those same rights. If a government cannot be held accountable for failing fully to protect those rights in the ordinary course, it will surely be even harder to hold it responsible for circumstances it did not create.[9]

Emergency conditions limit the application of human rights law. The most severe climate change impacts will be catastrophic—drought, floods, famines, mass migration, wars—and will affect large numbers of people. In such circumstances, a common response is to declare an emergency. International human rights treaties and most national constitutions typically allow for the suspension ("derogation") of many human rights in times of emergency.[10] Emergency regimes are habitually critical or dismissive of human rights constraints, tending instead to adopt an ends-oriented and charity-centred language of humanitarian relief. Governments are empowered to act expediently, with less regard to individual rights and interests that might act as a brake on achieving the greater good. Human rights, traditionally conceived as a bulwark against expansive state discretion, become less relevant as *legal* tools at such times (although their rhetorical force may increase). Indeed, many human rights traditionalists might be expected to oppose climate change action on precisely the grounds that it will empower government, both nationally and internationally, at the expense of individuals.[11]

Rights may conflict. Human rights protect others besides those who are potentially harmed by climate change. Economic actors are also rights-holders and it is foreseeable that some of them will invoke the human right to property or peaceful enjoyment of their possessions to prevent or reduce action on climate change. The right to property has been given a broad interpretation by international tribunals and could be asserted by those who have been licensed to act in ways that harm the environment. Other human rights claims too— such as to culture, or freedom of religion, or family reunion—may bring individuals into conflict with climate change policies. All of these rights, like other rights, may be limited for the public good, and struggles can be expected over exactly where the line should be drawn in such cases. Adversarialism is, of course, part of the ordinary human rights landscape. As climate change policies will necessarily generate choices about the distribution of costs and benefits, the invocation of human rights can be expected to produce struggles, pitting interest groups against one another in a way that is markedly different from the consensus-building and compromise that has traditionally guided climate negotiations.

The above objections are not negligible. But they nevertheless rely, perhaps excessively, on a *legalist* vision of human rights that, if frequently effective, is not necessarily definitive. Legal scholars will quickly recognise a long-standing dichotomy between formal and substantive justice: the hard rule-of-law formalism of human rights on one hand versus the soft law, policy orientation of the UNFCCC on the other. The ethical language of "equity" and "common but differentiated responsibilities" of the UNFCCC has a quite different texture to the moral certainty and universalism of statements like the Universal Declaration on Human Rights (UDHR) and the international human rights covenants. Indeed "equity", as it appears in the UNFCCC, might be thought difficult to reconcile with the formal equality that underpins human rights law, much as the UNFCCC's distinction between "Annex I" (wealthy or "developed") and "non-Annex I" ("developing") countries seemingly runs counter to the universal obligations held by all countries under human rights law.[12] Fortunately, however, as this report will show, the two approaches are not mutually exclusive.

POSSIBLE BENEFITS OF A HUMAN RIGHTS POLICY ORIENTATION

As harms due to climate change are increasingly felt, it is very likely that many of those affected will turn to the hard law language of human rights for protection. Indeed, this is already happening.[13] However, human rights can be articulated in registers other than law. In approaching climate change, a case might be made for a less legalist application of human rights principles to the climate change field, in favour of an approach better suited to the immense policy challenges that lie ahead. Five potential benefits of such a policy orientation are identified below.

Human rights prioritise harms to actual persons. As mentioned, human rights discourse cannot easily sustain discussion of hypotheticals: it reverts quickly to actual facts and outcomes. But this can be an advantage. In a debate necessarily steeped in scenarios and probabilities, human rights law requires that hard lines be drawn where possible. The important questions about impact scenarios would then be: *who*, precisely, is likely to suffer *what* and *why*? Human rights standards provide thresholds of minimum acceptability.[14] If an effect of climate change is to cause the living conditions of specific individuals to sink *below* these understood thresholds, it might be considered unacceptable (or even unlawful). This approach (discussed in more detail in the following chapter) is more modest than one that argues for equal rights to the atmosphere, or to a given level of aggregate prosperity, or to the notion of "utility maximisation" common in economic analysis. Because it is modest, achievable and fair, and uses a language to which few will object, a policy orientation based on human rights thresholds potentially provides a platform for broad-based dialogue on burden sharing of a kind that has frequently lacked in climate change debates.

Looking forward, mitigation and adaptation policies too might be framed or evaluated by reference to human rights thresholds. Deforestation, biofuel substitution, even emissions trading will all lead to outcomes that, like climate impacts themselves, can be reviewed in advance for their likely human rights effects. If specific policies are forecast to lead to faltering rights fulfilment, they could be altered or rejected. For vulnerable states, a focus on affected populations rather than (or in addition to) environmental damage may prove useful in mobilising international assistance.[15]

Ethical demands translate into legal obligations. Human rights thinking habitually resituates ethical imperatives within a legal framework. Observers of climate change negotiations have long noted that the distribution of climate change impacts is inherently unfair: the costs are carried less by those who created the problem than by innocent others elsewhere. One long-standing ethical worry has been that this original injustice will be reproduced throughout an international climate regime, allowing the beneficiaries of carbon overuse to pass their costs onto others distant in time or space. This hard ethical problem has always been close to the heart of climate change negotiations. It is unlikely that human rights law can resolve it. But human rights values might usefully refocus or perhaps help to ground the debate.

Accountability. The human rights preoccupation with accountability might be helpful in constructing a climate regime. In general, international environmental treaties have been slow to introduce judicial instruments or other mechanisms of direct accountability, preferring to emphasise collaborative action. However, as the climate regime extends, as the urgency of addressing the problem grows, and as the instruments involved increase in complexity, accountability is likely to become more important. Accountability mechanisms of some sort will be needed to underpin any functional climate regime, because compliance will be vital to credibility.[16] This is an area where human rights activists and lawyers have relevant experience—for example, of identifying and endeavouring to mend (albeit with limited success) the institutional gaps that obstruct the prosecution of transnational private actors for human rights violations. The incorporation of human rights assessments in policy projections could also help to determine who is accountable for what, and how accountability should be attributed.

Focus on the most vulnerable. Human rights analysis and advocacy have always paid particular attention to those who are on the margins of society as a result of poverty, powerlessness, or systemic discrimination. It is widely acknowledged that social and economic vulnerability greatly increases the risk of suffering from the impacts of climate change. Those who are less well off often lack the information or resources to make informed choices on adapting to or otherwise avoiding future damages.[17] They are also less likely to have a sustained voice in, or influence over, policy-making, and so in times of crises the vulnerability of marginalised groups can increase dramatically. A human rights focus can redirect attention to people who are otherwise likely to be ignored or unheard. Where communities are already living in precarious circumstances (shanty towns, polluted or otherwise fragile environments), posing human rights questions may help to locate some of the hazards posed by climate change—from desertification, water salination, sea level rise, and so on—as well as those who are most at risk from them. Particularly in countries and societies where poverty is linked to discrimination—ethnic, racial or religious—an analysis sensitive to the dynamics that drive exclusion is likely to foresee future trends and vulnerabilities more clearly.

Procedural guarantees. Various doctrines of procedural or process rights have evolved within human rights law, many of which have been adopted in international environmental law.[18] In principle these can help those harmed by climate change to influence policies that affect them, and

can assist policy-makers to understand and take account of public needs. These rights are particularly relevant to adaptation policy.

Taken together, these strengths suggest that human rights could play a valuable role during climate change negotiations and when implementing policies, particularly in ethically fraught areas. Human rights supply not only legal imperatives, but also a set of internationally agreed values around which common action can be negotiated and motivated. They provide a language of minimum thresholds, legally defined, about which there is already widespread consensus. They are potentially very relevant where the recent Bali roadmap, for example, speaks of "a shared vision for long-term cooperative action . . . taking into account social and economic conditions and other relevant factors".[19] The rule-of-law formalism of human rights practice might even provide backbone for the ethical aspirations and policy assumptions embedded in such language.

RIGHTS-BASED PERSPECTIVES ON CLIMATE CHANGE

Several attempts have been made to place rights at the centre of the future climate change regime. These have not, however, generally been human rights-focused: they have not been based upon or referred to human rights law, jurisprudence, policy experience or practice. When human rights have been invoked, it has been in a schematic fashion, as a set of background ethical assumptions that, for example, everyone has an equal entitlement to "fair treatment" in a "just" climate change regime, particularly in the context of mitigation options.

A general premise underlying many rights-based approaches to climate change mitigation is the distinction between "luxury emissions" and "subsistence" or "survival emissions" first put forward in 1991 by the India-based Centre for Science and the Environment, and further consolidated by the political philosopher Henry Shue.[20] Rather than assuming that everyone has an equal right to emit greenhouse gases in a world where overall emissions must be limited, the model distinguishes the use of carbon fuels (and other GHG sources) to fulfil *basic human needs* from use to perpetuate luxurious lifestyles. Whereas the former might be regarded as a fundamental (or human) right, the latter cannot be. This intervention has proved helpful by contrasting excess GHG use in some countries with continued need for future GHG use in others. The problem then becomes one of redressing an imbalance, which in turn involves inter-state obligations. This case might arguably be strengthened by linking "subsistence emissions" to the satisfaction of basic human rights, such as to food, health, water and so on—on the grounds that these rights are already widely accepted and governments are already bound by them. There have been curiously few attempts to explore this connection, however.[21]

The best known rights-based approach to climate change mitigation is the "contraction-and-convergence" (C&C) framework presented by the Global Commons Institute (GCI) at the second Conference of the Parties in 1996. The idea, very briefly, was to articulate a long-term mitigation regime that, while reducing the overall amount of greenhouse gas in use over time, would *also* equalise greenhouse gas emissions per person on a global scale over time. In such a regime, as overall global emissions dropped, the fall would be more precipitate in wealthy countries, while usage in poorer countries would continue to rise for a period in line with their greater development needs—towards convergence between rich and poor countries at some point in the future. Initially, GCI abjured the term "rights" in reference to C&C—

because they regarded the atmosphere as a global commons that "cannot be appropriated by any state or person".[22] Today, however, GCI claims that C&C "establishes a constitutional, global-equal-rights-based framework for the arrest of greenhouse gas emissions".[23] This appears to be in line with a general shift towards the language of rights in the climate change arena.

Whereas the "rights" at issue in models such as C&C amount to speculative universal "rights to emit", with no obvious basis in human rights law, they might be considered to derive from the "right to development", which is mentioned in the UNFCCC.[24] This would depend on demonstrating that "subsistence emissions" were in fact required to achieve basic human rights, a claim that is at least plausible. The right to development has declaratory (non-binding) status under international law, and has been a subject of protracted discussion within the United Nations.[25] Whatever its doctrinal status, discussion of this right has evolved with time, gradually providing elements of a bridge between the languages of development and human rights within the UN. It may therefore be helpful in any investigation of the human rights implications of climate change.

One recent model for GHG mitigation is explicitly based upon the right to development: the "greenhouse development rights" (GDR) framework put forward in 2007 by Tom Athanasiou, Paul Baer and Sivan Kartha.[26] They suggest that the climate change regime should give priority to violations of human rights (to food, water, health and shelter) associated with current low levels of development. In terms of allocating rights and duties, the GDR framework is less concerned with convergence towards equivalent emissions than with ensuring that all countries are permitted (and aided, where necessary) to reach a comparable "development threshold" at which basic rights might be fulfilled.[27]

The GDR framework offers pointers for determining the level at which different countries should cap their GHG emissions and emphasises the importance of technology transfer, swift and substantial adaptation funding, and other forms of assistance. These require levies on wealthy countries, which the authors calculate on the basis of excess GHG usage.

Finally, a rights-based approach has, in fact, been adopted at the heart of the climate change regime through the emissions market introduced by the Kyoto Protocol. Rights to buy or sell emission reductions amount in effect to rights to emit for those who obtain them. Questions might be raised about the appropriateness of allocating use rights to the atmosphere in an alienable—as opposed to inalienable—guise. As noted above, when rights to the atmosphere were put forward in the early climate change debates, they were consistently treated as fundamental, universal and inalienable. Their legal incarnation, however, has instead taken the form of exclusive tradable commodities. The ease with which this notion passed into international law (in the Kyoto Protocol) arguably demonstrates the comparative facility of establishing new property rights under international law as compared with new human rights.

Even though human rights play an increasingly prominent role in each successive rights-based appraisal of climate change, the latter have remained generally utilitarian, relying on cost-benefit and other economic analyses. They draw on human rights primarily for their normative value, to underpin distributional justice models, and give little weight to their achieved positive status under international law. Existing approaches mobilise human rights rhetoric in the interests of conceiving a just global regime for mitigating climate change, but do not examine specific human rights violations resulting from climate change or consider actions to address it. They speak about human rights as a means to spur climate change mitigation; they do not broach climate change policy in order to mitigate human rights violations that might result from it.[28] To note this is not, of course, to criticise these approaches. It is simply to register how few attempts have been made to apply international human rights tools to address harms resulting from climate change. The remainder of this report suggests what such an application might look like.

RIGHTS, NEEDS, DEVELOPMENT AND THE STATE

This report draws on the vocabularies of two different bodies of policy and law that do not always sit easily side by side. Certain terms familiar from one register sound jarring in the other. Human rights are presumptively universal. There is little obvious space for "equity" or for distinctions between countries along the lines of "developed" and "developing".[29] By contrast, climate change law and policy have striven to avoid absolute claims in favour of a flexible and discretionary "framework" language better suited to guiding compromise and consensus. This short section teases through some definitional issues that arise at the intersection of these discourses.

In this report, the term "human rights" refers to the core set of rights proclaimed under international law on behalf of all individuals, regardless of "race, colour, sex, language, religion, political or other opinion, national or social origin, property, birth or other status".[30] The primary source texts are the 1966 International Covenants on Civil and Political Rights (ICCPR) and on Economic, Social and Cultural Rights (ICESCR), both of which derive from the 1948 Universal Declaration on Human Rights. The two Covenants are legally binding on all states that have ratified them—the vast majority of the world's countries—and are supplemented by further binding treaties that protect the rights of children, migrant workers, and people with disabilities, and that prohibit torture as well as racial and gender discrimination. Regional binding human rights treaties also exist within Africa, the Americas and Europe. All these texts are further supported by the case law of international, regional and national courts, by a body of "soft law" (that is, non-binding resolutions and other texts from international bodies such as the UN General Assembly), and, to a lesser degree, by the doctrinal analyses of international lawyers and scholars.

The human rights laid out in these documents are generally referred to as "civil and political" on one hand and "social, economic and cultural" on the other. The former include rights to life, liberty, property, freedom of expression and assembly, political participation, a fair trial, privacy and home life, and protection from torture. The latter include rights to work, education, social security, to "enjoyment of the highest attainable standard of physical and mental health", and to "adequate food, clothing and housing, and to the continuous improvement of living conditions". Whereas the former rights are typically guaranteed through judicial mechanisms, including at international level, the latter have generally been dependent upon domestic welfare mechanisms in the absence of any dedicated international judicial machinery.[31]

Human rights therefore capture a range of concerns that are evidently relevant to climate change, including many that are elsewhere framed as "basic needs". For example, the assertion in both Covenants that "[i]n no case may a people be deprived of its own means of subsistence" is clearly relevant where a changing climate is having precisely this effect.[32] To speak of basic

subsistence needs (water, food, healthcare, shelter and so on) in terms of rights means more than merely to adopt a legal vocabulary in place of a charitable one. It also implies referral to a body of internationally agreed norms that have raised those needs to the level of entitlements for all. Under human rights treaty law, the duty to fulfil these entitlements lies with states (not with private actors or the "international community"). Each state that has ratified the ICESCR has a duty to "respect, protect and fulfil" the rights laid down in that treaty for those coming within their jurisdiction, and these duties have their own specific scope under the treaty. The obligation to *respect* a right means the state must take no steps that would violate that right; the obligation to *protect* requires states act to ensure that other actors, including private and international actors, are not permitted to violate the right; the obligation to *fulfil* requires that states take steps over time to "progressively realise" citizens' rights to food, shelter, health, education and so on.[33] The Committee on Social, Economic and Cultural Rights, which is the UN body that oversees the ICESCR, commonly requests that states demonstrate constant progress in the fulfilment of these rights. The Committee further provides guidelines on how human rights assessment can be integrated into development planning.[34]

States are thus the central actors in both regimes: they carry the primary responsibility for protecting human rights, and this responsibility extends into the negotiation of a solution to climate change. In the latter negotiations, states implicitly set in place global conditions that will affect the protection and fulfilment of human rights for which they are responsible at home. That responsibility should (and does) influence the negotiating positions states take. Resource poor countries have good reason to fear, for example, that emissions caps will adversely impact their obligation to respect, protect, or fulfil basic social rights. According to the ICESCR, states have an obligation to "undertake steps, individually and through international assistance and cooperation" to fulfil rights, and are required to use "the maximum of its available resources" to that end (Article 2). This would seem to indicate not only that recipient states must channel international assistance firstly to ends that will alleviate rights deficits, but also that they are obliged, in accepting aid, to refuse "conditionality" that might undermine those rights, including in climate change related funding. Indeed, on these grounds, recipient countries might themselves impose conditions on any funds accepted.

However, while the ICESCR, reinforced by the Committee's commentaries, encourages wealthier states to provide assistance to other states to fulfil social and economic rights, there is no binding obligation upon them to do so. A binding obligation to provide assistance does appear, however, in the climate change regime. The UNFCCC requirement on wealthy states to provide "new and additional" funding for adaptation is arguably stronger than the duty of international assistance under human rights law, and is applicable to broadly similar activities. There is presumably scope for mutual reinforcement between these complementary treaty obligations.

Although social and economic rights are clearly relevant to economic development in "developing countries", the language of rights has only been partially integrated in development discourse. The reasons for this are too complex to enter into here. While a number of bilateral development agencies and development nongovernmental organisations (NGOs) have explored a variety of "human rights-based approaches" and UN agencies have "mainstreamed" human rights, in practice their adoption has been uneven and international financial institutions, multilateral development banks and private foreign investors have largely refused to adopt a human rights methodology. Indeed the very applicability of international human rights law to these actors has often appeared uncertain, given that they are neither states nor, so it is argued in some cases, subject to specific territorial jurisdictions. Furthermore, international law provides no clear means to evaluate development activities for their rights outcomes or to hold the principal development actors to account on this basis.[35] The relationship between development and rights remains, as a result, complicated; and their integration in terms of practice is at best a work in progress. This partly explains, no doubt, the relative neglect of human rights in climate change discussions.

The present report follows the UNFCCC in speaking of "developed" and "developing" countries but recognises that these categories are simplistic. Neither category is monolithic: each contains countries that have very different characteristics in terms of those who need most protection from climate change harms and those who bear most responsibility. Similar differences exist within individual countries, both rich and poor. Elite groups in poor countries occupy a disproportionate share of the environmental space as they do in rich countries, and these groups are often allied. Powerful political and economic links exist between "North" and "South"; and the major companies in large developing countries are increasingly significant global producers in their own right. Finally, the responsibility and negotiating stances of outlier countries, particularly those that act with least apparent regard for the shared environment, such as the United States and China, need to be viewed in a distinct and nuanced manner. So whereas the report speaks of "developed" and "developing" countries because the terms are legally significant in the context of the UNFCCC, the language is used for convenience rather than for its precision.

REFERENCES

1. This chapter does not deal with all of these topics directly. On the rights of indigenous peoples under conditions of climate change, see IUCN, 2008. On migration, see IOM, 2008. On gender, see IUCN, 2007. On conflict, see German Advisory Council on Global Change, 2008; European Council Doc. 7249/08 Annex, *Climate Change and International Security*, Paper from the High Representative and the European Commission to the European Council (March 2008).

2. The vast literature on climate change vulnerability raises significant human rights concerns. See, for example, Brooks et al., 2005; Ribot, 1995; Guèye et al., 2007.

3. The situation is now changing. At its seventh session, in March 2008, the United Nations Human Rights Council passed a resolution on human rights and climate change. See UN Doc. A/HRC/7/L.21/Rev.1 (26 March 2008). The resolution calls on the Office of the High Commissioner of Human Rights to undertake "a detailed analytical study of the relationship between climate change and human rights" for consideration by the Council. A series of projects investigating the link have been initiated at universities and nongovernmental organisations and elsewhere.

4. Human rights are mentioned occasionally in IPCC AR4 (each volume is named after its relevant working group (WG)). The discussion of legal instruments for mitigation in Chapter 13 (IPCC AR4, WGIII, pp. 793–794) notes the existence of human rights litigation, without commentary. Passing references also appear, again without analysis, in IPCC AR4, WGII.

5. The Inuit case is the primary example. See the short discussion in IPCC AR4, WGIII.

6. These schematic points are not intended as expressions of legal doctrine.

7. Nevertheless, human rights bodies, notably the European Court of Human Rights, have found rights violations due to environmental impacts, including of the right to health. See Shelton, 2001, pp. 225–231; Robb, 2001. In a recent case, *Öneryıldız v. Turkey* (App. no. 48939/99, decision of 30 November 2004), the Court found against Turkey for failing to act on an environmental impact assessment, thereby contributing to deaths caused by a methane explosion at a rubbish tip.

8. Extraterritorial responsibility is a fraught area of international human rights law. Existing case law suggests that states have responsibility for (i) state actions taken in other countries, (ii) human rights protections in countries where they exercise "effective control", and (iii) some violations committed abroad by private actors who fall under their jurisdiction. See, for example, *Lopez Burgos v. Uruguay*, HRC Comm. No. R12/52 (1979), Views of 29 July 1981; *Legal Consequences of the Construction of a Wall in the Occupied Palestinian Territory*, ICJ Advisory Opinion of 9 July 2004; *Coard et al. v. United States*, IACHR Case No. 10.951, Reports no 109/99, 29 September 1999; *Bankovic v. Belgium* (App. 52207/99, Decision of 12 December 2001). However, the case law is sparse and its applicability to climate-related harms unclear. Alternative mechanisms involving "long-arm" domestic jurisdiction—such as the United States' Alien Tort Claims Act—may be of limited potential value. Although state responsibility for extraterritorial violations of social and economic rights has not been widely discussed, the particular harms caused by global warming may generate plausible claims of this kind.

9. Some vulnerable countries are themselves becoming significant emitters, of course. Examples include China and to a lesser extent India and Brazil. In such cases, the relevance of human rights law will depend increasingly on the legal expression and enforcement capacity of human rights norms in the countries in question.

10. For accounts of the applicability of human rights during emergencies see, Inter-Agency Standing Committee, 2006; and OHCHR, 2003, Chapter 16.

11. It has become increasingly common to adopt the language of emergency when referring not only to climate change effects but to the phenomenon in its entirety. Even if this language is intended to be emotive rather than literal, it tends to remove climate change impacts from the ordinary reach of human rights law, at least rhetorically.

12. The notion of human rights as thresholds is borrowed from the work of Simon Caney. See Caney, 2005, 2006 and forthcoming (2008).

13. Thinking of human rights as thresholds also has a bearing on the distribution of responsibilities when addressing climate change. Those who are extremely disadvantaged should not be required to pay the costs when doing so pushes them below a certain threshold.

14. See the discussion in Stern, 2006 ("The Stern Review"), Part VI, Chapters 21 and 27.

15. See text at note 2 above.

16. Notably Principle 10 of the 1992 Rio Declaration

on Environment and Development, and the 1998 Convention on Access to Information, Public Participation in Decision-Making and Access to Justice in Environmental Matters ("Aarhus Convention").

17. Decision-/CP.13, Bali Action Plan (Advance Unedited Version), Article 1(a). See also the Stern Review, 572–3. The Bali Action plan is online at

18. Agarwal and Narain, 1991; Shue, 1993.

19. A recent exception is the "greenhouse development rights" framework, discussed further below. One reason for caution in reading human (social and economic) rights into any right to "subsistence emissions" might be a concern that obligations would then be deflected from the governments of countries producing excess luxury emissions onto those in low-emission countries, who are less responsible.

20. AGBM/1.9.96/14, "Draft Proposals for a Climate Change Protocol based on Contraction and Convergence: A Contribution to Framework Convention on Climate Change," Ad Hoc Group on the Berlin Mandate, 1996, at www.gci.org.uk/contconv/protweb.html. The authors suggest using "quotas" rather than rights.

21. See www.gci.org.uk.

22. UNFCCC, Article 3(4): "The Parties have a right to, and should, promote sustainable development." In this ambiguous wording, however, the guaranteed right appears to be the state's "right to promote" development.

23. See, for example, Saloman, 2005. See contributions to Andreassen and Marks, 2006; Alston, 2001, p. 283.

24. Baer et al., 2007. The report was co-produced by the Stockholm Environmental Institute, EcoEquity and Christian Aid.

25. The "threshold" is schematically set at US$9,000 per capita at purchasing power parity.

26. Some organisations have called for adaptation transfers on the basis that adaptation funding should be viewed as "compensation" for harms inflicted by the actions of the rich world. This model too invokes human rights as an ethical rather than a legal imperative. See, for example, Oxfam International, 2007.

27. Common Article 2(1) of the International Covenant on Civil and Political Rights and the International Covenant on Social, Cultural and Economic Rights.

28. Social rights have increasing judicial traction. An Optional Protocol to the ICESCR, currently being developed, would create an international tribunal for these rights.

29. ICHRP would like to thank Kate Raworth of Oxfam for this point.

30. See, for example, UN Docs, E/C.12/1999/5, CESCR General Comment No. 12, The right to adequate food (Article 11) (12/05/99); E/C.12/2002/11, CESCR General Comment No. 15, The right to water (Articles 11 and 12) (2002); E/C.12/2000/4, CESCR General Comment No. 14, The right to the highest attainable standard of health (Article 12) (11/08/2000). There are 149 states parties to the ICESCR. The United States is not among them, having signed but not ratified it.

31. UN Doc. E/C.12/1991/1, Revised general guidelines regarding the form and contents of reports to be submitted by states parties under Articles 16 and 17 of the International Covenant on Eco-nomic, Social and Cultural Rights (17 June 2001).

32. The literature on the human rights obligations of the main development actors is voluminous. For a good recent overview, see Tan, 2008a.

33. See, for example, UN Docs, E/C.12/1999/5, CESCR General Comment No. 12, The right to adequate food (Article 11) (12/05/99); E/C.12/2002/11, CESCR General Comment No. 15, The right to water (Articles 11 and 12) (2002); E/C.12/2000/4, CESCR General Comment No. 14, The right to the highest attainable standard of health (Article 12) (11/08/2000). There are 149 states parties to the ICESCR. The United States is not among them, having signed but not ratified it.

34. UN Doc. E/C.12/1991/1, Revised general guidelines regarding the form and contents of reports to be submitted by states parties under Articles 16 and 17 of the International Covenant on Economic, Social and Cultural Rights (17 June 2001).

35. The literature on the human rights obligations of the main development actors is voluminous. For a good recent overview, see Tan, 2008a.

QUESTIONS

1. Three global changes were noted at the opening of the Rio+20 climate change meeting in June 2012: (1) increase in global interconnectedness among nations; (2) the recognition that humans have become the major driver of changes in the

earth's ecosystem; and (3) the emergence of countries like Brazil, China, Indonesia and India which hold the key to any global sustainability agenda. Why has it been so difficult to get the world's governments to accept the view of almost all scientists that we are in the midst of a massive, man-induced climate change that only concerted international effort and cooperation can possibly affect?

2. It has been suggested that governments may simply be unable to act effectively in the area of climate change. If this is true, where else must the world look for leadership and initiative in this arena? Is there a human right to a habitable planet?

3. As our climate changes, one major effect will be on access to clean water. The right to health is intimately tied to the right to water, usually referred to as the right to water and sanitation. What is the responsibility of the international community to make sure all inhabitants of the planet have access to clean drinking water and decent sanitation systems that can prevent the contamination of drinking water sources? What do you think are the major barriers to implementing a right to water? The slow recovery of Haiti after their earthquake presents a useful case study in how clean water is not just critical to day-to-day life, but can also help prevent major epidemics such as cholera.

4. Comment on the interconnectedness of human health and our environment. Do you think a healthful environment is a human right? Why or why not?

FURTHER READING

1. de Albuquerque, Catarina, *On the Right Track: Good Practices in Realising the Rights to Water and Sanitation.* New York: United Nations, 2012.
2. Sachs, Jeffrey, From Millennium Development Goals to Sustainable Development Goals. *Lancet,* 2012; 379: 2206–2212.
3. Haines, Andy, et al., From the Earth Summit to Rio+20: Integration of Health and Sustainable Development. *Lancet,* 2012; 379: 2189–2198.

POINT OF VIEW

Climate Change Is an Issue of Human Rights

Mary Robinson

In 1948, the UN General Assembly adopted the Universal Declaration of Human Rights, the cornerstone document created in the aftermath of unimaginable atrocities. This declaration, and the legal documents that stemmed from it, have helped us combat torture, discrimination and hunger. And now, this venerable document should guide us in the fight against one of the greatest challenges ever to face humankind: climate change.

Poor people are already coping with the impacts of global warming. From increasing droughts to increasing floods, from lower agricultural productivity to more frequent and severe storms, many rightly fear that things will only get worse. Their human rights—to security, health and sustainable livelihoods—are increasingly being threatened by changes to the earth's climate.

Indeed, the poorest who contributed the least to the problem of climate change are now bearing the brunt of the impacts. Ninety-seven per cent of deaths related to natural disasters already take place in developing countries. In South Asia, the 17 million people living on sandbanks in the river basins of Bangladesh could be homeless by 2030 as increasing Himalayan meltwater floods their homes. In Niger, changing rainfall patterns are contributing to increased desertification which, for the Tuareg and Wodaabe people, has caused massive losses of livestock and food insecurity. In South America, a loss of snow in the Andes in the next 15 to 20 years will pose a serious risk to the more than nine million people living in Lima, Peru's largest city.

Those who are already poor and vulnerable are and will continue to be disproportionately affected. Incrementally, land will become too dry to till, crops will wither, rising sea levels will undermine coastal dwellings and spoil freshwater, livelihoods will vanish. Carbon emissions from industrialised countries have human and environmental consequences. As a result, global warming has already begun to affect the fulfillment of human rights, and to the extent that polluting greenhouse gases continue to be released by large industrial countries, the basic human rights of millions of the world's poor to life, security, food, health and shelter will continue to be violated.

Our shared human rights framework provides a basis for impoverished communities to claim protection of these rights. We must not lose sight of existing human rights principles in the tug and push of international climate change negotiations. A human rights lens reminds us there are reasons beyond economics and enlightened self-interest for states to act on climate change.

Because climate change presents a new and unprecedented threat to the human rights of millions, international human rights law and institutions must evolve to protect the rights of these peoples. But, most importantly, states must take urgent action to avoid more serious and actionable violations of human rights.

The principles of human rights provide a strong foundation for policy-making and these principles must be put at the heart of a global deal to tackle global climate change. Urgently cutting emissions must be done in order to respect and protect human rights from being violated by the future impacts of climate change, while supporting the poorest communities to adapt to already occurring climate impacts is the only remedy for those whose human rights have already been violated.

As we passed the 60th anniversary of the Universal Declaration of Human Rights, it is worth remembering that climate change violates the declaration's affirmation that "everyone is entitled to a social and inter-national order in which [their] rights and freedoms . . . can be realised."

We must now grasp the opportunity to create the kind of international order that the framers of the UDHR dreamed of—even in a radically changed global context they never imagined.

Adapted with permission from *The Independent,* 10 December 2008.

Mary Robinson is President of the Mary Robinson Foundation—Climate Justice. She served as President of Ireland from 1990 to 1997 and UN High Commissioner for Human Rights from 1997 to 2002.

CHAPTER 35

Human Rights Implications of Governance Responses to Public Health Emergencies: The Case of Major Infectious Disease Outbreaks

Gian Luca Burci and Riikka Koskenmäki

INTRODUCTION

At the Fiftieth Anniversary of the Universal Declaration of Human Rights in December 1998, the Director-General of the World Health Organization (WHO) stated that "health security is a notion which encompasses many of the rights enlisted in the [Universal] Declaration", including the right "to live and work in an environment where known health risks are controlled".[1] Only a few years later, the multi-country outbreak of severe acute respiratory syndrome (SARS) in 2003, and the looming possibility of a catastrophic outbreak of pandemic influenza, prompted unprecedented attention to the threat of worldwide spread of emerging and re-emerging infectious diseases. These developments underlined the fact that an individual's health security must be founded upon global health security.[2]

The rapid international spread of SARS highlighted the insufficiency of domestic measures to tackle diseases that recognize no borders.[3] It also revealed the lack of preparedness of many countries, both developed and developing, to address large-scale public health emergencies.[4] Increased recognition of the need for an effective international prevention and control mechanism led to the revision of the WHO International Health Regulations (IHR) in 2005.[5] The IHR are the key international legal instrument designed to help protect all states from international public health risks and emergencies.

This chapter discusses human rights implications of selected governance responses, at both national and international levels, to public health emergencies. It focuses on major infectious disease outbreaks with potential to spread internationally, and on the IHR as the main international instrument for their control. While multiple state and non-state actors may be involved in responses to public health emergencies, this discussion focuses on responses by states at the national and international levels.

International human rights bodies and scholars have studied the limitations that can be imposed on the rights and freedoms of individuals for the purpose of controlling infectious diseases.[6] There has not been a comparable level of scrutiny regarding the impact of national and international disease prevention and control measures on the right to the highest attainable standard of health (hereafter "the right to health").[7] This chapter seeks to further understanding of such impact and links. For the purpose of this contribution, we will use as a normative reference for the right to health Article 12 of the International Covenant on Economic, Social and Cultural Rights (ICESCR),[8] as clarified by the Committee on Economic, Social and Cultural Rights in its General Comment No. 14 of 4 July 2000 (hereafter "General Comment").[9]

HUMAN RIGHTS IMPLICATIONS OF GOVERNMENTS' RESPONSES AT THE NATIONAL LEVEL

States have the duty to take measures to prevent and control epidemic and endemic diseases. This obligation exists under Article 12 of the ICESCR, as a step to achieve the full realization of the right to health, as well as under the IHR.[10] Disease control requires epidemiological surveillance, implementation of immunization programs and other disease control strategies, including pharmaceutical and non-pharmaceutical interventions during outbreaks. In addition to activities at the national level, disease control requires cooperation with other states and international agencies.[11]

Preparing for public health threats of unknown origin, such as SARS or Ebola hemorrhagic fever, is however particularly challenging since pharmaceutical interventions may not be available, at least during the first stages of the outbreak. Even when medication is available, states may face difficult questions such as ensuring access to treatment and prioritizing scarce resources in the face of widespread and acute needs of their populations. Non-pharmaceutical interventions, mostly applied in health emergencies where medication is not available (e.g., during the SARS outbreak) include testing and screening; notification and reporting of cases; mandatory medical examinations; social distancing;[12] isolation of persons with infectious conditions; and contact tracing and quarantine of persons who have been exposed to a public health risk.[13]

The widespread use of these measures during the SARS outbreak[14] and related advice by WHO,[15] drew renewed attention to the challenge of striking the proper balance between the protection of public health on the one hand and respect for individual rights and freedoms on the other.[16] It is well established that states are entitled to limit the exercise of certain human rights, or to derogate from some of their human rights obligations in particular circumstances. In serious communicable disease outbreaks, for example, states are permitted to apply health measures that may "limit" or "restrict" the right to freedom of movement (in case of isolation or quarantine), the right to physical integrity (in case of compulsory testing, screening, examination and treatment), or the right to privacy (in case of compulsory contact tracing or patient retrieval), under certain conditions.[17] The Siracusa Principles provide guidance concerning the question of when interference with human rights may be justified in order to achieve a public health goal. The Principles make clear that any limitation must be provided for by law and carried out in accordance with law; serve a legitimate aim and be strictly necessary to achieve that aim; be the least restrictive and intrusive means available; and not be arbitrary or discriminatory in the way it is imposed or applied.[18]

The burden of proof for assessing the legality and justifiability of measures limiting human rights for a common good normally falls on those who impose such restrictions.[19] State practice of resorting to such measures during the SARS outbreak makes an interesting study for assessing whether the above-mentioned human rights framework was actually followed. D. P. Fidler has noted that measures taken by states differed significantly, even in similar circumstances. While some states used compulsory and tightly monitored isolation and quarantine measures, others, by contrast, relied more on voluntary measures or no such measures at all.[20] These differences in policy, which may in part be explained by different factual circumstances, including the scientific knowledge available, as well as cultural and social contexts, raise questions concerning the application to the measures in question of the International Covenant on Civil and Political Rights (ICCPR), or comparable regional instruments, as well as the interpretive guidance contained in the Siracusa Principles. In particular, the question of whether such normative frameworks provide sufficient guidance on these complex issues is of central importance.

One of the important lessons of the SARS outbreak is the need for health emergency preparedness, including relevant legislation, policies, plans and programs, in line with human rights law.[21] All such strategies should be established and implemented through transparent and accountable processes, as the active and informed participation of individuals and communities in decision-making that bears upon their health is part of the right to health.[22] The strategies should address the rights of those affected and pay particular attention to the needs of the most vulnerable groups. For example, legal authority for quarantine and isolation, including that of recalcitrant individuals, needs to be established with clear criteria, including scientific assessment of public health risk and effectiveness of envisaged measures, due process guarantees and use of the least restrictive alternatives.[23] Legislation is also needed for protecting privacy in different contexts, for due process requirements and compensation when infected property may need to be destroyed, and for ensuring non-discriminatory practices and equal treatment, among other things. The strategies should

also ensure that individuals can access a full range of information on health issues affecting themselves and their communities.[24] The enactment of such policies, plans and legislation are essential tools for a balanced and accountable implementation of the right to health.[25]

Another important lesson from the SARS outbreak is the crucial role of well functioning national health systems for the control of epidemic diseases, capable of providing urgent medical care and relief.[26] Ensuring equitable access to health facilities, goods and services is essential for implementing the right to health but remains a challenge for many states, even in the absence of particular health emergencies.[27] Strengthening of health systems should thus be a high priority and based, according to the UN Special Rapporteur on the right to health, on a right-to-health approach.[28] The implementation of the core capacity requirements under the IHR provides an opportunity to reinforce work on surveillance and response capacities of health systems.[29]

HUMAN RIGHTS IMPLICATIONS OF THE WHO INTERNATIONAL HEALTH REGULATIONS

The IHR were initially adopted by the World Health Assembly in 1951,[30] and revised several times thereafter. They represent the culmination of a process of international cooperation begun in the mid-nineteenth century, which WHO was expected to continue and rationalize through centralized collective decision-making.[31] Under the WHO Constitution, regulations become legally binding for all member states unless they opt-out by a certain deadline.[32] This process and the constitutional basis of their legal effects make WHO regulations innovative international instruments, meant to address urgent regulatory needs in crucial public health areas.[33]

The IHR became progressively marginalized during the 1980s and 1990s, in particular since they were based on a number of assumptions that were overtaken by the development of public health and international law during that period.[34] The revision of the IHR languished, however, until 2003 when the collective scare caused by SARS and pandemic influenza made revision a top priority for the Organization. The World Health Assembly eventually adopted the revised IHR in May 2005 and they entered into force in June 2007. The IHR have 194 States Parties—the entire membership of WHO plus the Holy See—making them a truly global instrument.[35]

The IHR, as revised in 2005, are a complex and innovative instrument that opens a new era in international health law. The main features of the revised IHR include:

1. Expanded scope to address virtually all urgent and serious public health risks, regardless of origin or source, that might be transmissible across international borders—whether by travellers, trade, transportation or the environment. The IHR's scope of application goes well beyond the natural spread of infectious diseases, abandoning almost completely the approach based on a finite list of diseases. The IHR is consequently applicable to the public health aspects of diseases from biological, chemical or radionuclear sources, including in case of deliberate release of such agents;[36]

2. Detailed obligations requiring States Parties to develop national capacities for the surveillance of, and response to, diseases and events falling under the IHR and to report them to WHO;[37]

3. The central role of WHO in interacting with States Parties, providing information and supporting their prevention and control activities. In this context, WHO may rely on information obtained from nongovernmental sources, as provided in the Regulations;[38]

4. The Director-General of WHO may under certain circumstances determine that an event constitutes a "public health emergency of international concern" and issue temporary recommendations to respond to it, thus guiding the international response to grave public health risks as in the case of SARS.[39] The dramatic expansion of the scope and application of the IHR raises delicate issues as to their interaction with many other international rules, from trade and transportation to environmental protection and nuclear incidents.[40]

A major distinguishing feature of the revised IHR is that, unlike the predecessor Regulations, they contain provisions seeking to ensure that measures are applied consistent with human rights and freedoms, aiming to strike a balance between the protection of public health, interference with international traffic and trade,[41] and the protection of fundamental human rights.[42] While the protection of human rights is not an explicit component of the IHR's objectives, it figures prominently among their principles (Article 3) and thus provides fundamental interpretative guidance for their implementation.[43] Notwithstanding the reference to "persons" in that principle and the articles concerning WHO's recommendations, other IHR provisions mostly focus on "travellers",[44] thus significantly restricting their scope of protection ratione personae. The most important protective measures in the IHR include the requirement to apply the least intrusive and invasive medical examination that achieves the public health objective (Articles 17, 23, 31 and 43)[45] and the need for prior express informed consent except in special circumstances (Article 23). States Parties must treat travellers undergoing health measures with respect for their dignity and human rights, and provide certain facilities to minimize their discomfort (Article 32). The Regulations provide some protection as to confidentiality and lawful use of personal data collected under the IHR (Article 45) and introduce, most importantly, a general requirement of transparency and non-discrimination in the application of health measures (Article 42).

The aforementioned IHR provisions may seem narrow or skewed in favour of potentially coercive public health measures, and according to some commentators, they leave some important gaps.[46] At the same time, the IHR recognize in general terms that they and other international agreements should be interpreted so as to be compatible with each other, and the IHR clarify that the former shall not affect the rights and obligations of States Parties under the latter (Article 57). Consequently, over and above the specific protections summarized above, human rights obligations of States Parties may arguably prevail over incompatible IHR-based obligations. It has been suggested that, at the very least, the limitation or restriction of rights granted under the ICCPR in the implementation of the IHR should be subject to the balancing and interpretative test contained in the Siracusa Principles (explained above).[47] It is worth noting that the Principles state that "due regard shall be had to the International Health Regulations of the World Health Organization",[48] strengthening the importance of the IHR as a reference for achieving a balance between respect for human rights and protection of public health. The IHR have also been given the credit of contributing "to existing law on restricting human rights for health purposes" by providing greater detail for some of these principles.[49]

WHO provides guidance to states on measures in response to disease outbreaks, including those potentially affecting human rights and freedoms. For example, WHO advises countries neighbouring an area affected by cholera against the establishment of quarantine measures or a *cordon sanitaire* at borders; the introduction of travel restrictions, including requirement that travellers have proof of cholera vaccination; or the screening of travellers.[50]

In this connection, one may wonder whether the outbreak of an infectious disease with a potentially very serious public health impact—for example the virulence and lethality of current strains of avian influenza—may be invoked by States Parties to the ICCPR as a ground for the proclamation of a "public emergency which threatens the life of the nation" under Article 4. Even though the drafters of the Covenant probably had political situations in mind, the effects of an infectious disease may be equally devastating on the physical integrity of the population and the functioning of indispensable national institutions.[51] Furthermore, it may be questioned whether an event that has been determined to constitute a "public health emergency of international concern" by the Director-General of WHO under the IHR, could also qualify as a "public emergency" under the Covenant.

Even though explicit concerns about the protection or promotion of the right to health were absent from the negotiations on the revised IHR, an analysis of the IHR against the content and context of the right to health as articulated in General Comment No. 14 on the right to health reveals a number of synergies that could assist States Parties in pursuing the progressive realization of that right. The following aspects should be stressed in this regard:

1. Article 12 paragraph 2(c) of the ICESCR spells out "the prevention, treatment and control of epidemic … diseases" as an example of a core obligation of

the Parties to the Covenant. Through the very fact of implementing the IHR, therefore, States Parties take steps in fulfilling an important component of the right to health.

2. The General Comment on the right to health gives much importance to the enactment of policies and strategies as essential tools for a balanced and accountable implementation of the right to health.[52] This planning approach is also prominent in the case of the IHR, particularly through the obligation of States Parties in Articles 5 and 13 and Annex 1 to develop and implement plans of action to ensure the required core capacities to detect, report and respond to relevant public health risks.[53]

3. Ever since the 1978 Alma-Ata Declaration on Primary Health Care,[54] national health systems and their main components have been seen as the primary elements for the delivery of equitable public health outcomes and for fulfilling the right to health.[55] It is significant that the IHR follow and strengthen this approach by abandoning the traditional focus on ports and airports in favour of a more holistic vision to strengthen the components of national health systems crucial for the prevention of the international spread of disease. If based on a realistic and accountable process, including in terms of available resources, such an approach may usefully complement, and be integrated into, national health systems policies.[56]

4. Both the implementation of the IHR, and the realization of the right to health, rely substantially on international cooperation. The General Comment identifies a joint and individual responsibility of ICESCR Parties to cooperate, inter alia, in the international control of epidemic diseases, with particular regard to the needs of developing countries.[57] In view of the nature of infectious disease control as a global public good,[58] and the deep interdependence between states in this regard, there is arguably a collective responsibility of all States Parties to the ICESCR to cooperate in good faith with each other and with WHO in preventing and responding to the international spread of disease. The IHR provide a specific legal framework to enable such cooperation, which, at the same time, is instrumental in fulfilling a core dimension of the right to health. WHO in particular should play an important role in this respect, both directly and through the network of experts and institutions that it coordinates. WHO is not a financial institution and its main functions in this context would consist of technical advice and support, and the provision of reliable information and guidance. Among the networks at the disposal of WHO, particular mention should be made of the Global Outbreak Alert and Response Network (GOARN). GOARN is a technical collaboration of existing institutions and networks that pool human and technical resources for the rapid identification, confirmation and response to outbreaks of international importance. It enables WHO to rapidly mobilize highly specialized teams of experts from institutions around the world to support countries affected by an outbreak of infectious disease. GOARN has played a crucial role in several critical situations such as the 2007 outbreak of Ebola hemorrhagic fever in the Democratic Republic of the Congo.[59]

CONCLUDING REMARKS

As evidenced by the successful response to the SARS outbreak, responses at both national and international levels—and through the interplay of different governmental and nongovernmental actors—are essential requirements for public health emergency governance. While the IHR establish an international framework for this cooperation, formidable challenges remain, in particular as concerns resources for enabling States Parties to implement their capacity-building obligations at the national level. With the inclusion of human rights protection in their crucial provisions, the IHR underline the synergy between preparedness and response to health emergencies, on the one hand, and protection of fundamental rights on the other, both at the national and international levels.[60]

REFERENCES

1. Address by Dr. Gro Harlem Brundtland, Director-General of the WHO on the Fiftieth Anniversary of the Universal Declaration of Human Rights, Paris, France, 8 December 1998.

2. 'Global Health Security: Epidemic Alert and Response', World Health Assembly resolution WHA 54.14, 21 May 2001; WHO, *World Health Report 2007: A Safer Future* (Geneva: WHO, 2007). Global health security looks, through the public health lens, at "the collective health of populations living across geographical regions and international boundaries". Health security, at an individual level, includes universal access to adequate health care, access to education and information, the right to food in sufficient quantity and of good quality, the right to decent housing and to live and work in an environment where known health risks are controlled. Individuals' health security is affected by global health risks.

3. On the SARS outbreak, see, for example, WHO, *SARS: How A Global Epidemic Was Stopped* (Geneva: WHO, 2006), and D. P. Fidler, *SARS, Governance and the Globalization of Diseases* (New York: Palgrave Macmillan, 2004).

4. See, for example, T. Kian and F. Lateef, 'Infectious Diseases Law and Severe Acute Respirator y Syndrome—Medical and Legal Responses and Implications: The Singapore Experience' 7 *Asia Pacific League of Associations for Rheumatology Journal of Rheumatolog y* (2004), at 123–129.

5. The initial WHO International Sanitary Regulations of 1951 were revised and renamed the International Health Regulations (IHR) in 1969. The 58th World Health Assembly adopted the most recent revision of the Regulations on 23 May 2005. The text of the IHR (2005) is attached to World Health Assembly resolution WHA58.3 and is available at http://www.who.int/gb/ebwha/pdf_files/WHA58/WHA58_3-en.pdf. The revised IHR entered into force on 15 June 2007.

6. See, for example, WHO, *25 Questions & Answers on Health & Human Rights* (Geneva: WHO, 2002) and Lawrence Gostin, 'When Terrorism Threatens Health: How Far Are Limitations on Human Rights Justified', 31 *Journal of Law, Medicine & Ethics* (2003), at 521–528.

7. See, however, most notably, D. P. Fidler, *International Law and Infectious Diseases* (Oxford: Oxford University Press, 1999), at 179–197.

8. International Covenant on Economic, Social and Cultural Rights (ICESCR), adopted by UN General Assembly Resolution 2200A (XXI) of 16 December 1966.

9. Committee on Economic, Social and Cultural Rights, *General Comment No. 14 (2000) on the right to the highest attainable standard of health*, UN Doc. E/C.12/2000/4, 4 July 2000 (hereafter "General Comment No. 14").

10. ICESCR, Article 12(2)(c). According to the Committee on Economic, Social and Cultural Rights, the obligation is of comparable priority as the ICESCR's core obligations, i.e., a "minimum essential level[s]" of obligations for all states. General Comment No. 14, *supra* note 9, at paras. 43 and 44(c). See also IHR , in particular Articles 2, 5(1), 13(1) and Annex 1.

11. General Comment No. 14, *supra* note 9, paras. 16 and 40. For further analysis with regard to the IHR , see discussion below.

12. Social-distancing measures have been defined as "[a] range of community-based measures to reduce contact between people (e.g., closing schools or prohibiting large gatherings). Community-based measures may also be complemented by adoption of individual behaviours to increase the distance between people in daily life at the worksite or in other locations (e.g., substituting phone calls for face-to-face meetings, avoiding hand-shaking)." WHO, *Ethical considerations in developing a public health response to pandemic influenza*, WHO/CDS/EPR/GIP/2007.2 (Geneva: WHO, 2007), p. ix.

13. See on different measures in the context of pandemic influenza preparedness, ibid.

14. For an overview of the measures see J. W. Saspin, L. O. Gostin, J. S. Vernick et al., 'SARS and International Legal Preparedness' 77 *Temple Law Review* (2004) 155–173, at 158–163.

15. For advice issued by WHO in March–June 2003 relating to the SARS outbreak, see http://www.who.int/csr/sars/travel/en/index.html.

16. See, for example, Sofia Gruskin, 'SARS, Public Health and Global Governance: Is there a Government in the Cockpit: A Passenger's Perspective on Global Public Health: The Role of Human Rights' 77 *Temple Law Review* (2004) 313–333 at 322; and Fidler, *supra* note 3, at 152.

17. See ICCPR, Articles 12 and 17, and General Comment No. 14, *supra* note 9, at paras. 28–29 and 34.

18. United Nations Economic and Social Council, UN Sub-Commission on Prevention of Discrimination and Protection of Minorities, 'Siracusa Principles on the Limitation and Derogation of Provisions in the International Covenant on Civil and Political Rights', Annex, UN Doc E/CN.4/1985/4 (1985) (hereafter "Siracusa Principles"). See also, for example, Susan Marks and Andrew Clapham, *International Human Rights Lexicon* (Oxford: Oxford University Press, 2005), at 206.

19. General Comment No. 14, *supra* note 9, at para. 28.

20. Fidler, *supra* note 3, at 153.

21. For legal preparedness in particular see WHO, *Ethical considerations in developing a public health response to pandemic influenza*, *supra* note 12, p. 9, and J. W. Saspin, L . O. Gostin, J. S. Vernick et al., *supra* note 14, at 155–173.

22. General Comment No. 14, *supra* note 9, at para. 14. See also S. Gruskin and B. Loff, 'Do Human Rights have a Role in Public Health Work?' 360 *The Lancet* (2002), at 1880.

23. Lawrence O. Gostin, 'Public Health Strategies for Pandemic Influenza: Ethics and the Law' 295(14) *Journal of the American Medical Association* (2006) 1700–1704, at 1703.

24. General Comment No. 14, *supra* note 9, at para. 12.

25. See, inter alia, ICESCR, Article 2 and General Comment No. 14, *supra* note 9, paras. 36, 43 and 53.

26. See also accompanying text to notes 54–56 below.

27. General Comment No. 14, *supra* note 9, at para. 12.

28. Paul Hunt, 'Report of the Special Rapporteur on the right of everyone to the enjoyment of the highest attainable standard of physical and mental health', UN Doc. A/HRC/7/11, 31 January 2008.

29. IHR, Articles 5 and 13, and Annex 1. See also accompanying text to notes 54–56 below.

30. International Sanitary Regulations, adopted on 25 May 1951, reproduced in WHO *Technical Reports Series* No. 41, Geneva 1951, available at http://whqlibdoc.who.int/trs/WHO_TRS_41.pdf.

31. See, for example, D. P. Fidler, 'The Globalization of Public Health: the first 100 years of international health diplomacy' 79(9) *Bulletin of the World Health Organization* (2001) 842–849.

32. Articles 21 and 22 of the WHO Constitution, reproduced in WHO, *Basic Documents* (Fifty-sixth edition, Geneva: WHO, 2007), at 1.

33. For discussion see, for example, Laurence Boisson de Chazournes, 'Le pouvoir réglementaire de l'Organisation Mondiale de la Santé à laune de la santé mondiale: réflexions sur la portée et la nature du Règlement Sanitaire International de 2005' in *Droit du pouvoir, pouvoir du droit: mélanges offerts à Jean Salmon* (Bruxelles: Bruylant, 2007) 1157–1181.

34. Most notably, the IHR (1) only covered a limited list of diseases that had become scourges of the past; (2) they set maximum measures that states may apply to persons and conveyances, rather than relying on a contextual risk assessment—which placed them in conflict with international trade rules; and (3) they did not support WHO's active role in surveillance, coordination and cooperation.

35. A list of the States Parties to the IHR and related information is available at http://www.who.int/ihr/states_parties/en/index.html.

36. See IHR , Article 1(1) (in particular the expansive definitions of "disease", "event", "public health risk") and Article 2, according to which the purpose and scope of the Regulations are "to prevent, protect against, control and provide a public health response to the international spread of disease in ways that are commensurate with and restricted to public health risks, and which avoid unnecessary interference with international traffic and trade."

37. See IHR , Articles 5, 6, 13 and Annex 1.

38. See IHR in particular Articles 5(4), 9, 11 and 13(3).

39. IHR , Article 1(1) provides that "'public health emergency of international concern' means 'an extraordinary event which is determined, as provided in these Regulations: (I) to constitute a public health risk to other States through the international spread of disease and (II) to potentially require a coordinated international response'". See also IHR , Articles 12, 15–18, 48.

40. See, for example, information document prepared by the WHO Secretariat, 'Review and Approval of Proposed Amendments to the

International Health Regulations: Relations with other International Instruments', Intergovernmental Working Group on Revision of the International Health Regulations, A/IHR/IGWG/INF.DOC./1, 30 September 2004.

41. IHR , Article 11 defines the term "international traffic" as "the movement of persons, baggage, cargo, containers, conveyances, goods or postal parcels across an international border, including international trade."

42. For human rights related provisions in the IHR , see, for example, D. P. Fidler, 'From International Sanitary Conventions to Global Health Security: The New International Health Regulations' 4(2) *Chinese Journal of International Law* (2005) 325–392, Table 2; and B. Plotkin, 'Human Rights and Other Provisions in the Revised International Health Regulations (2005)' 121 *Public Health* (2007) 840–845.

43. IHR, Article 3(1) reads as follows: "The implementation of these Regulations shall be with full respect for the dignity, human rights and fundamental freedoms of persons".

44. Defined in Article 1(1) of the IHR as "a natural person undertaking an international voyage."

45. Under Article 17, the WHO Director-General also has an obligation to consider health measures "that, on the basis of a risk assessment appropriate to the circumstances, are not more ... intrusive to persons than reasonably available alternatives that would achieve the appropriate level of health protection."

46. D. P. Fidler, *supra* note 42; and Lawrence O. Gostin, 'The New International Health Regulation: An Historic Development for International Law and Public Health' 34(1) *The Journal of Law, Medicine and Ethics* (2006) at 85–94. The lack of the least intrusive measures approach in case of involuntary vaccination or other prophylaxis, isolation and quarantine, and the absence of specific due process requirements with regard to the application of public health measure are seen as important gaps by these authors.

47. H. L. Lambertson, 'Swatting a Bug without a Flyswatter: Minimizing the Impact of Disease Control on Individual Liberty under the Revised International Health Regulations' 25(2) *Penn State International Law Review* (2006) 531–555 at 554, and the Siracusa Principles, *supra* note 18.

48. Ibid., at para. 26.

49. States' determination of potential additional measures that may affect rights of persons in accordance with Article 43 of the IHR must be based, inter alia, on scientific principles and available evidence of a risk to health. As noted

by B. von Tigerstrom, this criterion is more specific than the relevant provisions concerning limitation of human rights for public heath pur poses under international human rights treaty law. For analysis, see B. von Tigerstrom, 'The Revised International Health Regulations and Restraint of National Health Measures' 13 *Health Law Journal* (2005) 35–76 at 63–64.

50. WHO statement relating to international travel and trade to and from countries experiencing outbreaks of cholera. 16 November 2007, available at http://www.who.int/cholera/choleratravel andtradeadvice161107.pdf.

51. Siracusa Principles, Part II, *supra* note 18.

52. General Comment No. 14, *supra* note 9, at paras. 36, 43 and 53.

53. Interestingly, D. P. Fidler considers that the surveillance and response capacity obligations in the IHR are more demanding than those under article 12 of the ICESCR because the IHR States Parties are required to have the capacities in place generally after the five-year grace period following the entry into force of the IHR as foreseen in the Regulations. The ICESCR's right to health is, by contrast, to be progressively realized. See further, Fidler, *supra* note 42, at 373.

54. 'Primary Health Care: Report of the International Conference on Primary Health Care' (Geneva: WHO, 1978) in particular the definition of primary health care at 3.

55. WHO has recently stated that "a health system consists of all organizations, people and actions whose primary intent is to promote, restore or maintain health". WHO, *Everybody's Business; Strengthening Health Systems to Improve Health Outcomes* (Geneva: WHO, 2007) at 1. The report identifies the building blocks of a health system as health services, health workforce, health information systems, medical products, health financing, as well as leadership, governance and stewardship. Ibid., at 3.

56. The UN Special Rapporteur on the right to health has reviewed this complex issue in 2008, recommended a right-to-health approach to strengthening health systems, and singled out planning, governance and accountability as aspects in particular need of strengthening. Paul Hunt, 'Report of the Special Rapporteur on the right of everyone to the enjoyment of the highest attainable standard of physical and mental health', UN Doc. A/HRC/7/11, 31 January 2008.

57. General Comment No. 14, *supra* note 9, at paras. 16 and 40.

58. See, for example, J. Giesecke, 'International

Health Regulations and Epidemic Control' in R. Smith, R. Beaglehole, D. Woodward, and N. Drager (eds.) *Global Public Goods for Health: Health Economics and Public Health Perspectives* (Oxford: Oxford University Press, 2003) 196–211.

59. For more information on GOARN, see http://www.who.int/csr/outbreaknetwork/en/.

60. Lance Gable, 'The Proliferation of Human Rights in Global Health Governance' 35 *Journal of Law, Medicine & Ethics* (2007) 534–544 at 539.

QUESTIONS

1. It is often asserted that "public health emergencies" require governments to balance public health and safety of the population with civil rights of the members of the population. Is this always true? What, exactly, is a public health emergency? Has the world become much more interested in possible pandemics after 9/11?

2. How was the SARS epidemic ultimately contained? What can be learned from the fact that all 28 affected countries applied different approaches, and each "succeeded"?

3. Why does state coercion of its citizens seem like the right thing to do in the face of a public health emergency? What procedures should be followed to ensure that state coercion is legitimate and not abusive?

4. Why do WHO and many other public health agencies now speak of epidemics in national security terms and metaphors? Is this useful? Comment on how using concepts of national security when applied to epidemics like SARS and influenza, and even HIV/AIDS, help (or hurt) efforts to prevent and respond to epidemics.

FURTHER READING

1. Fidler, David P., Germs, Governance and Global Public Health in the Wake of SARS, Emerging Infectious Diseases, *J Clinical Investigation*, 2004; 113: 799–804.

2. Rothstein, Mark, *Quarantine and Isolation: Lessons Learned from SARS.* Atlanta: CDC, 2003.

3. Barry, John M., *The Great Influenza: The Epic Story of the Deadliest Plague in History.* New York: Viking, 2004.

CHAPTER 36

Bioterror and "Bioart": A Plague o' Both Your Houses

George J. Annas

INTRODUCTION

Since September 11, 2001, the threat of bioterrorism has caused Congress and the President to dramatically increase research funding for countermeasures, including funding for new biosecurity laboratories. The new kind of war against non-state actors who use terror to intimidate populations has also made the creation of new ethical and legal rules for researchers seem critical. New laws have been passed, and there have been proposals for new codes of ethics for bioterrorism-related research. Almost five years after September 11, however, the outcome of the development of new research rules remains uncertain.

Ethical guidelines for life sciences research that could be related to bioterrorism are critical, and the scientific community should be actively engaged in setting the standards for such research.[1, 2] As the National Research Council of the National Academy of Sciences has stated, "biological scientists have an affirmative moral duty to avoid contributing to the advancement of biowarfare or bioterrorism."[1] It is reasonable for society to expect that scientists will adopt the equivalent of the physician's "do no harm" principle.[1] Arguing for such an oath well before September 11, literary scholar Roger Shattuck noted that it could

"help scientists scrutinize the proliferation of research in dubious areas" as well as "renew the confidence of ordinary citizens" in what is a potentially revolutionary endeavor.[3]

As the debate about the role of ethical standards proceeds, some legal standards have already been adopted. Even with their new legal powers, the Federal Bureau of Investigation (FBI) and Central Intelligence Agency (CIA) have been unable to discover the source of the anthrax attacks. The FBI investigations have, however, focused on two other biosafety cases that have become infamous. Neither of these cases involves bioterrorism, but both illustrate how—in a post–September 11 world—the federal government and the public can be expected to react and even overreact if new biosafety rules are broken in ways that may create a biohazard or public health problem.

THE CASE OF THOMAS BUTLER

Dr. Thomas Butler was the first and so far the only physician-scientist to stand trial in the United States on a bioterrorism-related charge after September 11. On January 2, 2006, Butler completed a two-year sentence that was imposed after a jury trial and upheld by a U.S. Circuit Court of Appeals.[4]

The bioterrorism-related facts no longer seem to be in serious dispute.

According to his colleagues in the field of infectious disease, Butler has had a long and successful career dating from completion of medical school and residency at Johns Hopkins University at the end of the 1960s and his service in Vietnam in the Naval Medical Research Unit. He was a faculty member at Johns Hopkins University Medical Center and Case Western Reserve University before becoming chief of infectious diseases at Texas Tech University Health Sciences Center in 1987, a post he held until his trial. His work on plague (*Yersinia pestis*) dates from his experiences treating civilians in the Vietnam War. Most recently, this work involved research in Tanzania, where he and a colleague there compared the efficacy of gentamicin with that of doxycycline in treating patients with plague infection.[5] The results of this research were published soon after Butler was released from prison.[6]

Butler traveled to Tanzania to help set up the study in 2001, and he returned in 2002 to collect samples of *Y. pestis* taken from the subjects. He returned to the United States with these samples without the required transport permits. In June, he drove to the laboratory of the Centers for Disease Control and Prevention (CDC) in Fort Collins, Colorado, to have the samples tested, again without the required government transport permits.

In September 2002, he sent a set of plague isolates back to Tanzania in a Federal Express box labeled "laboratory materials" without the required export permits, and in October, he flew from Lubbock, Texas, to Washington, D.C. (to the Army Medical Research Institute of Infectious Diseases), with plague samples without the required permit.

In November 2002, after a series of confrontations over timely documentation of complications and death among subjects in a study of antibiotics for the biotechnology company Chiron, Butler's local institutional review board prohibited him from performing research on human subjects. On January 9, 2003, the board, dissatisfied by his lack of cooperation, reiterated the suspension in an e-mail.[7] On January 10, he was notified by letter of a formal inquiry into his activities. On January 11, a Saturday morning, Butler noticed that a set of 30 tubes of *Y. pestis* cultures was missing, and he noted in his journal, "Set 5 missing!" The next day, he wrote, "Can't explain other than intentional removal, suspect theft."[8] On Monday, January 13, 2003, he reported to the biosafety officer at the health center that 30 vials of *Y. pestis* were missing from his laboratory. The next day, senior officials at the health center met and decided to notify the local police and the health department. The police notified the FBI, and more than 60 FBI agents and local police officers conducted an immediate investigation.

Butler was questioned by the FBI, and he waived his right to counsel (this waiver is almost always a mistake). He first insisted that he did not know what happened to the samples. However, after failing a lie-detector test (the failure was not admitted in court) and, he says, being told by an FBI agent that if he signed a statement that he had accidentally destroyed the samples (to reassure the public that there was no danger), that would be the end of the matter, he signed a statement to this effect.[4, 9] However, this statement was not the end of the matter. Butler was arrested, spent six days in jail, and then was placed under house arrest. In April 2003, a grand jury returned a 15-count indictment charging him with various crimes relating to his transport of *Y. pestis,* making false statements to the FBI, and tax evasion. Texas Tech also turned against Butler and helped the prosecution reframe the university's contract disputes with him as crimes. In

August 2003, after Butler refused to plead guilty in exchange for a six-month sentence, he was charged with 54 additional criminal counts; these included mail fraud, wire fraud, and embezzlement arising from Butler's research for two companies (Chiron and Pharmacia-Upjohn—now Pfizer) and concealment of two contracts with the Food and Drug Administration (FDA) from the university.[4]

As part of Butler's pay structure, a percentage of his income was provided by the state of Texas and the remainder came from the university's Medical Practice Income Plan, which included money earned from seeing patients, research grants, and clinical trials. All monies from these sources, with the exception of consulting contracts, were to be remitted to the Health Sciences Center. Butler entered into contracts with both Pharmacia and Chiron in which his fee per subject would be split between the Health Sciences Center and himself. These contracts, the first of which commenced in 1998, continued until August 2001, and they did not come to the attention of the Health Sciences Center until July 2002.[4]

Butler voluntarily gave up his medical license before the trial. After the three-week trial, which included testimony from 40 witnesses, a jury found Butler not guilty on almost all the plague-related charges (which included lying to the FBI) and not guilty of tax evasion. It did, however, find him guilty on most of the charges related to his split-fee contract arrangements (44 of the 54 fraud counts) and on 3 of the 18 charges relating to the transport of plague samples.[4] He was sentenced to 24 months in prison and 3 years of supervised release and was charged $15,000 in fines and $38,675 restitution to the university. He appealed.

Five issues were raised on appeal. The two most important of these issues dealt with the possibly prejudicial effect of combining the "plague counts" with the contract counts and whether there was sufficient evidence of criminal intent relative to the failure to file the required shipping forms for plague samples. Regarding the first issue, the appeals court ruled without much discussion (and arguably without much understanding of how medical research is conducted) that all these counts could be combined because they all had to do with Butler's "research efforts": "Butler's handling of plague bacteria as part of his research efforts was ultimately related to his scheme to defraud the Health Sciences Center by concealing both his contracts with the FDA and the split contracts Butler maintained with the two pharmaceutical companies."[4] If the Supreme Court agrees to hear his appeal, the possibly prejudicial effect of combining these counts is Butler's strongest argument.

The appeals court also had little sympathy for Butler's contention that the evidence was insufficient to show that he acted willfully in regard to the only 3 plague-related charges (of 18 charges) he was convicted of: first, exporting plague to Tanzania without a license; second, describing plague as "laboratory materials" on a Federal Express waybill; and third, violating federal hazardous materials regulations in shipping plague to Tanzania.[4] Regarding the first and third plague-related charges, the court was persuaded that because Butler "had successfully and legally shipped hazardous materials [during the 1990s] at least 30 times before making this particular shipment" there was sufficient evidence that he knew how to ship it properly and that "his infraction could not have been due to a good faith mistake or a misunderstanding of the law." As for Butler's contention that he did not intend to deceive anyone by labeling plague "laboratory materials," the court accepted the government's argument that he had also certified on the same label that he was "not shipping dangerous goods" and that the jury could reasonably conclude that he knew "that plague was a dangerous good requiring the proper identification."[4]

"BIOART" AND BIOTERRORISM

Shortly after Butler's trial, in another part of the country—Buffalo, New York—FBI agents were called in to investigate a suspected act of bioterrorism in the home of Steve Kurtz, a professor and artist at the State University of New York at Buffalo. Kurtz awoke on May 11, 2004, to find his wife dead beside him. Kurtz and his wife previously had cofounded the Critical Art Ensemble, an artists' collective "dedicated to exploring the intersections between art, technology, radical politics and critical theory."[10] Kurtz liked to distinguish what he did from the emerging field of "bio-art," which is perhaps best known to the public because of the notoriety of Alba, a rabbit that glowed green because of the insertion of a jellyfish gene. Kurtz thinks of bioart as consisting of stunts and his own art as an exploration of "the political economy of biotechnology."[10] He had previously argued against the introduction of genetically modified food, and he had encouraged activists to oppose it by means of "fuzzy biological sabotage"—for instance, by releasing genetically mutated and deformed flies at restaurants to stir up paranoia.[10]

The day after his wife's death, the FBI raided his home in full biohazard gear. Kurtz had been studying the history of germ warfare for a new project. In connection with this project, he was growing bacterial cultures that he was planning to use to simulate attacks with anthrax and plague. He had obtained the bacteria samples (*Serratia marcescens* and *Bacillus atrophaeus*) from a colleague, Professor Robert Ferrell, a geneticist at the University of Pittsburgh Medical Center, who had ordered them for him from the American Type Culture Collection. Kurtz and Ferrell were suspected almost immediately of being involved in a bioterror ring and were thoroughly investigated. Once the New York Department of Health determined that the bacteria were harmless and that Kurtz's wife had died of natural causes, the bioterrorism investigation was dropped. The Justice Department nonetheless charged both Ferrell and Kurtz with four counts of wire fraud and mail fraud. The allegation was that Ferrell, at Kurtz's request, defrauded the University of Pittsburgh and the American Type Culture Collection by representing that the bacteria samples he ordered would be used in his University of Pittsburgh laboratory.[11] Neither case has yet gone to trial.

Exactly what Kurtz was planning to do with the bacteria is unclear, but serratia, which is known for its ability to form bright red colonies, has been used in biowarfare simulations in the past. Perhaps its most well-known use was a 1950 simulation in which an offshore naval vessel blanketed a 50-square-mile section of San Francisco with an aerosol spray containing serratia to determine what dose could be delivered effectively to the population.[12] Whether using a similar technique as an art exhibit would constitute bioart, biotechnology, or biohazard (or even bioterrorism) may be in the eye of the beholder even more than in the eye of the artist or scientist.

Bioart is not bioterrorism, but the two are related politically. As bioart curator and commentator Jens Hauser has said, bioart aims "at the heart of our fears" and is meant to "disturb." He notes, "these artists expose the gulf between the apologetic official discourse about technoscience on the one hand, and paranoia on the other."[13] Like defensive and offensive bioweapons research, bioart and biotechnology may be impossible to distinguish by anything other than the researcher's or creator's intent. Thus, Alba, the bunny with the inserted jellyfish gene, is considered to be and is accepted as a creation of bioart, at least in the contemporary art community; whereas ANDi, the monkey with the inserted jellyfish gene, is considered to be a creation of science, at least in the biotechnology community. Hauser was referring to paranoia in the face of the "rapid acceleration of technical prowess."[13] On the basis of the reaction of federal law enforcement to the actions of Thomas Butler and Steve Kurtz, however, although the advances of biotechnology that have potential applications to bioterrorism and biowarfare are scary, even scarier are the responses—in the name of preventing bioterrorism—of law-enforcement agencies to legitimate scientists and artists whose actions pose no threat to the public.

Butler's arrest came about one year after a simulated bioterrorism event in Lubbock, Texas; this simulation involved the use of aerosolized plague at a civic center.[5] Simulations have been a centerpiece of efforts to prepare for acts of bioterrorism. As we should have learned from our obsession with building bomb shelters during the Cold War, however, simulations promote fear of worst-case scenarios and make them look much more likely. Bioterrorism simulations such as Dark Winter (smallpox) and Top Officials (TOPOFF) (plague) involve more art than science and are likely to provoke a response based more on fear than logic. They should probably be classified as bioart in the sense of performance art, and they should have their most socially useful outlet not in federal law-enforcement agencies or biosafety laboratories but in television dramas like *24*.

BIOTERRORISM AND SCIENCE

The case of physician-researcher Thomas Butler has been the subject of many commentaries—most arguing that his prosecution represents a gross overreaction on the part of federal authorities. Nonetheless, in an article in *Science,* Margaret A. Somerville and Ronald M. Atlas argued that Butler's prosecution "sent a clear signal to the research community, especially scientists and university researchers, that all ethical and legal requirements must be respected when undertaking research."[14] They continued, "Biosafety regulations are not merely legal technicalities. They constitute some of the terms of the pact between science and the public that establishes public trust."[14]

Somerville and Atlas are correct to argue that researchers must take law and ethics seriously, and their call for a new code of ethics is reasonable. It would be too broad, however, to suggest either that there are no such things as "legal technicalities" or that all such technicalities are reasonable. Jennifer Gaudioso and Reynolds M. Salerno of the Sandia National Laboratories, for example, have argued persuasively that not all pathogens and toxins pose the same risks and that risk in the laboratory should "be a function of an agent's weaponization potential and consequences of its use" (rather than the current assessment of biosafety risk, which focuses on "infectious disease dangers and the risk of accidental exposure in the laboratory").[15] They also note that under the regulations of the Uniting and Strengthening America by Providing Appropriate Tools Required to Intercept and Obstruct Terrorism (USA PATRIOT) Act and the Public Health Security and Bioterrorism and Response Act that require entities with certain agents to register with the CDC, only 323 of the 817 facilities that the CDC expected to register actually did.[15] Other facilities may register, but many research entities decided to discontinue their research projects, rather than conform to the new federal administrative and security rules for such research.[15] A 2006 National Academy of Sciences report rejects the use of an agent-specific threat list and instead recommends adoption of a "broader perspective on the 'threat spectrum' . . . to ensure regular and deliberate reassessments of advances in science and technology and identification of those advances with the greatest potential for changing the nature of the threat spectrum."[2]

Ethics and law are related, but they are not the same. Law draws the line we cannot cross without becoming "outlaws." Even if we do not like it, we must nonetheless follow it (while working to change it) or risk, as Butler did, being prosecuted for being an outlaw. All Americans, including physicians, should recognize that when the FBI wants to talk to them about their role in a possible bioterrorist event, they should not talk to the FBI without first speaking with a lawyer. Americans can go to jail for violating the law, but not for violating codes of ethics. We aspire to uphold ethics—we deserve praise (at least some) for behaving "ethically"; whereas we deserve none for simply following the law, some of which is in fact made up of "legal technicalities."

Because the differences between research on offensive biologic weapons and research on defensive biologic weapons are a matter of degree, not kind, and because biotechnology research is an international activity, any evidence that such research is doing more to put the public at risk than to protect the public will (and should) be especially damaging to the entire enterprise. This is one reason why Butler's report of missing plague bacteria (still unaccounted for) could not be tolerated by federal officials who support the expansion of research on countermeasures. It is also what makes Kurtz's bioart so disturbing—the public is confronted with the dark side of bioterrorism-related research, and it provokes a response. The inherent dual nature of biodefense research has been

dubbed "the Persephone effect," which refers to Demeter's daughter who was forced to spend six months every year with Pluto in Hell so she could live the other half of the year on Earth.[16]

One reasonable response to the dispute between Butler and the Justice Department and the dispute between Kurtz and the Justice Department could be Mercutio's retort in *Romeo and Juliet*: "A plague o' both your houses."[17] This is because the public is currently more victim and bystander than participant and seems much more likely to be harmed than helped by much of the research. Members of the public recognize this probability, and their skepticism of federal authorities, of the effectiveness of countermeasures, of the existence of weapons of mass destruction in Iraq, and of the entire bioterrorism scare is well illustrated by the few people who took drugs to treat anthrax that were offered after the anthrax attacks.[18] This same skepticism, combined with the lack of evidence of stockpiles of smallpox in Iraq and the certainty of side effects from the drugs, also explains the small number of health professionals who volunteered to take the smallpox vaccine immediately before and shortly after the commencement of the war in Iraq.[18]

Table 36.1 Seven Classes of Microbial Experiments That Should Require Review*

The experiments would:

    Demonstrate how to render a vaccine
        ineffective
    Confer resistance to therapeutically useful
        antibiotics or antiviral agents
    Enhance the virulence of a pathogen or
        render a nonpathogen virulent
    Increase transmissibility of a pathogen
    Alter the host range of a pathogen
    Enable the evasion of diagnostic and
        detection methods
    Enable the weaponization of a biologic agent
        or toxin

* Data are from the National Research Council.[1]

ETHICS, BIOTERRORISM, AND LIFE SCIENCES RESEARCH

Research directed at creating new pathogens or toxins that have direct bioterror or biowarfare applications deserves condemnation. The National Research Council, for example, has identified seven classes of microbial experiments (Table 36.1) that should "require review and discussion by informed members of the scientific and medical community before they are undertaken."[1] If such experiments are undertaken at all, I believe there also should be a requirement for publication of the protocol and public input into the decision. Research directed at individual pathogens and their weaponization potential also risks the diversion of scientific resources from more important public health concerns,[19] just as it has seemed to divert the FBI's attention from real terrorists.

There appears to be a consensus in the scientific community that the free and open exchange of information is ultimately the best defense to both naturally occurring pandemics and deliberate biologic attacks.[2, 20] There is also a growing recognition of the importance of developing an international code of ethics for scientists as well as a recognition that such a code must "become part of the lived culture" of scientists.[2, 20] Like bioart, the development of this code remains a work in progress.

REFERENCES

1. Committee on Research Standards and Practices to Prevent the Destructive Application of Biotechnology, National Research Council. Biotechnology research in an age of terrorism. Washington, D.C.: National Academies Press, 2004.
2. Committee on Advances in Technology and the Prevention of Their Application to Next Generation Biowarfare Threats, National Research Council. Globalization, biosecurity, and the future of the life sciences. Washington, D.C.: National Academies Press, 2006.
3. Shattuck R. Forbidden knowledge: from Prometheus to pornography. New York: St. Martin's Press, 1996:224.
4. United States v. Butler, 429 F.3d 140 (5th Cir. 2005).
5. Murray BE, Anderson KE, Arnold K, et al. Destroying the life and career of a valued physician-scientist who tried to protect us from plague: was it really necessary? Clin Infect Dis 2005; 40:1644–8.
6. Mwengee W, Butler T, Mgema S, et al. Treatment of plague with gentamicin or doxycycline in a randomized clinical trial in Tanzania. Clin Infect Dis 2006;42:614–21.
7. Gold R. With plague fears on rise, an expert ends up on trial. Wall Street Journal. April 14, 2003: A1.
8. Enserink M, Malakoff D. The trials of Thomas Butler. Science 2003;302:2054–63.
9. The case against Dr. Butler. 60 Minutes. October 19, 2003 (transcript).
10. Turner C. This is right out of Hitler's handbook. Guardian (London). October 20, 2005:18.
11. United States v. Steven Kurtz and Robert Ferrell, grand jury indictment 0-CR-155E (W.D.N.Y., June 2004).
12. Tansey B. Serratia has dark history in region: Army test in 1950 may have changed microbial ecology. San Francisco Chronicle. October 31, 2004:A7.
13. Hauser J. Genes, genius, embarrassment. In: Hauser J, ed. L'art biotech. Nantes, France: Editions Filigranes, 2003.
14. Somerville MA, Atlas RM. Ethics: a weapon to counter bioterrorism. Science 2005;307:1881–2.
15. Gaudioso J, Salerno R M. Biosecurit y and research: minimizing adverse impacts. Science 2004;304:687. [Erratum, Science 2004;305:180.]
16. Kwik G, Fitzgerald J, Inglesby TV, O'Toole T. Biosecurity: responsible stewardship of bioscience in an age of catastrophic terrorism. Biosecur Bioterror 2003;1:27–35.
17. Shakespeare W. Romeo and Juliet. Act III, Scene I, line 108.
18. Annas GJ. The statue of security: human rights and post-9/11 epidemics. J Health Law 2005;38:319–51.
19. Relman DA. Bioterrorism—preparing to fight the next war. N Engl J Med 2006;354:113–15.
20. Wheelif M, Rozsa L, Dando M. Deadly cultures: biological weapons since 1945. Cambridge, Mass.: Harvard University Press, 2006.

QUESTIONS

1. 9/11 didn't "change everything" but it did change a lot—including a fear of "bio-terrorism," the use of new or old pathogens to foment terror. Even top physician researchers became suspect, and at least one, Thomas Butler, was prosecuted and convicted of crimes related to his research on plague. Were his human rights violated? Did the prosecution of Butler help protect our health?

2. The late Roger Shattuck suggested that scientists adopt a version of the physicians' "do no harm" principle to guide their work. Are there experiments that simply should not be done because they pose too much danger to humanity? Who should decide this and on what basis?

3. In 2012 two studies were published that showed how H5N1 flu virus could be engineered to become more lethal and transmissible. Many objected that this study (which was funded by the US) should never have been done; others thought it was permissible to do the studies, but not to publish the results because terrorists could use them to create their own killer flu virus. The debate continues. What do you think? Should the WHO have a role in reviewing "dual use" research, or only in preparing for and responding to epidemics?

FURTHER READING

1. Levy, Barry & Sidel, Victor, eds, *Terrorism and Public Health*, 2nd ed. New York: Oxford University Press, 2012.
2. Wheelis, Mark, Rozsa, Lajos, & Dando, Malcolm, eds., *Deadly Cultures: Biological Weapons Since* 1945. Cambridge: Harvard University Press, 2006.
3. Shattuck, Roger, *Forbidden Knowledge*. New York: Harcourt Brace, 1996.
4. Editorial, Publishing Risky Research. *Nature*, 2012; 485: 5 and articles in a special issue of *Science* on the H5N1 controversy in *Science*, 2012; 336: 1522–1533.

Harm Reduction, HIV/AIDS, and the Human Rights Challenge to Global Drug Control Policy

Richard Elliott, Joanne Csete, Evan Wood and Thomas Kerr

The global HIV/AIDS pandemic has added to the list of harms associated with unsafe drug use and provided yet further evidence that the dominant, prohibitionist approach to illicit drugs is not only ineffective but also counter-productive. Embodying this approach, international drug control treaties cast a chill over—or in some cases, may prohibit, *de jure* or *de facto*—implementation of measures proven effective in reducing the spread of HIV. Furthermore, a prohibitionist paradigm engenders policies and practices that inhibit drug users' access to care, treatment, and support, be it for HIV disease, addiction, overdose, or other health concerns.

Consequently, the HIV/AIDS pandemic has intensified debate over the norms and institutions of the global drug control regime. In part because of the increasingly apparent devastation of injection drug use and associated spread of HIV, pressure is mounting for drug policy reform at the international as well as domestic level. AIDS has upped the ante; the sheer magnitude of the epidemic driven by unsafe drug use has meant greater pressure to confront issues that governments would often rather ignore. It is increasingly evident that a commitment to harm reduction—defined broadly as "policies and programs which attempt primarily to reduce the adverse health, social and economic consequences of mood altering substances to individual drug users, their families and their communities"—must entail some degree of reform of the dominant prohibitionist approach.[1,2] Simultaneously, the emergence of HIV/AIDS has catalyzed a movement of researchers and activists articulating the multi-dimensional, multi-directional relationship between health and human rights. Given that unsafe drug use, particularly by injection, is now one of the major factors fueling the global epidemic, it is only natural that the legal regime that affects drug use(rs) comes under human rights scrutiny.

A commitment to the human rights of drug users has marked the thinking and advocacy of many people concerned with harm reduction from the outset, and the principles, objectives, and initiatives that fall under the broad rubric of "harm reduction" can be characterized as reflecting or advancing human rights. Harm reductionists, therefore, in effect, are human rights advocates, contributing to a larger effort aimed at securing universal respect for, and observance of, fundamental human rights. Yet it is only in recent years that the language of human rights has begun to inform discussions about drug policy reform in international and intergovernmental fora beyond the circles of harm reduction proponents and/or human rights experts.[3]

There may be strategic reasons, in any given instance, to focus on either the "public health" rationale or a "human rights" argument for a specific reform in order to sway decision-makers in a particular direction. Combining the two approaches, however, may strengthen such a case: public health evidence can support principled legal arguments with a sound evidentiary basis, and the principles of human rights law strengthen statistical or other data with the normative claim that states have an ethical and legal obligation to act upon that evidence. We suggest that joining human rights law with public health evidence can help shift global drug control policy away from the current, failed emphasis on prohibition to a more rational, health-promoting framework that is both pragmatic and principled. As a contribution to this collective endeavor of "regime change," this chapter:[4]

- reviews briefly the global extent of injection drug use and the linked HIV/AIDS epidemic and the impact of prohibition and harm reduction on health and human rights, focusing on HIV/AIDS-related effects;
- outlines the basic elements of the international legal regime of illicit drug control;
- considers some of the conceptual and programmatic links between harm reduction and human rights as recognized in international law; and
- discusses strategies for reforming global drug control policy to reflect a more human rights-based approach that facilitates harm reduction.

INJECTION DRUG USE AND HIV/AIDS: GLOBAL HEALTH CHALLENGES

Recent estimates suggest that there are over 13 million people who inject illicit drugs in the world today, the majority of whom are from developing countries.[5] Injection drug use was first documented in North America, Australia, and Western Europe well before HIV/AIDS was first discovered, but evidence of the emergence and rapid diffusion of injection drug use has recently been documented in Eastern Europe, the former Soviet Union, South East Asia, China, India, the Middle East, and West Africa.[6] HIV prevalence higher than 20% among persons who inject drugs has been reported for at least 1 site in 25 countries and territories, from several different regions of the world.[7]

Injection drug use is a key risk factor for HIV infection, given the high-risk behavior of sharing injection equipment.[8] Of the 136 countries that reported injection drug use in 2003, 93 also reported HIV infection among users.[9] In Eastern Europe and the former Soviet Union, regions with two of the fastest growing HIV epidemics, injection drug use accounts for the majority of new infections.[10] In other countries, such as Thailand, high HIV incidence persists in this population.[11] Currently, injection drug use is estimated to account for 10% of HIV infections globally, although this proportion is likely increasing in light of the dual epidemics of injection drug use and HIV in Eastern Europe, the former Soviet Union, and Asia.[12] Experience demonstrates that HIV can spread rapidly once established within communities of drug users.[13] Other health-related harms among persons who inject drugs include high rates of hepatitis C infection, bacterial infections, multidrug-resistant tuberculosis, fatal and nonfatal overdoses, and high violence and suicide rates.[14]

Overall, the evidence suggests that while drug users generally do not enjoy adequate access to highly active antiretroviral therapy (HAART), the challenges of access and adherence to treatment regimens can be overcome with appropriate support, including the provision of drug treatment and various harm reduction services such as methadone maintenance therapy (MMT).[15, 16] International reviews also indicate that HIV epidemics driven by injection drug use can be prevented or reversed by instituting prevention measures while seroprevalence is still relatively low, including such measures as syringe exchange programs and outreach services.[17] Unfortunately, HIV prevention efforts remain inadequate in many countries with high rates of HIV incidence among drug users. For example, the Global HIV Prevention Working Group reported in 2003 that only 11% of injection drug users (IDUs) in the countries of the former Soviet Union and Eastern Europe have access to syringe exchange programs.[18]

THE DAMAGE OF DRUG PROHIBITION

The dominant approach, in both national and international responses to drug use, remains the attempt to reduce or prevent the supply and use of controlled substances by means of legal prohibitions on their cultivation, production, transport, distribution, and possession. Yet the available evidence suggests that drug law enforcement has not produced the purported benefits. Street-level drug policing has been shown to have little, if any, sustained effect on the price of illicit drugs, their availability, or the frequency of use.[19] Nor have law enforcement efforts produced greater use of addiction treatment by drug users.[20] Public order gains are generally time-limited and often simply result in displacement of drug markets and drug users into other areas, frequently away from HIV prevention services.[21] Such ineffective use of policing budgets also carries the opportunity cost of lost investments in other, more beneficial police work (for example, community policing).[22] Consider, for example, that the US federal government spends billions of dollars each year to fund the "war on drugs" yet spends nothing on syringe exchange programs, despite hundreds of thousands of documented cases of HIV infection among people who inject drugs.[23]

In some cases, prohibition actually fuels risky injection and drug storage practices, increasing the risk of overdose, viral and bacterial disease transmission, and other harms.[24] Policies of prohibition have prompted some drug users to switch to drug injection from other practices: drugs consumed by smoking (for example, opium and cannabis) can be harder to conceal than drugs regularly consumed by injection (for example, heroin), and injection may be a more efficient way to consume when the drug supply or time for consumption is limited. Evidence also indicates that law enforcement initiatives can displace drug users into less safe environments (for example, "shooting galleries") and disrupt relationships within illicit drug markets, leading to increased violence among users and dealers.[25] Similarly, policing practices can undermine users' access to health services, including harm reduction programs. Deterring drug users from visiting syringe exchanges encourages them to share syringes and dispose of syringes and related litter improperly rather than risk being found in possession of such items by police.[26] Harassment and arrest of syringe exchange workers, including for possession of material explaining safer injection practices, obviously undermines efforts to protect drug users against HIV and other risks of unsafe use.[27] Other reports indicate that fear of prosecution deters many drug users from seeking medical assistance during or following an overdose.[28]

HARM REDUCTION IS HEALTH PROMOTION

Harm reduction does not preclude abstinence as a worthy goal, but rather it accepts that illicit drug use has been, and will continue to be, a feature of cultures throughout the world and that efforts should made to reduce harms (including HIV infection) among individuals who continue illicit drug use. In practice, interventions aimed at promoting the health of drug users by reducing harms from unsafe drug use and/or facilitating access to care and support include:

- outreach programs;
- peer-driven interventions;
- empowerment through drug user organizations;
- syringe exchange programs;
- opioid substitution therapy (for example, methadone maintenance) and controlled heroin prescription; and
- safer injection facilities and other supervised drug consumption sites.

A large body of evidence indicates that harm reduction measures can have a positive impact in preventing HIV infection among people who use illicit drugs and their sexual and drug-sharing partners; can improve their access to health and other services; and are more respectful of their dignity and rights than other measures.[29] Globally, we observe that countries that have adopted comprehensive harm reduction measures have succeeded in preventing or stabilizing HIV epidemics among IDUs; while countries that have been slow to implement such measures and have focused instead on enforcing prohibition have suffered greater spread of HIV among IDUs and subsequent spread to non-drug using populations.[30]

Outreach programs have been demonstrated to reach marginalized populations, including out-of-treatment IDUs who may be at highest risk for HIV infection, creating an important link to testing, prevention, and treatment services. Peer-driven interventions have been an important

means of providing social networks of drug users, through "indigenous leaders," with HIV- and overdose-prevention measures.[31] Drug user-groups connect active users with health services but also play a more critical role in the self-empowerment of users by educating the public about issues facing drug users and effecting policy change through activism.[32, 33]

Syringe exchange programs, which have been found to reduce risk behavior and the incidence of HIV and hepatitis C, have not led to increases in drug use and have been associated with substantial savings in health care expenditures.[34, 35] These programs are widely regarded as the single most important factor in preventing HIV epidemics among IDUs.[36] An international investigation found that in cities with syringe exchange or distribution programs HIV seroprevalence decreased by 5.8% per year, while HIV prevalence increased by 5.9% per year in cities without such programs.[37] A more recent analysis has suggested an even greater impact on HIV prevalence of the presence or absence of syringe exchange programs.[38] Opioid substitution therapy (for example, methadone) has been shown to lead to reduction in, and even elimination of, illicit opiate use, as well as reductions in criminal activity, unemployment, and mortality rates.[39] It has also been associated with reduced risk behaviors (for example, needle sharing) and reduced rates of transmission of HIV and viral hepatitis.[40]

Safer injection facilities where IDUs can inject pre-obtained illicit drugs under medical supervision have been implemented in the Netherlands, Germany, Switzerland, Spain, Australia, and Canada.[41] Among other health benefits, they have been associated with reduced HIV-risk behavior and overdose deaths, although further evaluation is warranted.[42]

Despite evidence supporting the above measures, they often remain unpopular among many politicians; and instead of implementing such programs with proven or reasonably predictable health benefits, many governments have opted to rely on expensive, ineffective, and harmful enforcement policies and practices. In the next section, we consider whether such approaches are required by international drug control treaties and the extent to which governments may pursue more health-friendly alternatives.

DRUG CONTROL AND HARM REDUCTION IN INTERNATIONAL LAW

The current global system for illicit drug control rests upon three international conventions: the 1961 Single Convention on Narcotic Drugs, the 1971 Convention on Psychotropic Substances, and the 1988 Convention against Illegal Traffic in Narcotic Drugs and Psychotropic Substances ("Vienna Convention").[43–45] The treaties require signatory states to take various measures to criminalize drug-related activities such as cultivation, production, manufacture, export, import, distribution, trading, and possession of controlled substances except for "medical and scientific purposes."[46] The 1998 Convention (Article 3:2) specifically requires the criminalization of possession for personal consumption, casting drug users as criminals.[47] Three international bodies administer the treaties:

- The UN Commission on Narcotic Drugs (CND) consists of 53 UN member states and is the central policy-making body within the UN system in relation to drug control, with the authority to bring forward amendments to existing treaties or propose new treaties. At the insistence of the United States, the CND currently operates by consensus, meaning that any single country can block a resolution or other initiative.[48]

- The UN Office on Drugs and Crime (UNODC) "assist[s] UN member states in their struggle against illicit drugs, crime and terrorism." UNODC is a co-sponsor of the Joint UN Programme on HIV/AIDS (UNAIDS) and had begun to show some support for harm reduction measures, at least insofar as it relates to preventing HIV among drug users.[49] However, recent statements by the senior management have manifested overt hostility toward proven harm reduction measures, even as some parts of the agency support more harm reduction-friendly interpretations. Resolving the consequent internal tension, and contradictions with other "core values" of the UN, is necessary if the UNODC is to be a credible interlocutor in the response to the global AIDS pandemic.[50]

- The International Narcotics Control Board (INCB) is "the independent and quasi-judicial control organ for the implementation of the United Nations drug conventions," with the "responsibility to promote government compliance with the provisions of the drug control treaties."[51] Established by the 1961 Single Convention, the INCB consists of 13 individual experts and has manifested a general hostility toward harm reduction. Although the UN conventions enjoin states to ensure drug treatment programs in addition to law enforcement systems, a review of the Board's annual reports demonstrates that its monitoring activities have focused virtually exclusively on the latter. The INCB has lamented that harm reduction has "diverted the attention (and in some cases, funds) of Governments from important demand reduction activities such as primary prevention or abstinence-oriented treatment."[52] Although INCB interpretations of the conventions are not legally binding, they help shape the political climate in which decision-makers determine national drug policies.

The INCB and prohibitionist states have emphasized the provisions in the conventions requiring criminalization and penalties for drug-related activities. However, the treaties also contain important qualifications that can make some space for harm reduction initiatives, even if this "room for manoeuver" is limited.[53] Indeed, the legal advisory branch of UNODC has advised the INCB that most harm reduction measures are compatible with the UN drug control conventions, which can be interpreted to permit opioid substitution therapy, syringe distribution, and safer injection facilities.[54] As for treaty articles that may be at odds with harm reduction initiatives, the UNODC memorandum stated: "It could even be argued that the drug control treaties, as they stand, have been rendered out of synch with reality."[55]

So what flexibility currently exists within the drug control regime? The 1961 and 1971 treaties allow for the production, distribution, or possession of controlled substances for "medical and scientific purposes."[56] It is up to States parties to determine how they will interpret such provisions in their domestic legislation. The treaties also allow states to provide measures of treatment, rehabilitation, and social reintegration as alternatives, or in addition, to criminal penalties, meaning that states enjoy discretion in deciding whether or not to impose criminal penalties for the personal (non-medical) possession and consumption of drugs controlled by the treaties.[57, 58] In addition, the 1961 and 1971 conventions actually mandate states to "take all practicable measures" for the "treatment, ... rehabilitation and social reintegration" of drug users.[59]

It is true that the 1988 Convention expressly requires each state to criminalize possession of a controlled substance even for personal consumption. Some have suggested that the provision means that personal consumption is contrary to the 1961 and 1971 Conventions, thereby retrospectively interpreting those earlier treaties.[60] However, this interpretation is incorrect and should be rejected as it leads to the improper (and often draconian) application of criminal sanctions under domestic legislation that is not strictly required by the treaty. The 1988 Convention merely says that countries must criminalize possession for personal consumption if such consumption is contrary to the provisions of the two earlier treaties; the flexibility found in the earlier conventions is preserved, meaning that possession for personal consumption authorized by domestic law, in accord with the 1961 and 1971 Conventions, is permissible. Importantly, the 1988 Convention also acknowledges that the obligation to criminalize personal consumption is "subject to the constitutional principles and the basic concepts of its legal system."[61] Given this qualification, the provision is open to creative interpretation, affording some possible leeway for States parties willing to temper prohibition with some ethical concern for the welfare and human rights of drug users in their legal and policy approaches to drug use.

As this brief overview indicates, current international law on drug control is not entirely hostile toward harm reduction. It is, however, hardly satisfactory that any such measures rely upon exceptions, caveats, or particular interpretations of treaties whose overriding purpose is prohibition. In many instances, it is a matter of securing the political will to adopt such interpretations and act upon them in the face of great pressure to maintain a strict prohibitionist facade. We return to this in the last section of this chapter.

HARM REDUCTION AND HUMAN RIGHTS: CONCEPTUAL AND NORMATIVE LINKS

While the exact parameters of harm reduction may still be the subject of some debate, there is general agreement as to its core content. For present purposes, consider the following working definition, with its noteworthy explicit reference to human rights:

> Harm reduction is a pragmatic and humanistic approach to diminishing the individual and social harms associated with drug use, especially the risk of HIV infection. It seeks to lessen the problems associated with drug use through methodologies that safeguard the dignity, humanity and human rights of people who use drugs.[62]

As suggested by this definition, there is an obvious affinity between harm reduction and human rights. Yet there has been relatively little explicit discussion of the conceptual and normative links between harm reduction and the international law of human rights in academic journals devoted to either of the two fields.[63] This has begun to change, particularly as the harm reduction movement—or at least that part of it that articulates the need to change punitive drug laws—has intensified its efforts to reform global drug control policy and grapples with questions of international law.

How are human rights relevant to harm reduction? We suggest that there are a number of inter-connected ways in which harm reduction and human rights are, or can be, linked.

First, the harm reduction movement inherently entails a commitment to the human rights of drug users. Most obviously, as a movement aimed at reducing harms that are sometimes associated with the use of drugs, harm reduction's raison d'être is the fulfillment of the human right to enjoy the highest attainable standard of physical and mental health. In addition, harm reductionists are necessarily concerned not only with the direct adverse health consequences of drug use and laws related to drugs but also with the range of other harms experienced by drug users—including the denial or violation of other human rights. To put it at its most basic, "drug users are people too."[64] Although trite, the proposition is regularly disregarded in the ongoing dehumanization of drug users and the tragic daily violation of users' human rights by both states and non-state actors—from torture to the blatant denial of health care, from harsh sentences of imprisonment to extrajudicial execution. Sadly, therefore, it is a point that must still be made.

Second, from a purely pragmatic perspective, securing human rights is necessary for the success of harm reduction. In an earlier article, Alex Wodak explored how prohibitionist drug policy leads to infringements of various human rights, thereby contributing to the harms suffered by drug users:

> Reliance on criminal sanctions as the major response to illicit drug use inevitably results in the denial of human rights of the IDU population as drug use remains defined as a law enforcement rather than a health problem. Poor health outcomes in this population then follow, because health promotion and health care services are more difficult to provide to a now stigmatized and underground population. Protection of human rights is an essential precondition to improving the health of individual drug users and improving the public health of the communities where they live.[65]

Judit Fridli, chair of the Hungarian Civil Liberties Union, points out, similarly, that human rights are necessary preconditions to health improvements for drug users and their communities, suggesting that the political viability of harm reduction practice itself is human rights-dependent:

... Perhaps most importantly, [harm reduction] is about human rights.... Protection of human rights makes harm reduction—and thus life itself—possible. ... [Some harm reduction methods] will not be started or survive unless they are protected by a public culture of rights and liberties.[66]

Third, as suggested above, human rights norms point toward harm reduction, rather than prohibition, in policy responses to drug use. At the very least, states are required to remove obstacles to the implementation of such measures by others.[67] We expand on the human rights-based case for harm reduction—and hence for reform of the international drug control regime—in the next section.

In light of these connections, we suggest that harm reduction advocates can and should deploy human rights norms in making the case for international drug policy reform. But in order to make a human rights case for harm reduction, we first need to clarify what we mean by human rights and what role its principles, norms, and instruments can and should play in a harm reduction analysis.

Andrew Hathaway argues the harm reduction movement has adopted too strictly empirical a focus and has claimed to occupy the "middle-ground" on drug issues, articulating its principles as emerging from a "scientific public health model" but "unduly overlooking the deeper morality of the movement with its basis in concern for human rights."[68] In his call for a "morally invested drug reform strategy" (clearly characterizing drug reform as an essential aspect of harm reduction), he criticizes this strategic shortcoming:

As a multidisciplinary movement firmly grounded in the public health perspective ... harm reduction is wellsuited for revealing the logical flaws in prohibition by way of empirical analysis. The moral warrants behind the movement to which harm reduction might profitably lay claim, however, are the very principles that have yet to be firmly established and articulated. The greatest challenge for harm reduction, once again, lies in the promotion of its underlying ideals.... Preferring to keep such ideological, liberty-based values [as respect for free will and human adaptive potential] out of the analysis, harm reduction opts for a morally neutral form of inquiry wherein autonomy and rights have no apparent value in themselves.[69]

Sam Friedman and others have pointed out that the harm reduction movement was formed during a period marked by a "political economy of scapegoating" that targeted drug users, among others, as responsible for social ills; they suggest that "this climate shaped and limited the perspectives, strategies, and tactics of harm reductionists almost everywhere."[70] In a climate hostile to the notion that drug users are entitled to human rights, a pragmatic response to the immediate harms caused by prohibitionist excesses is to cast the problem in the language and data of public health. However, Hathaway is critical of "the rhetorical limitations of an empirical perspective lacking the moral capacity to challenge prohibition on principle, in terms of human rights of users."[71] Without a more fundamental challenge to the barriers blocking humane, rational drug policy, such as the dehumanization of drug users, short-term advances that are urgently needed to prevent and alleviate current suffering will not be sustainable over the long term. "Despite making inroads on pragmatic grounds alone, forsaking deeper principles is short-sighted."[72]

Hathaway's critique is grounded chiefly in a traditional civil libertarian emphasis on the civil and political rights that governments should refrain from infringing upon, such as liberty, equality, privacy, and freedom from cruel and unusual treatment or punishment—all rights recognized in the International Covenant on Civil and Political Rights.[73] While valid as far as it goes, this is but one dimension of a human rights-based understanding of harm reduction.

Equally important is a recognition of the economic and social rights recognized in international law. For example, Nadine Ezard has offered a detailed typology, mapping measures to reduce harm, the risk of harm, and the underlying vulnerabilities against the human rights in which such measures can be grounded.[74] She argues that our understanding of harm reduction must include not just the reduction of harm and of "risk," but also the reduction of "vulnerability" and the "complex of underlying factors" at the individual, community, and societal level that "constrain choices and limit agency" and thereby "predispose" one to the risk of drug-related harm.[75] The World Health Organization (WHO) makes the same basic point as Ezard but without explicit reference to human rights: "Successful harm reduction is based on a policy, legislative and social environment that minimizes the vulnerability of injecting drug users."[76] In public health parlance, these are among the "determinants of health." In legal terms, they are also questions of human rights as recognized in the Universal Declaration of Human Rights and the International Covenant on Economic, Social and Cultural Rights (ICESCR)—such as the rights to security of person, the right to just remuneration and to social security, the right to an adequate standard of living, and the right to enjoy the highest attainable standard of health. Ezard's call for linking harm reduction with human rights focuses more on the need for positive action by states to address economic and social rights as part of the response to drug use in order to reduce vulnerability to, and risk of, harm.

THE HUMAN RIGHTS CASE FOR HARM REDUCTION . . . AND FOR GLOBAL DRUG POLICY REFORM

What is the human rights case for harm reduction? And what are the implications of such a rights-based approach for drug policy, whether international or national? The discharge of states' human rights obligations under international law carries at least two obligations. First, states have a legal duty to implement harm reduction measures that are known to protect and promote health, or that can reasonably be expected to have such benefits.

Second, states must reform the current aspects of prohibitionist drug policy, globally and domestically, which either impede harm reduction measures or cause or contribute to the harms suffered by drug users. The application of international human rights law not only points to the duty of states to address the social exclusion and economic inequities that contribute to harmful drug use, but it also calls into question the prohibitionist legal regimes that cause or exacerbate the harms associated with drug use. Most importantly, if laws and policies aimed at controlling illicit drugs have adverse effects on the health of people who use those drugs, their right to health is jeopardized, and those laws and policies must be compared against the state's international legal obligations relating to health—including the law of human rights. Because the harms associated with drug use are inseparable from the environment in which drug use occurs,

> . . . policies that are intended to reduce drug related harms are most effective in supportive environments. This has resulted in increased attention being paid to public health and international human rights law in the attempt to create such an environment. In this context, it is widely agreed that human rights law should apply to drug policies as to all other public policies.[77]

Consider, then, the application of one specific human right. States that are parties to the ICESCR "recognize the right of everyone to the enjoyment of the highest attainable standard of physical and mental health."[78] Furthermore, states legally commit to taking steps to realize this right over time, including "those necessary for ... the prevention, treatment and control of epidemic ... diseases; [and] the creation of conditions which would assure to all medical service and medical attention in the event of sickness."[79] The UN committee tasked with monitoring state compliance with the ICESCR has clarified that states' obligations are threefold—namely, to respect, protect, and fulfill this right.[80]

This means that, absent sufficient justification, states may not adopt policies limiting individuals' ability to safe-guard their health, such as having access to needle exchanges or being able to have access to clean needles in prison. Similarly, states must take positive steps to protect drug users against discrimination by health care providers and to address users' health needs through facilities and programs.

States are also in breach of their obligation to respect the right to health through any actions, policies, or laws that "are likely to result in ... unnecessary morbidity and preventable mortality."[81] As described above, there is mounting evidence that enforcing drug prohibitions contributes to the spread of HIV/AIDS, let alone multiple other harms, including violations of various human rights. At what point will a body with sufficient standing draw the conclusion that such enforcement results in unnecessary disease and avoidable death, thereby amounting to an on-going and massive violation of the human right to health by any state that is party to the ICESCR?

This is but one cursory example of how states' human rights obligations should inform their actions in relation to drug control. It should be remembered that all member states of the UN have pledged to take action to achieve "solutions of international health problems" and "universal respect for, and observance of, human rights."[82] This is a binding obligation under the UN Charter. Health and human rights are among the apex objectives of the UN. The control of certain narcotic and psychotropic substances, except to the extent that it advances those objectives, is not. Thus, if the international law of human rights mandates a different approach than the prohibitions set out in the UN drug control treaties, how can the latter legal regime be reformed so as to be consonant with states' obligations under the former? We turn to some proposed strategies in the final section.

HUMAN RIGHTS AS NORMATIVE COUNTERWEIGHT

In considering those strategies, we see the chief function of human rights law as presenting a "normative counterweight" to those harmful aspects of the international legal regime of drug control. We draw here a parallel with recent instances of HIV/AIDS activism in which the law and language of human rights have played just such a role in resolving the conflict between the human rights and public health imperative of access to affordable medicines and the limitations imposed de jure or de facto by the World Trade Organization's (WTO) Agreement on Trade-Related Aspects of Intellectual Property Rights (TRIPS), which prescribes certain standards for all WTO members in relation to pharmaceutical patents. As with the case of drug policy reform, conflict over the interpretation and implementation of international intellectual property treaties plays out in both domestic and international arenas and demonstrates how an international legal regime can impede or delay state action that would advance human rights, even within a state's own bailiwick and in the presence of supposed flexibilities and safeguards in that international regime.

Recall, for example, the case of The Pharmaceutical Manufacturers' Association of South Africa and Others v. The President of the Republic of South Africa and Others, in which 39 multinational pharmaceutical companies initiated legal action to block the South African government from implementing legislative measures aimed at lowering the cost of medicines.[83] Notwithstanding that the South African statute was in conformity with its obligations as a WTO member, the TRIPS Agreement was invoked by countries (chiefly the US) in pressuring South Africa not to implement the legislation, as well as in the pharmaceutical companies' court papers. While the companies ultimately abandoned their application in response to public outrage—and, presumably, in recognition of its weakness on the legal merits—hundreds of thousands of South Africans had fallen ill or died in the interim because they lacked access to needed medicines.

On the international stage, consider the challenge at the WTO from developing countries and health activists that ultimately led to the adoption in November 2001 of the Doha Declaration on the TRIPS Agreement and Public Health (acknowledging the right of WTO members to give health primacy over exclusive patent rights) and the subsequent Decision of the WTO General Council on August 30, 2003 (permitting compulsory licensing of pharmaceutical products for export in significant quantities to countries in need of lower-cost generic medicines).[84] Even though a policy measure, such as compulsory licensing, is plainly available as a matter of WTO law, both resource-poor and some resource-rich countries have been reluctant to use it to increase access to lower-priced medicines, partly for fear of negative repercussions from powerful countries such as the US.[85] This reluctance, and the consequent need for an instrument such as the Doha Declaration, illustrate the chilling effect on human rights of an international legal regime whose primary paradigm is the enforcement of intellectual property claims and which powerful states have interpreted in a particularly restrictive manner. The parallel to the UN drug control treaties (or at least their interpretation and the politics of their implementation) should be evident.

The example of treatment activism also bears witness to the importance of deploying human rights norms, both as a matter of principle and as a matter of strategy. This tactic was particularly evident in the domestic context of South Africa. The Treatment Action Campaign (TAC), the grassroots activist organization leading the struggle for access to care for South Africans living with HIV/AIDS, effectively deployed the language and law of human rights in resisting the pharmaceutical companies' legal action, while simultaneously pressuring the government to develop and implement a national HIV/AIDS treatment plan. Supported by a global advocacy effort, TAC undertook a strategy of popular protest that invoked human rights in tandem with formal intervention, as amicus curiae, to advance legal arguments based on both South African and international human rights law. As Mark Heywood has explained, in so doing TAC consciously sought to "turn a dry legal contest into a matter about human lives," not only to place the impugned legislation in its proper context but also to influence public opinion.[86] Through its invocation of human rights, TAC altered both the public discourse and the issues at play in the court action, effectively counter-balancing a lopsided focus solely on intellectual property law.

Similarly, on the international stage, it was necessary to generate a political environment supportive of countries wishing to use the "flexibilities" in the WTO's TRIPS Agreement to implement measures such as compulsory licensing to facilitate access to more affordable medicines. Consequently, developing countries and health advocates created countervailing normative forces in other arenas of international law and diplomacy. In doing so, they succeeded in re-shaping international policy. For example, months before the 2001 WTO Ministerial Conference that adopted the Doha Declaration, Brazil succeeded in obtaining a resolution at the UN Commission on Human Rights, declaring that "access to medication is one fundamental element for achieving progressively the full realization of the right of everyone to the enjoyment of the highest attainable standard of physical and mental health."[87] The resolution specifically grappled with the conflict between the right to health and the patent rules of the WTO regime. Updated to reflect subsequent developments (such as the WTO Doha Declaration), the resolution has since been adopted at a number of Commission sessions (by consensus, including the US), thereby solidifying recognition in international law of the right to health and the specific aspect of access to medication.

The example of treatment activists challenging the international intellectual property regime is instructive for harm reduction advocates. Injecting human rights into the global debate over drug policy can bring to bear principles and norms that make visible the human suffering caused by a zealous insistence upon harmful prohibitionist approaches. As in the case of treatment activism, "rights talk" in the struggle for harm reduction asserts that concern for the welfare of those who are excluded and marginalized is not simply a matter of charitable humanitarianism. Rather, it establishes that drug users are rights-bearers, whose rights are disrespected through the deliberate application of policies known to produce avoidable suffering and death, and who have a moral and legal claim to the means of promoting and protecting their health. "Rights talk" also insists that states have an obligation, and not merely an option, to respect, protect and fulfill that right (and others) in developing and implementing legislation, policy, and other measures. The language and law of international human rights provide not only an underpinning for harm reduction's "moral warrants" but also a set of norms that states and others can invoke in making the case for more health-friendly global policies on drug control. This can complement the growing public health evidence demonstrating the damage of prohibition and the benefits of harm reduction. The pressure for reform of the UN drug control regime will grow over the coming years, and human rights analysis should, in our view, be part of revisiting the current treaties.

REGIME CHANGE: STRATEGIES FOR REFORMING GLOBAL DRUG POLICY[88]

We noted above that, at least in theory, States parties to the UN drug control conventions retain some flexibility to implement harm reduction measures and that challenges to strictly prohibitionist interpretations are growing. For example, under pressure, the INCB has accepted that both substitution therapy and needle exchange programs are "permissible" under international drug control treaties (although methadone remains classified on the schedule of the most tightly controlled drugs under the drug control treaties).[89] The Commission on Narcotic Drugs has "taken note" of this INCB position.[90] However, other important harm reduction measures remain contested. For example, in 2000, the INCB issued a statement decrying what it called "drug injection rooms"—which it equated with "shooting galleries" and "opium dens"—as "a step in the direction of drug legalization."[91] It ignores the fact that safer injection facilities serve "medical and scientific purposes," and has stated that any government that allows such sites "facilitates drug trafficking" and contravenes the UN conventions.[92] This criticism provides convenient cover for national governments opposed to such measures. Similarly, the widely accepted (albeit incorrect) view that the 1988 Convention requires States parties to criminalize even possession of illicit drugs for (non-medical) personal consumption—thereby rendering all drug users criminal offenders—further narrows the room for maneuver for states willing to treat drug use as primarily a health issue rather than a criminal one.

Furthermore, even if states have some interpretive leeway in complying with their obligations under the drug control treaties and can muster the political will domestically to forge ahead with harm reduction initiatives, the larger political environment limits the amount of "policy space" that they can open up. The structural inertia of the CND operating on consensus among member states, the internal contradictions within the UNODC, and the ideological opposition of the INCB hardly make for a supportive global framework. Finally, many powerful countries are committed to the prohibitionist agenda.[93] Consequently, as is often the case with international instruments, it is as much (or even more) a question of politics as it is law. As Robin Room puts it: "The impact of the system comes instead from the implementation of the treaties, and with the international politics that surrounds that."[94] He describes "an international environment where states have been reluctant to break openly with a governing orthodoxy describing drug control in terms of a war on drugs."[95]

Yet "cracks in the consensus" are emerging.[96] A number of countries are shifting away from, or at least tempering, criminalization as their dominant approach to illicit drugs. The UN General Assembly will next debate global drug policy in 2008, a decade after its Special Session on Drugs and the adoption of various declarations largely reaffirming the prohibitionist goal of eradicating "drug abuse." Therefore, the next few years call for strategies to reform the current regime. What might the options be?

Given the need for consensus, the chances of amending the existing conventions are slim at best. Advocates' limited time and resources are likely spent better elsewhere. Similarly, adopting a new convention on harm reduction would be a very long-term project facing the same challenges. Of course, such efforts would have the benefit of squarely engaging states in a discussion that can gradually shift political consciousness and call into question the sanctified status of prohibition. But millions of drug users across the globe are facing a current and ongoing health crisis; while longer-term strategies are important, they need to be complemented by more pragmatic, short-term steps.

In theory, some more progressive states might be convinced to denounce (that is, withdraw from) one or more of the conventions, but this is unlikely. Aside from domestic political considerations, any single state taking such a step "would have to be prepared to face not only US-UN condemnation but also the threat or application of some form of US sanctions" against what would be condemned as a "pariah narcostate."[97]

However, a more feasible and interim approach would be to promote a strategy of "collective withdrawal." A critical mass of like-minded states could form a coalition that would state, in some formal instrument introduced in relevant UN bodies, their interpretation of which harm reduction measures are permissible under the existing drug control conventions and, if necessary, identify those aspects of the treaties from which they are withdrawing.

Such a step by progressive states would be unlikely to happen without coordinated advocacy by civil society organizations. Support from UN bodies with relevant mandates would strengthen the position of such states, and therefore, harm reduction advocates need to engage with those bodies as well, focusing on those most likely to be sympathetic and those whose support would be most helpful.[98] For example, UNAIDS and WHO could bring to their governing boards, for endorsement, a policy that would encourage states to ensure the implementation of harm reduction measures. The committees that monitor the implementation of UN human rights treaties, the Office of the High Commissioner for Human Rights, and the special rapporteurs should incorporate concerns about the human rights impacts of the war on drugs and the human rights benefits of harm reduction measures into their work. Resolutions could be brought before the UN Commission on Human Rights and the World Health Assembly affirming the human rights of drug users and recognizing the right of sovereign states to implement harm reduction measures. Several of these UN agencies could jointly submit a report to the Commission on Narcotic Drugs, including strong support for harm reduction measures and for protecting and promoting the human rights of drug users, that could inform resolutions emanating from the Commission. Civil society advocates can intervene directly or indirectly in these various processes with evidence, arguments, and documentation that make the case for a more rational, human rights-friendly approach to drug policy. In addition, UNODC should be encouraged to manifest public support for harm reduction; and the UN Secretary General, who has stated his personal commitment to responding to the global AIDS crisis, should show leadership by speaking out publicly against violations of drug users' human rights.

CONCLUSION

The majority of the world's countries have ratified one or more of the UN drug control conventions that mandate drug prohibition and its enforcement as the dominant response to the use of certain drugs. Consequently, the international legal regime, backed by powerful states and some UN bodies, affects the possibilities for national-level reform across the globe. It is, therefore, of common concern to all those who can witness the human and economic devastation wreaked by the war on drugs. Harm reduction measures are an important component of the larger struggle to realize fully the human right to health of all people who use illicit drugs. A harm reduction approach to drugs must be pursued by pushing for more health-friendly interpretation and implementation of the existing drug control treaties and by pursuing complementary strategies for reforming them. The harm reduction and human rights movements enjoy a close kinship; further exploration of the conceptual links and the role that human rights advocates can play in the harm reduction movement would benefit each. Collaboration will increase the likelihood of effecting regime change at the global and domestic levels, and in turn, has the potential to greatly reduce the burden of HIV infection among injection drug users.

REFERENCES

1. International Harm Reduction Association. "What Is Harm Reduction?" http://www.ihra.net.
2. The term is still defined with some elasticity. Neil Hunt has noted that, although the term

came into use as early as 1987 and the principles of harm reduction can be traced back at least several decades earlier, there is still "no definitive definition" of the term, although a number of definitions have been proposed: N. Hunt, with contributions from M. Ashton, S. Lenton, L. Mitcheson, B. Nelles, and G. Stimson, "A Review of the Evidence-Base for Harm Reduction Approaches to Drug Use," Forward Thinking on Drugs (March 2003). For some such definitions, see the following, as referenced by Hunt: R. Newcombe, "The Reduction of Drug Related-Harm: A Conceptual Framework for Theory, Practice and Research," in P. O'Hare et al. (eds), The Reduction of Drug-Related Harm (London: Routledge, 1992); D. Riley et al., "Harm Reduction: Concept and Practice—A Policy Discussion Paper," Substance Use and Misuse 34/1v(1999): pp. 9–24; S. Lenton and E. Single, "The Definition of Harm Reduction," Drug and Alcohol Review 17 (1998): pp. 213–20; M. Hamilton, A. Kellehear, and G. Rumbold, "Addressing Drug Problems: The Case for Harm Minimisation," in G. Rumbold and M. Hamilton (eds), Drug Use in Australia: A Harm Minimisation Approach (Oxford: Oxford University Press, 1998). In an effort to synthesize some of the above definitions, the UK Harm Reduction Alliance has produced a statement on the meaning of harm reduction. http://www.ukhra.org/harm_reduction_definition.html.

3. A number of articles explicitly examining the relationship between international human rights law and the principles of the harm reduction movement have appeared in the International Journal of Drug Policy.

4. D. R. Bewley-Taylor and C. S. J. Fazey, "The Mechanics and Dynamics of the UN System for International Drug Control," Forward Thinking on Drugs (March 2003): p. 15. www.forward-thinking-on-drugs.org/review1-print.html.

5. C. Aceijas, G. V. Stimson, M. Hickman, and T. Rhodes, on behalf of the United Nations Reference Group on HIV/AIDS Prevention and Care among IDU in Developing and Transitional Countries. "Global Overview of Injecting Drug Use and HIV Infection among Injecting Drug Users," AIDS 18 (2004): pp. 2295–2303. For an earlier discussion, see: A. Ball, S. Rana, and K. Dehne, "HIV Prevention among Injecting Drug Users: Responses in Developing and Transitional Countries," Public Health Reports 133 (1998, Supp. 1): pp. 170–181.

6. UNAIDS, Drug Use and HIV/AIDS: UNAIDS Statement Presented at the [1998] United Nations General Assembly Special Session on Drugs (Geneva: 1999).

7. Aceijas et al. (see note 5).

8. UNAIDS, AIDS Epidemic Update: December 2003 (Geneva: 2003).

9. World Health Organization, Management of Substance Abuse: WHO Drug Injection Study (Geneva: 2003).

10. UNAIDS, AIDS Epidemic Update: December 2003 (Geneva: 2003). See also: T. Rhodes, A. Sarang, A. Bobrik, E. Bobkov, and L. Platt, "HIV Transmission and HIV Prevention Associated with Injecting Drug Use in the Russian Federation," International Journal of Drug Policy 15 (2004): pp. 1–16.

11. D. Celentano, "HIV Prevention among Drug Users: An International Perspective from Thailand," Journal of Urban Health 80/4 Supp. 3 (2003): pp. 7–14.

12. UNAIDS (see note 6).

13. S. A. Strathdee, D. M. Patrick, and S. L. Currie et al., "Needle Exchange Is Not Enough: Lessons from the Vancouver Injecting Drug Use Study," AIDS 11/18 (1997): pp. 59–65; D. Kitayaporn, C. Uneklabh, B. G. Weniger, et al., "HIV-1 Incidence Determined Retrospectively among Drug Users in Bangkok, Thailand," AIDS 8/10 (1994): pp. 1443–50.

14. A. Wodak, "Health, HIV Infection, Human Rights, and Injection Drug Use," Health and Human Rights 2/4 (1997): pp. 25–41; D. Vlahov et al., "Bacterial Infections and Skin Cleaning Prior to Injection among Intravenous Drug Users," Public Health Report 107/5 (1992): pp. 595–8; A. Palepu et al., "Hospital Utilization and Costs in a Cohort of Injection Drug Users," Canadian Medical Association Journal 165/4 (2001): pp. 415–20; P. A. Selwyn et al., "Clinical Manifestations and Predictors of Disease Progression in Drug Users with Human Immunodeficiency Virus Infection," New England Journal of Medicine 327/24 (1992): pp. 1697–703; R. R. Robles et al., "Risk Behaviors, HIV Seropositivity, and Tuberculosis Infection in Injecting Drug Users Who Operate Shooting Galleries in Puerto Rico" Journal of Acquired Immune Deficiency Syndromes and Human Retrovirology 17/5 (1998): pp. 477–83; M. W. Tyndall et al., "Impact of HIV Infection on Mortality in a Cohort of Injection Drug Users," Journal of Acquired Immune Deficiency Syndromes 28/4 (2001): pp. 351–7; European Monitoring Centre for Drugs and Drug Addiction, Annual Report on the State of the Drugs Problem in the European Union and Norway (Libson: EMCDDA, 2002). http://www.emcdda.eu.int.

15. K. Porter et al., "Determinants of Survival Following HIV-1 Seroconversion After the Introduction of HAART," The Lancet 362

(2003): pp. 1267–74; E. Wood, T. Kerr, M. Spittal et al., "An External Evaluation of a Peer-Run 'Unsanctioned' Syringe Exchange Program," Journal of Urban Health 80/3 (2003): pp. 455–64; S. J. Ferrando et al., "Psychiatric Morbidity, Illicit Drug Use and Adherence to Zidovudine (AZT) among Injection Drug Users with HIV Disease," American Journal of Drug and Alcohol Abuse 22/4 (1996): pp. 475–87; R. D. Muma et al., "Zidovudine Adherence among Individuals with HIV Infection," AIDS Care 7/4 (1995): pp. 439–47; N. Singh et al., "Determinants of Compliance with Antiretroviral Therapy in Patients with Human Immunodeficiency Virus: Prospective Assessment with Implications for Enhancing Compliance," AIDS Care 8/3 (1996): pp. 261–69; S. A. Strathdee et al., "Barriers to Use of Free Antiretroviral Therapy in Injection Drug Users," Journal of the American Medical Association 280 (1998): pp. 547–9; T. L. Wall et al., "Adherence to Zidovudine (AZT) among HIV-Infected Methadone Patients: A Pilot Study of Supervised Therapy and Dispensing Compared to Usual Care," Drug and Alcohol Dependence 37 (1995): p. 261.

16. M. N. Gourevith et al., "Successful Adherence to Observed Prophylaxis and Treatment of Tuberculosis among Drug Users in a Methadone Program," Journal of Addictive Diseases 15/1 (1996): pp. 93–104; E. Wood et al., "Expanding Access to HIV Antiretroviral Therapy among Marginalized Populations in the Developed World," AIDS 17 (2003): pp. 2419–27; A. Antela et al., "Influence of a Methadone Maintenance Programme on the Improved Outcome of a Cohort of Injecting Drug Users with Advanced HIV Disease" [letter], AIDS 11 (1997): pp. 1405–6; A. Moreno et al., "Long-Term Outcomes of Protease Inhibitor-Based Therapy in Antiretroviral Treatment-Naïve HIV-Infected Injection Drug Users on Methadone Maintenance Programmes," AIDS 15 (2001): pp. 1068–70.

17. S. F. Hurley et al., "Effectiveness of Needle-Exchange Programmes for Prevention of HIV Infection," The Lancet 349 (1997): pp. 1797–1800; D. C. Des Jarlais et al., "Maintaining Low HIV Seroprevalence in Populations of Injecting Drug Users," Journal of the American Medical Association 274 (1995): pp. 1226–31; G. Stimson, C. Des Jarlais, and A. Ball (eds), Drug Injecting and HIV Infection (London and New York: Routledge, 1998); N. Hunt (see note 2); S. A. Strathdee et al., "Can HIV Epidemics among Injection Drug Users Be Prevented?" AIDS 12/Supp. A (1998): pp. S71–9. See also: T. Rhodes, A. Sarang, A. Bobrik, E. Bobkov, and L. Platt, "HIV Transmission and HIV Prevention Associated with Injecting Drug Use in the Russian Federation," International Journal of Drug Policy 15 (2004): pp. 1–16 (reporting that evidence associates syringe distribution and exchange with reductions in risk behavior and concluding by noting the critical importance of policy interventions to maximize syringe distribution coverage among IDU populations).

18. Global HIV Prevention Working Group, Global HIV Prevention: Closing the Gap (Geneva: UNAIDS, 2003).

19. L. Maher and D. Dixon, "Policing and Public Health: Law Enforcement and Harm Minimization in a Street-Level Drug Market," British Journal of Criminology 39 (1999): pp. 488–512; C. Aitken et al., "The Impact of a Police Crackdown on a Street Drug Scene: Evidence from the Street," International Journal of Drug Policy 13 (2002): pp. 189–98; E. Wood et al., "Displacement of Canada's Largest Public Illicit Drug Market in Response to a Police Crackdown," Canadian Medical Association Journal 170 (2004): pp. 1551–56; D. Best et al., "Assessment of a Concentrated High-Profile Police Operation: No Discernible Impact on Drug Availability, Price or Purity," British Journal of Criminology 41 (2001): pp. 738–45.

20. Wood et al. (see note 19); D. Weatherburn and B. Lind, "The Impact of Law Enforcement Activity on a Heroin Market," Addiction 92 (1997): pp. 557–69.

21. D. Dixon and P. Coffin, "Zero Tolerance Policing of Illegal Drug Markets," Drug & Alcohol Review 18 (1999): pp. 477–86; L.W. Sherman and D.P. Rogan, "Deterrent Effects of Police Raids on Crack Houses: A Randomized Controlled Experiment," Justice Quarterly 12 (1995): pp. 755–81; D. Weisburd and L. Green, "Policing Drug Hotspots: The Jersey City Drug Market Analysis Experiment," Justice Quarterly 12 (1995): pp. 711–35; C. Aitken et al. (see note 19); Wood et al. (see note 19).

22. B. L. Benson, I. S. Leburn, and D. W. Rasmussen, "The Impact of Drug Enforcement on Crime: An Investigation of the Opportunity Cost of Police Resources," Journal of Drug Issues 31 (2001): pp. 989–1006.

23. S. R. Friedman, "The Political Economy of Scapegoating—and the Philosophy and Politics of Resistance," Drugs: Education, Prevention & Policy 5/1 (1998): pp. 15–32.

24. Maher and Dixon (See note 19); Aitken et al. (See note 19); R. S. Broadhead et al., "Safer Injection Facilities in North America: Their Place in Public Policy and Health Initiatives," Journal of Drug Issues 32 (2002): pp. 329–355.

25. Wood et al. (see note 19); S. Darke et al., "Geographical Injecting Locations among Injecting Drug Users in Sydney, Australia," Addiction 96/2 (2001): pp. 241–6.

26. F. I. Bastos and S. A. Strathdee, "Evaluating Effectiveness of Syringe Exchange Programmes: Current Issues and Future Prospects," Social Science & Medicine 51/12 (2000): pp. 1771–82; R. N. Blumenthal et al., "Collateral Damage in the War on Drugs: HIV Risk Behaviours among Injection Drug Users," International Journal of Drug Policy 10 (1999): pp. 25–38; T. Diaz et al., "Needle and Syringe Acquisition among Young Injection Drug Users in Harlem, New York City," National HIV Prevention Conference (1999): p. 654; J. P. Grund et al., "In Eastern Connecticut, IDUs Purchase Syringes from Pharmacies But Don't Carry Syringes," Journal of Acquired Immune Deficiency Syndromes and Human Retrovirology 10/1 (1995): pp. 104–5; T. Rhodes et al., "Situational Factors Influencing Drug Injecting, Risk Reduction and Syringe Exchange in Togliatti City, Russian Federation: A Qualitative Study of Micro Risk Environment," Social Science & Medicine 57/1 (2003): pp. 39–54; B. Weinstein et al., "Peer Education of Pharmacists and Supplying Pharmacies with IDU Packets to Increase Injection Drug Users' Access to Sterile Syringes in Connecticut," Journal of Acquired Immune Deficiency Syndromes & Human Retrovirology 18/Supp.1 (1998): pp. S146–7.

27. M. Struthers and J. Csete, Fanning the Flames: How Human Rights Abuses Are Fueling the AIDS Epidemic in Kazakhstan (New York: Human Rights Watch, 2003).

28. K. H. Seal et al., "Attitudes About Prescribing Take-Home Naloxone to Injection Drug Users for the Management of Heroin Overdose: A Survey of Street-Recruited Injectors in the San Francisco Bay Area," Journal of Urban Health 80 (2003): pp. 291–301; B. Sergeev et al., "Prevalence and Circumstances of Opiate Overdose Among Injection Drug Users in the Russian Federation," Journal of Urban Health 80 (2003): pp. 212–19.

29. For more detail regarding each of these interventions, see Hunt (note 2).

30. A. Wodak, "Can We Prevent HIV Transmission Among IDUs?" Annual Conference of Australasian Society for HIV Medicine 8 (1996): p. 463 (abstract no.17); A. Wodak, "Health, HIV Infection, Human Rights, and Injection Drug Use," Health and Human Rights 2/4 (1997): pp. 25–41.

31. L. B. Cottler et al., "Peer-Delivered Interventions Reduce HIV Risk Behaviours Among Out-of-Treatment Drug Abusers," Public Health Reports 113/Supp.1 (1998): pp. 31–41; R. S. Broadhead et al., "Harnessing Peer Networks As an Instrument for AIDS Prevention: Results from a Peer-Driven Intervention," Public Health Reports 113/Supp.1 (1998): pp. 42–57; C. A. Latkin, "Outreach in Natural Settings: The Use of Peer Leaders for HIV Prevention among Injecting Drug Users' Networks," Public Health Reports 113/Supp.1 (1998): pp. 151–9; R. S. Broadhead et al., "Increasing Drug Users' Adherence to HIV Treatment: Results of a Peer-Driven Intervention Feasibility Study," Social Science & Medicine 55/2 (2002): pp. 235–46; R. H. Needle et al., Evidence for Action: Effectiveness of Community-Based Outreach in Preventing HIV/AIDS among Injecting Drug Users (Geneva: World Health Organization, 2004).

32. J. P. Grund et al., "Reaching the Unreached: Targeting Hidden IDU Populations with Clean Needles Via Known User Groups," Journal of Psychoactive Drugs 24/1 (1992): pp. 41–7; E. Wood et al., "An External Evaluation of a Peer-Run 'Unsanctioned' Syringe Exchange Programme," Journal of Urban Health 80/3 (2003): pp. 455–64.

33. T. Kerr et al., Responding to an Emergency: Education, Advocacy and Community Care by a Peer-Driven Organization of Drug Users—A Case Study of the Vancouver Area Network of Drug Users (VANDU) (Ottawa: Health Canada, 2001). http://www.vandu.org/pdfs/casestudy.pdf.

34. D. C. Des Jarlais et al., "HIV Incidence Among Injecting Drug Users in New York City Syringe-Exchange Programmes," The Lancet 348 (1996): pp. 987–91; H. Hagan et al., "Reduced Risk of Hepatitis B and Hepatitis C among Injection Drug Users in the Tacoma Syringe Exchange Programme," American Journal of Public Health 85 (1995): pp. 1531–7; R. N. Bluthenthal et al., "The Effect of Syringe Exchange Use on High-Risk Injection Drug Users: A Cohort Study," AIDS 14/5 (2000): pp. 605–11; E. R. Monterroso et al., "Prevention of HIV Unfection in Street-Recruited Injection Drug Users," Journal of Acquired Immune Deficiency Syndromes 25/1 (2000): pp. 63–70.

35. D. G. Fisher et al., "Needle Exchange and Injection Drug Use Frequency: A Randomized Clinical Trial," Journal of Acquired Immune Deficiency Syndromes 33/2 (2003): pp. 199–205; J. Normand et al., Preventing HIV Transmission: The Role of Sterile Needles and Bleach (Washington, DC: National Academy Press, 1995).

36. D. C. Des Jarlais et al., "Maintaining Low HIV Seroprevalence in Populations of Injecting Drug Users," Journal of the American Medical Association 274 (1995): pp. 1226–31.

37. S. F. Hurley et al., "Effectiveness of Needle-Exchange Programmes for Prevention of HIV Infection," The Lancet 349 (1997): pp. 1797–1800.

38. M. MacDonald et al., "Effectiveness of Needle and Syringe Programmes for Preventing HIV Transmission," International Journal of Drug Policy 14/5/6 (2003): pp. 353–357.

39. R. P. Mattick et al., "Methadone Maintenance Therapy Versus No Opioid Replacement Therapy for Opioid Dependence," The Cochrane Database of Systematic Reviews 2 (2003) (Art. No.: CD002209. 10.1002/14651858.CD002209). R. P. Mattick et al., "Buprenorphine Maintenance Versus Placebo or Methadone Maintenance for Opioid Dependence," Cochrane Review 1 (2003); J. Ball and A. Ross, The Effectiveness of Methadone Maintenance Treatment: Patients, Programs, Services and Outcomes (New York: Springer-Verlag, 1991); R. L. Hubbard et al., Treatment Outcome Prospective Study (TOPS): Client Characteristics Before, During, and After Treatment (Washington, DC: NIDA, 1984); E. C. Strain et al., "Moderatevs High-Dose Methadone in the Treatment of Opioid Dependence: A Randomized Trial," Journal of the American Medical Association 281/11 (1999): pp. 1000–5; K. L. Sees et al., "Methadone Maintenance vs 180-Day Psychosocially Enriched Detoxification for Treatment of Opioid Dependence: A Randomized Controlled Trial," Journal of the American Medical Association 283/10 (2000): pp. 1303–10; S. Vanichseni et al., "A Controlled Trial of Methadone Maintenance in a Population of Intravenous Drug Users in Bangkok: Implications for Prevention of HIV," International Journal of Addiction 25/12 (1991): pp. 1313–20; W. S. Condelli and G. H. Dunteman. "Exposure to Methadone Programs and Heroin Use," American Journal of Drug and Alcohol Abuse 19/1 (1993): pp. 65–78; V. P. Dole et al., "Methadone Maintenance of Randomly Selected Criminal Addicts," New England Journal of Medicine 280 (1969): pp. 1372–5; F. Gearing and M. Schweitze, "An Epidemiologic Evaluation of Long-Term Methadone Maintenance Treatment for Heroin Addiction," American Journal of Epidemiology 100/2 (1974): pp. 101–12; R. G. Newman and W. B. Whitehill, "Double-Blind Comparison of Methadone and Placebo Maintenance Treatments of Narcotic Addicts in Hong Kong," The Lancet 2 (1979): pp. 485–8; R. G. Newman and N. Peyser, "Methadone Treatment: Experiment and Experience," Journal of Psychoactive Drugs 23/20 (1991): pp. 115–21; M. Stenbacka et al., "The Impact of Methadone on

Consumption of Inpatient Care and Mortality, with Special Reference to HIV Status," Substance Use & Misuse 33/14 (1998): pp. 2819–34; I. Sheerin et al., "Reduction in Crime by Drug Users on a Methadone Maintenance Therapy Programme in New Zealand," New Zealand Medical Journal 117/1990 (2004): p. U795.

40. WHO/UNODC/UNAIDS, Position Paper: Substitution Maintenance Therapy in the Management of Opioid Dependence and HIV/AIDS Prevention (Geneva and Vienna: 2004); WHO/UNODC/UNAIDS, Policy Brief: Reduction of HIV Transmission through Drug-Dependence Treatment (Geneva and Vienna: 2004); R. G. Newman et al., "DoubleBlind Comparison of Methadone and Placebo Maintenance Treatments of Narcotic Addicts in Hong Kong," The Lancet 2 (1979): pp. 485–8; D. Novick et al., "Absence of Antibody to Human Immunodeficiency Virus in Long-Term Socially Rehabilitated Methadone Maintenance Patients," Archives of Internal Medicine 150 (1990): pp. 97–9; D. M. Hartel and E. E. Schoenbaum, "Methadone Treatment Protects Against HIV Infection: Two Decades of Experience in the Bronx, New York City," Public Health Reports 113/Supp.1 (1998): pp. 107–15; D. S. Metzger et al., "Human Immunodeficiency Virus Seroconversion Among Intravenous Drug Users Inand Out-of-Treatment: An 18-Month Prospective Follow-Up," Journal of Acquired Immune Deficiency Syndromes 6/9 (1993): pp. 1049–56; R. Zangerle et al., "Trends in HIV Infection Among Intravenous Drug Users in Innsbruck, Austria," Journal of Acquired Immune Deficiency Syndromes 5/9 (1992): pp. 865–71; K. Wong et al., "Adherence to Methadone is Associated with a Lower Level of HIV-Related Risk Behaviours in Drug Users," Journal of Substance Abuse Treatment 24/3 (2003): pp. 233–239.

41. Hunt et al. (see note 1); E. Wood et al., "Rationale for Evaluating North America's First Medically Supervised Safer Injecting Facility," Lancet Infectious Diseases 4 (2004): pp. 301–6; R. S. Broadhead et al., "Safer Injection Facilities in North America: Their Place in Public Policy and Health Initiatives," Journal of Drug Issues 32/1 (2002): pp. 329–55.

42. European Monitoring Centre for Drugs and Drug Addiction, European Report on Drug Consumption Rooms (Lisbon: 2004); K. Dolan et al., "Drug Consumption Facilities in Europe and the Establishment of Supervised Injecting Centres in Australia," Drug and Alcohol Review 19 (2000): pp. 337–46; C. Ronco et al., "Evaluation for

Alley-Rooms I, II and III in Basel," Social and Preventive Medicine 41 (1996): pp. S58–68; W. de Jong and U. Wever, "The Professional Acceptance of Drug Use: A Closer Look at Drug Consumption Rooms in the Netherlands, Germany and Switzerland," International Journal of Drug Policy 10 (1999): pp. 99–108; R. P. Mattick et al., Six-Month Process Report on the Medically Supervised Injecting Centre (Sydney: National Drug and Alcohol Research Centre, 2001); J. Fitzgerald et al., "Health Outcomes and QuasiSupervised Settings for Street Injecting Drug Use," International Journal of Drug Policy 15 (2004): pp. 247–57.

43. 976 U.N.T.S. 105 (as amended by the 1972 Protocol Amending the Single Convention on Narcotic Drugs).

44. 1019 U.N.T.S. 14956.

45. UN Doc. E/CONF. 82/15 (1988), reprinted in 28 I.L.M. 493 (1989).

46. 1961 Convention (see note 43), Articles 4, 33, 35, and 36; 1971 Convention (see note 44), Articles 21 and 22; 1988 Convention (see note 45), Article 3.

47. See note 45.

48. United Nations Office on Drugs and Crime, The Commission on Narcotic Drugs: Its Mandate and Functions (Economic and Social Council in its resolution 9 (I) of February16, 1946). For a more detailed discussion, see Bewley-Taylor and Fazey (note 4).

49. See, for example, WHO/UNODC/UNAIDS, Position Paper: Substitution Maintenance ... (note 40).

50. D. R. Bewley-Taylor, "Emerging Policy Contradictions Between the UNODC "Universe" and the Core Values and Mission of the UN," Paper for the 2003 Lisbon International Symposium on Global Drug Policy (October 23–26, 2003). www.senliscouncil.net/documents/Taylor_paper.

51. See "Role of INCB" on INCB website at www.incb.org

52. INCB, Report of the International Narcotics Control Board for 2000, E/INCB/2000/1, http://www.incb.org.

53. N. Dorn and A. Jamieson, Room for Manoeuvre: Overview of Comparative Legal Research Into National Drug Laws of France, Germany, Italy, Spain, the Netherlands and Sweden and Their Relation to Three International Drugs Conventions (London: DrugScope, 2000).

54. "Flexibility of Treaty Provisions As Regards Harm Reduction Approaches," E/INCB/2002/W.13/SS.5, prepared by the Legal Affairs Section of the UN International Drug Control Programme (UNDPC—now the UNODC), September 30, 2002. http://www.tni.org/drugsreform-docs/un300902.pdf.

55. Ibid.

56. 1961 Single Convention, Article 4(c); 1971 Convention, Articles 5 and 7.

57. 1961 Single Convention, Article 36; 1971 Convention, Article 22; 1988 Convention, Article 4.

58. United Nations, Commentary on the Single Convention on Narcotic Drugs 1961 (New York: 1973) (see commentary on Article 4, paras 15ff).

59. 1961 Single Convention, Article 31; 1971 Convention, Article 20. Note that the 1988 Convention does not say that States parties "shall" take such measures, but rather that they "may." (Article 4).

60. Bewley-Taylor and Fazey (see note 4).

61. 1988 Convention, Article 3(2).

62. What Is Harm Reduction? (New York: International Harm Reduction Development Program, 2004).

63. We note that concern for human rights makes repeated appearances in much of the "grey" literature, and certainly in discussions within the harm reduction movement, including some analysis that explicitly references sources of international human rights law.

64. E. A. Nadelmann, "Progressive Legalizers, Progressive Prohibitionists and the Reduction of Drug-Related Harm," in N. Heather, A. Wodak, and E. Nadelmann (eds), Psychoactive Drugs and Harm Reduction: From Faith to Science (London: Whurr Publishers, 1993), pp. 34–45.

65. A. Wodak, "Health, HIV Infection, Human Rights, and Injecting Drug Use, Health and Human Rights 2/4 (1998): pp. 24–41, 38–9.

66. J. Fridli, "Harm Reduction Is Human Rights," Harm Reduction News 4/1 (2003): p. 3.

67. For a more detailed discussion of this point, specifically as it relates to removing barriers to experimenting with one particular harm reduction measure, see I. Malkin, R. Elliott, and R. McRae, "Supervised Injection Facilities and International Law," Journal of Drug Issues 33/3 (2003): pp. 538–78.

68. A. D. Hathaway, "Shortcomings of Harm Reduction: Toward a Morally Invested Drug Reform Strategy," International Journal of Drug Policy 12 (2001): pp. 125–37.

69. Ibid.: pp. 135–36.

70. S. R. Friedman et al., "Harm Reduction—A Historical View from the Left," International Journal of Drug Policy 12 (2001): pp. 3–14.

71. Hathaway (see note 67): p. 133.

72. Ibid.: p. 126.

73. In this same libertarian vein, one author has proposed a new article in the UDHR affirming the right to use psychotropic substances of

one's own choice. Van Ree invokes standard liberal utilitarian principles, arguing that only limited restrictions on the individual freedom to use drugs may be justified, in the interests of preventing harms to others. Taken to its logical conclusion, he suggests that recognition of such a right would inevitably require an end to the war on drugs: E. van Ree, "Drugs As a Human Right," International Journal of Drug Policy 10 (1999): pp. 89–98. Hathaway does not take his analysis this far, although such a position certainly seems consistent with, and perhaps even implicit, in his call for respecting personal autonomy.

74. N. Ezard, "Public Health, Human Rights and the Harm Reduction Paradigm: From Risk Reduction to Vulnerability Reduction," International Journal of Drug Policy 12 (2001): pp. 207–219.

75. The framework of harm, risk, and vulnerability applied by Ezard builds on models developed in: R. Newcombe, "The Reduction of Drug Related Harm: A Conceptual Framework for Theory, Practice and Research." In: P. O'Hare et al. (eds). The Reduction of Drug Related Harm (London: Routledge, 1992); J. Mann, D. Tarantola, and T. Netter (eds) (Cambridge: Harvard University Press, 1992); J. Mann and D. Tarantola, AIDS in the World II (New York: Oxford University Press, 1996); D. Tarantola and S. Gruskin, "Children Confronting HIV/AIDS: Charting the Confluence of Health and Rights," Health and Human Rights 2/4 (1998): pp. 163–181.

76. Health Organization, "Harm Reduction Approaches to Injecting Drug Use" http://www.who.int/hiv/topics/harm/reduction/en/.

77. D. Riley, Drugs and Drug Policy in Canada: A Brief Review and Commentary (November 1998). http://www.cfdp.ca/sen1841.htm.

78. ICESCR, Article 12.

79. Ibid.

80. UN Committee on Economic, Social and Cultural Rights, General Comment No. 14: The Right to the Highest Attainable Standard of Heath, UN Doc E/C.12/2000/4 (2000).

81. Ibid.: para. 50.

82. Charter of the United Nations, Articles 55 and 56.

83. Materials from The Pharmaceutical Manufacturers' Association v. The President of the Republic of South Africa, Case No. 4183/98, High Court of South Africa (Transvaal Provincial Division) are available at http://www.tac.org.za (under "Medicines Act court case").

84. Declaration on the TRIPS Agreement and Public Health, World Trade Organization Ministerial Conference, Fourth Session, Doha, November 9–14 2001, WT/MIN(01)/DEC/2; WTO General Council. Decision on the Implementation of Paragraph 6 of the Doha Declaration on the TRIPS Agreement and Public Health, IP/C/W/405 (August 30, 2003). Both available at http://www.wto.org.

85. R. Weissman and A. Long, "Strange TRIPS: The Pharmaceutical Industry Drive to Harmonize Global Intellectual Property Rules, and the Remaining WTO Legal Alternatives Available to Third World Countries," University of Pennsylvania Journal of International Economic Law 17 (1996): p. 1069; E. 't Hoen, "TRIPS, Pharmaceutical Patents, and Access to Essential Medicines: A Long Way from Seattle to Doha" Chicago Journal of International Law 3 (2002): p. 27; F. Abbott, "The WTO Medicines Decision: World Pharmaceutical Trade and the Protection of Public Health," American Journal of International Law 99 (2005): p. 317.

86. M. Heywood, Debunking 'Conglomo-talk': A Case Study of the Amicus Curiae As an Instrument for Advocacy, Investigation and Mobilisation (Presented at Health, Law and Human Rights: Exploring the Connections—An International Cross-Disciplinary Conference Honoring Jonathan M. Mann: Philadelphia, PA, September 29-October 1, 2001): p. 12.

87. UN Commission on Human Rights Res. 2001/33 (April 23, 2001). Available via www.unhchr.ch. The resolution was adopted by a vote of 52 in favor with one abstention (United States).

88. Bewley-Taylor and Fazey (see note 4).

89. INCB, Report of the International Narcotics Control Board for 2003, E/INCB/2003/1, paragraphs 221–222. http://www.incb.org.

90. Res. 47/2 (2004), UN Doc. E/CN.7/2004/13, at 22.

91. INCB, "Drug Injection Rooms—Not in Line with International Conventions," (February 23, 2000). http://www.incb.org.

92. INCB (see note 88): paras. 223–224.

93. M. Jelsma, "Drugs in the UN System: The Unwritten History of the 1988 United Nations General Assembly Special Session on Drugs," International Journal of Drug Policy 14 (2003): pp. 188–195; H. G. Levine, "Global Drug Prohibition: Its Uses and Crises," International Journal of Drug Policy 14 (2003): pp. 145–153; D. Wolfe and K. MalinowskaSempruch, Illicit Drug Policies and the Global HIV Epidemic: Effects of UN and National Government Approaches (Open Society Institute: New York, 2004).

94. R. Room, Impact and Implications of the International Drug Control Treaties on IDU and HIV/AIDS Prevention and Policy (Paper prepared for 2nd International Policy Dialogue on HIV/AIDS, Warsaw, Poland, November 12–14, 2003).

95. Ibid.

96. M. Jelsma and P. Metaal, "Cracks in the Vienna Consensus: The UN Drug Control Debate," in Drug War: A WOLA Briefing Series (Washington, DC: Washington Office on Latin America, 2004).

97. D. R. Bewley-Taylor, "Challenging the UN Drug Control Conventions: Problems and Possibilities," International Journal of Drug Policy 14 (2003): pp. 171, 176–7.

98. For more discussion of such a proposal, see D. Spivack, Conclusions from Workshop III: International Cooperation on Drug Policy (Presented at the Lisbon International Symposium on Drug Policy, October 23–26, 2003). http://www.senliscouncil.net/documents/ Spivack_paper.

QUESTIONS

1. What do we mean by "harm reduction" as a public health strategy? Compare the use of harm reduction strategies applied to tobacco smoking to dealing with cocaine or marijuana. What are the political, policy and policing issues involved with each of these substances? Define the commonalities and differences.

2. What are the major arguments that have been used to obstruct clean needle exchange programs? Compare the human rights implications of public health measures that deal with physical things (like airbags, road design, labeling) rather than with people by trying to modify their behavior (such as through criminal penalties or education campaigns).

3. Has the "war on drugs" been lost? From both a public health and a human rights perspective, should governments treat currently illegal drugs more like alcohol and tobacco, and regulate them rather than attempt to outlaw them?

FURTHER READING

1. Marlatt, G. Alan, Larimer, Mary E., & Wilkiewtz, Katie, eds, *Harm Reduction*, 2nd ed. New York: Guilford Press, 2012.

2. Kozlowski, L. T., Harm Reduction, Public Health, and Human Rights: Smokers have a Right to Be Informed of Significant Harm Reduction Options. *Nicotine & Tobacco Research*, 2002;S55-S60.

3. Glantz, L. H., Mariner, W. K., & Annas, G. J., Risky Business: Setting Public Health Policy for HIV-infected Health Care Professionals. *Milbank Quarterly*, 1992; 70: 43–79.

CHAPTER 38

Tuberculosis Control and Directly Observed Therapy from the Public Health/Human Rights Perspective

Anna-Karin Hurtig, John D. H. Porter and Jessica A. Ogden

INTRODUCTION

The enjoyment of the highest attainable standard of health is one of the fundamental rights of every human being.
—Preamble to the WHO
Constitution UN, 1948

THE 1980s AND 1990s have seen a resurgence of interest in tuberculosis. Increasing cases world-wide led to the World Health Organization (WHO) declaring a global emergency in April 1993.[1, 2] Despite the availability of 'tools' for controlling TB, programmes have been unable to sustain high cure rates.[3] As a consequence of this, and the increasing problems of drug resistance, the international community, through the WHO, has developed and launched the directly observed therapy short course (DOTS) strategy.[4, 5] This strategy is described as: government commitment to a national TB programme; case detection through 'passive' case finding (sputum smear microscopy for pulmonary tuberculosis suspects presenting at a health facility); short course chemotherapy for all smearpositive pulmonary TB cases (under direct observation for, at least, the initial phase of treatment [DOT]); regular, uninterrupted supply of all essential anti-TB drugs; and a monitoring system for programme supervision and evaluation.[4–6]

The DOTS strategy has achieved excellent results in New York and other parts of the US[7–10] and in China.[11] However, from other parts of the world voices have been raised asking if DOTS is the most effective way to control tuberculosis,[12, 13] if DOTS can and should be perceived as a panacea,[14] and if the DOTS strategy is ethical.[15, 16]

The control of infectious diseases like tuberculosis lies within the broad framework of public health. A currently accepted definition of public health is 'providing the conditions in which people can be healthy'.[17] Although public health contains within it many perspectives and disciplines, it is the biomedical perspective, the realm of medicine based on knowledge and practice from the natural sciences, which currently dominates thinking and approaches to health care and control of disease. Increasingly, it is being appreciated that biomedicine can benefit from working with other disciplines and perspectives. This interdisciplinarity encourages change and flexibility in approaches to health care and disease control.

A perspective which can complement and improve current approaches to the control of tuberculosis has been developed in recent years at the Harvard School of Public Health.[18, 19] This approach looks at control of disease through the human rights framework, using the Declaration of Human Rights as a basis for analysing public health programmes.[19] This framework enables a broader, more socially contextualised perspective on public health programmes. In this paper the current international strategy for tuberculosis control will be analysed using the health and human rights framework.

BACKGROUND

Infectious Disease Control

Current public health control strategies are predominantly framed by the biomedical model and its associated methodologies.[20] Of particular influence is public health's core discipline, epidemiology, which, in investigating infectious diseases, looks primarily at interactions between 'agent', 'host' and 'environment'. Interventions are designed to treat patients, ensure the protection of the population and prevent the occurrence of epidemics. The main strategies for control are to attack the source (e.g., treatment of cases/carriers of the isolation of cases); to interrupt transmission (e.g., environmental and personal hygiene, vector control); and to protect the susceptible population (e.g., immunisation, chemoprophylaxis).[21]

Tuberculosis Control

Current TB control strategies include the following components: case finding and treatment, chemoprophylaxis, vaccination with BCG and the improvement of socioeconomic conditions.[22] The biomedical focus for TB control concentrates on reducing the transmission of pulmonary tuberculosis by targeting the most contagious persons (sputum-positive cases), by finding cases of sputum-positive TB and treating them until they become sputum-negative and are eventually cured.

Compliance

Compliance is an important part of TB control and can be defined as the extent to which a person's health-related behaviour coincides with medical advice.[23] It can be a problem for many infectious disease control programmes. The direct observation of treatment (DOT) contained within the DOTS strategy is designed to enhance patient compliance. The strategy requires that the patient take his or her medications in the presence of a health care worker or other 'responsible' third party. In the biomedical/public health terms described above, DOT is part of the strategy for 'attacking the source' of infection and rendering the person non-infectious by treating him/her with the appropriate drugs for an appropriate period of time. DOT is fast becoming the standard approach for control of many infectious diseases, including sexually transmitted diseases, leprosy and tuberculosis.[16] Nevertheless, recent observers have noted that the intervention may be ethically problematic.[16] Embedded within it is the imbalance of power and capacity between the public health profession and the infected person. An uncritical application of DOT may also create problems by placing the onus for cure on the patient, while masking the responsibility of the health care professionals and health care structures to 'provide the conditions in which people can be healthy'.[16] Others have acknowledged the shared obligations of the patient in the need to comply with biomedical treatment, and of society in the need to provide the patient with the necessary treatment facilities.[24, 25]

Sumartojo has recently called for the development of an approach to improving compliance which engages with the responsibility of health care structures to provide an appropriate service and which '. . . recognise(s) the needs and dignity of patients'.[26] Similarly, Farmer has noted that '[t]hroughout the world, those least likely to comply are those least able to comply . . . these settings are crying out for measures to improve the quality of care, not the quality of patients'.[27]

Potential Problems with the DOTS Strategy

The increasing use of DOT in infectious disease programmes and the development of the DOTS strategy for TB control have coincided with a reappraisal (in some quarters) of the principles underlying public health interventions.[16, 28, 29] Also under renewed consideration is the need to understand the interaction and balance between the health needs of the individual and the health needs of the society. The kinds of questions being asked are: Is public health too paternalistic? Is there an imbalance of power and capacity between the public health profession and the infected person? If so, are these imbalances being reinforced by public health control measures? Are there alternative ways of approaching public health interventions that would redress, rather than reinforce, these kinds of imbalances and inequalities?[15, 20, 24]

HUMAN RIGHTS AND PUBLIC HEALTH: A FRAMEWORK FOR NEGOTIATION

Human Rights

In 1948 the Universal Declaration of Human Rights was accepted and adopted by the participating members of the United Nations.[30, 31] Today these principles continue to be relevant, and are being applied to considerations of health. It has recently been suggested, for example, that the extent to which human rights are realised may represent a better and more comprehensive index of well-being than traditional health status indicators.[18] From a public health perspective, while the availability of medical and other health care constitutes one of the essential conditions for health, the availability of these technologies and services does not in itself create 'health'. Indeed only a small fraction of health status variations between populations can be attributed to health care: clearly, then, adequate health care[32] is a necessary, though not sufficient, constituent of health.

The Health and Human Rights Analysis

Public health and human rights can be considered as two complementary, though often conflicting, ways of looking at human well-being. Even when they address similar, or even identical problems their language and underlying assumptions differ. Public health, for example, is built on the principle of seeking the greatest good for the greatest number of people: health is important and public health is considered a valid reason for limiting individual rights under some circumstances. The principles on which the human rights discourse is based, on the other hand, are concerned with promoting the well-being of *individuals* by ensuring respect for their rights and dignity. Interweaving these perspectives, then, it becomes clear that public health aims and interventions must be the least intrusive and least restrictive measures available to accomplish the public health goal.[19] Any ensuing compromise of an individual's rights must apply equally to all those affected.

In order to explore, negotiate and debate the potential tensions between human rights and public health policies, programmes and practices an approach known as the Health And Human Rights Framework has been developed.[33] The framework can be used to analyse public health programmes in order to provide 'new' ways of intervening which embrace both of these two complementary, but again sometimes conflicting, ways of looking at health issues.

The framework involves: 1) assessing the extent to which the proposed policy or programme represents 'good public health'; 2) discerning whether the proposed policy or programme is respectful and protective of human rights; 3) finding how the best possible combination of public health and human rights quality can be achieved; and finally 4) asking if the proposed policy or programme still appears to be the optimal approach to the public health problem (Figure 38.1).[33] To ensure that the full range of potential burdens on human rights is identified, each of the rights listed in the Universal Declaration of Human Rights should be considered.[33]

TUBERCULOSIS CONTROL FROM A HUMAN RIGHTS PERSPECTIVE

To What Extent Does the Proposed Policy or Programme Represent 'Good Public Health'?

As already stated, public health strategies for the control of infections concentrate on disease rather than 'well-being'. From a biomedical perspective, TB control strategies are 'rational' approaches developed from good science. As only people with sputum-positive pulmonary tuberculosis are regarded as being infectious to others, and because control needs to prevent transmission to the wider public, public health interventions are targeted at cases of *infectious* TB only (primarily sputum-positive pulmonary tuberculosis). Forms of TB that are considered non-infectious,

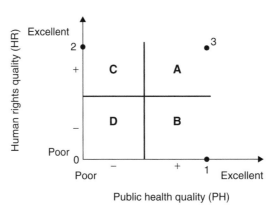

Sector explanation:
A: Best case
B: Need to improve HR quality
C: Need to improve PH quality
D: Worst case, need to improve both PH and HR quality

Points explanation:
0: Poor quality
1: Ideal PH quality
2: Ideal HR quality
3: Ideal PH and HR quality

Figure 38.1 A framework for negotiation: human rights and public health. (Reproduced with kind permission from AIDS, Health and Human Rights, the International Federation of Red Cross and Red Crescent Societies, and Francois-Xavier Bagnoud Center for Health & Human Rights, Harvard School of Public Health, Boston, 1995.)

such as extrapulmonary TB or TB in children, are not, therefore, seen to be public health issues. While 'rational' from a positivist, biomedical point of view, the human rights approach would question this perspective. What message does this give to the parents of children with tuberculosis? What message does it give to people with extra-pulmonary disease?

There is an inherent contradiction in the public health approach to the control of infectious diseases like tuberculosis. While the interest of a programme is ultimately the good of the population, the strategy focuses on the individual patient, who is treated without reference to the social conditions that frame his or her life. Take, for example, a TB programme that simply focuses on the act of directly observing patients take their medication, without taking into account the economic and social factors that are associated with the disease. A patient in this situation may be forced to discontinue treatment because a) she cannot travel to the clinic every other day for DOT, either because she lacks resources herself or because her household has refused to support her; b) she may not be able to tell her family that she has TB (and therefore cannot ask for support) because a TB diagnosis may precipitate divorce or obviate her marriage chances; c) she is feeling too unwell to travel the sometimes long distances over difficult roads; and/ or d) she simply cannot afford to take the time out of daily life (work, responsibilities for child care, etc.). Such a programme is unlikely to achieve the hoped for results. Barnhoorn and Adriaanse note that before the obstacles to a particular treatment regimen can be cleared away, patients have to understand the system, and the system must be consistent with the underlying health beliefs and social norms of the community.[34] The programme will also need to take account of the practical realities of everyday life which play a role in the ability of people to adhere to any treatment regimen.

Is the Proposed Policy or Programme Respectful and Protective of Human Rights?

In reviewing the human rights articles from the perspective of current TB control activities, several broad concepts will be considered: stigma, treatment, adherence to medication, limitations of freedom, education and living conditions. Seeing TB control from a different perspective and addressing these issues with greater sensitivity will lead to better care of TB patients.

Stigma

In many cultures the social stigma of tuberculosis contributes to the abandonment of treatment and lengthy delays in seeking professional care.[35] Human rights article 12 states: "*No one shall be subjected to arbitrary interference with his privacy, family, home nor to attacks upon his honour and reputation...*" DOT affects the TB patient's private life and must therefore be conducted with sensitivity. If treatment takes place at home, the privacy of the patient and his or her family is being jeopardised, whereas if treatment occurs in a public place known for the treatment of TB, there may be stigma or discrimination.[36] A recent study in the West Cape Region of South Africa showed that 6 months of continuous daily attendance at a site of supervision of administering the drugs was considered 'unreasonably long'. Many patients spoke about more pressing issues that they needed to attend to in their daily lives. Participants illustrated how the duration of treatment impacted on their duties to care for children and to provide an income for their families. These feelings appeared to contribute to a temptation to cease treatment once symptoms had abated.[37]

Many TB patients hide knowledge of their illness from employers, friends and family members. Some interpret supervised treatment as the system's distrust of them.[37] These feelings were compounded by the blasé manner in which health professionals informed them of their diagnosis. A lack of empathy exhibited by members of the health team appeared to have an impact on the patient's subsequent relationship with the clinical staff.[38]

Human rights article 16 states: *"Men and women of full age, without any limitation due to race, nationality or religion, have the right to marry and to found a family . . ."* In Pakistan, divorce and broken engagements occurring as a consequence of tuberculosis are seen more often in female than male patients.[39] In India a diagnosis of TB can be a hindrance to marriage.[40] Parents of girls of marriageable age may be reluctant to send their daughters to the clinic.[34] The belief that pregnancy enhances the risk for relapse also decreases their marriage prospects, and pregnancy is also seen to be a reason for stopping TB treatment.[39]

The voices of two women from Sialkot, Pakistan tell how this right to marry and found a family can be violated by being diagnosed with TB: *"When I go home, people will talk about me. People will say 'She was a TB patient and you should not accept her for your son to marry.' Even if we get well the effect will be the same."*

"We are two sisters and marriage arrangements have been made with men from one family. If my (future) family-in-law knows that I have TB they will be sure to break the engagement. I am not worried for me, but I'm worried for my sister. Her engagement also could break off because of my sickness."[39]

Human rights article 23 states: *"Everyone has the right to work, . . . to just and favourable conditions of work and to protection against unemployment . . ."* and article 25 continues; *"Everyone has the right to. . .*

medical care and necessary social services, and the right to security in the event of unemployment, sickness, disability. . .". For people with tuberculosis, it is common to avoid informing employers about the diagnosis, due to fear of the 'consequences' in the workplace and the risk of losing their jobs.[41] In Pakistan TB patients mentioned that they face difficulties in obtaining sick leave, and even in government service they are at risk of losing their jobs. Those who depend on seasonal work for income are particularly affected at certain times of the year like planting and harvesting time.[39] The need to support the family, fear of having to ask for support from employers to buy medicines due to stigmatisation and possible loss of job were factors mentioned by patients in Vietnam.[41]

Treatment

Human rights article 25 (HRA 25) states: *". . . motherhood and childhood are entitled to special care and assistance."* Two patient categories are excluded from the current international TB control strategy: children and extra-pulmonary TB cases. Between 10% and 20% of new tuberculosis cases occur in children, and approximately 450,000 deaths per year are in children less than 15 years of age.[42] Most children acquire their infection from a smear-positive adult case, but they themselves develop smear-negative disease and are therefore considered to be a relatively unimportant source of infection.[24] In the case of extrapulmonary TB, it is estimated that there are 1.[22] cases of smear-negative and extra-pulmonary tuberculosis for every case of smear-positive tuberculosis in developing countries,[43] and the case fatality rate for untreated smear-negative tuberculosis is between 40 and 50%.[43]

Human rights articles 18 and 19 state: *"Everyone has the right to freedom of thought, conscience and religion . . .*

Everyone has the right to freedom of opinion and expression; this right includes freedom to hold opinions without interference ..." TB patients need to be treated with dignity and respect. Effective care and a productive health worker–patient relationship require an understanding that different communities may have different perceptions of the disease and its treatment.[34, 44] In some societies, for example, attitudes to suffering are profoundly affected by religious beliefs.[45] In addition it is important to recognise that in most societies a range of health care options are now available to people. It cannot be assumed any more that patients will visit the local government health clinic in the first instance. Many patients may choose to visit private practitioners, NGOs (non governmental organisations), or practitioners of alternative kinds of treatment. In countries with a thriving private health care sector, the success of tuberculosis control strategies will depend on the effective involvement of this sector.[12, 40, 46, 47]

Adherence

Human rights article 21 states that *"Everyone has the right to equal access to public service in his country ..."* and human rights article 25 adds *"Everyone has the right to ... medical care and necessary social services ..."*

The act of giving DOT is seen as an essential part of control activities within the tuberculosis control structure currently advocated by the WHO. As noted above, however, this process has the effect of placing the primary responsibility for adherence onto the patient, and obscures the role of policy and health care practice. As Chaulet has noted, *"adherence is nothing more or less than the outcome of a process involving a long chain of responsibilities, extending from the decision-makers at the Health Ministry to the treating physician."*[48]

Others, too, have recognised the need for a 'creative array' of services that go well beyond the observation of drug ingestion.[36, 49] The accessibility (social, economic and physical) of a tuberculosis programme is essential for the success of the treatment it offers.[50]

In many countries only parts of the population have access to some kind of TB treatment, and even fewer to DOTS. Estimates suggest that fewer than half of patients with tuberculosis in developing countries are in contact with treatment services.[2, 51]

Empirical observations of TB patients in Kumasi, Ghana, suggest that non-adherence is largely due to lack of funds for transport to the clinic, non-availability of drugs at the TB clinic, and the refusal of staff in peripheral health posts to inject TB patients with streptomycin supplied at the central TB clinic.[52] In the developing world, self-medication is encouraged through a combination of low quality, unaffordable health services coupled with a lack of effective regulation of the sale of drugs, and aggressive marketing by the pharmaceutical industry.[53] Many patients can only afford to buy a small amount of medication at a time. This inevitably results in the interruption of treatment and often means that patients consume an inadequate or inappropriate combination of drugs.[41] Strengthening of the public sector as well as improving communication with the private sector are therefore crucial elements for improving adherence.

Limitations of Freedom

Human rights article 29 states: *"In the exercise of his right and freedom, everyone shall be subjected only to such limitations as are determined by law solely for the purpose of securing due recognition and respect for the rights and freedom of others. ..."*

Within liberal democracies, it is generally accepted that the state may intervene when the exercise of one person's freedom may result in harm to another.[54] This is known as the 'harm principle'. The nineteenth century philosopher John Stuart Mill defined this principle in the following way: *"The only purpose for which power can be rightfully exercised over any member of a civilised community, against his will, is to prevent harm to others. His own good, either physical or moral, is not a sufficient warrant."* This principle provides the ethical foundation for establishing public health programmes designed to require those with communicable diseases like tuberculosis to behave in ways that are likely to reduce the risk of transmission.

In some industrialised countries, an important question for TB control activities is: When may DOT be imposed by the state? In the United States, universal DOT has been challenged as an unethical intrusion upon autonomy and as a violation of the constitutional requirements that the least restrictive intervention be used.[15]

Education

Human rights article 26 states: *"Everyone has the right to education. . . ."*

Some studies have shown that public health education contributes to the success of tuberculosis control programmes, especially when peers and family members were also exposed to education.[55] The relation between educational background and knowledge of the symptoms and significance to health of tuberculosis, however, varies from region to region, and greater education and knowledge of tuberculosis does not necessarily lead patients to present earlier to the appropriate medical services.[45] Despite the fact that unemployed coloured women in Ravensmead, Cape Town, exhibited a good knowledge of tuberculosis, for example, this knowledge

did not necessarily result in biomedically appropriate/predictable health behaviour. In the event of developing symptoms or disease, individuals either did not seek medical care or failed to complete treatment.[38]

The Indian literature supports these findings. In India it appears that the general public have fairly good 'knowledge' regarding the cause, symptoms and spread of tuberculosis,[40, 56–59] although understanding of its diagnosis and treatment does not appear to be present to the same extent.[12, 41, 56–60] Uplekar and Rangan indicate, however, that even where knowledge regarding the consequences of irregular treatment is good, it does not affect treatment adherence.[40] Narayan and Srikantaramu report that there is no difference in awareness levels between regular and irregular patients.[61] A recent review of this literature notes that education and information regarding tuberculosis must go hand in hand with the provision of a service that 'makes sense' in terms of the realities and priorities of the everyday lives of patients and their families.[50]

Living Conditions

Human rights article 25 states: *"Everyone has the right to a standard of living adequate for the health and well-being of himself and his family . . ."* Tuberculosis is a disease that is closely associated with poverty.[20] Control of TB can not, and should not, be separated from the development of measures to reduce inequity and poverty.

How Can We Achieve the Best Possible Combination of Public Health and Human Rights Quality?

As already stated, TB control programme structures have been developed from the biomedical perspective. Either as an affect or effect of this, there continues to be a dearth of useful qualitative information on the social and behavioural aspects of TB and other infectious diseases. Available information indicates that there are problematic disjunctions between TB patients and providers, and between the population and the policy makers. The non-medical factors that determine health such as behaviour, the environment, human biology and socio-economic status, remain the most important factors affecting people's health. After the dramatic successes of the sanitary revolution, however, less attention has been paid to these critical, if non-medical, health determinants.[62]

This analysis of TB control from the health and human rights perspectives has highlighted the importance of a wider concept of health and of the need to understand tuberculosis within the context of people's everyday lives. A 'healthy' interaction between patients and providers, another critical element, can only be achieved when health care structures are themselves functioning efficiently and effectively.[44] The best possible approach to TB control will include a consideration of these issues, and will incorporate a complementarity of public health and human rights principles.

Does the Proposed Policy or Programme Still Appear to be the Optimal Approach to the Public Health Problem?

The positive aspects of the current international TB control strategy are that it has been well constructed from scientific studies and is a rational approach to TB control. It is important to remember that 'DOTS' is more than DOT alone. DOTS as a whole emphasises providing an efficient programme which is able to maintain and sustain high quality laboratory diagnostics, regular drug supplies and a well-trained cadre of health workers who are responsive to patient needs.

The negative aspects of the programme stem largely from its narrowly biomedical orientation. It falls short of embracing the social, economic and cultural dimensions of tuberculosis. Taken in isolation from the rest of the structure, a singular focus on the direct observation component of DOTS has the effect of placing the focus on patient behaviour, highlighting patient 'failures', while effectively masking the failures of the system to enable patients to comply. Managers and others developing TB policy and organising TB control structures need to be more aware of the process of developing appropriate and 'healthy' programmes.

DISCUSSION

The human rights/public health framework encourages a different perspective on the standard biomedical approach to disease control in order to develop improved ways of dealing with diseases like tuberculosis. A concentration on the individual, without an understanding of the wider socio-economic and cultural issues that frame their lives, is likely to create ineffective interventions—interventions which fail to 'provide the conditions in which people can be healthy'. TB patients can only be expected to comply with treatment if they are able to do so. Therefore, in any given setting, the key dimensions of social, economic and physical access to TB services need to be assessed and accounted for in programme design. Shifting the burden of ensuring programme effectiveness from the patient to the programmers will have the added benefit of enabling patients to obtain appropriate treatment whilst retaining their dignity and social and self-respect.

This change in perspective will require more qualitative research and the development of broader outcome indicators than are currently used in TB control programmes. It will entail a shift in focus from DOT alone to DOTS as a process/management structure. Control programmes need to ensure that there is a quality laboratory service and a regular sustained drug supply, but in addition, they need to develop a managerial system that respects the needs of TB patients and takes the importance of the health care worker/patient relationship into account. This can not be achieved with internationally fixed strategies, but rather in locally developed programmes recognising the specific needs and resources of the community.

This analysis also indicates that it is time to view TB control within a wider concept of health. Diseases such as tuberculosis are a reflection of underlying societal conditions of inequity and poverty. They are indicators of wider social, environmental and global conditions, and they need to be seen within the broad context of globalisation and intersectoral collaboration. The health and human rights framework enables us to view public health programmes from a perspective that takes these factors into account. If this perspective leads to changes in practice commensurate with improved human rights, then the framework will have achieved its goal.

REFERENCES

1. World Health Organisation. TB. A global emergency. WHO Report on the TB Epidemic. WHO/TB/94.177. Geneva: WHO, 1994.

2. Raviglione M C, Dye C, Schmidt S, Kochi A. Assessment of worldwide tuberculosis control. Lancet 1997; 350: 624–629.

3. Porter J D H, McAdam K P W J. The re-emergence of tuberculosis. Ann Rev Public Health 1994; 15: 303–323.

4. World Health Organization. WHO Tuberculosis Programme. Framework for effective tuberculosis control. WHO/TB/ 94.179. Geneva: WHO, 1994.

5. World Health Organization. WHO Report on the Tuberculosis Epidemic, 1995. DOTS Stops TB at the Source. WHO/TB/95.183. Geneva: WHO, 1995.

6. Harries A D, Maher D. TB/HIV. A clinical manual. WHO/TB/ 96.200. Geneva: WHO, 1996.

7. Morse D I. Directly observed therapy for tuberculosis: spend now or pay later. BMJ 1996; 312: 719–720.

8. Chaulk P, Moore-Rice K, Rizzo R, Chaisson R E. Eleven years of community-based directly observed therapy for tuberculosis. JAMA 1995; 274: 945–951.

9. Frieden T R, Fujiwara P I, Washko R M, Hamburg M A. Tuberculosis in New York City: Turning the tide. N Engl J Med 1995; 333: 229–233.

10. McKenna M T, McCray E, Jones J L, Onorato I M, Castro K G. The fall after the rise: tuberculosis in the United States, 1991 through 1994. Am J Public Health 1998; 88: 1059–1063.

11. Zhao Feng-Zeng, Murray C, Spinaci S, Styblo K, Broekmans J. Results of directly observed short-course chemotherapy in 112 842 Chinese patients with smear positive tuberculosis. Lancet 1996; 347: 358–362.

12. Juvekar S K, Morankar S N, Dalal D B, et al. Social and operational determinants of patient behaviour in lung tuberculosis. Indian J Tuberc 1995; 42: 87–94.

13. Gangadharam P R J. Chemotherapy of tuberculosis under program conditions. [editorial]. Tubercle Lung Dis 1994; 75: 241–244.

14. Makubalo L E. [editorial]. Epidemiol Comments 1996; 23: 1.

15. Bayer R, Dupuis L. Tuberculosis, public health, and civil liberties. Ann Rev Public Health 1995; 16: 307–326.

16. Porter J D H, Ogden J A. Ethics of directly observed therapy for the control of infectious diseases. Bull Inst Pasteur 1997; 95: 117–127.

17. Institute of Medicine. Future of Public Health. Washington DC: National Academy Press, 1988: pp 1–7.

18. Mann J M. Human rights and the new public health. Health Hum Rights 1994; 1: 229–233.

19. Mann J M, Gostin L, Gruskin S, Brennau T, Lazzarini Z, Fineberg H V. Health and human rights. Health Hum Rights 1994; 1: 7–23.

20. Porter J D H, Ogden J A. Social inequalities in the re-emergence of infectious disease. In: Strickland S S, Shetty P S, eds. Human biology and social inequality. Cambridge, UK: Cambridge University Press, 1998: pp 96–113.

21. Vaughan J P, Morrow R H. Manual of epidemiology for district health management. Geneva: WHO, 1989.

22. Rodrigues L C, Smith P G. Tuberculosis in developing countries and methods for its control. Trans Roy Soc Trop Med Hyg 1990; 84: 739–744.

23. Snider D E. General view of problems with compliance in programmes for the treatment of tuberculosis. Bull Int Union Tuberc 1982; 57(3–4): 55–260.

24. Bayer R, Neveloff Dubler N, Landesman S. The dual epidemic of tuberculosis and AIDS: ethical and policy issues in screening and treatment. Am J Public Health 1993; 83: 649–654.

25. The tuberculosis revival: individual rights and societal obligations in a time of AIDS. New York, NY: Publications Program, United Hospital Fund of New York, 1992: 1–75.

26. Sumartojo E. When tuberculosis treatment fails. A social behavioral account of patient adherence. Am Rev Respir Dis 1993; 147: 1311–1320.

27. Farmer P. Social scientists and the new tuberculosis. Soc Sci Med 1997; 44: 347–358.

28. Lupton D. Risk as moral danger: the social and political functions of risk discourse in public health. Int J Health Services 1993; 23: 425–435.

29. Cole P. The moral bases for public health interventions. Epidemiology 1995; 6: 78–83.

30. Bilder R B. An overview of International Human Rights Law. In: H Annum, ed. Guide to International Human Rights Practice. Philadelphia, PA: University of Pennsylvania Press, 1994.

31. Universal Declaration of Human Rights. Adopted and proclaimed by UN General Assembly Resolution 217 A(III), Dec 10, 1948.

32. McGinnis J M, Foege W H. Actual causes of death in the United States. JAMA 1996; 270: 2207–2212.

33. International Federation of Red Cross and Red Crescent Societies and Francois-Xavier Bagnoud Center for Health and Human Rights. The public health-human rights dialogue in AIDS, health and human rights. An explanatory manual. Boston, MA: Harvard School of Public Health, 1995.

34. Barnhoorn F, Adriaanse H. In search of factors responsible for non-compliance among tuberculosis patients in Wardha district, India. Soc Sci Med 1992; 34: 291–306.

35. Rubel A J, Garro L C. Social and cultural factors in the successful control of tuberculosis. Public Health Rep 1992; 107: 626–636.

36. Gostin L O. Controlling the resurgent tuberculosis epidemic. A 50-state survey of TB statutes and proposals for reform. JAMA 1993; 269: 255–261.

37. Dick J, Schoeman J H, Mohammed A, Lombard C. Tuberculosis in the community: 1. Evaluation of a volunteer health worker programme to enhance adherence to anti-tuberculosis treatment. Tubercle Lung Dis 1996; 77: 274–279.

38. Dick J, Schoeman J H. Tuberculosis in the community: 2. The perceptions of members of a tuberculosis health team towards a voluntary health worker programme. Tubercle Lung Dis 1996; 77: 380–388.

39. Liefooghe R, Michiels N, Habib S, Moran M B, De Muynck A. Perception and social consequences of tuberculosis: a focus group study of tuberculosis patients in Sialkot, Pakistan. Soc Sci Med 1995; 41: 1685–1692.

40. Uplekar M, Rangan S. Tackling TB: the search for solutions. Bombay: Foundation for Research in Community Health (FRCH), 1996.

41. Johansson E, Diwan V K, Huong N D, Ahlberg B M. Staff and patient attitudes to tuberculosis and compliance with treatment: an exploratory study in a district in Vietnam. Tubercle Lung Dis 1996; 77: 178–183.

42. Raviglione M C, Snider D E, Kochi A. Global epidemiology of tuberculosis. JAMA 1995; 273: 220–226.

43. Murray C J L, Styblo K, Rouillon A. Tuberculosis. In: Jamison D T, Mosley W H, eds. Disease control priorities in developing countries. New York: Oxford University Press/World Bank, 1993.

44. Wingerd J. Communication and credibility: Little Haiti and the public health clinic. 94th Annual Meeting, American Anthropological Association, San Francisco, November 20–24, 1996.

45. Grange J M, Festenstein F. The human dimension of tuberculosis control. Tubercle Lung Dis 1993; 74: 219–222.

46. Brugha R, Zwi A. Improving the quality of private sector delivery of public health services: challenges and strategies. Health Policy and Planning 1998; 13: 107–120.

47. Bennett S, McPake B, Mills A, eds. Private health providers in developing countries: serving the public interest? London: Zed Press, 1997.

48. Chaulet P. Compliance with chemotherapy for tuberculosis: responsibilities of the Health Ministry and of physicians. Bull Int Union Tuberc 1990–1991; 66 (Suppl): 33–35.

49. Bloch A B, Sumartojo E, Castro K G. Directly observed therapy for tuberculosis in New York City [letter]. JAMA 1994; 272: 435–436.

50. Rangan S, Uplekar M, Brugha R, et al. Tuberculosis control: a state of the art review. Delhi, India: UK Department for International Development (DFID), 1997.

51. Anon. The global challenge of tuberculosis. [editorial] Lancet 1994; 344: 277–279.

52. Twumasi P A. Non compliance with tuberculosis treatment: the Kumasi experience. Tropical Doctor 1996; 26: 43–44.

53. Homedes N, Ugalde A. Patients' compliance with medical treatments in the third world: what do we know? Health Policy Planning 1993; 8: 291–314.

54. Shindell S. Legal and ethical aspects of public health. In: J M Last, ed. Maxcy Roseany Public Health and Preventive Medicine. 11th ed. New York: Appleton-Century-Crofts 1980: pp 1834–1845.

55. Uplekar M, Rangan S. Alternative approaches to improve treatment adherence in tuberculosis control programme. Indian J Tuberc 1995; 42: 67–74.

56. Purohit S D, Gupta M L, Arun Madan, Gupta P R, Mathur B B, Sharma T N. Awareness about tuberculosis among general population: a pilot study. Indian J Tuberc 1988; 35: 183.

57. Geetakrishnan K, Pappu K P, Roychowdhury K. A study on knowledge and attitude towards tuberculosis in a rural area of West Bengal. Indian J Tuberc 1988; 35: 83.

58. Goyal S S, Mathur G P, Pamra S P. Tuberculosis trends in an urban community. Indian J Tuberc 1978; 25: 77.

59. Ramachandran Rajesawari, Diwakara A M, Ganapathy Sudha, Sudarsanam N M, Rajaram K, Prabhakar R. Tuberculosis awareness among educated public in two cities in Tamil Nadu. Lung India 1995; 13: 108.

60. Nair Dinesh M, George A, Chacko K T. Tuberculosis in Bombay: new insights from poor urban patients. Health Policy and Planning 1997; 12: 77–85.

61. Narayan Radha, Srikantaramu N. Significance of some social factors in the treatment behaviour of tuberculosis patients. NTI Newsletter 1987; 23: 76.

62. Lee P, Paxman D. Re-inventing public health. Ann Rev Public Health 1997; 18: 1–35.

QUESTIONS

1. TB is the second leading killer in the world, accounting for more than 2 million deaths a year. Public health has historically been concentrated on prevention at the population level, and has not been overly concerned with human rights. Why? How does taking human rights seriously affect how TB screening and treatment is done?

2. Directly observed treatment (DOT) has become the international gold standard for treating TB, even in the absence of evidence that it is the most effective approach. Why? Does the added epidemic of multiple drug resistant TB require a more aggressive public health response and more drastic derogations of human rights?

3. Are you persuaded that applying a human rights approach to the treatment of TB will be as effective as an approach that ignores or marginalizes the human rights dimensions of this disease, e.g., with mandatory quarantine for those who cannot be trusted to take their drugs or stay at home while contagious?

FURTHER READING

1. Daniel, Thomas, *Captain of Death: The Story of Tuberculosis.* Rochester: University of Rochester Press, 1997.

2. Singh, J. A., Upshar, R., & Padayatchi, N., XDR-TB in South Africa: No time for Denial or Complacency, *PLOS Medicine,* 2007; 4: e50; 0019–0025.

3. Annas, G. J., Control of Tuberculosis and the Law. *New Engl J Med,* 1993; 328: 585–590.

4. Gostin, L., Controlling the Resurgent Tuberculosis Epidemic *JAMA,* 1993; 296: 255–259.

CHAPTER 39

A Human Rights-Based Approach to Non-Communicable Diseases

Helena Nygren-Krug

SCOPE, MAGNITUDE AND RISK FACTORS

In recent years, the global public health community has increasingly been calling for intensified action to prevent and control non-communicable diseases (NCDs).[1] NCDs represent 60% of all deaths globally, with 80% of deaths due to non-communicable diseases occurring in low- and middle-income countries, and approximately 16 million deaths involving people less than 70 years of age.[2] Total deaths from NCDs are projected to increase by a further 17% over the next 10 years.[3] NCDs, principally cardiovascular diseases, diabetes, cancers, and chronic respiratory diseases, caused an estimated 35 million deaths in 2005.[4] These NCDs, often considered "life-style epidemics", have a number of common modifiable risk factors—tobacco use, unhealthy diet and physical inactivity and the harmful use of alcohol. These risk factors are mainly behavioural and are on the rise everywhere due to the "nutrition transition" with diets rich in saturated fats and poorer in complex carbohydrates and dietary fibre, fruit and vegetables; the growth of urban lifestyles involving less physical exertion; and the promotion and rising consumption of tobacco and alcohol.[5] While some of these risk factors, such as tobacco consumption, have received attention in recent years, others have been much neglected. Obesity, for example, is one of today's most blatantly visible—yet most neglected—public health problems.[6]

A HUMAN RIGHTS APPROACH TO NON-COMMUNICABLE DISEASES

The most recent World Health Assembly adopted a draft action plan to prevent and control non-communicable diseases (NCDs), recognizing that the global burden continues to grow.[7] This plan sets out three strategic directives as follows:

1. Map the epidemics and analyze their social, economic, behavioural and political determinants as the basis for providing guidance on effective interventions;

2. Reduce the level of exposure of individuals and populations to the common modifiable risk factors and their determinants while strengthening the capacity of individuals and the population to make healthier choices and follow lifestyle patterns that foster good health;

3. And strengthen health care for people with NCDs.[8]

Human rights are relevant to each of these strategic directives. Overall, integrating a human rights-based approach to the efforts to address NCDs means that the realization of health-related human rights[9] becomes the overall goal of these efforts and that human rights principles[10] guide all actions towards this goal. Moreover, a human rights-based approach supports action to build the capacity of rights-holders to claim their rights, and duty-bearers to meet their obligations.[11] There are two main rationales for using a human rights approach to address NCDs. The intrinsic rationale, acknowledging that a human rights-based approach is the right thing to do, morally or legally; and the instrumental rationale, recognizing that a human rights-based approach leads to better and more sustainable human development outcomes.[12]

The human right to health is the right to the enjoyment of a variety of facilities, goods, services and conditions necessary for the realization of the highest attainable standard of health.[13] It provides a universal normative framework to design and assess health-care and health determinants in relation to NCDs. Other human rights that guide and support action to address NCDs include equality and non-discrimination and the rights to information, education and participation.

Specific human rights instruments have been adopted over the years that have articulated rights in relation to specific groups of populations that have been exposed disproportionately to human rights violations, including the enjoyment of the right to health. Indigenous peoples; persons with disabilities; migrant workers; prisoners; ethnic, religious and linguistic minorities; women; children; are examples of population groups addressed in specific human rights instruments. Addressing the health of these population groups effectively requires an approach, which begins from their perspective, keeping in mind their needs and situations and with their full participation.

In addition to normative and analytical guidance, the human rights framework contains a number of international, regional and national mechanisms that can support monitoring and accountability in relation to action to address NCDs.

ANALYZING AND ADDRESSING NCDS

A human rights-based approach provides not only a conceptual framework but also a practical methodology for analyzing and addressing the determinants of NCDs.[14] It involves various steps of analysis, starting with a causal one, to identify the immediate, underlying and root causes of NCDs. This helps to go beyond the behavioural risk factors, such as smoking and overeating, to consider underlying and root causes, such as the enjoyment of a range of health-related human rights such as freedom from discrimination and the rights to safe and healthy working conditions, nutritious food, information and education. Secondly, a pattern (also called role/obligation) analysis aims at identifying who are the rights-holders and duty-bearers and their corresponding entitlements and obligations. This step in the analysis maps the various stakeholders involved in promoting or undermining actions to address NCDs. Under international human rights law, the government is the prime duty-bearer; it is under an obligation to promote and protect human rights across all sectors. Within government, in the context of NCDs, specific duty-bearers identified will range across sectors such as agriculture, finance and taxation, education, recreation and sports, media and communication, transportation, and urban planning. However, beyond the government, a range of other duty-bearers can be identified that have specific responsibilities. These may range from family members to multinational corporations and donors. In the area of NCDs, moreover, the private sector plays a significant role, including the tobacco, food, sugar, and alcohol industries. This does not, however, absolve the obligations of the government, which must protect human rights by regulating the private sector so that it acts in conformity with human rights.[15] Some identified stakeholders may be both duty-bearer and rights-holder. For example, a teacher is a duty bearer vis-à-vis children who should be educated on healthy eating habits, but is also a rights-holder in relation to local and national authorities that should give him or her the authority and resources to carry out health-promotion activities in schools.[16]

In a human rights-based approach to programming, human rights principles guide all stages of the analysis, including the principles of equality and the right to participation. The latter means that those groups identified as most affected should be involved in decisions about possible interventions. The human rights-based approach is concerned with the population groups most exposed to human rights violations: This stems from the focus on equality and non-discrimination in human rights discourse.[17] Focusing the analysis on individuals and groups experiencing a disproportionate burden of exclusion, marginalization and discrimination will help unveil further underlying and root causes of NCDs. As such, the identity of the rights-holder(s) becomes an important and central feature in analyzing why the right to health is not being enjoyed. Addressing NCDs from a human rights perspective thus requires collecting disaggregated data on the prevalence of NCDs, to identify which population groups are most affected. Where there is no systematic collection of disaggregated data, efforts should nevertheless be made to identify the most vulnerable and/or marginalized population groups through research and interviews with those knowledgeable about the national and local context. Such an analysis usually reveals that some populations groups suffer consistently poorer health than others in the same country. For example, across countries, available mortality and morbidity data provide scientific evidence of significant inequalities in the health status of indigenous populations.[18] Smoking, alcoholic and substance abuse are serious health and social problems, along with cardiovascular diseases, diabetes and cancer.[19] Many of these illnesses are associated with lifestyle changes resulting from land displacement and acculturation, which constitute underlying and root causes of NCDs in indigenous communities. In this context, the UN Committee on Economic, Social and Cultural Rights has recognized that development-related activities that lead to the displacement of indigenous peoples against their will from their traditional territories and environment, denying them their sources of nutrition and breaking their symbiotic relationship with their lands, has a deleterious effect on their health.[20] To improve indigenous health, therefore, a holistic approach is required, considering the range of underlying, structural and root causes, and with full participation of the indigenous communities affected.

The third, and final, step in a human rights analysis is the capacity gap analysis, to reveal why rights are not realized, paying particular attention to why duty-bearers are not living up to their human rights obligations or responsibilities. This involves considering questions such as the authority, motivation, commitment, ability to communicate and leadership of duty-bearers, as well as their access to, and control over, resources. This analysis will reveal where interventions will be most effective and how they can be designed so as to enhance the capacities of rights-holders to claim their rights and duty-bearers to meet their obligations. The involvement of rights-holders in all stages of a rights-based analysis is not only a question of safeguarding the right to participation, but also has instrumental value, ensuring that interventions are culturally appropriate and sustainable. Anchored in human rights law, interventions should span across government actors and other stakeholders and generate change at different levels synergistically, from the local and community level to the national and international levels. At all these levels, a priority focus for a human rights-based response is how to enhance accountability of the duty-bearers so that they live up to, and deliver on, their obligations and responsibilities.

HOLDING THE DUTY-BEARERS TO ACCOUNT

A human rights analysis of NCDs reveals those required to take action and what human rights obligations and responsibilities they have assumed. Accountability is one of the most important features of human rights and requires effective monitoring. To facilitate the monitoring of State Parties' performance in realizing the various rights enshrined in the core UN human rights treaties, the human rights treaty bodies have been engaged in identifying appropriate indicators. Indicators proposed for the monitoring of the right to health include some particularly relevant to monitoring the commitment of governments to address NCDs. Such indicators include: Death rates associated with and prevalence of NCDs (an "outcome indicator"); the proportion of school-going children educated on health and nutrition issues (a "process indicator") and, finally, the timeframe and coverage of national policy on child health and nutrition (a "structural indicator").[21]

Human rights law focuses on state obligations and thus mechanisms at international, regional and national levels focus on monitoring government performance. Since the 1990s, however, there has been an ongoing debate regarding the roles and responsibilities of the private sector in promoting and violating human rights. This debate has focused predominantly on labour standards, with a plethora of initiatives unfolding, mainly in the form of self-regulation and voluntary codes of conduct. In recent years, moreover, attempts are being made at clarifying duties and roles of the private sector specifically in relation to the right to health.[22] Meanwhile, work in public health is increasingly engaging the private sector to attract resources, attention and increase outreach and impact of public health interventions. This poses inherent risks, particularly when there are tremendous commercial interests involved and there is no common framework to address human rights and businesses. The Special Representative of the Secretary-General on the issue of human rights and transnational corporations and other business enterprises, John Ruggie, has sought to address the lack of a framework by proposing three foundational principles: Protect, respect and access to remedy.[23] The first element aims to underscore the role of the state as the steward and prime-duty bearer. Governments need to mainstream the business and human rights agenda across all sectors and ensure adequate domestic policy coherence in order to ensure policy coherence at the international level.[24] The second principle—the principle to respect—is directed at companies themselves, recognizing a corporate responsibility to "do no harm". This poses particular challenges in the context of NCDs and tobacco in particular. How can the tobacco industry operate in a way consistent with human rights? Can a tobacco company respect the right to life—the most fundamental of all human rights—or is there a contradiction given that the substance that it produces, tobacco, kills a third to a half of all those who use it?[25] Application of this principle in practice challenges the very raison-d'être of some businesses. The third and final principle in the framework proposed is that of effective remedy.

It is the first principle—to protect—that has evolved most substantively in international law given that states are the principal actors in this field. As far back as in the 70s, high profile nongovernmental organizations' (NGO) campaigns sought to protect and promote breast-feeding for babies and prevent the inappropriate marketing of breast milk substitutes.[26] Supported by UNICEF and the WHO, these campaigns led governments in the World Health Assembly to adopt the International Code of Marketing of Breast-Milk Substitutes (1981) which constitutes a set of recommendations to regulate the marketing of breast-milk substitutes, feeding bottles and teats.[27] Breastfeeding has long-term benefits associated with NCDs. Adults who were breastfed as babies often have lower blood pressure and lower cholesterol, as well as lower rates of overweight, obesity and type-2 diabetes.[28] Although most of the countries that have adopted the Code have put in place some implementing measures, frequently by enforceable legislation, voluntary means are also being used. Despite this now long-standing code, however, manufacturers of infant formula milks are still accused of using manipulative marketing techniques that have an adverse affect on breastfeeding rates around the work.[29] According to Save the Children, an international treaty on Baby Milk marketing is required, based on the WHO code but with much stronger state obligations and institutional oversight.[30] Others argue that the Code has become a flexible, clear and authoritative reference and contains more

detailed standards than could have been expected in a binding convention.

Accountability is closely linked to the need for legal standards that bind duty bearers to take action. General Comment No. 14 notes that "(t)he realization of the right to health may be pursued through numerous, complementary approaches, such as the formulation of health policies, or the implementation of health programs developed by the World Health Organization (WHO), or the adoption of specific legal instruments . . ."[31] As such, the General Comment assumes that WHO focuses on policies, guidelines and other non-binding instruments to address health challenges, rather than legally binding instruments. Indeed, despite extensive powers to establish health-related standards and adopt treaties under its constitution, WHO has not been notably active in using such instruments to address public health challenges.

The first treaty negotiated under the auspices of WHO was the WHO Framework Convention on Tobacco Control (FCTC).[32] Mergers and trade liberalization, and the resulting globalization of the tobacco epidemic, generated support for the development of global legal norms for tobacco control.[33] Moreover, clear evidence demonstrated that tobacco kills. With strong leadership from the WHO secretariat, the WHO FCTC was developed and adopted. It helps governments to live up to their right-to-health obligations. The UN Committee on Economic, Social and Cultural Rights has specifically identified "the failure to discourage production, marketing and consumption of tobacco" as a violation of the obligation to protect the right to health in General Comment No. 14.[34] This follows from the failure of a state to take all necessary measures to safeguard persons within their jurisdiction from infringements of the right to health by third parties, and includes such omissions as the failure to regulate the activities of individuals, groups or corporations to prevent them from violating the right to health of others.[35] From a human rights perspective, regulation is often a necessity, particularly when it comes to protecting vulnerable groups. To protect young people, for example, WHO has urged governments to ban all tobacco advertising, promotion and sponsorship, in light of recent studies that prove that the more young people are exposed to tobacco advertising, the more likely they are to start smoking.[36]

Arguments are being put forward for the development of international legal standards in select areas of diet and nutrition, as a strategy for ensuring that the health of future generations does not become dependent on corporate charity and voluntary commitments.[37] However, in the area of diet and nutrition, a voluntaristic approach has so far dominated. In 2004, the member states of the FAO agreed upon the Voluntary Guidelines on the Right to Food, which encourage states "to take steps, in particular through education, information and labeling regulations, to prevent over-consumption and unbalanced diets that may lead to malnutrition, obesity and degenerative diseases".[38] The same year, 2004, the World Health Assembly adopted a Global Strategy on Diet, Physical Activity and Health to address non-communicable diseases. Ironically, the paragraph in the resolution that adopted the Strategy, containing the strongest language, is the one which urges member states to avoid trade-restrictive or trade-distorting impact of public policies adopted in the context of implementation of the Strategy.[39] In reviewing food labels and their impact on free trade, the WTO extensively relies on a decision of the Codex Alimentariaus Commission.[40] A WTO Dispute Resolution Panel has distinguished between foods that pose a danger to the life or health of the consumer, and foods that were nutri-

tionally disadvantageous due to the quality or quantity of their nutrients, but without necessarily presenting a danger to the health of the consumer.[41] The implications of this distinction are that health warnings about nutritional quality of food are likely to be treated under the Agreement on Technical Barriers to Trade ("TBT Agreement").[42] The TBT Agreement states that "technical regulations shall not be more trade-restrictive than necessary to fulfill a legitimate objective, taking account of the risks non-fulfillment would create. Such legitimate objectives are, inter alia: . . . protection of human health or safety".[43] To address NCDs, arguments have been made for global standards in relation to labelling of product constituents, fair warning of health risks, and health claims to enable consumers to make informed and healthy food choices.[44] Such standards would support the realization of the right to information as well as the empowerment of rights-holders to demand healthier choices and hold duty-bearers more accountable.

EMPOWERING THE RIGHTS-HOLDERS

Under international human rights law, the government is under the obligation to protect the right to health and thus must regulate non-state actors—companies and other stakeholders—to act in a way consistent with this right. This raises the question as to how far the state can regulate, particularly in relation to the enjoyment of other human rights. The aforementioned Special Representative refers to the UN human rights treaty monitoring bodies for guidance on how far the duty to protect human rights applies.[45] In general terms, the Human Rights Committee has underscored that the protection of the right to life requires that states adopt positive measures to increase life expectancy.[46] But how far do individuals have a free choice to overeat, smoke or consume alcohol in a way harmful to their own health? In the case of tobacco, the courts have been willing to limit the interpretation of the right to privacy to safeguard public health. In this context, the British courts held that preventing a person from smoking did not generally involve such adverse effect upon his physical or moral integrity as would amount to an interference with the right to respect for private or home life within the meaning of Article 8 of the European Convention on Human Rights.[47] However, denying a job or dismissing qualified persons solely on the basis of their obesity or because they are off-duty smokers would amount to discrimination and constitute an undue intrusion in their private life.[48] An important test in reviewing the balance between the right to privacy and measures taken to safeguard public health are the Siracusa Principles.[49] These can protect individuals against punitive, discriminatory and disproportionate measures taken by governments to ostensibly protect the public's health. Unfortunately, however, many societal measures adopt punitive approaches to NCDs on the assumption that those affected are solely responsible for their predicament. Some argue, and some health insurance companies maintain, that people who overeat and become obese should not burden society by having others pay for their health care costs. Indeed, the tobacco industry managed to avoid compensating any of its victims for the first 40 years of litigation not only by persistently refusing to admit that smoking caused any disease, but also by convincing judges and juries that the smoker was entirely at fault for "choosing" to smoke in the face of known risks as well as government mandated health warnings included on cigarette packs since 1966.[50] These arguments fail to consider the underlying and root causes of ill-health, which are as important to determining someone's level of health as the immediate causes. These

underlying causes go beyond the immediate risk factors and implicate a broad range of duty-bearers that may play a role in influencing a person's health throughout his or her life-cycle, ranging from local communities, private companies and international actors. The government needs to act as the steward to ensure that society as a whole acts coherently and in a way that is health enhancing. International human rights instruments thus focus on the state as the prime duty-bearer, and these treaties may contain explicit duties to encourage individual responsibility for health. For example, the original European Social Charter (1961) and its revised form (1996) sets out the obligation of the state to ensure that the population is adequately informed and educated about health matters in order to encourage individual responsibility in health matters.[51]

Greater awareness among the general public of health-related human rights is generating increased demand for transparency and accountability from duty-bearers, particularly governments, to take action for better health. Significantly, under international human rights law, rights-holders are able to hold duty-bearers to account. In recent years, there has been an upsurge in litigation in the area of health rights in general. Increasingly, people are demanding access to medicines, treatments and care before the courts. However, in relation to NCDs, which are often chronic, courts have been reluctant to review decisions taken by political organs and medical authorities as to how to allocate budgets and decide on priorities. For example, in 1997, the Constitutional Court of South Africa held that a hospital that had refused renal dialysis treatment to a patient suffering from terminal illness had not violated the constitutional right not to be "refused emergency medical treatment" as the treatment did not amount to an "emergency" in the sense of a sudden catastrophe, but rather an "ongoing state of affairs".[52] However, the increased recognition of health rights and some successful claims being brought before the courts, are empowering claim-holders to secure treatment even without going to the courts. For example, in 2006, a woman with breast cancer shamed Somerset Primary Care Trust in the United Kingdom into providing a drug, Herceptin, after threatening to take her case to the European Court of Human Rights.[53]

CONCLUSION

Analysing and addressing NCDs from a human rights perspective brings to the forefront the most challenging and pressing issues in public health, such as how to ensure a more intersectoral and coherent response to address upstream determinants of health; how far the private sector can be held responsible and accountable; the nature and scope of state obligations under international law; the extent of the role of the state in protecting public health versus allowing individual freedom and choice; and how to empower people affected by ill-health to demand action from powerful actors to promote and protect health.

Human rights provide an internationally recognized legal framework under which governments have concrete obligations relevant to NCDs. However, these obligations should be further articulated to better address the challenges posed by NCDs, not only in relation to specific applicable human rights norms such as the rights to life, health, food and education, but also in relation to the human rights responsibilities of the private sector. Although some industries are engaged in an ongoing and constructive dialogue on how to address NCDs,[54] they, along with many governments that benefit from their profits, are generally adverse to international legal standards, particularly in areas dominated by powerful commercial interests. In the absence of specific, internationally binding standards to address NCDs, beyond the WHO FCTC, human rights norms should be further and better articulated to incorporate the risk factors and underlying determinants of NCDs. This would ensure that the accountability mechanisms dedicated to human rights monitoring at the international, regional and national levels pay greater attention to NCDs.

Moreover, the emerging "health rights movement" should forge stronger alliances with the public health community. The health rights movement brings with it the skills of the international human rights movement including advocacy, litigation, social mobilization and societal transformation skills. The public health community has the authoritative tools of epidemiology, which are revealing causal links not only between smoking and death, but also between unhealthy diets and a range of chronic diseases, including cardiovascular diseases, cancer, diabetes and other conditions linked to obesity. Together, the human rights and public health communities can generate stronger leadership from governments and international organizations to address NCDs through a human rights-based approach.

REFERENCES

1. Although WHO does not have an official definition of what is meant by non-communicable diseases, diseases within this category are generally those diseases which are not caused by infectious agents (excluding diseases of pregnancy and gynaecological diseases).
2. See Sixty-First World Health Assembly, 'Prevention and Control of Non-communicable Diseases: Implementation of the Global Strategy', Resolution A61/8, 18 April 2008.
3. Ibid.
4. Ibid.
5. Ibid.
6. WHO, 'Controlling the Global Obesity Epidemic', http://www.who.int/nutrition/topics/obesity/en/index.html.

7. See World Health Assembly Resolution, *supra* note 2.

8. Ibid.

9. Health-related human rights include the rights to health, information, food, education, equality and non-discrimination.

10. Key human rights principles that guide all actions which are rights-based are: Universality and inalienability; indivisibility; interdependence and interrelatedness; equality and non-discrimination; participation and inclusion; and accountability and the rule of law. See UN Common Understanding on a Human Rights-Based Approach to Development Cooperation 2003, http://www.undg.org/?P=221.

11. Ibid.

12. Office of the High Commissioner for Human Rights (OHCHR), 'Question 17: What Value Does A Human Rights-Based Approach Add To Development?' in *Frequently Asked Questions on a Human Rights-Based Approach to Development Cooperation* (Geneva: OHCHR, 2006), at 16.

13. Committee on Economic, Social and Cultural Rights (CESCR), *General Comment No. 14 on the right to the highest attainable standard of health*, 11 August 2000, UN Doc. E/C.12/2000/4, para. 9.

14. UN Common Learning Package on a Human Rights-Based Approach, http://www.undg.org/index.cfm?P=531.

15. See 'Question 10' in *25 Questions and Answers on health and human rights*, at 15, http://www.who.int/hhr/NEW37871OMSOK.pdf.

16. For more detailed analysis of how to operationalize a human rights-based approach to programming, see Urban Jonsson, 'Human Rights Approach to Development Programming' (UNICEF, 2003).

17. According to General Comment No. 14 discrimination is prohibited "on the grounds of race, colour, sex, language, religion, political or other opinion, national or social origin, property, birth, physical or mental disability, health status (including HIV/AIDS), sexual orientation and civil, political, social or other status".

18. See *The Lancet*, volume 367, 17 June 2006, www.thelancet.com.

19. WHO, *The Health of Indigenous Peoples*, WHO publication No. WHO/SDE/HSD/99.1, available at http://whqlibdoc.who.int/hq/1999/WHO_SDE_HSD_99.1.pdf.

20. Paragraph 27 of General Comment No. 14 specifically discusses health as it relates to indigenous peoples.

21. See 'List of Illustrative Indicators on the Right to Enjoyment of the Highest Attainable Standard of Physical and Mental Health', UN Doc. HRI/MC/2008/3, at 25.

22. See, for example, Draft Guidelines for Pharmaceutical Companies, open for consultations until 15 May 2008, http://www2.ohchr.org/english/issues/health/right/.

23. John Ruggie, Report of the Special Representative of the Secretary-General on the issue of human rights and transnational corporations and other business enterprises, 7 April 2008, UN Doc. A/HRC/8/5.

24. John Ruggie, 'Next Steps in Business and Human Rights', speech at Chatham House, London, 22 May 2008, http://www.reports-and-materials.org/Ruggie-speech-Chatham-House-22-May-2008.pdf.

25. WHO, World Health Statistics 2008: *Reducing Deaths from Tobacco* (Geneva: WHO, 2008), at 18.

26. International Council of Human Rights Policy (ICHRP), *Beyond Voluntarism: Human Rights and the Developing International Legal Obligations of Companies* (Versoix: ICHRP, 2002) http://www.ichrp.org/files/reports/7/107_report_en.pdf.

27. World Health Assembly Resolution 34.22, 21 May 1981, http://www.ibfan.org/english/resource/who/whares3422.html.

28. See WHO, '10 Facts on Breast-Feeding: Long-Term Benefits for Children', http://www.who.int/features/factfiles/breastfeeding/en/index.html.

29. Save the Children, 'Case Study 7: "Baby milk" Marketing' in Jennifer A. Zerk, *Corporate Abuse in 2007: A Discussion Paper on What Changes in the Law Need to Happen* (London: The Corporate Responsibility (COHE) Coalition, 2007), http://www.corporate-responsibility.org/module_images/corporateabuse_discussionpaper.pdf.

30. This would harmonize corporate obligations, requiring disclosure by companies of policies regarding marketing, research, lobbying and promotional activities, and provide for effective enforcement at the state level.

31. *General Comment No. 14, supra* note 13, para. 1.

32. See http://www.who.int/fctc/en/index.html.

33. Roger S. Magnusson, 'Short Report: Non-Communicable Diseases and Global Health Governance: Enhancing Global Processes to Improve Health Development' 3(2) *Globalization and Health* (2007), at 6, available at http://www.globaliza tionandhealth.com/content/3/1/2.

34. *General Comment No. 14, supra* note 13, para. 1.

35. Ibid.

36. 'WHO Wants Total Ban on Tobacco Advertising', News Release, 30 May 2008, http://www.who.int/mediacentre/news/releases/2008/pr17/en/index.html.

37. Magnusson, *supra* note 33.

38. Guideline 10, Voluntary Guidelines to Support the Progressive Realization of the Right to Adequate Food in the Context of National Food Security, Adopted by the 127th Session of the FAO Council, November 2004, http://www.fao.org/docrep/meeting/009/y9825e/y9825e00.htm.

39. Global Strategy on Diet, Physical Activity and Health, adopted by the Fifty-Seventh World Health Assembly, 22 May 2004, WHO Doc. No. WHA57.17, Operative paragraph 4(7).

40. http://www.codexalimentarius.net.

41. *EC-Biotech Products Case* (European Communities—Measures Affecting the Approval and Marketing of Biotech Products), WT/DS291, WT/DS292, WT/DS293.

42. http://www.wto.org/english/docs_e/legal_e/17-tbt.pdf.

43. Article 2.2 of the TBT Agreement.

44. Magnusson, *supra* note 33, at 11.

45. Ruggie, *supra* note 23, para. 18.

46. Human Rights Committee, *General Comment No. 6 on the right to life*, 30 April 1982, UN Doc. HRI/GEN/1/Rev.1, at para. 5.

47. See further, 'Smoking Is Not a Right Protected by Law' in *The Times*, 28 May 2008, http://business.timesonline.co.uk/tol/business/law/reports/article4015677.ece, discussing the case of *Regina (G) v Nottingham Healthcare NHS Trust; Regina (N) v Secretary of State for Health; Regina (B) v Nottingham Healthcare NHS Trust*, Queen's Bench Divisional Court.

48. ILO, 'Declaration on Fundamental Principles and Rights at Work', ILO Fact Sheet series, available at www.ilo.org/public/english/region/eurpro/budapest/download/pressrelease/european_fact_sheet_eng.pdf.

49. See WHO, 'Question 13' in *25 Questions and Answers on health and human rights*, WHO Health and Human Rights Publication Series, Issue No. 1, July 2002, at 18.

50. Richard A Daynard, Clive Bates, Neil Francey, 'Tobacco Litigation Worldwide', 320 *British Medical Journal* (2000), at 111–113.

51. European Social Charter, Article 11 on the right to protection of health, and Revised European Social Charter (which reads that among appropriate measures to be taken by the contracting parties is the provision of "advisory and educational facilities for the promotion of health and the encouragement of individual responsibility in matters of health").

52. *Soobramoney v Minister of Health (KwaZulu Natal)* CCT32/97 (1997) ZACC 17; 1998 (1) SA 765 (CC).

53. See further http://www.independent.co.uk/life-style/health-and-wellbeing/health-news/breast-cancer-drug-hailed-as-stunning-breakthrough-511695.html.

54. See, for example, 'WHO Talks Held With Members Of The Alcohol Industry', http://www.who.int/substance_abuse/openconsultalcind/en/.

QUESTIONS

1. How should public health prioritize diseases? Noncommunicable diseases do constitute a majority of what people die from, but they are a "threat" only to the people who have them (unlike communicable diseases, which threaten others). What should be done to ensure that non-communicable diseases prevention and control occupy a rightful place on public health agendas?

2. Should the age at which most people die of a disease matter in determining how many resources states should devote to the treatment and prevention of the disease? Do you think that governments should adopt a cost-effectiveness analysis for treatments based on quality-of-life adjusted years that the sick person has remaining (so-called QUALYs)? Why or why not? How could you bring cost-effectiveness and human rights arguments together to determine resource allocation in this area?

3. What is meant by a "life-style disease"? What does Nygren-Krug mean when she says, "governments must protect human rights by regulating the private sector

so that it acts in conformity with human rights"? Specifically, what can governments do about tobacco advertising and food labeling? What are the potential pitfalls of an over-regulated environment?

FURTHER READING

1. Brown, P., & Calnan, M., Political Accountability of Explicit Rationing: Legitimacy Problems Faced by NICE, *J Health Services Research Policy*, 2010; 15: 65–66.
2. Calabresi, Guido & Bobbitt, Philip, *Tragic Choices.* New York: Norton, 1978.
3. Sandel, Michael, *Justice: What's the Right Thing to Do?* New York: Farrar, Straus & Giroux, 2009.

POINT OF VIEW

Economic Globalization: A Human Rights Approach to Occupational Health

Anand Grover

In my April 2012 report to the UN Human Rights Council on the right of everyone to the enjoyment of the highest attainable standard of physical and mental health, I considered occupational health as an integral component of the right to health. My report outlines international human rights and other instruments related to occupational health, and addresses occupational health in the informal economy, focusing on the needs of vulnerable and marginalized groups. It also addresses the obligation of States to formulate, implement, monitor and evaluate occupational health laws and policies, as well as the requirement for the participation of workers at all stages of those activities. The discussion of State obligations is followed by the analysis of such occupational health issues as environmental and industrial hygiene; prevention and reduction of the working population's exposure to harmful substances; challenges posed by emerging technologies; minimization of hazards in the workplace; and availability and accessibility of occupational health services. I then elaborate on the prospective and retrospective components of accountability, as well as remedies for violations related to occupational health. The report concludes with a number of recommendations aimed at strengthening occupational health, as a component of the right to health.

Since the establishment of the International Labour Organization (ILO), the landscape of work and the relationships between workers and employers have deteriorated dramatically as a result of, amongst other things, globalization and the growth of transnational corporations. The quest for cheaper labour, particularly when skills are not requisites to employment; the growing reliance on workforce mobility both within national boundaries and across countries; and the frequent relocation of productiuon sites to meet the unabated pressures of the global market have all created new employment opportunities for some, losses of jobs for others, and a fragilized relationship between workers and employers. These phenomena have had significant impacts on the occupational health of workers. At the same time, the contemporary understanding of work has been greatly enriched by the recognition and examination of the informal economy as a persistent and substantial portion of the modern, globalized economy, and the source of work for millions of individuals. This has been cause for the re-evaluation of traditional approaches to the promotion and protection of occupational health.

As a result of economic pressure, volatility of the labour market and transient employment opportunities, a growing numbers of workers are employed in workplace environments lacking adequate protections for their occupational health. At the same time, workers in high income countries, particularly migrants and workers in emerging technologies, are exposed to workplace hazards that are inadequately regulated or outside the purview of existing occupational health regimes.

A right to health approach to occupational health is particularly critical in light of these developments. This approach requires States to intervene directly in order to fulfil their obligations towards the right to occupational health of workers in both the formal and informal economy; facilitate the direct participation of workers in the formulation, implementation, monitoring and evaluation of occupational health laws and policies; implement regulation towards the detection, prevention and treatment of occupational disease, control or prohibit of harmful substance in the work place; pay special attention to the situation of vulnerable and marginalized workers; and ensure adequate accountability mechanisms are in place and remedies are available to workers. In all of these approaches, States should focus on the most vulnerable populations and be attentive to gender differentials in occupational health hazards and coping mechanisms. To illustrate this point, women employed in the garment industry and put under heavy pressure to meet manufacturing quotas are highly exposed to extreme mental and physical stress which affect them as well as potentially members of their household. These hazards are exacerbated in the informal economy due to the lack of legal protection, formal financial services, social protection health insurance afforded to formal sector employees, exposure to harsh law enforcement, job insecurity and discrimination. Moreover, workers in the informal sector often face greater risk of occupational disease and injury than their peers working in the formal economy. As a result, informal workers are among the least secure and most vulnerable of all workers, and thus require special attention under the right

to occupational health. Approximately two-thirds of the female labour force is working in the informal economy (not including agriculture) and in less skilled jobs and with lower earnings than men. A lower employment status is often granted to migrant workers, particularly when they are undocumented and thus exposed to exploitation by employers. The resulting vulnerability to occupational ill-health of these populations is exacerbated by structural and institutional racism while social, cultural and linguistic barriers may prevent them from knowing, demanding and enjoying the legal rights they do possess.

The right to health requires that occupational health services are available, accessible, acceptable to the entire work force—formal and informal—and of good quality. The State, therefore, has an obligation to ensure that such services are put in place either through the establishment of occupational health outreach, and/or through social and health insurance that covers all workers, regardless of their employment status, level of skills, country of origin, gender or any other attribute that may result in disparity in access, exposure to occupational risks or health outcomes.

Alarmed by the gravity of the situation, I call upon States to extend existing occupational health laws and policies to cover more effectively the formal workforce and equitably extend protection to the informal workforce, including when they are employed by sub-contractors. Occupational health services must reach these two populations and include primary health care interventions that are designed to train informal workers about occupational health. A human rights-based approach to occupational health and sound public health practice must ensure the active and informed participation of workers, particularly informal workers, in the formulation and implementation of occupational health laws and policies in a fair and transparent fashion. This requires mechanisms of complaints without exposure to termination or prosecution, and remedies when abuses have been evidenced. Monitoring and evaluation processes, including Health Impact Assessments, should accompany the formulation and implementation of occupational laws and polices. The State has the obligation to ensure that its own workforce as well as those employed by the private and informal sector receive equal attention, protection and support in the workplace and that the health effects of technologies or exposure to potentially hazardous agents are accurately assessed, communicated to workers and controlled. The State has an equal obligation to establish legal and political mechanisms through which transnational corporations are held accountable for the violations of the right to occupational health, either in the host country or in the country where the corporation is domiciled. The right to occupational health should become a permanent feature of all trade agreements and prioritize the occupational health of workers over trade concerns.

Several other recommendations presented in my report provide action-oriented opportunities for change. Protecting the human right to occupational health is a question of justice, global public health, and makes economic sense. It is only when these conditions are met that the globalization of the economy can regain a human face.

This Point of View is an abridged version of the report submitted by the author to the Human Rights Council on April 12, 2012: www.ohchr.org/Documents/HRBodies/HRCouncil/RegularSession/Session20/A-HRC-20-15_en.pdf.

Anand Grover is a Senior Advocate practicing in the Supreme Court of India, the UN Special rapporteur on the Right of Everyone to the Enjoyment of the Highest Attainable Standard of Physical and Mental Health, and the founder of the Lawyers Collective in India. The Collective has been on the forefront of litigationin suppport of the right to health and other human rights, prominently as these relate to people living with HIV.

CHAPTER 40

Bias, Discrimination and Obesity

Rebecca Puhl and Kelly D. Brownell

INTRODUCTION

It has been said that obese persons are the last acceptable targets of discrimination.[1-4] Anecdotes abound about overweight individuals being ridiculed by teachers, physicians, and complete strangers in public settings, such as supermarkets, restaurants, and shopping areas. Fat jokes and derogatory portrayals of obese people in popular media are common. Overweight people tell stories of receiving poor grades in school, being denied jobs and promotions, losing the opportunity to adopt children, and more. Some who have written on the topic insist that there is a strong and consistent pattern of discrimination,[5] but no systematic review of the scientific evidence has been done.

Some anecdotes relevant to this issue have become highly visible. One reported by National Public Radio is that of Gina Score, a 14-year-old girl in South Dakota sent in the summer of 1999 to a state juvenile-detention camp.[6] Gina was characterized as sensitive and intelligent, wrote poetry, and was planning to skip a grade when she returned to school. She was sent to the facility for petty theft—stealing money from her parents and from lockers at school "to buy food." She was said to have stolen "a few dollars here, a few dollars there" and paid most of the money back.

The camp, run by a former Marine and modeled on the military, aimed, in the words of an instruction manual, to "overwhelm them with fear and anxiety." On July 21, a hot humid day, Gina was forced to begin a 2.7-mile run/walk. Gina was 5 feet 4 inches tall, weighed 224 pounds, and was unable to complete even simple physical exercises such as leg lifts. She fell behind early but was prodded and cajoled by instructors. A short time later, she collapsed on the ground panting, with pale skin and purple lips. She was babbling incoherently and frothing from the mouth, with her eyes rolled back in her head. The drill instructors sat nearby drinking sodas, laughing, and chatting, accusing Gina of faking, within 100 feet of an air-conditioned building. After 4 hours with Gina lying prostrate in the sun, a doctor came by and summoned an ambulance immediately. Gina's organs had failed and she died.

There are many more examples, from teachers weighing children in front of a class and announcing the weights, to doctors belittling patients because of their weight, to Dr. Kenneth Walker, who said in his nationally syndicated newspaper column that for their own good and the good of the country, fat people should be locked up in prison camps.[5] However, anecdotes of bias and discrimination could represent isolated events and do not prove that discrimination occurs in a systematic and widespread manner. It is important, therefore, to document whether discrimination does exist. Discrimination is harmful to its victims in many ways and can have enduring effects.[7-8] With 54% of the U.S. population now overweight and 34% obese and with the prevalence still increasing in the United States and around the world, the health and well-being of many millions of people might be affected.[9]

Perhaps the first commentary on widespread discrimination toward obese individuals was offered by Allon[10] over two decades ago. Since then, obesity is becoming increasingly recognized as a "social liability in Western society."[11] The purpose of this chapter is to examine existing literature on this topic, with special attention to areas of major importance to well-being. Legal remedies sought by obese individuals accusing institutions of discrimination will be discussed, areas in need of further research will be noted, and conclusions will be drawn about the state of this field. This chapter is organized in sections on discrimination in areas of employment, medical and health care, education, and areas we believe are in need of additional research.

There are a number of important related topics, such as theoretical models underlying stigma, psychological processes and social origins leading to discrimination of obese people, effects of this stigma on obese individuals, and possible discrimination against obese people in social relationships. All are important and require attention but will not be addressed here because systematic review would be lengthy. Our first priority is to document whether discriminatory attitudes and behaviors occur.

EMPLOYMENT SETTINGS

Hiring Prejudice

The workplace is one sphere where overweight people may be vulnerable to discriminatory attitudes and fat bias. A number of studies have investigated weight-based discrimination in employment. The results point to prejudice, insensitivity, and inequity in work settings.

Experimental studies addressing stereotypic attitudes in employers suggest that overweight people may be at a substantial disadvantage even before the interview process begins. Experimental studies have investigated hiring decisions by manipulating perceptions of employee weight, either through written description or photograph. Participants (most often college students) are randomly assigned to a condition in which a fictional job applicant is described or pictured as overweight or average weight (but with identical résumé) and are asked to evaluate the applicant's qualifications.

An example is a study using written descriptions of hypothetical managers.[12] Managers described as average weight were rated as significantly more desirable supervisors, and overweight managers were judged more harshly for undesirable behaviors (such as taking credit) than were average weight managers. Similarly, in a study by Klassen et al.,[13] women students (N 216) read employee summaries of nine fictitious women employees, varying in weight and in stereotypical descriptions associated with obesity and thinness. Participants indicated the most desire to work with thin targets and the least desire to work with obese targets, although participants did not rely on stereotypical perceptions of weight in recommending harsh discipline to employees.

A study of job applicants for sales and business positions reported that written descriptions of target applicants resulted in significantly more negative judgments for obese women than for non-obese women.[14] Participants (N 104) rated obese applicants as lacking self-discipline, having low supervisory potential, and having poor personal hygiene and professional appearance. In general, participants held these negative stereotypes for obese applicants for sales positions but not for business positions. Interestingly, the study's findings were not mirrored when photographs were used instead of written descriptions of weight. The authors proposed several confounding factors to explain this outcome, such as differing applicant information accompanying the photographs, and concluded that obese applicants remain vulnerable to negative evaluations because of their weight.[14]

Several studies have manipulated applicant weight with videotapes. This was done over two decades ago by Larkin and Pines[15] in which participants (N 120) viewed a video of a job applicant in a simulated hiring setting. The scenario involved an applicant completing written screening tests for work requiring logical analysis and eye-hand coordination. Overweight applicants were significantly less likely to be recommended for hiring than average-weight applicants, and overweight applicants were judged as significantly less neat, productive, ambitious, disciplined, and determined.[15] Another study using a simulated hiring interview for a receptionist position found that the obese applicant was less likely to be hired than the non-obese applicant.[16] This study was able to rule out the extraneous factor of facial attractiveness by masking the faces of both applicants.

A more recent and impressive study used videotaped mock interviews with the same professional actors acting as job applicants for computer and sales positions in which weight was manipulated with theatrical prostheses.[17] Subjects (N 320) indicated that employment bias was much greater for obese candidates than

for average-weight applicants; the bias was more apparent for women than for men. There was also a significant effect reported for job type; obese applicants were more likely to be recommended for a systems analyst position than for a sales position.[17] Other evidence also demonstrates employer perceptions of obese persons as unfit in public sales positions and more appropriate for telephone sales involving little face-to-face contact.[18, 19] Jasper and Klassen[20] instructed participants (N 135) to evaluate a hypothetical salesperson's résumé that included a written manipulation of the employee's weight. Obesity led to more negative impressions of the applicant and made the applicant significantly less desirable to work with. Participants who viewed the obese applicant description said directly that the obesity led to their judgments.

Excess weight may be especially disadvantageous in some settings. In a recent study of hiring preferences of overweight physical educators, most hiring personnel sampled (N 85) reported that being 10 to 20 pounds over-weight would handicap an applicant, regardless of qualifications.[21] The authors concluded, "our hope is that these findings may serve to motivate some of these individuals to improve their health behaviors and in turn become better professional role models."[21]

Inequity in Wages, Promotions, and Employment Termination

A comprehensive literature review by Roehling[22] summarizes numerous work-related stereotypes reported in over a dozen laboratory studies. Overweight employees are assumed to lack self-discipline, be lazy, less conscientious, less competent, sloppy, disagreeable, and emotionally unstable. Obese employees are also believed to think slower, have poorer attendance records, and be poor role models.[23] These stereotypes could affect wages, promotion, and termination.

There is evidence of a significant wage penalty for obese employees. This takes several forms: lower wages of obese employers for the same job performed by non-obese counterparts, fewer obese employees being hired in high-level positions, and denial of promotions to obese employees. A study of over 2,000 women and men (18 years of age and older) reported that obesity lowered wage growth rates by nearly 6% in 1982 to 1985.[24]

Although both obese men and women face wage-related obstacles, they experience discrimination in different ways. An analysis from the National Longitudinal Survey Youth Cohort examined earnings in over 8,000 men and women 18 to 25 years old and reported that obese women earned 12% less than non-obese women[25] Like studies to follow, this investigation indicated that the economic penalty of obesity seems to be specific to women. More recently, research based on earnings of 7,000 men and women from the National Longitudinal Survey of Youth indicated that women face a significant wage penalty for obesity and that obese women are much more likely than thin women to hold low-paying jobs.[26] Another longitudinal study following young adults over 8 years found that overweight women earned over $6,000 less than non-obese women.[26] Gortmaker et al.[27] and Stunkard and Sorensen[4] attribute lower wages to social bias and discrimination. Obese men do not face a similar wage penalty but are underrepresented and paid less than non-obese men in managerial and professional occupations and are over-represented in transportation occupations, suggesting that obese men engage in occupational sorting to counteract a wage penalty.[26]

Experimental research indicates that obese employees are rated to have lower promotion prospects than average weight counterparts.[28] A recent study instructed supervisors and managers (N 168) to evaluate the promotion potential of a hypothetical employee in a manufacturing company with one of eight disabilities or health problems, including obesity, poor vision, depression, colon cancer, diabetes, arm amputation, facial burns, or no disability.[29] The obese candidate received lower promotion recommendations (despite identical qualifications) than a nondisabled peer and was rated to be less accepted by subordinates than the other promotion candidates.

Little research has addressed the issue of employment benefits for obese workers. Employers may demand that overweight employees pay higher premiums for the same benefits as non-overweight employees.[23] One self-report study of 445 obese individuals found that among those 50% or more above their ideal weight, 26% indicated that they were denied benefits such as health insurance because of their weight, and 17% reported being fired or pressured to resign because of their weight.[30]

As the work by Rothblum et al.[30] suggests, some obese employees perceive that they have been fired and suspended due to their weight. Legal case findings suggest that termination against obese persons can result from prejudiced employers and arbitrary weight standards.[30] For example, in the case of *Civil Service Commission v. Pennsylvania Human Relations Commission*, a man was suspended without pay because he exceeded the required weight standards for city laborers.[31, 32] Similarly, in *Smaw v. Commonwealth of Virginia Department of State Police*, an obese state trooper of 9 years was demoted to a dispatcher position for failing a weight-loss program.[33, 34] Formal employment termination cases on the basis of weight have also reached the courts. For example, in *Nedder v. Rivier College*, a morbidly obese woman was removed from her teaching position because of her weight, and in *Gimello v.*

Agency Rent-a-Car Systems, an office manager was fired due to his obesity despite his excellent employment records and commendations of high performance.[35, 36]

Airline industry weight regulations for flight attendants have also posed problems for employees above average weight. In *Tudyman v. Southwest Airlines*, a flight attendant was terminated and his reinstatement was denied because his weight exceeded airline requirements.[37] Courts have accepted airline weight restrictions, even though most weight maximums have been arbitrarily chosen and make no exceptions for age or body frame.[38] Airlines have claimed that weight maximums are necessary for job performance and attendants' health and abilities to perform duties, although physical fitness or actual tests of job-related abilities would be more appropriate standards.[38] Flight attendants are required to be certified yearly through evaluations of their abilities, and weight policy methods for evaluation and termination are difficult to justify on grounds other than appearance.[38]

The existence of legal cases does not establish that weight discrimination occurs in great numbers, only that some employees believe that they have been treated unfairly due to weight. Courts will decide whether a legal basis exists for such claims, but additional research is needed to determine the prevalence of the problem, the people who will most likely be affected, and the consequences on the health and well-being of the people who experience discrimination. From the evidence presented here, it seems that discrimination does occur.

Summary and Methodological Limitations

There are multiple sources of evidence suggesting that discrimination against obese employees may be significant, and that certain occupations may be especially

affected. At least some obese employees may receive inequitable treatment with respect to promotions and benefits. Additional research is needed to support these preliminary findings and to provide more confident conclusions that these are indeed real-life problems. Table 40.1 presents a general summary of topics which we believe are priorities for further research.

Several methodological limitations are also evident in this research. First, studies have primarily used written description, videotapes, and self-report measures to assess whether or not an obese person would be hired, and have done less examination of real-life hiring practices. Second, many studies have failed to address possible confounds such as age, race, and gender in attempting to examine weight-related discrimination. Third, many studies have relied on college-student samples, which may not provide an adequate understanding of hiring and interviewing processes used by employers and managers. Fourth, few studies have surveyed obese employees about their discriminatory experiences. In one self-report study, 16% of obese adults (*N* 55) reported being discriminated against because of their weight, which resulted in difficulties at work and in social relationships.[39] Additional research is necessary to determine whether the prevalence of discriminatory experiences is indeed this common.

MEDICAL AND HEALTH SETTINGS

Attitudes of Medical Professionals Toward Obese Individuals

Anti-fat attitudes among health care professionals, if they exist, could potentially affect clinical judgments and deter obese persons from seeking care. A number of studies have addressed this topic. A study of over 400 physicians identified patient characteristics that aroused feelings of

Table 40.1 Summary of Research Needs to Be Addressed in Domains of Weight Discrimination

Domain	Research Needs
General methodological issues	Inclusion of obese persons in study samples. Increased use of randomized designs and ecologically valid settings. Evaluation of reliability and validity of measures assessing weight discrimination. Development of assessment methods to examine discriminatory practices.
Theoretical issues	Evaluation of predictive power among obesity-stigma models. Further exploration of why negative attitudes arise. Examination of psychological and social origins of weight prejudice. Experimental manipulation of proposed components of stigmatizing attributions. Assessment of attitudinal and behavioral expressions of weight bias. Cross-cultural examinations of anti-fat attitudes and weight-related attributions.
Legal questions	Clarification of definitions of disability and impairment relevant to obesity. Examination of legislative approaches used to counter discriminatory practices.
Employment	Increased attention to hiring, promotion, and benefits discrimination against obese employees. Closer examination of which occupations are most vulnerable to weight bias.
Health care	Experimental assessment of physician/nurse attitudes towards obese patients. Examination of how negative professional attitudes influence health care. Examination of coverage practices by insurance providers to obese individuals. Evaluation of health care costs associated with small weight losses. Address cost-effectiveness of various weight-loss treatments.
Education	Documentation of weight discrimination/bias among educators and peers. Development and testing of curricula to promote weight acceptance.
Unstudied topics	Documentation of weight discrimination in areas of public accommodations (seating in restaurants, theatres, planes, buses, trains), housing (raised rental fees for obese persons), adoption (weight-based criteria for parents), jury selection practices (biased against overweight jurors), health club memberships (raised fees for obese people), and others.
Prevention/ intervention	Identification of theoretical components to guide stigma-reduction strategies. Development and testing of stigma-reduction strategies on anti-fat attitudes. Clarification of psychological/social consequences of weight discrimination. Examination of coping strategies used by obese persons to combat aversive stigma experiences.

discomfort, reluctance, or dislike.[40] Physicians were mailed anonymous questionnaires and asked to specify five diagnostic categories and social characteristics of patients to which they responded negatively. One third of the sample listed obesity as one of these conditions, making it the fourth most common category listed (among dozens of other categories), and ranked behind only drug addiction, alcoholism, and mental illness. Physicians associated obesity and other negatively perceived conditions with poor hygiene, noncompliance, hostility, and dishonesty. The authors concluded that physicians' responses may reflect Protestant ethic values, which emphasize self-discipline, persistence in the face of adversity, and achievement—characteristics that physicians believed were low or absent in patients with conditions like obesity and alcoholism.[40] Similarly, a study of 318 family physicians using anonymous questionnaires found that two-thirds reported that their obese patients lacked self-control, and 39% stated that their obese patients were lazy.[41]

Another study examined attitudes about obese patients in health care professionals specializing in nutrition (N 52) and found that 87% believed that obese persons are indulgent, 74% believed that they have family problems, and 32% believed that they lack willpower.[42] Furthermore, 88% said that obesity was a form of compensation for lack of love or attention, and 70% attributed the cause to emotional problems.

These negative attitudes are not new. In 1969, Maddox and Liederman[43] addressed fat biases using self-report measures among 100 physicians and student clerks from a medical clinic. Obese patients were viewed as unintelligent, unsuccessful, inactive, and weak-willed. In addition, physicians indicated that they preferred not to treat overweight patients and that they did not expect success when they were responsible for their management.

Some research has also examined perceptions of nurses. A study of 586 nurses investigated beliefs about obesity and found that patient noncompliance was rated as the most likely reason for obese patients' inability to lose weight[44] and that ineffectiveness of weight loss programs as the least important reason for lack of success. Yet, the nurses reported confidence in giving weight loss advice regardless of the outcome and despite spending 10 minutes or less discussing weight loss with patients.

In a similar study, nurses agreed that obesity can be prevented by self-control (63%) and that obese persons are unsuccessful (24%), overindulgent (43%), lazy (22%), and experience unresolved anger (33%).[45] In addition, 48% of nurses agreed that they felt uncomfortable caring for obese patients, and 31% would prefer not to care for an obese patient at all.

These findings parallel another investigation of women registered nurses (N 107), where 24% of nurses agreed or strongly agreed that caring for an obese patient repulsed them, and 12% reported that they preferred not to touch an obese patient.[46] Older nurses had less favorable attitudes than younger nurses, and dissatisfaction with their own weight was positively correlated with negative stereotypes.

Only two studies have examined attitudes toward obesity among dietitians. One study of 439 registered dietitians showed ambivalent attitudes toward obese clients.[47] In contrast, a study examining attitudes among dietetic students (N 64) and registered dietitians (N 234) reported negative attitudes toward obesity among both groups.[48] This is an important area for further inquiry because dietitians are often in a position to influence patients' attitudes toward food and eating.

In addition to professionals already working in the medical field, studies have also surveyed medical students regarding their attitudes toward the obese. Blumberg and Mellis[49] reported substantial prejudice by medical students toward obese patients. On characteristics of personality, humanistic qualities, body image, and qualities related to medical management, students rated morbidly obese individuals significantly more negatively than average weight persons, who were rated neutrally or positively. Adjectives thought to apply to obese patients included worthless, unpleasant, bad, ugly, awkward, unsuccessful, and lacking self-control.[49] Negative attitudes did not change after students worked directly with obese patients during an 8-week psychiatry rotation. These results support other research documenting stigma and stereotyping among students.[50, 51]

The most recent study on practices of health professionals queried obese individuals in treatment about their experiences with physicians. The subjects were generally satisfied with their care for general health issues and their physicians' medical expertise. They were, however, significantly less satisfied with the care they received for their obesity. Nearly one-half reported that their physicians had not recommended common methods for weight loss, and 75% reported that they look to their physicians a "slight amount" or "not at all" for help with weight.[52]

Only one study has attempted to intervene by reducing stigma toward obese patients, this among medical students.[53] Before random assignment to a control group or education intervention involving videos, written materials, and role playing exercises, the majority of medical students in this study (N 75) characterized obese individuals as lazy (57%), sloppy (52%), and lacking in self-control (62%), despite indicating an accurate scientific understanding of the cause of obesity. After the educational course, students demonstrated significantly improved attitudes and beliefs about obesity compared with the control group. The effectiveness of the intervention was still supported 1 year later.

Implications of Prejudice for Health Care of Obese Persons

It is important to address the impact of negative professional attitudes on clinical judgment, diagnosis, and care for obese individuals. Several studies have indicated that obesity may influence judgments and practices of professionals. Young and Powell[54] assessed clinical judgments among mental health workers using an analog approach in which participants evaluated a case history of a patient in one of three weight conditions. The obese patient was most frequently assigned negative symptoms compared with the overweight and average weight clients and was rated more severely on a variety of dimensions of psychological functioning.[54]

A more recent investigation of over 1,200 physicians (representing specialties of family practice, internal medicine, gynecology, endocrinology, cardiology, and orthoped-

ics) indicated poor obesity management practices.[55] Physicians completed self-report surveys addressing attitudes, intervention approaches, and referral practices for obese patients. Although physicians recognized the health risks of obesity and perceived many of their patients to be overweight, they did not intervene as much as they should, were ambivalent about how to manage obese clients, and were unlikely to formally refer a client to a weight loss program. Only 18% reported that they would discuss weight management with overweight patients, which increased to 42% for mildly obese patients.

Similar results were reported by Price et al.[41] Among 318 physicians surveyed, many referred obese patients to commercial weight loss programs with questionable success. Although the majority felt obligated to treat their obese patients, 23% did not recommend treatment to any of their obese patients and 47% said that counseling patients about weight loss was inconvenient.[41]

Another study suggests that physicians may be ambivalent in treating obesity. In a sample of 211 primary care physicians, only 33% reported being centrally responsible for managing their patient's obesity, where 39% perceived their role to be cooperative to other providers.[56] Although attitudes were not reported in this study, physicians indicated that insufficient time, lack of medical training, and problems of reimbursement were difficulties in managing obesity effectively.

A final study surveying attitudes and practices of 752 general practitioners in weight management reported mixed results.[57] These physicians reported holding positive views about their roles in obesity management but underused practices that promote lifestyle changes in patients, described weight management as professionally unrewarding, and noted their most common frustrations in treating obesity were perceptions of poor patient compliance and motivation.

Negative attitudes and reluctance in physicians may lead obese persons to hesitate to seek health care,[58] although as we mention below, other factors may also contribute. In one study of physician and patient behaviors, 290 women and over 1300 physicians responded to anonymous questionnaires to determine the influence of obesity on the frequency of pelvic examinations.[59] Reluctance to have examinations increased from average weight to moderately overweight to very overweight women, where the very overweight women were significantly less likely to report annual pelvic examinations. Body image was associated with pelvic exams; 69% of women who had a positive body image vs. 55% of those who had negative body image reported obtaining examinations. Among physicians, 17% reported reluctance in providing pelvic exams to very obese women, and 83% indicated reluctance when patients were reluctant themselves. The youngest physicians were most reluctant to perform pelvic exams, and among the oldest physicians a gender difference emerged where men physicians were more reluctant to provide exams than women physicians. Considering that overweight women feel hesitant to obtain exams because of their negative body image and that physicians are reluctant to perform exams on obese or reluctant women, many overweight women may not receive necessary treatment.[59]

Two other studies have documented delay in seeking medical care by obese women. One investigation of self-reports of 310 hospital-employed women (such as nurses and nursing assistants) found that body mass index (BMI) was significantly related to appointment cancellations.[60] Over 12% of women indicated that they delayed or canceled physician appointments due to weight concerns, and of the 33% of women who had discussed weight with their physicians, discussions were described as negative.[60] In addition, 32% of women with a BMI > 27 kg/m², and 55% of those with a BMI over 35 kg/m² delayed or canceled visits because they knew they would be weighed; the most common response for delaying appointments was embarrassment about weight.[60]

Another recent self-report study of women (N 6891) included in the 1992 National Health Interview Survey reported that increased BMI was associated with decreased preventive health care services.[61] Obese women were significantly more likely than non-obese women to delay breast examinations, gynecologic examinations, and papanicoloau smears, despite an increase in physician visits as BMI increased. The authors concluded that even when obese women have more frequent physician appointments, they seem least likely to use preventive services.[61]

Most available studies have assessed physician attitudes and beliefs, which may or may not affect their practice, and, other health care professionals have not been studied in detail. Research has failed to account for the fact that obese patients may delay or cancel medical appointments for a variety of reasons, such as anxiety about being weighed or disrobing regardless of how supportive health care professionals may be. Still, it is clear that health professionals share general cultural anti-fat attitudes. Considering that bias affects many of the ways individuals interact with stigmatized groups, it would be surprising if medical practices were immune.

The hope is that care for obese individuals will improve as bias decreases. Some health care professionals perceive obesity to be a social problem and systematically avoid it in their practices[62] For those who consent to treat obese patients, removing prejudice and blame may be crucial. As Yanovski[63] notes, "The primary care physician who provides sensitive and compassionate care for severely obese patients without denigrating them for their inability to lose weight performs a much needed service." Other suggested changes include recognition of obesity as a chronic medical condition, improved knowledge of nutrition and multidisciplinary treatments, familiarity with community resources, creating more accessible environments for obese persons by providing armless chairs and larger examination gowns, and treating patients with respect and support.[63, 64]

INSURANCE AND HEALTH CARE COST OBSTACLES

Controversies in Coverage for Obesity

Treatment and prevention have seldom been emphasized by insurance providers, despite spiraling health care costs attributed to obesity. With more Americans overweight, obesity has become a leading cause of preventable death.[65] Direct costs associated with obesity represent 6% to 7% of the National Health Expenditure;[66, 67] 99.2 billion dollars were attributed to obesity in 1995, of which 51.6 billion dollars were direct medical costs.[67]

A study examining the 25-year health care costs for overweight women over age 40 years using an incidence-based analysis, predicted that 16 billion dollars will be spent in the next 25 years treating overweight middle-aged women alone.[68] Other investigations have suggested a relationship between BMI and health care expenditures. In one study, medical and health care use records of obese women (N 83) belonging to a health maintenance organization were compared with records of non-obese women.[69] As BMI increased, so did the number of medical diagnoses and the use of health care resources. In another analysis of employees of 298 companies

(N 8822), obesity was directly and significantly related to higher health care costs (an 8% higher cost), even when adjusting for age, sex, and a number of chronic conditions.[70] A longitudinal observational of obese individuals (N 383) covered by the same insurance plan reported that the probability of health care expenditures increased at BMI extremes.[71]

A study of over 17,000 respondents to a 1993 health survey reported a strong association between BMI and total inpatient and outpatient costs.[66] Compared with individuals with a BMI of 20 to 24.9 kg/m², there was a 25% to 44% increase in annual costs in moderately and severely overweight people, adjusted for age and sex. Wolf and Colditz[67] reported an 88% increase in the number of physician appointments attributed to obesity from 1988 to 1994, and a total of 62.6 million obesity-related physician visits in 1994. A recent review of the scant literature on access to and usage of health care services suggests that obese persons use medical care services more frequently than do non-obese people and that they tend to pay higher prices for these services.[72]

Beliefs that obesity treatment is unsuccessful and too costly have been challenged.[73] Weight losses as small as 10% are associated with substantially reduced health care costs, reduced incidence of obesity-related comorbid conditions, and increased lifetime expectancy.[73, 74] Recent research has addressed the cost-effectiveness of drug treatments and surgery for obesity. In 1999 Greenway et al.[75] found that weight losses produced by medications (fenfluramine with mazindol or phentermine) reduced costs more than standard treatment of comorbid conditions. Gastric bypass surgery has demonstrated even more impressive effects, with lower costs and greater long-term weight loss maintenance in comparison to low-calorie diets and behavior modification,[76] as well as significant reductions in BMI, incidence of hypertension, hyperinsulinemia, hypertriglyceridemia, and hypo-high density lipoprotein cholesterolemia, and sick days from work compared with matched controls.[77, 78]

Current Coverage Practices

Even with some evidence of cost-savings for some weight-loss methods, medical coverage is inconsistent. Surgical treatment is often not reimbursed even though diseases with less supported treatments are compensated.[79] Some have explicitly pointed to prejudice against obesity surgery by insurance providers who are preventing its broader acceptance and use in practices.[80] As Frank[81] concludes, "... no claim to justify the denial of benefits for the treatment of obesity has any validity when held to the standards of health insurance otherwise available in the United States. It should be obvious that such a judgment is ethically unconscionable."

It is typical for health insurance plans to explicitly exclude obesity treatment for coverage.[82] Physicians often have difficulties receiving reimbursement for their services.[79] Many reimbursement systems do not categorize obesity as a disease, leading physicians to report comorbid disorders as the reason for their services.[79]

In 1998, the Internal Revenue Service excluded weight-loss programs as a medical deduction, even when prescribed by a doctor. In response, several organizations such as the American Obesity Association[83] filed petitions for a ruling to allow the costs of obesity treatment to be included as a medical deduction. As of 2000, the Internal Revenue Service policy changed its criteria, allowing costs for weight-loss treatments to be deducted by taxpayers for certain treatment programs under a physician's direction to treat a specific disease.[84]

The Social Security Administration has eliminated obesity from its list of impairments, which is used to determine eligibility for disability payments.[65] Because individuals who receive social security disability benefits are also eligible for Medicare after 2 years, those who are denied disability also forgo opportunities for medical coverage.[65]

Although few studies have addressed this issue, a recent cross-sectional analysis of third-party payer reimbursement for weight management for obese children reported low reimbursement rates.[85] Despite the medical necessity of weight management for obese children in the study, no reimbursement was given to 35% of the children enrolled in weight-management programs, and no association existed between the severity of obesity and the reimbursement rate.[85]

Although this chapter does not intend to examine all of the potential factors that may underlie these coverage policies, one likely contributor are perceptions that obesity is a problem of willful behavior and that treatment is unsuccessful and expensive.[81] Although health insurance typically covers treatment for substance abuse and sexually transmitted diseases, which are also considered to be problems of willful behavior, obese persons may not receive the services they need.[81]

Denying obese people access to treatment may have medical consequences, but also denies people an opportunity to lose weight, which itself may reduce exposure to bias and discrimination. For example, Rand and MacGregor[58] assessed perceptions of discrimination among morbidly obese patients (N 57) before and after weight-loss surgery. Before their operations, 87% of patients reported that their weight prevented them from being hired for a job, 90% reported anti-fat attitudes from co-workers, 84% avoided being in public because of their weight, and 77% felt depressed on a daily basis. Fourteen months after surgery, every patient reported reduced discrimination, 87% to 100% of patients reported that they rarely or never perceived prejudice or discrimination, and 90% reported feeling cheerful and confident almost daily. A further study indicated that 59% of patients requested surgery for social reasons such as embarrassment, and only 10% for medical reasons.[86] After the operation, patients reported improved interpersonal functioning (51%), improved occupational functioning (36%), and more positive changes in leisure activities (64%). Although these studies are based on self-reports from selected samples and, therefore, have limitations, it is interesting to note the dramatic reduction in postsurgical perceptions of prejudice and discrimination, and the power of social perceptions in motivating surgery decisions.

Summary and Methodological Limitations

A "fat is bad" stereotype exists in the medical field.[87] Further study is needed to test the degree to which this affects practice. It seems that obese persons as a group avoid seeking medical care because of their weight. One barrier to drawing further conclusions, however, is that much of the research relies on self-report measures of variable reliability and validity. There is a need to move beyond reports of attitudes to actual health care practices.

EDUCATIONAL SETTINGS

Peers in the School Environment

Peer rejection may be an overweight individual's first challenge in educational settings. Anecdotes have been noted where harsh treatment from peers has resulted in suicide.[88, 89] Such anecdotes are extreme, but research does show substantial rejection of obese children by peers at school. An often cited example is a study conducted in the early 1960s in which children in public school and summer camp settings (N 600) ranked six pictures of children varying in physical characteristics and disabilities in order of who they would like most for a friend.[90] The majority of children ranked a picture of an obese child last among children with crutches, in a wheelchair, with an amputated hand, and with a facial disfigurement. A recent replication of this study among fifth- and sixth-grade students (N 458) reported that the strongest bias was against the obese child and that there was an increase in prejudice against the obese child compared with the findings from 40 years earlier.[91]

Other recent studies showing photographs of obese and non-obese persons to schoolchildren showed negative stereotypes and suggested that bias is formed by 8 years of age.[92] Some work shows anti-fat attitudes in 3-year-old pre-schoolchildren.[93] Research addressing children's attitudes toward thinness and ideal body size indicate the same trend. One study of fourth-grade children (N 817) found that 49% of girls and 30% of boys chose ideal figures thinner than themselves when shown a number of different body types.[94] Only 10% of boys and 11% of girls selected an ideal body size larger than their own.

Other work has demonstrated that children in grades four through six endorse negative stereotypes for both obese children and adults, and regardless of the child's own weight, age, and gender.[95] Children reported that they believed that obesity was under personal control; this belief was positively related with negative stereotyping. Another study examined knowledge about obesity among third and sixth graders who were randomly assigned to watch a videotape of a peer who was average weight, obese, or obese with a medical explanation for the obesity.[96] Obese children received the most negative judgments, and although children attributed less blame to the obese child with the medical explanation, this knowledge did not improve attitudes among children toward obese peers. This parallels findings from a study attempting to change negative attitudes about obesity among undergraduate students where an increase in knowledge did not alter attitudes.[97] Authors of both studies,[96, 97] concluded that more powerful means are necessary to foster positive attitude changes toward obese individuals. For children, this might involve broad educational approaches to increase weight tolerance, which reduced teasing toward overweight peers and increased acceptance of diverse body types among fifth-grade students in a recent study.[98]

One study assessed personal descriptions of perceived stigmatization among overweight adolescent girls.[99] Ninety-six percent reported negative experiences because of their weight, the most frequent being hurtful comments such as weight-related teasing, jokes, and derogatory names. Peers were the most common critics and school was the most common venue. Many reported being teased continually about their weight throughout elementary school, middle school, and high school and indicated that they had not yet learned how to cope with stigmatizing encounters with peers. Some research has examined the long-term impact of weight-based teasing in a clinical sample of obese women and found that more frequent teasing during childhood and adolescence was related to more negative self-perceptions of attractiveness and greater body dissatisfaction in adulthood.[100]

The psychological and social consequences of these experiences have been addressed in the literature for many years.[101–103] Although obese pre-school children seem to have similar levels of self-esteem as non-obese pre-schoolers,[104] this drastically changes once children begin school. A study of children 9 to 11 years of age (*N* 67) reported that clinically overweight children had significantly lower self-esteem than non-overweight children.[105] Self-esteem was lowest among overweight children who believed that they were responsible for their over-weight and who believed that weight was the reason for few friends and exclusion from games and sports. In addition, 91% of the overweight children felt ashamed of being fat, 90% believed that teasing and humiliation from peers would stop if they lost weight, and 69% believed that they would have more friends if they lost weight.[98] These findings parallel other reports of low self-esteem and poor social and athletic competence among obese children 9 to 12 years of age.[106–107]

Weight Stigmatization in High School and College

In addition to continued endorsement by college students of negative stereotypes about obese individuals as lazy, self-indulgent, and even sexually unskilled and unresponsive,[108, 109] weight stigmatization can be more overt at higher levels of education. There are reports of overweight students receiving poor evaluations and poor college acceptances and facing dismissal due to their weight.[5, 110] Most studies have addressed these issues at the college level. Canning and Mayer[111] examined school records and college applications of high school students and found that obese students were significantly less likely to be accepted to college despite having equivalent application rates and academic performance to non-obese peers. Moreover, obese women were accepted less frequently (31%) than were obese men (42%).

Crandall[112] examined reasons for the lower college acceptance of obese women. In studies assessing issues of weight, financial aid, and college income among undergraduate students (*N* 833), a reliable relationship emerged between BMI and financial support for education. Normal-weight students received more family financial support for college than over-weight students, who depended more on financial aid and jobs; this effect was especially pronounced for women. Differences in family support remained despite controlling for parental education, income, ethnicity, and family size.

In a study of overweight women, Crandall[113] again demonstrated parental bias. High school seniors (N 3386) completed questionnaires about their weight, college aspirations, financial support, grades, and parental political attitudes. Both overweight men and women were underrepresented in those who attend college, and overweight women were least likely to receive financial support from families. Politically conservative attitudes of parents predicted who paid for college, where conservative ideological attitudes among parents (characterized by values of self-discipline and the tendency to perceive people as responsible for their own fate), were positively correlated with BMI of students. Crandall[114] theorized elsewhere that anti-fat attitudes are related to Protestant work ethic values of self-determination and the ideology that people deserve what they get. Thus, individuals with such ideological beliefs may be more likely blame their obese children for their weight.[114]

There have been celebrated cases of obese students being dismissed from college because of their weight; one reached the U.S. Supreme Court. In 1985 an obese nursing student named Sharon Russell was dismissed from Salve Regina College 1 year before obtaining her nursing degree for failing to lose weight.[110, 115, 116] Although the school did not object to Russell's obesity at admission to the program, her weight became an issue of public scrutiny and harassment by students and faculty.[110] Russell demonstrated good academic performance

in her courses, though in her junior year she received a failing grade in one course (which was determined to be the result of her weight and not her academic performance).[110] Instead of expulsion, Russell was asked to sign a contract agreeing that she could remain if she lost 2 lb/wk. A year later and several credits shy of her degree, Russell was dismissed from the school for her inability to lose weight.[115]

Once successfully obtaining her degree at another college and obtaining her nursing license, Russell sued her previous college for wrongful dismissal, intentional infliction of emotional distress, and discrimination in violation of the Rehabilitation Act.[115] Six years later she was granted monetary damages and the case was concluded.[117] In a nursing journal, Weiler and Helmes[110] noted, ". . . what should be particularly troublesome for nurse educators, is that the nursing profession prides itself on providing caring and compassionate treatment for all patients, yet in this case it failed to extend this same sensitivity to a future colleague."

It is possible that negative attitudes by educators toward obesity are more widespread than has been documented. Solovay[5] notes, "Many fat kids exist on a diet of shame and self-hatred fed to them by their teachers." One study reported that junior and senior high school teachers and school health care workers (N 115) believed that obesity was primarily under individual control.[118] Although approximately one-half of the teachers did recognize biological factors in the etiology of obesity, teachers agreed that obese persons are untidy (20%), more emotional (19%), less likely to succeed at work (17.5%), and more likely to have family problems (27%). Forty-six percent agreed that obese persons are undesirable marriage partners for non-obese people, and fully 28% agreed that becoming obese is one of the worst things that could happen to a person.[118]

These findings support the 1994 Report on Discrimination Due to Physical Size by the National Education Association, which stated that "for fat students, the school experience is one of ongoing prejudice, unnoticed discrimination, and almost constant harassment" and that "from nursery school through college, fat students experience ostracism, discouragement, and sometimes violence."[119]

Summary and Methodological Limitations

Rejection, harassment, and stigmatization of obese children at school is an important social problem. The severity and frequency of this treatment by peers and teachers is disturbing, but, again, the literature must be strengthened to understand the entire picture. Self-reports are the most common method used. It is essential to collect both peer ratings and teacher ratings and to conduct behavioral observations in the classroom and schoolyard. College admission data are old, so it is necessary to determine the extent to which discriminatory practices now occur. Finally, some reports are anecdotal. Anecdotes can lead to needed research but do not prove discrimination.

UNDERSTUDIED DOMAINS OF POTENTIAL OBESITY DISCRIMINATION

Public Accommodations

Obese individuals can experience problems in public settings, such as restaurants, theaters, airplanes, buses, and trains because of inadequate seat size and inadequate sizes of features such as seat belts. Although no research has documented the extent of these problems and few litigated cases exist, a recent law review highlights several legal cases that may signal growing concern.[3]

In the case of *Sellick v. Denny's Inc.*, an obese man sued Denny's restaurants for inadequate seating.[3, 120] His claim was dismissed, although negotiations between the National Association for the Advancement of Fat Acceptance (NAAFA) and Denny's restaurants led Denny's to agree to make bigger seats.[3] In *Birdwell v. Carmike Cinemas*, an obese woman filed suit against a national theater chain for unequal access.[121] Birdwell knew that she could not fit in the theater seats and requested to bring her own chair to sit in the row for disabled individuals. Her request was accepted, but when Birdwell arrived at the theater, she was told her chair would create a safety hazard.[3] This case was settled out of court.

Transportation services have also received similar complaints. In the case of *Hollowich v. Southwest Airlines*, an obese woman waiting to board a flight was told that she had to buy an additional seat and that she would be escorted off the plane by armed guards if she boarded.[122] She sued the airline for intentionally inflicting emotional distress and discrimination against a disabled person.[3] Similarly, in *Green v. Greyhound*, an obese woman was told to leave the bus because her weight necessitated two seats.[123] After refusing to leave, she was arrested, although the charge of disorderly conduct was dropped and she instead sued Greyhound for emotional distress.[3]

Current conditions are consistent with social attitudes that obese people take up more space than they deserve.[3] O'Hara[3] notes that airlines accommodate seating for individuals with wheelchairs and for pregnant women, but obese people are expected to purchase two seats.

Jury Selection

Jury selection is another area needing research. When choosing a jury, attorneys are provided peremptory challenges, allowing them to dismiss potential jurors for unstated reasons. Jurors can be dismissed for displaying bias, although attorneys must state their reasons for doing so.[5] Although courts have not formally recognized this, obese persons can be dismissed as jurors because of their weight, and attorneys may be able to mask other types of racial or gender discrimination through peremptory challenges against obese individuals.[5]

With the negative attributions applied to obese persons (e.g., lazy and stupid), systematic exclusion of jurors is possible. The lack of representation of obese individuals in juries would mean the absence of a large segment of the population in the justice system and potentially biased cases where obesity is a central or even peripheral issue.

Housing

One small study suggests that weight discrimination may exist for obese tenants seeking apartment rentals.[124] Obese and non-obese student confederates each visited 11 available rental units, pretending to be seeking each apartment for rent. All 11 landlords offered the units to the non-obese confederate, but 5 landlords would not rent to the obese confederate.[124] Three of these five actually increased the rental price with the obese confederate.[124] Because this study is both dated and limited in its small sample, additional research replicating these findings would be valuable and could broaden the present insufficient knowledge of this potentially discriminatory issue.

Adoption

Obesity could potentially be a basis for denying individuals the right to adopt a child. This issue has not been addressed in research, but several countries outside of North America may be using parental weight criteria in adoption procedures.[125] Anecdotal evidence suggests that this may occur in the United States, where obese women have reported being turned down by adoption agencies and told that they would be unfit mothers due to their weight.[58]

NAAFA believes that weight discrimination in private American adoption agencies is a reality and has formulated an official position advocating equal access to adoption services for obese individuals and couples.[126] NAAFA has resolved to improve education about size discrimination in adoption, provide support to obese individuals facing such discrimination, and assist plaintiffs in litigation.[126] Because the issue has not been studied, research documenting whether this discrimination exists is important.

Research

It is critical that research itself not exclude obese persons. Overweight people have been underrepresented in research unless studies have focused on obesity.[5] As an example, the National Institute of Health funded the Women's Health Initiative for over 600 million dollars to investigate cancer, heart disease, and osteoporosis in women. Although tens of thousands of women are participating in this longitudinal study, and despite overweight women having increased vulnerability for some of the diseases being investigated, the study excluded obese women.[5, 127]

Limitations of Existing Research

Laboratory studies addressing discriminatory attitudes and behaviors rely primarily on student samples, so generalization must be examined. Second, most studies on anti-fat attitudes among medical, educational, and hiring professionals have used nonrandom designs, self-report methods, and a variety of attitudinal assessment measures that may not have been tested for validity and reliability. Third, the literature is not sufficiently large or mature to draw conclusions across all areas in which discrimination has been claimed. For instance, there are hints but not documentation of obese individuals being denied children in adoption proceedings, the assumption being that weight reflects personal failings that would make people unfit parents. Finally, it is not clear whether the severity and frequency of discrimination increases as an individual becomes more obese.

Many theoretical questions about weight stigma have yet to be studied. Although a few preliminary models have been proposed, theories have not been compared and there is no consensus of which factors best predict who will stigmatize obese people. Despite evidence of various cultural attributions toward obesity throughout history, there is also a need to examine the cultural factors that affect this population.[128] As research better documents weight discrimination, conceptual frameworks for understanding weight stigma can be refined, and hypotheses can be increasingly guided by theory. Ultimately, the integration of theory and empirical studies should be used to derive stigma reduction strategies and interventions to eliminate discrimination.

LEGAL CHALLENGES TO WEIGHT-BASED DISCRIMINATION

Current Weight-Specific Legislation

No federal laws exist to prohibit discrimination against obese individuals, and only Michigan's civil rights legislation prohibits employment discrimination on the basis of weight at the state level.[34] The District of Columbia forbids discrimination on the basis of appearance including weight, and Santa Cruz, California includes weight in its definition of unlawful discrimination.[129] In the spring of 2000, San Francisco passed legislation to ban weight discrimination, adding weight and height to existing characteristics (such as gender, ethnicity, age, and sexual orientation) that are protected.[130] Advocates in San Francisco gained support for this legislation when a health club created a billboard with a space alien saying, "When they come, they'll eat the fat ones first." Overall, few locations have weight-specific legislation, so most obese persons are forced to use existing human rights statutes for legal protection. In particular, overweight individuals have depended on the Rehabilitation Act (RA) of 1973 and the American Disabilities Act (ADA) of 1990.[131] Employment discrimination cases encompass the vast majority of such actions.

The RA was the first effort to prohibit federal employee discrimination against individuals with disabilities.[32] A person with a disability is one who has a physical or mental impairment that substantially limits at least one major life activity (activities such as walking, breathing, self-care, and working), has a record of such an impairment, or is perceived as having an impairment.[34, 129] The RA does not actually include obesity as a specific protected impairment.[32]

The ADA expanded federal disability discrimination legislation by extending mandates to private employers, state and local employment agencies, and labor unions.[23, 131] Like the RA, the ADA protects disabled but qualified employees who can perform essential aspects of employment.[131] The Equal Employment Opportunity Commission (EEOC) implemented regulations for more flexible interpretation of ADA impairments, allowing obesity to be included in its broader definitions.[129, 132] The guidelines of the EEOC do not consider obesity alone to be an impairment. However, obesity can meet impairment definitions if one's weight can be attributed to or results in a physiological disorder, or if a person's weight is severe as in cases of morbid obesity.[132]

Under the ADA two kinds of cases can be pursued: those involving actual disabilities, and those of perceived disabilities. An actual disability claim requires that an individual's obesity be substantially limiting in at least one major life activity. A perceived disability occurs when one is regarded by others as having an impairment.[131] Here, the obese individual must demonstrate either an actual impairment that does not limit life activities but is perceived to be limiting by others or that there is no impairment at all but that the individual is perceived as having one. As many courts do not recognize obesity as an actual impairment, obese individuals must often use perceived impairment claims.[131]

Inconsistent Rulings

Although alleged discrimination is being met with lawsuits, the overall picture of cases pursued under these statutes is one of mixed results. The majority of courts have ruled that obesity, per se, is not a disability.[32] In *Krein v. Marian Manor Nursing Home*, for instance, an obese nurse's aid was discharged because of her weight. The court held that her obesity was not a disability and, thus, was inadequate to qualify the plaintiff for discrimination protection.[131, 133] Similar court rulings were held for a flight attendant in *Tudyman v. Southwest Airlines* and for a labor worker *in Civil Service Commission v. Pennsylvania Human Relations Commission*, where both plaintiffs failed to show that their obesity caused, or was caused by, a condition that would qualify them for state protection.[31, 37]

Later cases continue to follow this trend. In *Cassista v. Community Foods Inc.*, an obese woman was denied a cashier/stocking position because of her weight.[131, 134] In the case of *Philadelphia*

Electric Co. v. Pennsylvania Human Relations Commissions, an obese woman was refused employment in a customer service position due to her obesity, despite having passed pre-employment evaluation. The court ruled that her obesity did not impair her job performance and, thus, could not constitute a disability and receive protection.[37, 135]

Although few cases have held that obesity on its own constitutes a disability, several court rulings have demonstrated circumstances in which obese plaintiffs have been successful. In the case of *New York Division of Human Rights v. Xerox Corporation*, an obese plaintiff was denied a computer programming position because her obesity made her medically unsuitable for the job, according to the company's physician.[32, 136] The state court recognized broader definitions of disability under New York law and ruled that her obesity was an impairment as defined by Xerox's medical staff, although she had no other medical conditions and could perform the duties of the position.[32, 37] In the case of *King v. Frank*, a postal worker alleged that he was fired because his supervisor perceived his obesity to be an impairment.[137] The commission ruled that because the employer perceived the worker to be substantially limited in work (one of the major life activities of the RA), he was granted protection under the RA.[32] Finally, the case of *Gimello v. Agency Rent-a-Car Systems* also accepted a disability claim in which the court concluded that the plaintiff's obesity was a physical disability because he had sought medical treatment for his condition.[36]

Unresolved Issues: Blame and Disability

The legal issue of whether obesity is a disability has not been decided. Very obese persons or individuals whose obesity is attributed to an underlying medical condition may have the most success under the ADA,[131] but it is difficult to predict which cases will be successful. Court decisions of whether obesity is an impairment may be the result of many factors besides ADA guidelines, such as court beliefs, cultural perceptions, academic views, previous case rulings, and weight bias in judges.

Inconsistent court decisions will likely continue until ambiguities in existing legislation are resolved. Under the ADA there is no standard for determining how obese a person must be for weight to be considered a disability.[37, 132] Being moderately fat will only be considered a disability if accompanied by an additional impairment, whereas obesity on its own does not meet ADA impairment definitions. Morbid obesity can meet disability requirements. Korn[138] notes that limiting the protection of the ADA to morbid obesity ignores the majority of the obese population and reinforces misperceptions that anything less than morbid obesity can be personally controlled.

Courts have generally viewed overweight as voluntary and mutable and, therefore, have disqualified it as a disability.[131, 138] The ADA does not actually require a condition to be immutable or involuntary to be considered a disability.[32] The RA and ADA protect other mutable conditions like alcoholism, drug addiction, and acquired immune deficiency syndrome, all of which involve voluntary behavior.[32] Although the EEOC states that being voluntary is irrelevant in the definition of impairment, the fact that obesity is rarely considered an impairment without an underlying medical condition suggests that the EEOC sees obesity as controllable.[138]

Another unsettled issue is the applicability of the perceived disability theory. Because courts are unlikely to accept obesity as an impairment, overweight persons can stand on this section of the law. Yet successfully applying this theory to obese individuals may be unlikely, because the plaintiff must prove that the employer perceived weight to be an impairment, not just that the employee was perceived to be overweight.[131]

Legal pursuits are not necessarily easier for obese individuals proceeding under actual disability claims. Successfully proving that one's condition substantially limits a major life activity does not necessarily satisfy legal requirements. Both the ADA and RA can deny protection even if one's obesity does impair life activities.[34] The obese plaintiff must also prove that he or she can satisfy the essential functions of the position, and those who cannot perform job duties with or without reasonable accommodation will not be protected.[34]

Whether it is advantageous for obesity to be considered a disability is a matter of debate. Despite the legal advantages of the disability label, considering obese persons disabled may have unwanted ramifications. For example, it may be undesirable for overweight children to consider themselves "disabled." Because weight is a disabling condition in only a minority of cases, it may be harmful to attach a disability label to a condition already severely stigmatized.

A key problem is that existing statutes were not intended to protect against weight discrimination.[129] Categorizing discrimination claims under current disability definitions makes less sense than finding other strategies to fight weight discrimination. Several suggestions have proposed revising the ADA. One option may be to change definitions of disability in the ADA to explicitly include obesity.[37, 138] Doing this would allow individuals uniform protection for having limiting conditions due to obesity, although this option would also mean attaching a disability label.[37] Others have concluded that the EEOC should declare issues of voluntariness and mutability as irrelevant to decisions determining impairment and enforce that they be excluded.[131]

An alternative is to create new legal options for obese employees other than the RA and ADA. Adamitis[129] suggests that the most appropriate alternatives are state and local laws for protection from weight discrimination. It may be more realistic to consider state statutes, which often provide broader coverage, than to focus on federal laws.[129] As mentioned earlier, legal cases prove only that discrimination based on weight is perceived and that legal justification for seeking relief is growing. One cannot infer that discrimination is widespread from such cases. Prevalence studies are necessary.

DISCUSSION

There is a clear and consistent scientific literature showing pervasive bias against overweight people. It is logical that the bias begets discrimination. There is now sufficient evidence of discrimination to suggest it may be powerful and occurs across important areas of living.

Studies on employment have shown hiring prejudice in laboratory studies. Subjects report being less inclined to hire an overweight person than a thin person, even with identical qualifications. Individuals make negative inferences about obese persons in the workplace, feeling that such people are lazy, lack self-discipline, and are less competent. One might expect these attributions to affect wages, promotions, and disciplinary actions, and such seems to be the case.

Overweight women, for the same work, receive less pay than their thin counterparts. This does not seem to be the case for men, but overweight men sort themselves into lower-level jobs. There is evidence that promotion prospects are dimmer for overweight individuals, and there are many examples of people being fired on account of excess weight. Rarely would the physical demands of the job make weight an issue.

Health care is another arena in which biased attitudes are an issue. Very negative attitudes about overweight individuals have been reported in physicians, nurses, and medical students, much the same as in general society. Overweight individuals can be reluctant to seek medical care, especially for their obesity, because they believe that they will be scolded and even humiliated, hence screening and treatment for diseases may be delayed. It is important to know whether the bias seen in health care professionals affects the quality of care that they provide.

Stigmatization in educational settings seems to take place at all ages. From teasing of obese children to college acceptance, an overweight individual faces serious challenges. We would expect this to affect self-esteem, intellectual self-efficacy, and very tangible outcomes like where one attends college and employment opportunities. One telling study found that parents of overweight children provided them less support for college than parents did for their thin children.[113] It is strong prejudice indeed when parents discriminate against their own children.

Individuals believing that they have been victims of discrimination have sought legal relief, typically by asking that obesity be considered a disability, thereby protecting those affected under the ADA. This has been successful in some cases but raises questions about whether it is desirable for obese persons to be considered disabled. We believe that legislation, similar to what was passed in 2000 by the city of San Francisco, that prohibits discrimination based on weight, is the most direct and logical approach. Except for the rare cases in which excess weight makes it impossible for a person to perform a job, overweight individuals deserve the same access to employment possibilities as do thin people and deserve to earn as much for their work.

Discriminatory attitudes as powerful and consistent as these belie fundamental stigma, bias, and prejudice. These in turn are determined by beliefs that individuals and society have about obese people. These beliefs, it seems, are the confluence of several factors. First, overweight people are assumed to have multiple negative characteristics, ranging from flaws in personal effort (being lazy), to more core matters such as intelligence and being a good or bad person.[139] Second, overweight individuals are believed to be responsible for their condition and that an imperfect body reflects an imperfect person.[140] Finally, whatever bad comes from the bias and discrimination is acceptable, even merited, based on the common belief that people get what they deserve and deserve what they get. In cases where explicit attitude measures show little or no bias, implicit measures show significant bias, even in health professionals who specialize in the treatment of obese persons.[141] Further research on the origins of weight stigma and methods for countering the negative attitudes is important to foster.

It is important to know whether the increasing prevalence of obesity will lead to more or less discrimination. The two have not been tracked in tandem. Latner and Stunkard[91] suggested that prejudice has increased over the past several decades. One might also guess that more people being obese will reduce societal biases because more people will become victims of stigma and awareness of inequity will increase.

Certainly more work is needed to understand fully the degree and consequences of stigmatization against obese persons. Table 1 outlines areas of research that we believe are necessary directions in which to take these efforts. In general, we believe that there are several compelling directions to move, in research, education, and policy:

1. Methodological and theoretical gaps in the literature require attention. Necessary improvements in methodology include the use of random assignment, evaluation of reliability and validity of measures used to assess weight discrimination, and the generalization of studies across segments of the population. A second priority for research is to better understand why and how such negative attitudes arise toward obese people and then to develop conceptual frameworks for understanding the stigma.

2. The extent to which discriminatory attitudes become acts of discrimination and the processes by which this occurs, must be better understood.

3. A great number of important research questions must be addressed. The areas of living in which discrimination occurs must be documented, the psychological and social origins of the discrimination must be better understood, and the consequences of the discrimination must be clarified. Subtle forms of discrimination affecting daily life, such as body language and eye contact, should be studied.

4. Means must be developed and tested to temper society's negative attitudes. Vast numbers of people stand to be affected by weight discrimination, with the numbers growing steadily.

5. Attention must be paid to the social action, legal, and legislative approaches that might best be used to counter discriminatory practices. Considering obesity a disability is one possible approach using existing laws, but the legal relief achieved by selected individuals may be more than offset with the social liability of obese persons being considered disabled. Legislation directly addressing weight discrimination might be more beneficial.

In summary, discrimination against obese individuals is very real. It occurs in key areas affecting health and well-being. Although all important research questions have not yet been addressed, there is a sufficient body of information to justify aggressive treatment of this topic in research, legal settings, and the real world.

REFERENCES

1. Falkner NH, French SA, Jeffery RW, Neumark-Sztainer D, Sherwood NE, Morton N. Mistreatment due to weight: prevalence and sources of perceived mistreatment in women and men. *Obes Res.* 1999; 7:572–6.
2. Kilbourne J. Still killing us softly: advertising and the obsession with thinness. In: Fallon P, Katzman MA, Wooley SC, eds. *Feminist Perspectives on Eating Disorders.* New York, NY: Guilford Press; 1994, pp. 395–418.
3. O'Hara MD. Please weight to be seated: recognizing obesity as a disability to prevent discrimination in public accommodations. *Whittier Law Rev.* 1996; 17:895–954.
4. Stunkard AJ, Sorensen TI. Obesity and socioeconomic status: a complex relation. *N Engl J Med.* 1993; 329:1036–7.
5. Solovay S. *Tipping the Scales of Injustice: Fighting Weight-Based Discrimination.* Amherst, NY: Prometheus Books; 2000.
6. National Public Radio. Jailhouse abuse, 2000. http://search.npr.org/cf/cmn/cmnps05fm.cfm?SegID76587.
7. Kessler RC, Mickelson KD, Williams DR. The prevalence, distribution, and mental health correlates of perceived discrimination in the United States. *J Health Soc Behav.* 1999; 40:208–30.
8. Perlmutter P. *Legacy of Hate: A Short History of Ethnic, Religious, and Racial Prejudice in America.* New York, NY: M. E. Sharpe; 1999.
9. Rippe, JM. The obesity epidemic: challenges and opportunities. *J Am Diet Assoc.* 1998; 98(suppl 2): S5.
10. Allon N. The stigma of overweight in everyday life. In: Wolman BB, ed. *Psychological Aspects of Obesity.* New York, NY: Van Nostrand Reinhold; 1982.
11. Rothblum ED. The stigma of women's weight: social and economic realities. *Feminism Psychol.* 1992; 2:61–73.
12. Decker WH. Attributions based on managers' self-presentation, sex, and weight. *Psychol Reports.* 1987; 61:175–81.
13. Klassen ML, Jasper CR, Harris RJ. The role of physical appearance in managerial decisions. *J Bus Psychol.* 1993; 8:181–98.
14. Rothblum ED, Miller CT, Garbutt B. Stereotypes of obese female job applicants. *Int J Eating Disord.* 1988; 7:277–83.
15. Larkin JC, Pines HA. No fat persons need apply: experimental studies of the overweight stereotype and hiring preference. *Sociol Work Occupations.* 1979; 6:312–27.
16. Klesges RC, Klem ML, Hanson CL, et al. The effects of applicant's health status and qualifications on simulated hiring decisions. *J Obes Relat Metab Disord.* 1990; 14: 527–35.
17. Pingitoire R, Dugoni R, Tindale S, Spring B. Bias against overweight job applicants in a simulated employment interview. *J Appl Psychol.* 1994; 79:909–17.
18. Bellizzi JA, Hasty RW. Territory assignment decisions and supervising unethical selling behavior: the effects of obesity and gender as moderated by job-related factors. *J Person Selling Sales Manage.* 1998; 18:35–49.
19. Everett M. Let an overweight person call on your best customers? Fat chance. *Sales Market Manage.* 1990; 142:66–70.
20. Jasper CR, Klassen ML. Perceptions of salespersons' appearance and evaluation of job performance. *Percept Mot Skills.* 1990; 71:563–6.
21. Melville DS, Cardinal BJ. Are overweight physical educators at a disadvantage in the labor market? A random survey of hiring personnel. *Physical Educator.* 1997; 54:216–22.
22. Roehling MV. Weight-based discrimination in employment: psychological and legal aspects. *Personnel Psychol.* 1999; 52:969–1017.
23. Paul RJ, Townsend JB. Shape up or ship out? Employment discrimination against the overweight. *Employee Responsibilities Rights J.* 1995; 8:133–45.
24. Loh ES. The economic effects of physical appearance. *Soc Sci Quart.* 1993; 74:420–37.
25. Register CA, Williams DR. Wage effects of obesity among young workers. *Soc Sci Quart.* 1990; 71:130–41.
26. Pagan JA, Davila A. Obesity, occupational attainment, and earnings. *Soc Sci Quart.* 1997; 78:756–70.
27. Gortmaker SL, Must A, Perrin JM, Sobol AM, Dietz WH. Social and economic consequences of overweight in adolescence and young adulthood. *N Engl J Med.* 1993; 399: 1008–12.
28. Brink TL. Obesity and job discrimination: mediation via personality stereotypes? *Percept Mot Skills.* 1988; 66:494.
29. Bordieri JE, Drehmer DE, Taylor DW. Work-life for employees with disabilities: recommendations

for promotion. *Rehab Counseling Bullet.* 1997; 40:181–91.

30. Rothblum ED, Brand PA, Miller CT, Oetjen HA. The relationship between obesity, employment discrimination, and employment-related victimization. *J Vocational Beh.* 1990; 37:251–66.

31. *Civil Service Commission v. Pennsylvania Human Relations Commission,* 591 A. 2d 281 (Pa. 1991).

32. Perroni PJ. Cook v. Rhode Island, Department of Mental Health, Retardation, Hospitals. The First Circuit tips the scales of justice to protect the overweight. *N Engl Law Rev.* 1996; 30:993–1018.

33. *Smaw v. Virginia Department of State Police,* 862 F. Suppl. 1469 (E. D. Va. 1994).

34. Frisk AM. Obesity as a disability: an actual or perceived problem? *Army Lawyer.* 1996; 3–19.

35. *Nedder v. Rivier College,* 908 F. Suppl. 66 (D. N H. 1995).

36. *Gimello v. Agency Rent-A-Car Systems, Inc.,* 594 A. 2d 264 (N.J. Super Ct. App. Div. 1991).

37. Garcia J. Weight-based discrimination and the Americans with Disabilities Act: is there an end in sight? *Hofstra Labor Law J.* 1995; 13:209–37.

38. Post R. Brennan Center Symposium Lecture. Prejudicial appearances: the logic of American anti-discrimination. *California Law Rev.* 2000; 88:1–40.

39. Harris MB, Waschull S, Walters L. Feeling fat: motivations, knowledge, and attitudes of overweight women and men. *Psychol Reports.* 1990; 67:1191–202.

40. Klein D, Najman J, Kohrman AF, Munro C. Patient characteristics that elicit negative responses from family physicians. *J Fam Practice.* 1982; 14:881–8.

41. Price JH, Desmond SM, Krol RA, Snyder FF, O'Connell JK. Family practice physicians' beliefs, attitudes, and practices regarding obesity. *Am J Prev Med.* 1987; 3:339–45.

42. Maiman LA, Wang VL, Becker MH, Finlay J, Simonson M. Attitudes toward obesity and the obese among professionals. *J Am Dietetic Assoc.* 1979; 74:331–6.

43. Maddox GL, Liederman V. Overweight as a social disability with medical implications. *J Med Educ.* 1969; 1969:44: 214–20.

44. Hoppe R, Ogden J. Practice nurses' beliefs about obesity and weight related interventions in primary care. *Int J Obes Relat Metab Disord.* 1997; 21:141–6.

45. Maroney D, Golub S. Nurses' attitudes toward obese persons and certain ethnic groups. *Percept Mot Skills.* 1992; 75: 387–91.

46. Bagley CR, Conklin DN, Isherwood RT, Pechiulis DR, Watson LA. Attitudes of nurses toward obesity and obese patients. *Percept Mot Skills.* 1989; 68:954.

47. McArthur L, Ross J. Attitudes of registered dietitians toward personal overweight and overweight clients. *J Am Dietetic Assoc.* 1997; 97:63–6.

48. Oberrieder H, Walker R, Monroe D, Adeyanju M. Attitudes of dietetics students and registered dietitians toward obesity. *J Am Dietetic Assoc.* 1995; 95:914–6.

49. Blumberg P, Mellis LP. Medical students' attitudes toward the obese and morbidly obese. *Int J Eating Disord.* 1980: 169–75.

50. Keane M. Contemporary beliefs about mental illness among medical students: implications for education and practice. *Academic Psychiat.* 1990; 14:172–7.

51. Lyons M, Ziviani J. Stereotypes, stigma, and mental illness: learning from fieldwork experiences. *Am J Occupation Ther.* 1995; 49:1002–8.

52. Wadden TA, Anderson DA, Foster GD, Bennett A, Steinberg C, Sarwer DB. Obese women's perceptions of their physicians' weight management attitudes and practices. *Arch Fam Med.* 2000; 9:854–60.

53. Wiese HJ, Wilson JF, Jones RA, Neises M. Obesity stigma reduction in medical students. *Int J Obes Relat Metab Disord.* 1992; 16:859–68.

54. Young LM, Powell B. The effects of obesity on the clinical judgments of mental health professionals. *J Health Soc Beh.* 1985; 26:233–46.

55. Kristeller JL, Hoerr RA. Physician attitudes toward managing obesity: differences among six specialty groups. *Prev Med.* 1997; 26:542–9.

56. Pratt CA, Nosiri UI, Pratt CB. Michigan physicians' perceptions of their role in managing obesity. *Percept Mot Skills.* 1997; 84:848–50.

57. Campbell K, Engel H, Timperio A, Cooper C, Crawford D. Obesity management: Australian general practitioners' attitudes and practices. *Obes Res.* 2000; 8:459–66.

58. Rand CW, MacGregor AM. Morbidly obese patients' perceptions of social discrimination before and after surgery for obesity. *South Med J.* 1990; 83:1390–5.

59. Adams CH, Smith NJ, Wilbur DC, Grady KE. The relationship of obesity to the frequency of pelvic examinations: do physician and patient attitudes make a difference? *Women Health.* 1993; 20:45–57.

60. Olson CL, Schumaker HD, Yawn BP. Overweight women delay medical care. *Arch Fam Med.* 1994; 3:888–92.

61. Fontaine KR, Faith MS, Allison DB, Cheskin LJ. Body weight and health care among women in

the general population. *Arch Fam Med*. 1998; 7:381–4.

62. Frank A. Futility and avoidance: medical professionals in the treatment of obesity. *JAMA*. 1993; 269:2132–3.

63. Yanovski SZ. A practical approach to treatment of the obese patient. *Arch Fam Med*. 1993; 2:309–16.

64. Grace DM. Waiting for weight loss. *Can J Surg*. 1991; 34: 416–7.

65. American Obesity Association. AOA fights social security plan to keep obese from benefits. *Am Obes Assoc Rep*.1999; 2:6.

66. Quesenberry CP, Caan B, Jacobson A. Obesity, health services use, and health care costs among members of a health maintenance organization. *Arch Intern Med*. 1998; 158:466–72.

67. Wolf AM, Colditz GA. Current estimates of the economic cost of obesity in the United States. *Obes Res*. 1998; 6: 97–106.

68. Gorsky RD, Pamuk E, Williamson DF, Shaffer PA, Koplan JP. The 25-year health care costs of women who remain overweight after 40 years of age. *Am J Prev Med*.1996; 12:388–94.

69. Sansone RA, Sansone LA, Wiederman MW. The relationship between obesity and medical utilization among women in a primary care setting. *Int J Eating Disord*. 1998; 23: 161–7.

70. Pronk NP, Tan AWH, O'Connor P. Obesity, fitness and health care costs. *Med Sci Sports Exerc*. 1999; 31:S66.

71. Black DR, Sciacca JP, Coster DC. Extremes in body mass index: probabilities in healthcare expenditures. *Prev Med*. 1994; 23:385–93.

72. Fontaine KR, Bartlett SJ. Access and use of medical care among obese persons. *Obes Res*. 2000; 8:403–6.

73. Goldstein DJ. Beneficial health effects of modest weight loss. *Int J Obes Relat Metab Disord*. 1992; 16:397–415.

74. Oster G, Thompson D, Edelsberg J, Bird AP, Colditz GA. Lifetime health and economic benefits of weight loss among obese persons. *Am J Public Health*. 1999; 89:1536–42.

75. Greenway FL, Ryan DH, Bray GA, Rood JC, Tucker EW, Smith SR. Pharmaceutical cost savings of treating obesity with weight loss medications. *Obes Res*. 1999; 7:523–31.

76. Martin LF, Tan TL, Horn JR, et al. Comparison of the costs associated with medical and surgical treatment of obesity. *Surgery*. 1995; 118:599–606.

77. Sjöström CD, Lissner L, Wedel H, Sjöström L. Reduction in incidence of diabetes and lipid disturbances after intentional weight loss induced by bariatric surgery: the SOS Intervention Study. *Obes Res*. 1999; 7:477–84.

78. Narbo K, Agren G, Jonnson E, et al. Sick leave and disability pension before and after treatment for obesity: a report from the Swedish Obese Subjects (SOS) study. *Int J Obes Relat Metab Disord*. 1999; 23:619 24.

79. Martin LF, White S, Lindstrom W. Cost-benefit analysis for the treatment of severe obesity. *World J Obes*. 1998; 22:1008–17.

80. Baxter J. Obesity surgery—another unmet need: it is effective but prejudice is preventing its use. *Br Med J*. 2000; 321:523–4.

81. Frank A. Conflicts in the care of overweight patients: inconsistent rules and insufficient money. *Obes Res*. 1997; 5:268–70.

82. Gibbs WW. Treatment that tightens the belt: is insurance part of America's obesity problem? *Sci Am*. 1995; 272:34–5.

83. American Obesity Association. IRS target of AOA action. *Am Obes Assoc Rep*. 2000; 4:1–8.

84. American Obesity Association. A taxpayer's guide on IRS policy to deduct weight control treatment. http://www.obesity.org/taxguide.htm.

85. Tershakovec AM, Watson MH, Wenner WJ, Marx AL. Insurance reimbursement for the treatment of obesity in children. *J Pediatr*. 1999; 134:573–8.

86. Peace K, Dyne J, Russell G, Stewart R. Psychological effects of gastric restriction surgery for morbid obesity. *N Zealand Med J*. 1989; 102:76–8.

87. Nordholm LA. Beautiful patients are good patients: evidence for the physical attractiveness stereotype in first impressions of patients. *Soc Sci Med*. 1980; 14:81–3.

88. Lederer EM. Teen-ager takes overdose after years of 'fatty' taunts. London: Associated Press; October 1, 1997.

89. Solovay S. Fat doesn't kill, fat hatred does. Fat!So? 1999; 2:19.

90. Richardson SA, Goodman N, Hastorf AH, Dornbusch SM. Cultural uniformity in reaction to physical disabilities. *Am Sociol Rev*. 1961: 241–7.

91. Latner JD, Stunkard AJ. The stigmatization of obese children: 40 years and counting. 2001. (in press).

92. Counts CR, Jones C, Frame CL, Jarvie GJ, Strauss CC. The perception of obesity by normal-weight versus obese school-age children. *Child Psychiatry Hum Dev*. 1986; 17: 113–20.

93. Cramer P, Steinwert T. Thin is good, fat is bad: how early does it begin? *J Appl Dev Psychol*. 1998; 19:429–51.

94. Thompson SH, Corwin SJ, Sargent RG. Ideal body size beliefs and weight concerns of fourth-grade children. *Int J Eating Disord*. 1997; 21:279–84.

95. Tiggermann M, Anesbury T. Negative

stereotyping of obesity in children: the role of controllability beliefs. *J Appl Soc Psychol.* 2000; 30:1977–93.

96. Bell SK, Morgan SB. Children's attitudes and behavioral intentions toward a peer presented as obese: does a medical explanation for the obesity make a difference? *J Pediat Psychol.* 2000; 25:137–45.

97. Harris MB, Walters LC, Waschull S. Altering attitudes and knowledge about obesity. *J Soc Psychol.* 1991; 131:881–4.

98. Irving L. Promoting size acceptance in elementary school children: the EDAP puppet program. *Int J Eating Disord.* 2000; 8:221–32.

99. Neumark-Sztainer D, Story M, Faibisch L. Perceived stigmatization among overweight African-American and Caucasian adolescent girls. *J Adolesc Health.* 1998; 23:264–70.

100. Grilo CM, Wilfley DE, Brownell KD, Rodin J. Teasing, body image, and self-esteem in a clinical sample of obese women. *Addict Behav.* 1994; 19:443–50.

101. Friedman MA, Brownell KD. Psychological correlates of obesity: Moving to the next research generation. *Psychol Bull.* 1995; 117:3–20.

102. Stunkard AJ. *The Pain of Obesity.* Palo Alto, CA: Bull Publishing Co.; 1976.

103. Wadden TA, Stunkard AJ. Social and psychological consequences of obesity. *Annals Intern Med.* 1985; 103:1062–7.

104. Klesges RC, Haddock CK, Stein RJ, Klesges LM, Eck LH, Hanson CL. Relationship between psychosocial functioning and body fat in preschool children: a longitudinal investigation. *JCCP.* 1992; 60:793–6.

105. Pierce JW, Wardle J. Cause and effect beliefs and self-esteem of overweight children. *J Child Psychol Psychiat.* 1997; 38:645–50.

106. Braet C, Mervielde I, Vandereycken W. Psychological aspects of childhood obesity: a controlled study in a clinical and non-clinical sample. *J Pediat Psychol.* 1997; 22:59–71.

107. Phillips RG, Hill AJ. Fat, plain, but not friendless: self-esteem and peer acceptance of obese pre-adolescent girls. *Int J Obes Relat Metab Disord.* 1998; 22:287–93.

108. Tiggermann M, Rothblum ED. Gender differences in social consequences of perceived overweight in the United States and Australia. *Sex Roles.* 1988; 18:75–86.

109. Regan PC. Sexual outcasts: the perceived impact of body weight and gender on sexuality. *J Appl Soc Psychol.* 1996; 26:1803–15.

110. Weiler K, Helms LB. Responsibilities of nursing education: the lessons of Russell v Salve Regina. *J Prof Nurs.* 1993; 9:131–8.

111. Canning H, Mayer J. Obesity—its possible effect on college acceptance. *N Engl J Med.* 1966; 275:1172–4.

112. Crandall CS. Do heavy-weight students have more difficulty paying for college? *Pers Soc Psych Bull.* 1991; 17:606–11.

113. Crandall CS. Do parents discriminate against their heavy-weight daughters? *Pers Soc Psych Bull.* 1995; 21:724–35.

114. Crandall CS. Prejudice against fat people: ideology and self-interest. *J Pers Soc Psych.* 1994; 66:882–94.

115. *Russell v. Salve Regina,* 649 F. Suppl. 391 (D. R. I. 1986).

116. Schweitzer TA. Academic challenge cases: should judicial review extend to academic evaluations of student? *Am Univ Law Rev.* 1992; 41:267–367.

117. *Russell v. Salve Regina,* 938 F. 2d 315 (1st Cir. 1991).

118. Neumark-Sztainer D, Story M, Harris T. Beliefs and attitudes about obesity among teachers and school health care providers working with adolescents. *J Nutr Educ.* 1999; 31:3–9.

119. National Education Association. Report on discrimination due to physical size. 1994; 11.

120. *Sellick v. Denny's, Inc.,* 884 F. Suppl. 388 (D. Or. 1995).

121. *Birdwell v. Carmike Cinemas,* No. 940014 (M. D. Tenn. 1994).

122. *Hollowich v. Southwest Airlines,* No. BC035389 (Ca. 1991).

123. *Green v. Greyhound,* No. 92VS55226H (N.D. Ga. 1992).

124. Karris L. Prejudice against obese renters. *J Soc Psychol.* 1977; 101:159–60.

125. Katz LM. A modest proposal? The convention on protection of children and cooperation in respect of intercountry adoption. *Emory Int Law Rev.* 1995; 9:283–328.

126. National Association for the Advancement of Fat Acceptance. NAAFA policy on adoption discrimination. http://www.naafa.org/documents/policies/adoption.html.

127. Anderson G, Cummings S, Freedman LS, et al. Design of the women's health initiative clinical trial and observational study. *Control Clin Trials.* 1998; 19:61–109.

128. Stunkard AJ, LaFleur WR, Wadden TA. Stigmatization of obesity in medieval times: Asia and Europe. *Int J Obes Relat Metab Disord.* 1998; 22:1141–4.

129. Adamitis EM. Appearance matters: a proposal to prohibit appearance discrimination in employment. *Washington Law Rev.* 2000; 75:195–223.

130. Epstein E. Fat people get a positive hearing in San Francisco: supervisors set vote on protected status. *San Francisco Chronicle.* May 4, 2000.

131. Ziolkowski SM. Case comment: the status of weight-based employment discrimination under the Americans with Disabilities Act after Cook v. Rhode Island Department of Mental Health, Retardation, and Hospitals. *Boston Univ Law R ev.* 1994; 74:667–86.

132. Crossley M. The disability kaleidoscope. *Notre Dame Law R ev.* 1999; 74:621–716.

133. *Krein v. Marian Manor Nursing Home*, 425 N. W. 2d 793 (N.D. 1987).

134. *Cassista v. Community Foods Inc.*, 856 P. 2d 1143 (Ca. 1993).

135. *Philadelphia Electric Company v. Pennsylvania Human Relations Commission*, 448 A 2d 701 (Pa. 1982).

136. *New York Division of Human Rights v. Xerox Corp.*, 480 N.E. 2d 695 (N.Y. 1985).

137. *King v. Frank*, E.E.O.C. Appeal No. 01893939 at 1 (1990).

138. Korn JB. Fat. *Boston Univ Law Rev.* 1997; 77:25–67.

139. Teachman B, Gapinski K, Brownell K. Stigma of obesity: implicit attitudes and stereotypes. Poster presented at the Society for Personality and Social Psychology, San Antonio, TX, February 2001.

140. Brownell KD. Dieting and the search for the perfect body: where physiology and culture collide. *Behav Ther.* 1991; 22:1–12.

141. Teachman BA, Brownell KD. Implicit anti-fat bias among health professionals: is anyone immune? *Int J Obes Relat Metab Disord.* 2001; 25:1525–31.

QUESTIONS

1. The authors write that "obese persons are the last acceptable targets of discrimination." Do you agree? Why or why not?

2. What would it mean to say that obesity is a disability under the Americans with Disabilities Act? Should obesity be considered a disability?

3. When, if ever, is it permissible for physicians to treat people with a specific condition different from people without it? For example, can physicians treat extremely obese people differently from those with a "normal" weight? How is obesity similar and different from race, sex or other prohibited categories of discrimination?

FURTHER READING

1. World Health Organization, *Obesity: Preventing and Managing the Global Epidemic.* Geneva: World Health Organization, 2000.

2. Pendo, Elizabeth, Reducing Disparities through Health Care Reform: Disability and Accessibility of Medical Equipment. *Utah Law Rev,* 2010; 4: 1057–1083.

3. Welch, Gilbert, Schwartz, Lisa, & Woloshin, Steven, *Overdiagnoses: Making People Sick in the Pursuit of Health.* Boston: Beacon Press, 2011.

CHAPTER 41

Human Rights: A New Language for Aging Advocacy

Russell E. Morgan, Jr. and Sam David

Growing older should not be a disability in itself. But for many, it entails a struggle to maintain a decent standard of living.

The high costs of health care and the frequent bias against seniors in the workplace contribute to the difficulties of those approaching advanced age. As the United States experiences *population aging*—the steep rise in number of seniors, as well as their proportion of the total population—the problem may indeed worsen. Aging baby boomers, medical advances, and declining birth rates are swelling the number of seniors, thus increasing how many people will encounter these struggles.

Advocates for aging adults need a convincing argument that will establish broad political support for maintaining a high quality of life for all seniors throughout their lives. The platform for establishing these values, too much ignored thus far, is human rights (a concept that is understandable to those of all ages and for which they can also be passionate). Educating the general population about the universality of human rights concepts and their direct relevance to the most important policy issues impacting seniors can inspire public support for all segments of the population. Advocates could then use the newfound support and perhaps activism in lobby-ing for changes that would help the elderly population, while helping humanity in general.

WHY HUMAN RIGHTS?

Like women or members of racial or ethnic minorities, the aging too are part of a unique minority, a minority that cuts across all other social divisions because we all eventually join it. And there are inherent difficulties that accompany the process of aging. The question becomes one of how to address the inevitable quality-of-life issues with concrete results.

Human rights principles, emerging into an international movement half a century ago, have evolved into a political force. Various treaties spell out standards and rights both for certain segments of the population and for everyone. But these documents are not well known by most of the U.S. population. For example, a 1997 poll commissioned by the National Center for Human Rights Education, in Atlanta, Georgia, showed that 92% of the American public has never heard of the Universal Declaration of Human Rights (UDHR), written in 1948 (National Center for Human Rights Education, 2001). Ironically, this was developed by a committee chaired by Eleanor Roosevelt and adopted by the United Nations on December 10th of that year. Although the human rights standards that the UDHR lays out, and which are enforced through the various human rights treaties, have not been fully recognized in the United States, they establish a basic foundation for supporting moral values for all societies.

Using human rights standards to advocate for seniors would characterize their needs within a framework that includes all other social and age groups. The right to health care, for example, applies to everyone, regardless of age or social status. Advocating for seniors' rights to accessible and universally affordable health care is thus an argument for good health care for all. If advocates for seniors depict the pursuit of health care for elders as a broader struggle (i.e., a struggle for our entire society, which is based on human rights and the fundamental values they establish), they would likely command wide, intergenerational support.

But convincing those who formulate aging-related policies to consciously recognize and respect the collective rights of seniors is crucial. And the means to that end lies in educating the general public about the rights of all citizens. If the majority of American people knew and understood that a healthy 80-year-old may be capable of working at the same level as his 40-year-old counterpart but won't earn as much, or that a 75-year-old's medicine for her age-related illness may cost her three times as much as her daughter's chronic illness drugs, then a typical policy maker might respond to the louder and more pervasive outcry for help. This education must include bringing about public awareness of the values incorporated in the UDHR (1948)—an understanding that will help Americans to digest the incontrovertible truth that all people are entitled to human rights, no matter who they are or where they live.

The concept of human rights has recently been catapulted into the forefront of American minds, as the events of September 11, 2001, and their aftermath keep the country saturated with media coverage of rights abuses. The horrors in various areas of the world have never gone away, but citizens are now more attuned to and informed of the realities that lie beyond their immediate vision. The inequities in the United States that result from national policies that treat young and old people differently create a significant issue of human rights as well and merit the attention of those of all ages. Why should a person lose the high quality of health care received 30 years earlier, and why should anyone encounter obstacles upon trying to learn the new skills required for his or her career?

There is potential public support: In a poll sponsored by the National Center for Human Rights Education (2001), Peter Hart found that 54% of Americans believe elderly people need support through government programs to maintain a basic standard of living. The Center aptly states that "our compassion for those in need is greater than our understanding about how to use human rights to end their suffering." That lack of understanding must be remedied.

THE HUMAN RIGHTS FRAMEWORK

What are internationally recognized human rights and how do they pertain to seniors? Human rights standards are enshrined in a variety of international treaties and covenants, which are legally binding upon those nations that ratify them. Other documents and declarations also specify such rights, but are without the force of law behind them. They nevertheless represent a moral consensus of the international community.

Three documents comprise the International Bill of Rights: (a) UDHR (1948), (b) the

International Covenant on Civil and Political Rights (ICCPR; 1966), and (c) the International Covenant on Economic, Social, and Cultural Rights (ICESCR; 1966). The ICESCR (1966) enunciates rights to work (Article 6) and to just and favorable working conditions that provide workers with "a decent living for themselves and their families" (Article 7). Article 9 attests to a right to Social Security—essential for those in retirement and to those in need of long-term assistance. The right to "the enjoyment of the highest attainable standard of physical and mental health" is enunciated (Article 12), while recognizing limitations imposed by biological and socioeconomic preconditions and the government's available resources.

Three other human rights documents pertinent to seniors are (a) the Convention on the Elimination of All Forms of Discrimination Against Women (CEDAW; 1979), (b) the International Convention on the Elimination of All Forms of Racial Discrimination (CERD; 1993) and (c) the Convention Against Torture and Other Cruel, Inhuman or Degrading Treatment or Punishment (CAT; 1984).

CEDAW (1979) and CERD (1993) make clear the obligation of governments to work toward abolishing all gender and race discrimination. They offer a sweeping definition of discrimination, clarifying that policies and practices that have an unjustifiably disparate gender- or race-based impact may constitute discrimination, even if the result was unintended. This understanding of discrimination is important for seniors, because gender and race are often relevant in examining the causes of preexisting inequalities in areas such as income and health care (Muller, 1999).

The ICCPR (1966), part of the International Bill of Rights, establishes a right to freedom from "cruel, inhuman, or degrading treatment or punishment" (Article 7). These injustices are understood in CAT (1984) to be acts "committed by or at the instigation of or with the consent or acquiescence of a public official or other person acting in an official capacity" (Article 16[1]). Although the meanings of these terms remain the subject of some debate, the prohibition against abusive treatment could be used to argue for more protection for seniors in nursing homes and facilities. As many of these homes are government funded, the residents—vulnerable because of a reliance on others for their care—could benefit from effective advocacy based on the stated prohibitions.

Seniors' advocates must also be aware of the United Nations (U.N.) Principles for Older Persons (1991). Although the guidelines therein do not have the legal force of the international human rights treaties, they are drawn directly from the principles established in the International Bill of Rights. Central to the U.N. Principles are the standards of independence, participation, care, self-fulfillment, and dignity for seniors, to be incorporated into government programs whenever possible.

The fundamental rights enunciated in the international treaties and their further exploration in the U.N. Principles for Older Persons (1991) provide the foundation for seniors' advocates to formulate their issues as society-wide human rights concerns. The United States, however, has not yet agreed to abide by all the treaties. It has signed and ratified the ICCPR (1966), CERD (1993), and CAT (1984), obliging the nation to meet those treaties' standards and to report on compliance with them to the relevant U.N. treaty bodies. But neither the ICESCR (1966) nor the CEDAW (1979) has been ratified by the United States. Unfounded congressional fears and arrogance may well play a part in this shameful disregard, but advocates must go beyond those politicians determined to keep the treaties off their senatorial desks. It must be articulated also to the public that there are core values shared by most Americans, and it is in the best interest of each citizen to stand up for the rights of others—strangers or not.

Thus, instead of focusing only on the unfortunate U.S. legal status of these two human rights accords, advocates should emphasize the accords' moral power and organizing potential. The ICESCR (1966) and CEDAW (1979) are the outcome of extensive consideration of economic, social, cultural, and gender-based issues, and represent wide agreement in the international community: 142 countries are a party to the ICESCR and 165 to CEDAW (United Nations, Office of the United Nations High Commissioner for Human Rights, 2000). Used carefully yet assertively by seniors' advocates, these agreements can become a mobilizing tool that enhances the movement to protect seniors—and all other members of society as well.

APPLYING HUMAN RIGHTS STANDARDS TO SENIORS' ISSUES

Four key areas in the lives of seniors exemplify how the integration of human rights values could improve the creation of public policies, federal and state, that address the needs of the growing senior population in communities across America: (a) work, (b) retirement security, (c) health care, and (d) long-term care.

The Workplace

Jeff is in his 60s and lost his high-level marketing job a decade ago. His difficulty finding a new job is typical for seniors: the years of experience didn't matter, once employers noticed his age. Some employers even admitted that his age led them not to hire him. He started his own business, earning a decent living although it was itself a demotion: he went from the upper $80,000s to the upper $30,000s. "I enjoy my work. I've stayed on the cutting edge of technology and computers and get a great deal of enjoyment from it; there is still software I would like to create and market," he says.

Jeff is entitled to the same just and favorable working conditions that are easily accepted and expected by those in other minority groups. But age-based discrimination is unfortunately not unusual.

Although mandatory retirement is less of a problem now than in previous years because of the Age Discrimination in Employment Act (1967), the issue of age discrimination in hiring and firing decisions has not improved to the same degree. The ability of seniors to realize equality in the workplace has been hurt by their limited access to training and employers' negative views of older workers. Stereotypes continue to convince many employers that older workers are inflexible and not easily adaptable to new technologies (Rix, 1999).

Although stereotypes cannot be changed by policies and laws, they can be gradually molded by education. The public can be made more aware, through effective advocacy efforts, that a person in Jeff's predicament is as entitled to and as capable of performing a good job as someone 20 years his junior. Not only might this new understanding mean that many employers would take older workers more seriously, but the workers themselves may stand up for their rights with more confidence and public support behind them.

Older women and minorities are particularly affected by these inequalities, as their training and income have been historically disproportionate to the rest of the senior population (Muller, 1999). Thus, they are especially vulnerable to the prospect of low-income jobs with limited benefits, exacerbating the preexisting problem.

Policy makers are pursuing reforms to encourage seniors to remain in the workforce longer. But some of the attempts to lengthen seniors' participation in the working world could result in jeopardizing their ability to secure just and favorable working conditions.

Employers' convincing seniors to keep working (e.g., by increasing eligibility ages for pensions or creating new incentives such as flexible schedules) does not expand their opportunities for decent employment. New training programs, however, would help to burst the myths that older workers (a) cannot learn new procedures as well as younger workers, and (b) are not interested in the latest technologies and methods. As stated in the U.N. Principles for Older Persons (1991), "Older persons should have access to appropriate educational and training programs."

By highlighting the fact that older workers are indeed entitled to the same opportunities and working conditions as members of other minorities, simply because both groups have the same rights, advocates can pressure policy makers to focus on finding solutions to the problem of age discrimination in hiring decisions—not on creating reforms that make it harder for aging workers to leave where they are.

Retirement Security

Susan, in her mid-70s, kept working until 2 years ago when she became ill. For three decades she has taken care of her mother, father-in-law, mother-in-law, and husband, who died in 1980. She is paying off her mortgage, has never had a job that provided a pension, and relies on Social Security as her lifeline. She spends about $25 per week on groceries, and cannot afford to really become sick.

Susan's situation is not that different from many seniors who rely on Social Security benefits for the majority of their retirement income. Nearly 60% of older Americans rely on Social Security benefits for 50% or more of their income, and nearly one third rely on Social Security benefits for 80% or more of their income (Dauster, 1996). Population aging threatens this crucial source of retirement support.

As the 76 million baby boomers leave the workforce, fewer workers will support an increasing number of retirees through Social Security investments. In the short term, Social Security trust fund balances will grow, but these balances may reach their limit in 2022 (Meyers, 1999).

There is considerable dispute over the extent to which Social Security is imperiled. Several new economic and social policies have been proposed that may help counterbalance these effects of population aging. For example, people working beyond age 65 would contribute longer to Social Security; or, new government employees, at the state and local levels, could be included in the expanded pool of workers supporting Social Security. Thus valid questions have been raised about assumptions regarding the potential bankruptcy of Social Security and the degree to which the costs of providing it will rise (Meyers, 1999). But most analysts agree that there is a need for some modifications in order to maintain a financially healthy social insurance program that benefits all Americans.

One unacceptable alteration would be a dramatic reduction of Social Security benefits: This would result in clear discrimination against women and minorities. Two of the human rights documents, powerful in their morality, prohibit gender and race discrimination: CEDAW (1979) and the CERD (1993). As women and minorities are over-represented in the elderly poor population, any harmful effects to that population in general are therefore disproportionately harmful to women and minorities. Seniors' advocates can invoke these documents to highlight how curtailments of Social Security would hurt women and minorities more than non-minorities. A successful explanation of this problem to politicians and citizens may illustrate the fundamental inequalities, and voters too may voice their concerns for a more equitable Social Security program.

Health Care

Sandra, covered by Medicare, pays for her prescription drugs out of her Social Security check, since neither Medicare nor her supplemental insurance covers them. She is finding that she can no longer afford the expense. Mary and her husband are $8,000 in debt because they have been forced to pay for prescription drugs out of pocket.

Health care financing for seniors clearly needs to be changed. As the number of seniors rises, their main health insurance program—Medicare—will be increasingly challenged. Just as the integrity of Social Security is disputed, the extent to which Medicare is endangered is also debated.

Aside from population aging, other health care-related developments have contributed to the increased demands on Medicare (Binstock, 1999). The onset of new diseases, the increase in the number of people living into old age, and the costs of medicine and long-term care all put more demand on health insurance for elders. But according to government projections, the rapid rise in beneficiaries after the first baby boomers turn 65 is what will usher in Medicare's financial shortfall. (This shortfall refers to Medicare's Part A, which is a trust fund in much the same way as Social Security. In the 1999 annual report on the solvency of Medicare's Part A, the Hospital Insurance Trustees projected that the trust fund will remain solvent until 2015. In 1998 they projected solvency until 2008; see Caplan, Brangan, & Gross, 1999.) Measures under consideration to alleviate the problem include relying more heavily on health maintenance organizations (HMOs; a scenario under way for some years now), raising the eligibility age for Medicare, creating medical savings accounts, supplying health care vouchers, and rationing, or restricting, health care for seniors.

Examining these proposals through a human rights lens will demonstrate how such plans are inadequate and damaging for seniors. A human rights-based discussion could help close these gaps in access to health care. By focusing on everyone's right to the best possible health care, advocates for aging adults can point out to policy makers exactly how seniors are being left behind in this regard—seniors are not provided with the options or range of choices for adequate health care.

As access to health care is woefully insufficient for seniors, it may become even more problematic with the growth of population aging. Medicare does not cover prescription drugs, nor does it require its participating HMOs to do so. Approximately one third of Medicare beneficiaries have no drug coverage whatsoever (Pear, 2000). The remaining two thirds receive some degree of drug coverage through medigap policies, Medicare HMOs, or employer retirement packages. But these plans do not preclude high out-of-pocket medicine expenses, nor do they protect against fluctuations in coverage due to policy profits and market trends. Some seniors are traveling to Canada, where pharmaceutical prices are lower because of the government's commitment to equity in aging.

Medicare does cover mental health costs, but copayments for mental health care remain significantly higher than those for physical health care. This is an ongoing obstacle to seniors' access to mental health treatment and increases the financial burden on their caregivers. HMOs fall short as well in providing adequate and consistent coverage for mental health care (Katz, 1999).

But for seniors, mental health care is indispensable. Mental health problems, especially depression, occur at high rates among the elderly population (National

Institutes of Health, 1991). There are also clear links between depression and declining physical health, including malnutrition, worsening disabilities, and even increased mortality (U.S. Office of the Surgeon General, 1999).

The comorbidity factor often arises in seniors who suffer from depression; one disease may impede recovery from another. A stroke victim, for example, may not want to take the medication that is essential for his or her recovery if an underlying clinical depression is lurking. That depression, hidden or not, must then be treated in order for the patient to have a good chance at recovery from the stroke.

Advocates for aging adults also need to encourage medical researchers to be aware of special health concerns of seniors. Ethicists and legal professionals, as well as medical researchers, must watch for any bias against seniors in their case work and analysis and be vigilant in incorporating the health care challenges of seniors into any decisions and studies.

A rising problem in the senior population is one usually thought of as affecting only young adults: AIDS. But at least 10% of all cases are in patients aged older than 50. And a quarter of those are aged older than 60 (National Association on HIV Over Fifty, 2001). From 1991 to 1996, cases in those aged older than 50 increased by 22%—a much larger increase than the 9% that occurred in those aged 13–49 (Hirschhorn, 2001).

Health care providers and seniors themselves are not conditioned to be wary of the disease—they do not necessarily realize that this age group is at risk just as other age groups are. Educational campaigns about AIDS and HIV are not targeted at seniors: "How often does a wrinkled face appear on a prevention poster?" (National Association on HIV Over Fifty, 2001, p. 1). According to the National Association on HIV Over Fifty, the senior population

has been, for the most part, omitted from research, clinical drug trials, educational prevention programs, and intervention efforts. Thus outreach, education, and research on AIDS and HIV infection should be undertaken and encouraged by seniors' advocates, making it clear to both doctors and patients that thousands of people of a certain age are becoming infected each year. Facing that reality and taking steps to alleviate the problem will not only improve many lives in the older population, but save them.

The rights of seniors to good health care are mandated by human rights standards that apply to other segments of society— whether those standards concern equal opportunity in the workplace for women or access to public buildings for disabled people.

Long-Term Care

LaShawn, 84, was living in independent senior housing but became quite ill following an incorrect diagnosis of a medical problem. At 90 pounds, she moved in with her daughter, herself 65, who takes care of her. LaShawn's granddaughter also helps out, but worries that she could end up being the caregiver for both her mother and grandmother. LaShawn cannot be left alone, but day care costs and health expenses are high.

The problems of LaShawn and her family are common. The caregivers of frail seniors struggle to ensure that their loved ones receive the care they need in a supportive environment. Public funding for care is difficult to obtain: Medicare-funded home care, for example, is generally provided only for short, post-acute care needs and has restrictive rules for eligibility (Bergquist, 1999). Medicaid's requirements are less stringent, but not all services are provided.

Financially, the system is set for seniors to lose. To qualify for long-term care, one cannot have more than $2,000 in assets, except for his or her home. A spouse's assets are considered as well, although a higher limit is set. A spend-down process often ensues, in which all assets are drained until eligibility is reached (Rein, 1996). The consequence is financial hardship and further dependency, both of which are socially and psychologically debilitating. Private insurance, if held, rarely covers long-term care: In 1995 it covered less than 6% of the national cost of nursing home and home care costs (Stone, 1999).

The demand for long-term assistance will dramatically increase with the rising number of seniors and with medical advances allowing people with chronic illnesses to live longer and with lower levels of pain (Stone, 1999). At the same time, other demographic factors may decrease the resources available for long-term care. For example, fewer children have been born to baby boomers than to those of previous generations, creating a shortage of people available to provide informal care and financial support for formal care to those entering old age in 25 years (Stone, 1999). Higher rates of divorce among baby boomers may further weaken the informal care networks. Women, the traditional providers of informal long-term care, now enter the labor force with higher frequency and duration than in previous years, limiting their ability to care for older relatives (U.S. Bureau of Labor Statistics, 2000). Finally, the enormous geographic range of many contemporary families makes the provision of informal care and familial supervision of formal care more difficult (Barnes, 1995).

Thus, the necessity for high-quality formal care institutions is as high as it has ever been. Advocacy efforts based on human rights could have an impact on those who see no problem with limiting the number of students in a public school class—if a certain number of teachers is required by law for a given number of students, why is a nursing home allowed to be understaffed? A study by the Department of Health and Human Services reveals appalling conditions in many residential facilities, in part because of inadequate staffing levels (U.S. Department of Health and Human Services, 2000). People who are 85 years old have the same basic rights as the school children who are 8 years old.

The growing need for long-term care heightens the potential for elder abuse. Many seniors have a limited ability to voice real concerns regarding their care, depending on the extent of their physical or mental incapacitation. Some analysts estimate that 1.5 million seniors are the victims of elder abuse each year (Baron & Welty, 1999). Although elder abuse laws have been approved, the human rights education programs to prevent the abuse have been ignored. Thus abuse may be underreported because of dependency, lack of awareness of legal protection, or lack of competency, precluding the recognition of abuse. Both seniors and their caregivers must hear and digest the assertions of advocates who can explain why basic human rights are neglected in many of the policies that affect seniors.

New research into alternative long-term care options, increased support for families providing long-term care, and new monitoring mechanisms for private care facilities are important potential improvements in the lives of elderly people. Advocates should stress, through public-relations and educational efforts, that these issues are likely to affect almost everyone at some point.

AN ACTION AGENDA

Human rights standards can be a mighty long-term force in protecting the welfare of seniors in an era of population aging. In the crucial areas of work, retirement, health, and long-term care, these standards can be used to voice a principled defense of the rights of seniors, operating as a baseline for establishing the values that underlie new public policies. By framing seniors' issues as an integral component of a rights-based society, advocates could forge a broad consensus among all segments of society to support the improvement of living conditions for seniors.

The importance of seniors' issues must be emphasized not only to policy makers but to other human rights-based advocacy groups as well, whose positions would only be strengthened by incorporating these senior-related issues into their arguments. Human rights are a life span issue, affecting each person for his or her entire life, from birth through death. Seniors' issues affect a significant portion of one's lifetime, just as children's issues are relevant for many years of one's life. If each advocacy group bases its arguments on the universality of human rights, a new network of partnerships can then be built, gaining strength from the sharing of a fundamental concept: Everyone has the same rights throughout life. Everyone will, at some point, be personally involved with human rights concerns—directly or indirectly.

Advocates for aging adults can take many steps to promote better conditions for seniors, in their communities and collectively at the national level, basing their efforts on a human rights-based approach:

1. Establish a clear statement of nonnegotiable values on which grassroots education and public marketing campaigns can be based.
2. Create formal human rights education programs for children and adults.
3. Promote national awareness of aging problems from the standpoint of human rights by identifying a set of fundamental principles to be communicated to all Americans. These principles would demonstrate that all seniors have the right to (a) adequate food, clothing, and shelter; (b) full benefits of social security, including long-term care; (c) just and favorable working conditions; (d) access to health care to maintain or regain an optimum level of physical, mental, and emotional well-being, and to prevent or delay the onset of illness; (e) live in dignity with respect to personal privacy; (f) freedom from exploitation and physical and mental abuse; (g) the pursuit of opportunities for the full development of their potential; and (h) remain integrated into society, and to participate actively in the formulation and implementation of policies that directly affect their well-being, sharing their knowledge and skills with younger generations.
4. Develop human rights education programs for caregivers and for seniors themselves, empowering them to be active on their own behalf and in cooperation with younger generations.
5. Form alliances with mainstream human rights and advocacy groups, encouraging specific review of issues relevant to seniors.
6. Form alliances with other social groups that focus on the common interest of fundamental human rights, such as civil rights groups, children's advocacy organizations, and public health groups that fight against inadequate health care coverage.
7. Publicize the standards outlined in the Universal Declaration of Human Rights (1948) and its related treaties and covenants, including the U.N. Principles for Older Persons (1991). Use them explicitly in both domestic and international education and advocacy efforts, while encouraging U.S. government ratification of all human rights documents.

By incorporating the powerful ideas behind the principle of human rights, advocates for aging adults can assist in fashioning a society that recognizes the dignity of all people, from the beginning of life until its end—a society, in the words of the United Nations, "for all ages" (United Nations Program on Aging, 2002).

REFERENCES

Age Discrimination in Employment Act, 29 U.S.C. §621 (1967).

Barnes, A. (1995). The policy and politics of community-based long-term care. *Nova Law Review, 19,* 487–531.

Baron, S., & Welty, A. (1999). Elder abuse. In L. A. Frolik (Ed.), *Aging and the law* (pp. 581–584). Philadelphia: Temple University Press.

Bergquist, M. L. (1999). Home health care: What it is and who pays for it. In L. A. Frolik (Ed.), *Aging and the law* (pp. 410–414). Philadelphia: Temple University Press.

Binstock, R. H. (1999). Older persons and health care costs. In R. N. Butler, L. K. Grossman, & M. R. Oberlink (Eds.), *Life in an older America* (pp. 75–96). New York: Century Foundation Press.

Caplan, C., Brangan, N., & Gross, D. (1999). *The trustees' annual report on the status of Medicare hospital insurance (HI) trust fund: 1999.* Washington, DC: Public Policy Institute, AARP.

Convention Against Torture and Other Cruel, Inhuman or Degrading Treatment or Punishment, adopted December 10, 1984, G.A. Res. 39/46, U.N. GAOR, 39th Sess., Supp. No. 51, at 197, U.N. Doc. A/39/51 (1984) (entered into force June 26, 1987), reprinted in 23 I.L.M. 1027 (1984), substantive changes noted in 24 I.L.M. 535 (1985).

Convention on the Elimination of All Forms of Discrimination Against Women, G.A. Res. 34/180 December 18, 1979, Art. 1.

Dauster, W. G. (1996, Summer). Protecting Social Security and Medicare. *Harvard Journal on Legislation, 33,* 461–509.

Hirschhorn, L. (2001). HIV in the aging population: Partnerships in clinical care. Slide presentation from the 2001 National Association on HIV Over Fifty National Conference.

Katz, I. R. (1999). Prepared statement before the Senate Special Committee on Aging. In L. A. Frolik (Ed.), *Aging and the law* (pp. 568–580). Philadelphia: Temple University Press.

Meyers, R. J. (1999). Dispelling the myths about Social Security. In R. N. Butler, L. K. Grossman, & M. R. Oberlink (Eds.), *Life in an older America* (pp. 9–24). New York: Century Foundation Press.

Muller, C. (1999). The distinctive needs of women and minorities. In R. N. Butler, L. K. Grossman, & M. R. Oberlink (Eds.), *Life in an older America* (pp. 97–120). New York: Century Foundation Press.

National Association on HIV Over Fifty. (2001). *Educational tip sheet.*

National Center for Human Rights Education. (2001). Bringing human rights home: Linking individual dignity with mutual destiny. *1996–2000 Report of Program Activities.* Atlanta: Author.

National Institutes of Health. (1991). *Consensus statement online 9* (3), 1–27.

Pear, R. (2000, June 27). 17 percent increase in prescription drug costs hit elderly hardest, study finds. *New York Times,* p. A16.

Rein, J. E. (1996, Spring). Misinformation and self-deception in recent long-term care policy trends. *Journal of Law and Politics, 12,* 195–340.

Rix, S. E. (1999). The older worker in a graying America. In R. N. Butler, L. K. Grossman, & M. R. Oberlink (Eds.), *Life in an older America* (pp. 187–216). New York: Century Foundation Press.

Stone, R. (1999). Long-term care: Coming of age in the twenty-first century. In R. N. Butler, L. K. Grossman, & M. R. Oberlink (Eds.), *Life in an older America* (pp. 49–74). New York: Century Foundation Press.

United Nations Program on Aging. (2002). *Mission statement.*

Universal Declaration of Human Rights, G.A. Res. 217 A (III), U.N. GAOR 3d Sess., Pt. 1, at 71, U.N. Doc. A/810 (1948).

U.S. Bureau of Labor Statistics. (2000, February 16). Changes in women's labor force participation in the 20th century. *Monthly Labor Review: The Editor's Desk.*

U.S. Department of Health and Human Services. (2000). *Report to congress: Appropriateness of minimum nurse staffing ratios in nursing homes.*

United States, Office of the Surgeon General. (1999). Consequences of depression. In *Mental health: A report of the surgeon general* (Chap. 5). Washington, DC: Government Printing Office.

QUESTIONS

1. The authors remark that the senior population has been, for the most part, omitted from research, clinical drug trials, educational prevention programs and intervention efforts. Why? Do you believe there are any instances in which this omission is justified? Should we spend more research dollars on trying to lengthen life and "enhance" it? How long do you want to live?

2. In the chapter, it is stated that "some seniors are traveling to Canada . . . because of the government's commitment to equity in aging." In your opinion, what would be appropriate national evidence of a "commitment to equity in aging"? Using additional resources, compare the US and Canadian approaches to the care of seniors. Do you agree that Canada shows a greater commitment to equity in aging? Consider differences between Medicare in the US, and health care programs for the elderly in Canada.

3. All of us will die, usually following a long illness that increasingly takes away our ability to function. It has been argued that this final disease can be "compressed" so that we die quicker and use fewer health resources. Others have argued that we should authorize physicians to assist their patients to commit suicide. What do you think should be done to improve the last years of life of the elderly? What would be the human rights implications of adopting this approach?

FURTHER READING

1. Callahan, D., Must We Ration Health Care for the Elderly? *J Law, Med. & Ethics*, 2012; 40: 10–16.
2. Parker, M. G., & Thorslund, M., Health Trends in the Elderly Population: Getting Better and Getting Worse. *Gerontologist*, 2007; 47: 150–158.
3. Deaton, A., Income, Aging, Health and Well-Being around the World: Evidence from the Gallup World Poll, in David A. Wise, ed., *Research Findings in the Economics of Aging*, Chicago: University of Chicago Press, 2010, 235–255.
4. Stock, Gregory, *Redesigning Humans: Our Inevitable Genetic Future*. Boston: Houghton Mifflin, 2002.
5. Mehlman, Maxwell, *The Price of Perfection: Individualism and Society in the Era of Biomedical Enhancement*. Baltimore: Johns Hopkins Press, 2009.

Concluding Note

Health and Human Rights has moved beyond its infancy. It is now an adolescent in development. As such, there is a body of knowledge to react to, as well as to grapple and struggle with as it matures. In this book we have documented what is known about the links between health and human rights to date. This text covers areas of theory, concept, method and practice. This has been accomplished through a collection of chapters and commentaries addressing the spectrum of challenges and concerns in the field. The chosen texts reflect a broad conceptualization of the use of a human rights framework in addressing the health and well-being of populations, and the nascent evidence being built through research and evaluation to document the synergies between health and human rights.

The textbook has presented a historical perspective and thematic analysis of the many and growing dimensions of health and human rights. Readers have had an opportunity to engage with the subject not only through presented texts, but through directed questions, suggested discussion points and additional readings often presenting dissenting perspectives. In each case, it is active engagement with the subject that matters, whether within the walls of a classroom or outside. It is our hope that after closing this textbook, you will choose to revisit it from time to time when you feel a need to refresh your memory or rekindle your commitment. We trust in the fact that readers will contribute to advancing understanding and the practice of health and human rights. Such action may be big or small and may take the form of advocacy, programming, projects, use of courts and law, engaging civil society, helping to build the evidence, as well as promoting and sharing knowledge with those who have not had privileged access to this education, and on a personal note, living as individuals enjoying more fully their own health and their human rights and helping others to achieve the same.

The text has identified successes and failures in the domain of health and human rights, and suggested ways to determine how these outcomes came about. Knowledge of the true, multifarious and reciprocal impacts of health and human rights must be expanded through reflection and debates, systematic evaluation and multi-disciplinary research. The research agenda for health and human rights is becoming more pressing, sophisticated and broader as demands are explicitly voiced by political leaders and policy makers, in particular, to demonstrate the "added value" of health and human rights approaches over those that favor on notions of economic growth, cost-efficiency and cost effective-ness. New ways to define individual and societal well-being must be invented that factor this range of outcomes into the human development agendas. To this end, methods and tools are needed to under-take scientifically sound empirical studies the results of which can be used to support further advocacy and action.

One of the challenges and dilemmas faced by the editors in compiling the pieces for this textbook has been the fact that much of the evidence, and the perspec-tives presented herein, come from indus-trialized countries, in particular the United States and European nations. When pieces concerned other countries, where more than two-thirds of the world's popula-tion lives, articles were mostly *about* them rather than *from* them. No country in the world can legitimately claim to serve as a model for others in health and human rights terms. No issue in this field should be obscured or remain silent because of insuf-ficient production and sharing of knowl-edge. We hope that in the future this text-book will include pieces from communities and nations around the world that are too often absent from the literature so that not only their suffering, but their knowledge, resilience and capacity to act—a reality of many developing countries and oppressed communities that is insufficiently docu-mented—are written-up by them and shared for others to learn from.

What will the field of Health and Human Rights look like in ten years? We believe there will be better designed and more widely applied methods evidencing the synergy between health and rights. Health and social development strategies will be more systematically evaluated, docu-mented and publicized, whether they have been successful or not. As the goal posts of health and human rights are bound to be endlessly moved forward, new issues will emerge, new aspirations will be voiced, new demands will be expressed, and new responses will be brought to bear on bla-tant injustices, inequality and inequity. There will be greater linkages to other disci-plines, and more disciplines yet to be born, as the issues at stake evolve and the social and structural roots of human disparity are better exposed. As a result, there will be a wider range of data and more robust evi-dence on what works and what does not. There will be an increased use of social and electronic connectors. Education will change, as will the media, both in the class-room and on the ground. The world will have moved a little step, but we hope take a giant leap towards realizing its health and human rights aspirations.

The future of Health and Human Rights is in your hands. You will take up the chal-lenge of research, education, service and advocacy that promote the health and human rights of everyone who lives on this planet. You will not be passive witnesses or silent bystanders. Borrowing from Martin Luther King: "Our lives begin to end the day we become silent about the things that matter."

Researching Health and Human Rights

We strongly encourage readers to seek out original documents referenced in the text, as well as additional resources to support their areas of study. The following links to intergovernmental, academic and non-governmental institutions, the list of which is by no means exhaustive, are convenient starting places for researching health and human rights.

INTERNATIONAL INSTITUTIONS

Office of the High Commissioner of Human Rights
http://www.ohchr.org/EN/Issues/Pages/ListOfIssues.aspx

The World Health Organization
http://www.who.int/hhr/en/

ACADEMIC CENTERS

Georgetown University , O'Neill Institute for National and Global Health Law
http://www.law.georgetown.edu/oneillinstitute/

Harvard School of Public Health, FXB Centre for Health and Human Rights
www.harvardfxbcenter.org

Johns Hopkins Bloomberg School of Public Health, Center for Public Health and Human Rights
http://jhsph.edu/humanrights

New York University, Center for Health and Human Rights
http://medicine.med.nyu.edu/dgim/sections/primary-care/health-and-human-rights-overview

Suffolk University, Center for Women's Health and Human Rights
http://www.suffolk.edu/college/10649.html

UCLA School of Law, Health and Human Rights Law Project
http://www.law.ucla.edu/centers-programs/international-human-rights-law-program/Pages/Health-and-Human-Rights-Law-Project.aspx

University of California Human Rights Center, Berkeley Law
http://www.law.berkeley.edu/hrc.htm

University of Cape Town Health and Human Rights Program
http://www.hhr.uct.ac.za/about/about.php

University of Southern California, Program on Global Health and Human Rights
http://globalhealth.usc.edu/ghhr

UNIVERSITY RESOURCES

The Institute of Human Rights (IHR) at Emory University
http://humanrights.emory.edu

University of Iowa
http://international.uiowa.edu/uichr/learn-about-human-rights

University of Minnesota
http://www1.umn.edu/humanrts/links/health.html

University of Toronto
http://www.law-lib.utoronto.ca/diana/mainpage.htm

NONGOVERNMENTAL ORGANIZATIONS

Amnesty International
www.amnesty.org

Center for Reproductive Rights
http://reproductiverights.org/

Global Lawyers and Physicians
http://www.globallawyersandphysicians.org

Human Rights Watch
www.hrw.org

International Federation of Health and Human Rights Organizations
www.ifhhro.org

Open Society Foundations
http://www.soros.org/about/programs/public-health-program

Physicians for Human Rights
www.physiciansforhumanrights.org

Credit Lines

R. Andorno, "Global bioethics at UNESCO: In defence of the Universal Declaration on Bioethics and Human Rights" from *Journal of Medical Ethics* 33 (2007): 150–154. Copyright © 2007 by British Medical Journal. Reprinted with the permission of the British Medical Journal Group.

G. J. Annas and H. J. Geiger, "War and Human Rights" from *War and Public Health*, edited by B. S. Levy and V. W. Sidel. Copyright © 2008. Reprinted with the permission of Oxford University Press, Ltd.

G.J. Annas, "American Vertigo: 'Dual Use', Prison Physicians, Research, and Guantanamo" from *Case Western Reserve Journal of International Law* 43 (2011): 43: 631–650. Reprinted with permission.

G.J. Annas, "Assisted Reproduction—Canada's Supreme Court and the 'Global Baby'," *New England Journal of Medicine* (2011): 365: 459–463. Reprinted with the permission of the Massachusetts Medical Society.

G.J. Annas, "Bioterror and 'Bioart'—A Plague o' Both Your Houses," from the *New England Journal of Medicine* 2006; 354: 2715–2720. Reprinted with the permission of the Massachussetts Medical Society.

G. J. Annas, "Global Health" from *Worst Case Bioethics: Death, Disaster, and Public Health*, G.J. Annas. Copyright © 2010. Reprinted with the permission of Oxford University Press, Ltd.

S. R. Benatar, S. Gill & I. Bakker, "Global health and the global economic crisis" from *American Journal of Public Health* 101 (2011): 646–53. Copyright © 2011. Reprinted with the permission of the American Public Health Association.

C. Bruderlein, and J. Leaning, "New challenges for humanitarian protection" from *British Medical Journal* 319 (1999): 430–435. Copyright © 1999 British Medical Journal Publishing Group. Reprinted with the permission of the British Medical Journal Group.

G. L. Burci and Koskenmäki, "Human Rights Implications of Governance Responses to Public Health Emergencies: The Case of Major Infectious Disease Outbreaks" from *Realizing the Right to Health*, edited by Andrew Clapman. Copyright © 2009. Reprinted with the permission of Rüffer & Rub, Zurich.

J. K. Burns, "Mental health and inequity: A human rights approach to inequality, discrimination, and mental disability" from *Health and Human Rights* 11 (2009): 19–31. Copyright © 2009 by the François-Xavier

Bagnoud Center for Health and Human Rights. Reprinted with permission.

R. J. Cook, "Gender, Health and Human Rights" from *Health and Human Rights* 1, no 4 (1995): 350–366. Copyright © 1995 by the François-Xavier Bagnoud Center for Health and Human Rights. Reprinted with permission.

J. Cottingham, A Germain, and P. Hunt, "Use of Human Rights to Meet the Unmet Need for Family Planning," *Lancet* (2011): 172–80. Reprinted with permission of Elsevier Science Ltd.

S. Davies, "Reproductive Health as a Human Right: A Matter of Access or Provision?" from *Journal of Human Rights—London* 9 (2010): 387–408. Copyright © 2010 by Taylor & Francis Group LLC. Reprinted by permission of Routledge/Taylor & Francis, Ltd.

C. Dresler, H. Lando, N. Schneider, and H. Sehgal, "Human Rights-Based Approach to Tobacco Control," *Tobacco Control* 21 (2012): 208–11. Reprinted with permission of BMJ Publishing Group Ltd.

R. Elliott et al., "Harm reduction, HIV/AIDS, and the human rights challenge to global drug control policy" from *Health and Human Rights* 8 (2005): 104–138. Copyright © 2005 by the François-Xavier Bagnoud Center for Health and Human Rights. Reprinted with permission.

M. Flaherty and J. Fisher, "Sexual Orientation, Gender Identity and International Human Rights Law: Contextualising the Yogyakarta Principles" from *Human Rights Law Review* 8 (2008): 207–248. Reprinted by permission of Oxford University Press, Ltd.

E. A. Friedman and L. O. Gostin, "Pillars for progress on the right to health: Harnessing the potential of human rights through a Framework Convention on Global Health" from *Health and Human Rights* 14, no. 1 (2012). Copyright © 2012 by the François-Xavier Bagnoud Center for Health and Human Rights. Reprinted with permission.

C. Garcia-Moreno and H. Stöckl, "Protection of sexual and reproductive health rights: addressing violence against women" from *International Journal of Gynecology and Obstetrics* 106 (2009): 144–147. Copyright © 2009 by the International Federation of Gynecology and Obstetrics. Reprinted by permission of Elsevier Science Limited.

R. Gay, "Mainstreaming wellbeing: An impact assessment for the right to health" from *Australian Journal of Human Rights* 13 (2008): 33–63. Copyright © 2008. Reprinted with permission.

S. Gruskin and L. Ferguson, "Using indicators to determine the contribution of human rights to public health efforts" from *Bulletin of the World Health Organization* 87 (2009): 714–719. Copyright © 2007 by the World Health Organization. Reprinted with permission.

S. Gruskin, E.J. Mills, and D. Tarantola, "History, Principles, and Practice of Health and Human Rights," from *The Lancet* 370 2007: 449–455. Copyright © 2007. Reprinted with permission of Elsevier Science Limited.

S. Gruskin and D. Tarantola, "What Does Bringing Human Rights into Public Health Work Actually Mean in Practice" from., *International Encyclopedia of Public Health*, Vol. 3, edited by Heggenhougen, Kristian and Quah, Stella. Copyright © 2008 Elesvier, Inc. Reprinted with permission of Elsevier Science Limited.

H. V. Hogerzeil et al., "Is access to essential medicines as part of the fulfilment of the right to health enforceable through the courts?" from *The Lancet* 368 (2006): 305. Copyright © 2006. Reprinted with permission of Elsevier Science Limited.

About the Contributors

Roberto Andorno, LLB, JD, is Senior Research Fellow, School of Law, University of Zurich, Switzerland, and was a former member of UNESCO's International Bioethics Committee from 1998 to 2005.

George J. Annas, JD, MPH, is William Fairfield Warren Distinguished Professor and Chair, Department of Health Law, Bioethics & Human Rights, Boston University School of Public Health, and Professor, Boston University School of Medicine, and Boston University School of Law.

Gunilla Backman, MSc, MA, is former Senior Research Officer to Paul Hunt, UN Special Rapporteur on the Right to the Highest Attainable Standard of Health (2002–2008), and is currently studying at the London School of Hygiene and Tropical Hygiene and Medicine, London, UK.

Isabella Bakker, PhD, FRSC, is Professor, Department of Political Science, York University, Toronto, Ontario, Canada, and a Trudeau Fellow.

Laurel Baldwin-Ragaven, MD, is Professor of Family Medicine, University of the Witwatersrand, Johannesburg, South Africa.

Solomon R. Benatar, MBChB, DSc (Med), FRSSAfr, is Emeritus Professor of Medicine, University of Cape Town, Western Cape, South Africa, and Professor, Dalla Lana School of Public Health and Joint Centre for Bioethics, University of Toronto, Toronto, Ontario, Canada.

Chris Beyrer, MD, MPH, is Director, Johns Hopkins Fogarty AIDS International Training and Research Program, Johns Hopkins Center for Public Health and Human Rights; Associate Director of Public Health and Professor, Johns Hopkins Center for Global Health; and Associate Director, Center for AIDS Research at the Johns Hopkins University, Baltimore, MD, USA.

Troyen Brennan, MD, JD, MPH, is Executive Vice President and Chief Medical Officer, CVS Caremark, and Adjunct Professor of Law and Public Health, Harvard School of Public Health, Boston, MA, USA.

Kelly D. Brownell, PhD, is Professor, Department of Psychology and Department of Epidemiology and Public Health, and Director, Rudd Center for Food Policy and Obesity, Yale University, New Haven, CT, USA.

Claude Bruderlein, LLM, is a Strategic Advisor to the President of the International Committee of the Red Cross, and Senior Researcher, Program on Humanitarian Policy and Conflict Research, Harvard School of Public Health, Boston, MA,

USA. He holds teaching appointments at the Harvard School of Public Health and Kennedy School of Government, Cambridge, MA, USA.

Gian Luca Burci, LLM, is Legal Counsel, World Health Organization, and Adjunct Professor of Law, Graduate Institute for International and Development Studies, Geneva, Switzerland.

Jonathan Kenneth Burns, MBChB, MSc, FCPsych, PhD, is Professor and Head, Department of Psychiatry, Nelson R. Mandela School of Medicine, University of KwaZulu-Natal, Durban, South Africa.

Andrew Byrnes is Professor of Law and Chair, Steering Committee of the Australian Human Rights Centre, Faculty of Law, The University of New South Wales, Sydney, Australia.

Tom Calma, HonDLitt, HonDSc, is Aboriginal Elder of the Kungarakan tribal group and a member of the Iwaidja tribal group; National Coordinator, Tackling Indigenous Smoking; Deputy Chancellor, University of Canberra Australia; and former Australian Aboriginal and Torres Strait Islander Social Justice Commissioner.

Jaume Vidal Casanovas, BA, has collaborated with the Centro de Investigación y Documentación Internacionales, worked as a Researcher and Consultant at the World Health Organization and the Pan American Health Organization.

Rebecca J. Cook, MA, MPA, JD, LLM, JSD, is Professor, Faculty of Law and Faculty of Medicine, University of Toronto, Toronto, Ontario, Canada.

Jane Cottingham, MSc, is an independent consultant and researcher in sexual and reproductive health and rights, focusing on the intersection of laws and policies, sexual health and human rights. She was former (1994–2009) Team Coordinator, Gender, Reproductive Rights, Sexual Health and Adolescence, Department of Reproductive Health and Research, World Health Organization, Geneva, Switzerland.

Sondra Crosby, MD, is Associate Professor, Department of Medicine, Boston University School of Medicine, and Associate Professor, Department of Health Law, Bioethics & Human Rights, Boston University School of Public Health, Boston, MA, USA.

Joanne Csete, MPH, PhD, is Senior Program Officer, Global Drug Policy Program, Open Society Foundations, London, United Kingdom.

Sam David, is former Research Assistant, SPRY Foundation, Chevy Chase, MD, and former Research Assistant, Human Rights Watch, New York, NY, USA.

Sara E. Davies, PhD, is Senior Research Fellow, Human Protection Hub, Griffith Asia Institute and Centre of Governance and Public Policy, Griffith University, Nathan, Australia.

Mandeep Dhaliwal, is Cluster Leader: Human Rights and Governance, HIV/AIDS Group, Bureau for Development Policy, United Nations Development Programme. She is also a physician and a lawyer with over 17 years' experience in HIV, health and human rights.

Carolyn Dresler, MD, MPA, is Medical Director, Arkansas Department of Health, Little Rock, Arkansas, USA, and is on the Board of Directors for the International Human Rights and Tobacco Control Network.

Richard Elliott, LLB, is Executive Director, Canadian HIV/AIDS Legal Network, Toronto, Ontario, Canada.

Paul Farmer, MD, PhD, is a founding director of Partners In Health (PIH);

Kolokotrones University Professor, Harvard University; Chair of the Department of Global Health and Social Medicine, Harvard Medical School; and Chief of the Division of Global Health Equity, Brigham and Women's Hospital, Boston, MA, USA.

Jamie Fellner, Esq., is Senior Advisor, US Program, Human Rights Watch, New York, NY, USA.

Laura Ferguson is an Assistant Professor, Department of Preventive Medicine, University of Southern California, CA, USA. She works within the Program on Global Health and Human Rights, Institute for Global Health, University of Southern California. In addition, Professor Ferguson is a Research Associate, University of Nairobi Institute for Tropical and Infectious Diseases, Nairobi, Kenya.

Harvey V. Fineberg, MD, PhD, is President, Institute of Medicine of the National Academy of Sciences, Washington, DC, USA.

John Fisher, LLB (Hons), LLM, is Codirector, ARC International. As ARC's representative, he has worked in Geneva since 2005 to better facilitate NGO engagement with United Nations human rights mechanisms. He is also former (1994–2002) founding Executive Director, Egale Canada (Canada's national LGBT equality organization).

Eric A. Friedman, JD, is Project Leader, Joint Action and Learning Initiative on National and Global Responsibilities for Health (JALI), Georgetown University Law Center, and former Senior Global Health Policy Advisor, Physicians for Human Rights, Washington, D.C., USA.

Claudia García-Moreno, MD, works in the Department of Reproductive Health and Research, World Health Organization, Geneva, Switzerland, with a special focus on women's health and gender in health.

Rebekah Gay, LLM, LLB, BSc, is Partner, Shelton IP, Sydney, Australia.

H. Jack Geiger, MD, MSciHyg, ScD, is Arthur C. Logan Professor Emeritus of Community Medicine, City University of New York Medical School, New York, NY, USA. He is also Founding Member and Past President, Physicians for Human Rights; Founding Member and Past President, Physicians for Social Responsibility; Founding Member and Past President, The Committee for Health in South Africa; and Founding Member and National Program Coordinator, Medical Committee for Human Rights.

Adrienne Germain, MA, is President Emerita, International Women's Health Coalition, New York, NY, USA. She has worked for women's health, development and human rights in low and middle income countries since 1970, with the Population Council, the Ford Foundation and the Coalition.

Stephen Gill, MA, PGCE, PhD, is Distinguished Research Professor of Political Science, Communications and Culture, Department of Political Science, York University, Toronto, Ontario, Canada.

David Gordon, BSc, PhD, FRSA, is Director, Townsend Centre for International Poverty Research, and Professor of Social Justice, University of Bristol, Bristol, UK.

Lawrence O. Gostin, JD, LLD, is University Professor and Faculty Director, O'Neill Institute for National and Global Health Law, Georgetown University Law Center, Washington, D.C., USA, and Director, World Health Organization Collaborating Center on Public Health Law and Human Rights.

Michael A. Grodin, MD, is Professor of Health Law, Bioethics & Human Rights, Department of Health Law, Bioethics & Human Rights, Boston University School of Public Health, and Professor of both Family

Medicine and Psychiatry, Boston University School of Medicine, Boston, MA, USA.

Anand Grover is United Nations Special Rapporteur on the Right to the Highest Attainable Standard of Health. He is also a Practicing Senior Advocate in the Supreme Court of India, and Director, Lawyers Collective HIV/AIDS, India.

Sofia Gruskin, JD, MIA, is Director, Program on Global Health and Human Rights, Institute for Global Health, University of Southern California, CA, USA. She holds a joint appointment as Professor of Preventive Medicine at the USC Keck School of Medicine and Professor of Preventive Medicine and Law at the USC Gould School of Law. In addition, Professor Gruskin is an Adjunct Professor of Global Health, Department of Global Health and Population, Harvard School of Public Health, MA, USA.

Michele Heisler, MD, MPA, is Associate Professor, Internal Medicine and Health Behavior and Health Education, University of Michigan Schools of Medicine and Public Health, and Research Scientist, Center for Clinical Management Research, Ann Arbor Veterans Affairs Health Services Research and Development Center of Excellence, Ann Arbor, MI, USA.

Zakhe Hlanze, MA, is Research Associate, Women and Law in Southern Africa, Lusaka, Zambia.

Hans V. Hogerzeil, MD, PhD, FRCP, Edin, is Professor of Global Health, University Medical Center Groningen, The Netherlands, and former Director, Department of Essential Medicines and Pharmaceutical Policies, World Health Organization, Geneva, Switzerland.

Stephen Humphreys, PhD, is Lecturer in International Law, London School of Economics, London, UK, and former Research Director, International Council on Human Rights, Geneva, Switzerland.

Paul Hunt, MA, MJur, served as Rapporteur, UN Committee on Economic, Social and Cultural Rights (1999–2002), UN Special Rapporteur on the Right to the Highest Attainable Standard of Health (2002–2008), and is currently Professor of Law, Essex University, UK, and Adjunct Professor, Waikato University, New Zealand.

Anna-Karin Hurtig, MD, DTM&H, DrPH, is Professor in Public Health and Clinical Medicine, Department of Epidemiology and Global Health, Umeå University, Umeå, Sweden. The article was written during her doctoral studies at London School of Hygiene and Tropical Medicine, UK.

Vincent Iacopino, MD, PhD, is Senior Medical Advisor, Physicians for Human Rights, Boston, MA, USA; Adjunct Professor, University of Minnesota Medical School, Minneapolis, MN, USA; and Senior Research Fellow, Human Rights Center, University of California at Berkeley, CA, USA.

Michael Johnson is Associate Professor, School of Social Sciences, The University of New South Wales, Sydney, Australia, and Deputy Chair of the Board of The Fred Hollows Foundation, an Australian based not-for-profit development organization addressing avoidable blindness operating in 20 countries.

Lynn Kemp is Associate Professor and Director, Centre for Health Equity Training Research and Evaluation, Centre for Primary Health Care and Equity, The University of New South Wales, Sydney, Australia.

Denali Kerr, is former Research Assistant, Department of Health Law, Bioethics, and Human Rights, Boston University School of Public Health, Boston, MA, USA.

Thomas Kerr, PhD, is Co-director, Addiction and Urban Health Research Initiative, British Columbia Centre for Excellence in HIV/AIDS, and Associate Professor, Department of Medicine, University of British Columbia, Vancouver, British Columbia, Canada.

Michael Kirby, AC, CMG, retired from the High Court of Australia in 2009 with the honor of being Australia's longest serving judge. He has been a member of the World Health Organisation's Global Commission on AIDS (1988–92); President of the International Commission of Jurists, Geneva (1995–8); UN Special Representative on Human Rights, Cambodia (1993–96); a member of the UNESCO International Bioethics Committee (1995–2005); a member of the UNAIDS Reference Group on HIV and Human Rights (2004–); and a member of the High Commissioner for Human Rights' Judicial Reference Group (2007–).

Riikka Koskenmäki, LLM, DEA, is in the Office of the Legal Advisor, International Labor Organization, which is a specialized agency of the United Nations.

Harry Lando, PhD, is a Distinguished International Professor, Division of Epidemiology and Community Health, School of Public Health, University of Minnesota, Minneapolis, MN, USA, and is on the Board of Directors for the International Human Rights and Tobacco Control Network.

Malcolm Langford, PhD, is Research Fellow and Director of the Socio-Economic Rights Programme, Norwegian Centre for Human Rights, Faculty of Law, University of Oslo, Oslo, Norway. He is also an advisor to the UN Office of the High Commissioner for Human Rights on Millennium Development Goals and Human Rights.

Zita Lazzarini, JD, MPH, is Associate Professor and Director, Division of Public Health Law and Bioethics, Department of Community Medicine and Health Care, University of Connecticut School of Medicine, Farmington, CT, USA.

Jennifer Leaning, MD, SMH, is François-Xavier Bagnoud Professor of the Practice of Health and Human Rights, Harvard School of Public Health; Associate Professor of Medicine, Harvard Medical School; and Director, François-Xavier Bagnoud Center for Health and Human Rights, Harvard University, Boston, MA, USA.

Karen Leiter, JD, MPH, is Human Rights Researcher, Center for Reproductive Rights, New York, NY, USA.

Leslie London, MB, ChB, BSc Hons, DOH, MD, MMed, is Professor, School of Public Health and Family Medicine; Head, Health and Human Rights Programme; and Associate Director, Centre for Occupational and Environmental Health Research, University of Cape Town, Cape Town, South Africa.

Jonathan M. Mann, MD, MPH, was Dean, School of Public Health, Allegheny University of Health Sciences, Philadelphia, PA, USA, and Founding Director, WHO Global Program on AIDS (deceased).

Jeffrey L. Metzner, MD, is Clinical Professor of Psychiatry, University of Colorado School of Medicine, Denver, CO, USA.

Alice M. Miller, JD, is Associate Adjunct Professor of Law and Associate Research Scientist in Law, Yale Law School; Assistant Clinical Professor, Yale School of Public Health; and Lecturer in Global Affairs, Jackson Institute for Global Affairs and Whitney and Betty MacMillan Center for International and Area Studies, Yale University, New Haven, CT, USA.

Edward J. Mills, PhD, MSc, LLM, is Canada Research Chair in Global Health and Associate Professor, University of Ottawa, Ottawa, Ontario, Canada. He holds adjunct faculty positions at Stanford University, CA,

USA, and National University of Rwanda, Butare Province, Rwanda.

Russell E. Morgan, Jr., DrPH, is President, SPRY Foundation, Chevy Chase, MD, USA, and Chair, International Human Rights Committee, American Public Health Association, Washington, D.C., USA.

Shailen Nandy, MSc, PhD, is Research Associate, Centre for the Study of Poverty and Social Justice, School for Policy Studies, University of Bristol, Bristol, UK.

Helena Nygren-Krug, LLB, LLM, is Health and Human Rights Advisor, Department of Ethics, Trade, Human Rights and Law, World Health Organization, Geneva, Switzerland. She has also held positions at the United Nations Centre for Human Rights and the United Nations High Commissioner for Human Rights, and was Adjunct Professor, Emory Law School, Atlanta, Georgia, USA.

Michael O'Flaherty, BCL, BPh, STB, MA, MPhil, FRSA, Solicitor, is Chief Commissioner of the Northern Ireland Human Rights Commission, Professor of Applied Human Rights, and Co-Chair, Human Rights Law Centre, School of Law, University of Nottingham, Nottingham, UK, and Vice-Chair, United Nations Human Rights Committee.

Jessica A. Ogden, PhD, is a consultant through her own company, Ogden Health & Development Connections. She has been working as a social anthropologist in public health for over 25 years, with a focus on structural approaches to infectious disease programming, equity, gender and the politics of public health.

Jeffrey O'Malley, MA, is Director, Policy and Strategy for UNICEF. When this commentary was written, he was Director, HIV, Health and Development, United Nations Development Programme.

Christina Pantazis, is Senior Lecturer, Centre for the Study of Poverty and Social Justice, School for Policy Studies, University of Bristol, Bristol, UK.

Simon Pemberton, LLB, MA, PhD, is a Birmingham Fellow jointly appointed to the School of Social Policy and School of Law, University of Birmingham, Birmingham, UK.

Nthabiseng Phaladze, PhD, is Professor, Department of Nursing Education, University of Botswana, School of Nursing, Gaborone, Botswana.

Helen de Pinho, MBBCh, FCCH, MBA, is Assistant Professor, Mailman School of Public Health, and Associate Director, Averting Maternal Death and Disability Program, Columbia University, New York, NY, USA.

Linda Piwowarczyk, MD, MPH, is Assistant Professor, Department of Psychiatry, Boston University School of Medicine, Boston, MA, USA, and Director, Boston Center for Refugee Health and Human Rights. She is current President of the National Consortium of Torture Treatment Programs, and has served on its Executive Committee since 2002.

John D. H. Porter, MBBS, MD, MPH, FRCP, FFPH, is Professor of International Health, Departments of Clinical Research and Global Health and Development, London School of Hygiene and Tropical Medicine, London, UK.

Rebecca Puhl, MS, PhD, is Director, Research and Weight Stigma Initiatives, Rudd Center for Food Policy and Obesity, and Senior Research Scientist, Yale University, New Haven, CT, USA.

Ladan Rahmani-Ocora, PhD, was a student intern under Hans V. Hogerzeil at the time their article was published.

Mary Robinson is President of the Mary

Robinson Foundation—Climate Justice. She served as President of Ireland from 1990 to 1997 and UN High Commissioner for Human Rights from 1997 to 2002.

Leonard Rubenstein, JD, is a lawyer and Senior Scholar, Center for Public Health and Human Rights, Johns Hopkins Bloomberg School of Public Health, Baltimore, MD, USA.

Melanie Samson, LLM, was a student intern under Hans V. Hogerzeil at the time their article was published.

Nick Schneider, MD, is Science Manager, German Cancer Research Center, Unit Cancer Prevention and WHO Collaborating Centre for Tobacco Control, Heidelberg, Germany, and is on the Board of Directors for the International Human Rights and Tobacco Control Network.

Claudio Schuftan, MD, is a Founding Member, People's Health Movement, and former Associate Professor, Department of International Health, Tulane School of Public Health and Tropical Medicine, Tulane University, New Orleans, USA.

Hitakshi Sehgal, MPH, is Coordinator, India Programs, School of Public Health, University of Minnesota, Minneaplois, MN, USA.

Kate Shannon, is Director, Gender and Sexual Health Initiative, British Columbia Centre for Excellence in HIV/AIDS, and Assistant Professor, Department of Medicine, University of British Columbia, Vancouver, British Columbia, Canada.

Pablo Solón worked as an activist for many years with different social organizations, indigenous movements, workers' unions, student associations, human rights and cultural organizations in Bolivia before becoming the Ambassador for the Plurinational State of Bolivia to the United Nations. In this capacity, he spearheaded successful resolutions on the Human Right to Water,

International Mother Earth Day, Harmony with Nature, and the Rights of Indigenous Peoples. He is currently Executive Director of Focus on the Global South, Chulalongkorn University, Bangkok, Thailand.

Heidi Stöckl, MSc, PhD, is Research Fellow, Social and Mathematical Epidemiology Group and the Gender Violence and Health Centre, Department of Global Health and Development, London School of Hygiene and Tropical Medicine, London, UK.

Daniel Tarantola, MD, is Visiting Professorial Fellow and former Professor of Health and Human Rights, School of Public Health and Community Medicine, The University of New South Wales, Sydney, Australia.

Keith Taylor, BSc, MPC, MRCGP, FHEA, GP, was Clinical Fellow, Dundee University Medical School, Dundee, Scotland, at the time his article was published.

Aminata Touré, is Minister of Justice in the Government of the Republic of Senegal and former senior staff of the United Nations Population Program.

Peter Townsend was Emeritus Professor of Social Policy at the University of Bristol, UK, and Professor of International Social Policy, London School of Economics, London, UK (deceased).

Alexander C. Tsai, MD, PhD, is Assistant Professor in Psychiatry, Chester M. Pierce, MD Division of Global Psychiatry; Assistant Professor, Health Decision Sciences, Center for Global Health, Massachusetts General Hospital; and Lecturer in Psychiatry, Harvard Medical School, Boston, MA, USA.

Sheri Weiser, MD, MA, MPH, is Assistant Adjunct Professor of Medicine, Division of HIV/AIDS, San Francisco General Hospital and the Center for AIDS Prevention Studies, University of California at San Francisco, San Francisco, CA, USA.

William Wolfe, MD, is Assistant Clinical Professor, Department of Psychiatry, University of California at San Francisco, and Medical Doctor, Posttraumatic Stress Disorder Program, San Francisco Veterans Affairs Medical Center, San Francisco, CA, USA.

Evan Wood, MD, PhD, ABIM, FRCPC, is Co-Director, Addiction and Urban Health Research Initiative, British Columbia Centre for Excellence in HIV/AIDS, and Clinical Associate Professor, Department of Medicine, University of British Columbia, Vancouver, British Columbia, Canada.

Alicia Ely Yamin, JD, MPH, is a Lecturer on Global Health and Director, Health Rights of Women and Children Program, François-Xavier Bagnoud Center for Health and Human Rights, Harvard School of Public Health, Boston, MA, USA. She is also a Senior Associated Researcher, Christian Michelson Institute, Bergen, Norway.

Anthony Zwi is Professor of Global Health and Development, School of Social Sciences, Faculty of Arts and Social Sciences, The University of New South Wales, Sydney, Australia.

About the Editors

Michael A. Grodin, MD, is Professor of Health Law, Bioethics and Human Rights at the Boston University School of Public Health and Family Medicine and Psychiatry at the Boston University School of Medicine. He has edited or co-edited: *The Nazi Doctors and the Nuremberg Code: Human Rights in Human Experimentation; Children as Research Subjects: Science, Ethics, and Law; Meta-Medical Ethics: The Philosophical Foundations of Bioethics; Health and Human Rights: A Reader; and Perspectives on Health and Human Rights.* He is co-founder of Global Lawyers and Physicians and co-director of the Refugee and Immigrant Health Program at Boston Medical Center.

Daniel Tarantola, MD, is a Visiting Professorial Fellow and former Professor of Health and Human Rights at the School of Public Health and Community Medicine, UNSW Medicine, The University of New South Wales, Sydney, Australia. He has occupied senior leadership positions in the World Health Organization, including that of a Senior Policy Advisor to the Director General. At the Harvard School of Public Health, and more recently at the University of New South Wales, his work focuses on the application of human rights principles, norms and standards to public health policy and programs.

George J. Annas, JD, MPH, is William Fairfield Warren Distinguished Professor and Chair, Department of Health Law, Bioethics and Human Rights, Boston University School of Public Health, and Professor, Boston University School of Medicine, and Boston University School of Law. He is the author or editor of more than a dozen books on health law and bioethics, including *American Bioethics: Crossing Human Rights and Health Law Boundaries, The Rights of Patients, Judging Medicine, Standard of Care,* and *Some Choice,* and writes a regular feature on "Legal Issues in Medicine" for the *New England Journal of Medicine.* He is the co-founder of Global Lawyers and Physicians.

Sofia Gruskin, JD, MIA, Professor Gruskin is director of the Program on Global Health and Human Rights at the USC Institute for Global Health. She holds a joint appointment as Professor of Preventive Medicine at the USC Keck School of Medicine and Professor of Preventive Medicine and Law at the USC Gould School of Law. She is Adjunct Professor in Global Health in the Department of Global Health and Population at the Harvard School of Public Health and serves as an associate editor for *The American Journal of Public Health, Global Public Health,* and *Reproductive Health Matters.* Gruskin's work has been instrumental in the conceptual, methodological, policy and practice development of linking health and human rights, with a focus on HIV, sexual and reproductive health, child and adolescent health, gender-based violence and health systems.

Global Lawyers and Physicians (GLP) is a non-profit, nongovernmental organization that focuses on health and human rights issues.

Global Lawyers and Physicians was founded in 1996 at an international symposium on health at the United States Holocaust Memorial Museum to commemorate the 50th anniversary of the Nuremberg Doctors' Trial. As one of the earliest and most important health and human rights documents, the Nuremberg Code was developed by lawyers and physicians working together. GLP was formed to reinvigorate the collaboration of the legal and medical/public health professions to protect the human rights and dignity of all persons. Lawyers and physicians, by virtue of their privileged position and their commitment to life, health, social justice and equality, have special obligations to all people. GLP was founded on the premise that these professions, working together transnationally, can be a much more effective force for human rights than either profession can working separately. http://www.globallawyersandphysicians.org/

PROGRAM ON GLOBAL HEALTH AND HUMAN RIGHTS, INSTITUTE FOR GLOBAL HEALTH, USC

The Program on Global Health & Human Rights (GHHR) is at the forefront of expanding research in the field of health and human rights, and a leader in developing tools for analysis, programmatic intervention, monitoring and evaluation. At this juncture in the history of the health and human rights field, GHHR is committed to strengthening health systems and demonstrating the effectiveness of using human rights to address public health challenges. The work of GHHR is to document examples of how human rights-based approaches to health make a greater positive difference to the lives of individuals and populations in a variety of areas, including HIV/AIDS, sexual and reproductive health, child and adolescent health and health systems strengthening. GHHR emphasizes the conceptual, methodological, policy and practice implications of linking health to human rights, with particular attention to women, children, gender issues, and vulnerable populations. http://globalhealth.usc.edu/

THE SCHOOL OF PUBLIC HEALTH AND COMMUNITY MEDICINE, UNSW MEDICINE, THE UNIVERSITY OF NEW SOUTH WALES, SYDNEY, AUSTRALIA

Capabilities The School of Public Health and Community Medicine seeks to contribute to the ongoing efforts, both within Australia and internationally, to promote health, prevent disease and ensure that health care is made available through the organized efforts of society. Its teaching and research aim to develop expertise, reduce unfair and unjust inequalities and improve access and participation in services and decision making. From 2005–2010, the School hosted the UNSW Initiative for Health and Human Rights (IHHR), a multidisciplinary research, teaching, service and advocacy initiative founded collectively by the Faculties of Arts and Social Sciences, Law and Medicine. The IHHR advanced Health and Human Rights as both an area of study and a new, composite method of research applicable to exploring the interface between health, development, human rights, poverty and globalization with a particular focus on vulnerable populations. http://www.sphcm.med.unsw.edu.au/SPHCMWeb.nsf/page/

Index

Locators in italics refer to tables and diagrams.